Editors

RICHARD A. BALDERSTON, M.D.
Clinical Professor, Orthopaedic Surgery
Thomas Jefferson University and the Rothman Institute of
*   Pennsylvania Hospital*
Philadelphia, Pennsylvania

RICHARD H. ROTHMAN, M.D., PH.D.
The James Edwards Professor and Chairman
Department of Orthopaedic Surgery
Thomas Jefferson University
and
Director, Rothman Institute of Pennsylvania Hospital
Philadelphia, Pennsylvania

ROBERT E. BOOTH, JR., M.D.
Clinical Professor and Vice Chairman
Department of Orthopaedic Surgery
Thomas Jefferson University
and
CoDirector, Rothman Institute of Pennsylvania Hospital
Chief of Physical Medicine and Rehabilitation, Pennsylvania Hospital
Philadelphia, Pennsylvania

WILLIAM J. HOZACK, M.D.
Assistant Professor of Orthopaedic Surgery
Thomas Jefferson University and the Rothman Institute of
*   Pennsylvania Hospital*
Philadelphia, Pennsylvania

The Hip

LEA & FEBIGER

PHILADELPHIA • 1992 • LONDON

Lea & Febiger
200 Chester Field Parkway
Malvern, Pennsylvania 19355-9725
U.S.A.
(215) 251-2230

Library of Congress Cataloging-in-Publication Data

The Hip / edited by Richard A. Balderston . . . [et al.].
   p. cm.
   Includes index.
   ISBN 0-8121-1302-0
   1. Hip joint—Diseases. 2. Hip joint—Surgery. I. Balderston,
Richard A.
   [DNLM: 1. Bone Diseases. 2. Hip Joint. 3. Hip Joint—injuries.
4. Hip Joint—surgery. 5. Hip Prosthesis. 6. Joint Diseases. WE
860 H666]
RD772.H55 1992
617.5'81—dc20
DNLM/DLC
for Library of Congress

91-14159
CIP

PRINTED IN THE UNITED STATES OF AMERICA

Print number: 5 4 3 2 1

Reprints of chapters may be purchased from Lea & Febiger in quantities of 100 or more.

Preface

It has been 30 years since Charnley's revolutionary article "Arthroplasty of the Hip—A New Operation." Charnley crystalizes the reasoning behind his thought processes from the very beginning of the article:

"In considering how arthroplasty of the hip can be improved, two facts stand out:

1) After replacement of the head of the femur by a spherical surface of inert material, the failures are essentially *long-term*. At first the patient may notice no difference between the artificial head and the living one which preceded it. Our problem is to make this temporary success permanent.

2) Objectives must be reasonable. Neither surgeons nor engineers will ever make an artificial hip joint which will last thirty years and at some time in this period enable the patient to play football." (Charnley J: Arthroplasty of the hip—a new operation. Lancet 1:1129, 1969.)

From the beginning Charnley emphasized the requirement of long-term followup, and indeed his numerous studies were exhaustive in their efforts to record data on each patient who had his operation. At the same time Charnley was specific with respect to the goals of surgery. He probably had no idea of the great impact his technology would have for hip patients over the next 30 years.

Charnley also recognized that no implant remains static within the human organism. The tissue response at both the local and organism level were central to Charnley's thinking:

"The capacity of the living organism to react favorably to sound mechanical design, and its capacity to reveal incipient mechanical failure by deterioration of function, even before the appearance of frank pain, is a fundamental guide in developing any arthroplasty." (Ibid.)

Charnley's description of his "present operation" introduced the concept of low-friction arthroplasty.

"Resistance to movement of the head in the socket is greatly reduced by reducing the radius of the ball and, therefore, reducing the "moment" of the frictional force. If at the same time the radius of the exterior of the polytetrafluroethylene socket is made as large as possible, the "moment" of the frictional force between the socket and bone will be increased, and this will lessen any tendency for the socket to rotate against the bone." (Ibid.) Thus, his femoral head design was reduced from 1 and five-eighths in., which was at that time standard for a Moore prosthesis, down to the seven-eighth in. or 22 mm head that has been used for the last 30 years. At the time of this original article, Charnley's 10-month followup showed negligible wear of the thickened socket by the femoral head.

In 1961, Charnley was using an uncemented acetabular component with a cemented femoral side. In the article Charnley does not discuss the specifics of his methylmethacrylate technique, however, he does mention that in three cases reexploration for a failed socket produced evidence of "absolutely rigid" fixation of the femoral prosthesis within the femur.

Charnley was careful when he detailed the indications for his surgery: "While the long-term results are still awaited, the method has been restricted to cases of gross disablement by (1) rheumatoid arthritis, (2) severe osteoarthritis in patients over 65, and occasionally (3) bilateral arthritis in middle age." The indications for total hip arthroplasty remained exactly these for at least a decade.

An overwhelming majority of the procedures performed on adults by hip surgeons today are descended from principles described in this article. The focus of this book is a comprehensive approach to problem solving for the hip surgeon. The text is divided into six major sections including basic science, pediatrics, trauma, clinical syndromes, nonarthroplasty surgical techniques, and primary and revision total hip arthroplasty.

The initial section includes chapters concerning anatomy, biomechanics, and surgical approaches. Without this basic, fundamental knowledge, the treatment of patients with hip disease is impossible.

The second section includes five chapters relating to pathology of the pediatric hip. Many of these conditions are not resolved by the end of adolescence and require medical care during the adult years. The surgeon must understand these pediatric disorders because surgical management greatly depends upon the understanding of their fundamentals.

The third section of the book includes three chapters defining the management of acetabular, intracapsular, and extracapsular fractures of the hip. Over the last several years dramatic improvements in the surgical management of fractures about the hip, particularly the acetabulum, have evolved to allow an increased long-term clinical success with concomitant diminution in morbidity.

The clinical presentation of various syndromes about the hip is the subject of part four. The focus of this group of chapters is to enable the clinician to obtain a history and physical and roentgenographic evaluation, and to determine the proper diagnosis. The final chapter in this section is a discussion of the differential diagnosis of hip pain.

The fifth section of the book includes chapters relating to nonarthroplasty operations. Twenty years ago this section would have had much greater relevance for hip surgery and would have been much longer. Arthroscopy, techniques of biopsy, and the decompression surgeries relating to osteonecrosis are surgical procedures that have increasingly relevant application in modern hip surgery. Hip fusion and cup arthroplasty are techniques that are used occasionally at our institution, but they demand technical excellence for successful execution.

The final section of *The Hip* is dedicated to those surgical techniques that have evolved from Charnley's article of 30 years ago. The chapters in this section include primary hip replacement, uncemented total hip, total hip replacement in rheumatoid arthritis, proximal femoral replacement, the infected total hip, and four chapters related to revision surgery. The theme of this section continues to reflect Charnley's concerns of three decades ago: (1) precision of surgical technique, (2) relentless pursuit of long-term followup, (3) goal definition for each surgical procedure, and (4) an appreciation for the relationship between human biology and the mechanical performance of each prosthesis.

RICHARD A. BALDERSTON, M.D.
ROBERT E. BOOTH, JR., M.D.
WILLIAM J. HOZACK, M.D.
RICHARD H. ROTHMAN, M.D., PH.D.

Contributors

RICHARD A. BALDERSTON, M.D.
Clinical Professor, Orthopaedic Surgery
Thomas Jefferson University and the
  Rothman Institute of Pennsylvania
  Hospital
Philadelphia, Pennsylvania

ARTHUR R. BARTOLOZZI, M.D.
Instructor, Orthopaedic Surgery
Thomas Jefferson University Hospital
Philadelphia, Pennsylvania

GEORGE S. BASSETT, M.D.
Assistant Professor of Orthopaedics
University of Southern California School of
  Medicine
Childrens' Hospital, Los Angeles
Los Angeles, California

ROBERT E. BOOTH, JR., M.D.
Clinical Professor and Vice Chairman
Department of Orthopaedic Surgery
Thomas Jefferson University
and
CoDirector, Rothman Institute of
  Pennsylvania Hospital
Chief of Physical Medicine and
  Rehabilitation, Pennsylvania Hospital
Philadelphia, Pennsylvania

J. RICHARD BOWEN, M.D.
Department of Medical Education
Alfred I. duPont Institute
Wilmington, Delaware

R. MICHAEL BUCKLEY, JR., M.D.
Chief of the Division of Infectious Diseases
Pennsylvania Hospital
and
Clinical Associate Professor of Medicine
University of Pennsylvania
Philadelphia, Pennsylvania

WILLIAM P. BUNNELL, M.D.
Professor and Chairman
Department of Orthopaedic Surgery
Loma Linda University School of Medicine
Loma Linda University Medical Center
Loma Linda, California

JOHN J. CALLAGHAN, M.D.
Assistant Professor
Department of Orthopaedics
University of Iowa Hospital
Iowa City, Iowa

JAMES C. COHEN, M.D.
Department of Orthopaedics
Michael Reese Hospital
and
Associate Professor
University of Illinois College of Medicine
Chicago, Illinois

ANTHONY F. DEPALMA, M.D.
Professor Emeritus, Orthopaedic Surgery
Jefferson Medical College
Philadelphia, Pennsylvania
and
University of Medicine and Dentistry of New
  Jersey
Newark, New Jersey

STEPHEN J. GLUCKMAN, M.D.
Chief, Division of General Internal Medicine
Professor of Clinical Medicine
University of Medicine and Dentistry of New
  Jersey
Robert Ward Johnson Medical School at
  Camden
and
Program Director, Internal Medicine
  Residency Program
Cooper Hospital/University Medical Center
Camden, New Jersey

DANNY GURBA, M.D.
Dickson Diveley Clinic
Assistant Clinical Professor
Department of Orthopaedics
University of Missouri at Kansas City
Kansas City, Missouri

WILLIAM J. HOZACK, M.D.
Assistant Professor of Orthopaedic Surgery
Thomas Jefferson University and the
    Rothman Institute of Pennsylvania
    Hospital
Philadelphia, Pennsylvania

ERIC L. HUME
Assistant Professor
Department of Orthopaedic Surgery
Thomas Jefferson University
Philadelphia, Pennsylvania

TIMOTHY H. IZANT, M.D.
Staff Surgeon, Crouse Irving Memorial
    Hospital
and
Clinical Instructor, SUNY Health Science
    Center
Syracuse, New York

JAMES KELLAM, M.D.
Division of Orthopaedic Surgery
Carolinas Medical Center
Charlotte, North Carolina

RICHARD D. LACKMAN, M.D.
Associate Clinical Professor
and
Chief of the Musculoskeletal Tumor Service
at Thomas Jefferson University Hospital
Philadelphia, Pennsylvania

RANDALL J. LEWIS, M.D.
Clinical Associate Professor
Department of Orthopaedic Surgery
George Washington University Medical
    Center
Washington, D.C.

WILLIAM McCLUSKEY, M.D.
Department of Orthopaedics
The Nemours Children's Clinic
Jacksonville, Florida

GARY MILLER, M.D.
Department of Orthopaedic Surgery
Washington University School of Medicine
St. Louis, Missouri

WESLEY W. PARKE, PH.D.
Professor and Chairman
Department of Anatomy
University of South Dakota
School of Medicine
Vermillion, South Dakota

GEORGE R. PAYNE III, M.D.
Department of Orthopaedics
Virginia Beach General Hospital
Virginia Beach, Virginia

PAUL M. PELLICCI, M.D.
Associate Attending Orthopaedic Surgeon
Acting Chief of Spine Service
Co-Director of Hip Service
Hospital for Special Surgery

PETER PIZZUTILLO, M.D.
Professor, Department of Orthopaedic Surgery
Jefferson Medical College at Thomas Jefferson
    University
Philadelphia, Pennsylvania

CHITRANJAN S. RANAWAT, M.D.
Professor of Orthopaedic Surgery
Cornell University Medical Center
and
The New York Hospital
and
The Hospital for Special Surgery
New York, New York

NEAL L. ROCKOWITZ, M.D.
Joint Implant and Reconstructive
    Orthopaedic Surgeon
Private Practice
Phoenix, Arizona

RICHARD H. ROTHMAN, M.D., PH.D.
The James Edwards Professor and Chairman
Department of Orthopaedic Surgery
Thomas Jefferson University
and
Director, The Rothman Institute of
    Pennsylvania Hospital
Philadelphia, Pennsylvania

EDUARDO A. SALVATI, M.D.
Clinical Professor of Orthopaedic Surgery
Cornell University Medical College
and
Director of the Hip Clinic
The Hospital for Special Surgery
New York, New York

CHARLES I. SCOTT, JR., M.D.
Chief, Division of Genetics
Alfred I. duPont Institute
Wilmington, Delaware

JEFFREY L. STAMBOUGH, M.D.
Associate Professor of Orthopaedic Surgery
Assistant Professor of Neurologic Surgery
Director, Giannestras Spine Service
University of Cincinnati School of Medicine
Cincinnati, Ohio

WILLIAM G. STEWART, JR., M.D.
Clinical Associate Professor
Department of Orthopaedics
Thomas Jefferson University
Philadelphia, Pennsylvania
and
Chief, Department of Orthopaedics
The Bryn Mawr Hospital
Bryn Mawr, Pennsylvania

ANTHONY UNGER, M.D.
Clinical Assistant Professor
Department of Orthopaedic Surgery
George Washington University Medical
  Center
Washington, D.C.

JOSEPH V. VERNACE, M.D.
Assistant Attending Orthopaedist
The Bryn Mawr Hospital
Bryn Mawr, Pennsylvania
and
Instructor, Department of Orthpaedics
Thomas Jefferson University Hospital
Philadelphia, Pennsylvania

RUSSELL E. WINDSOR, M.D.
Assistant Attending Orthopaedic Surgeon
Hospital for Special Surgery
and
Assistant Professor of Surgery (Orthopaedics)
Cornell Medical College
New York, New York

Contents

PART 4. CLINICAL SYNDROMES

PART 5. SURGICAL TECHNIQUES

PART 6. TOTAL HIP

PART I

Basic Science

CHAPTER ONE

The Anatomy of the Hip

WESLEY W. PARKE

Introduction

The hip joint is the polyaxial articulation between the body and the lower extremity. Because both the upper and lower limbs are proximally connected by ball and socket (enarthrodial) joints, but with differing emphasis on functional requirements, a general understanding of either one may be enhanced by a brief comparison of their structural similarities and differences. In both the shoulder and the hip, the distal component of the joint is the cartilage-covered spheroidal head of a long bone that is received by a concavity in the proximal component. This allows the limbs to be moved through a variety of motion axes that permit flexion-extension, abduction-adduction, circumduction (a combination of the foregoing); and medial-lateral rotation. In the shoulder, the joint has been structured to allow the greatest range of motion at the sacrifice of stability. The receiving proximal concavity, the glenoid fossa, contacts only a small fraction of the humeral head surface and relies on the relatively loosely arranged joint capsule and the closely attached tendons of the rotator cuff and biceps to provide stability. The proximal bones of the shoulder are only remotely connected to the axial skeleton and much enhancement to the range of motion is provided by the additional mobility of the scapula.

In contrast to the above, the hip joint must transfer the weight load of all body structure to the lower extremity and, in return, transfer the propulsive thrusts of the lower extremity to the body. Thus, the pelvis is firmly fixed to the vertebral column, and the anatomic design of the hip joint has been developed for stability at an expense to the universal range of motion. Whereas the glenoid fossa of the shoulder embraces but a small part of the humeral head, the head of the femur, which comprises nearly two-thirds of a sphere, is more than half encompassed by the acetabulum and its fibrocartilagenous extension of the labrum. This mechanical stability of the joint structure itself relieves the muscles of that responsibility and allows them and the capsular ligaments to be attached at some point more distal to the margin of the head. The hip joint is thus designed to favor the flexion-extension axis of motion by the angulation of the neck, but the presence of the elongated neck significantly limits abduction.

The following descriptive sections have been organized to provide an anatomic basis for the understanding diagnosis and treatment of hip disorders.

Osteology of the Hip

The Hip Bone (os coxae)

The two hip bones (Figs. 1–1, 1–2, 1–3) comprise the greater part of the pelvis. Their attachments posteriorly to the sacrum and anteriorly to each other at the pubic symphysis complete the bony ring that supports the abdominopelvic organs and transfers the thrust of weight-bearing and locomotion from the spine to the lower extremity. The configuration of the individual hip bone suggests a marine propeller as its central axial area; the acetabulum supports two flared and flat expansions that are pitched in opposite directions. To establish the proper anatomic relations of the isolated bone, it should be positioned with the acetabular opening directed laterally and the acetabular notch facing inferiorly and slightly anteriorly.

Although the hip bone is structurally and functionally a single osseous entity, developmentally and topographically it represents the fusion of three separate bones: the ilium, the ischium, and the pubis. These bones are joined in the formation of the acetabulum and, until approximately the seventeenth year, were connected by synchondroses. They are fused in the adult without any indication of their former developmental boundaries.

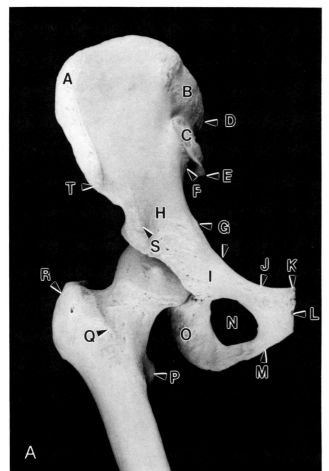 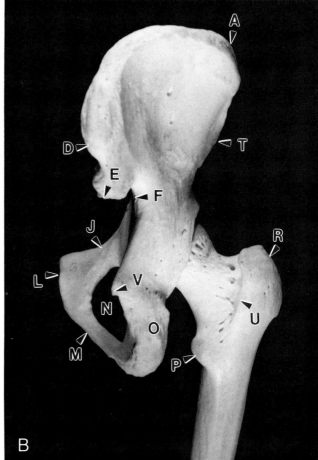

Fig. 1–1.

Figs. 1–1, 1–2, and 1–3 are photographs of the osseous components of the right hip joint of an adult female. The list of labels given below is common to all three figures.

Fig. 1–1A. Anterior view of articulated hip bones. B. Posterior view of articulated hip bones.
Fig. 1–2A. Lateral view of the os coxae. B. Medial view of the os coxae.
Fig. 1–3A. Anterior view of the proximal femur. B. Posterior view of the proximal femur.

List of labels for figures 1–1–1–3.
A. Iliac tuberosity of iliac crest
B. Tuberosity of ilium
C. Articular (auricular) surface
D. Posterior superior iliac spine
E. Posterior inferior iliac spine
F. Greater sciatic notch
G. Arcuate line
H. Body of Ilium
I. Body of pubis
J. Superior ramus of pubis
K. Pubic tubercle
L. Articular surface for pelvic symphysis

M. Inferior ramus of pubis
N. Obturator foramen
O. Ischial tuberosity
P. Lesser trochanter
Q. Intertrochanteric line
R. Greater trochanter
S. Anterior inferior iliac spine
T. Anterior superior iliac spine
U. Intertrochanteric crest
V. Ischial spine
W. Pubic crest
X. Body of ischium
Y. Posterior obturator tubercle
Z. Iliopectineal eminence
AA. Head of femur
BB. Fovea
CC. Fossa of greater trochanter
DD. Gluteal tuberosity
EE. Pectineal line
FF. Linea aspera
1. Lunate surface of acetabulum
2. Acetabular fossa
3. Acetabular notch

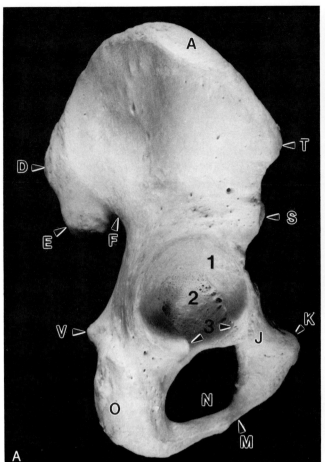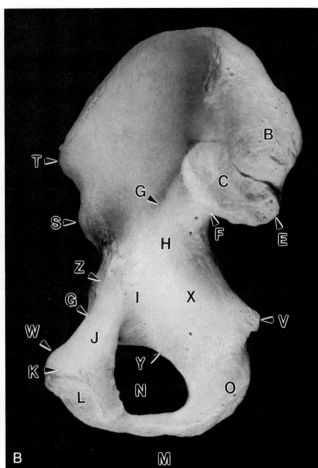

FIG. 1–2.

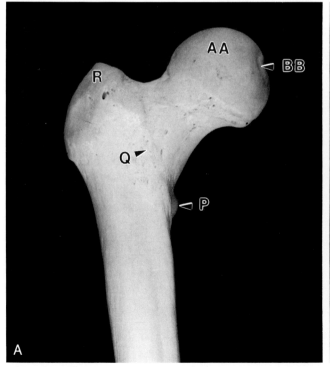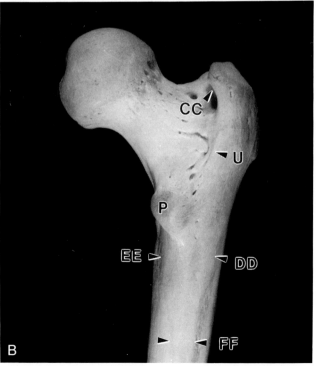

FIG. 1–3.

The Ilium

The body of the ilium forms the upper two-fifths of the acetabulum and superiorly bears a prominent fan-like expansion, the ala, which for the most part is concave medially and convex laterally. The superior border of the ala is surmounted by the iliac crest which, when viewed from above, is recurved. The anterior two-thirds of the crest follows the concavity of the iliac fossa, but the posterior one-third turns laterally where the inner surface of the ala bears the roughened tuberosity. The linear extent of the crest is bounded anteriorly by the anterior superior spine and posteriorly by the posterior superior spine. Its superior surface is rounded and expanded to form an external lip and a less marked internal lip. At the junction between the middle and anterior thirds of the crest, the external lip shows an expanded tubercle.

The posterior one-third of the external lip provides origin for the latissimus dorsi muscle, whereas the anterior part receives the insertion of the external abdominal oblique muscle and gives rise to the tensor fascia latae. The fascia latae is attached to the most lateral extreme of the entire external lip. The internal lip of the crest is the superior boundary of the iliac fossa and gives attachment to the iliac fascia and origin to the transversus abdominis muscle along its anterior two-thirds and to the quadratus lumborum on the posterior one-third. To the surface between the lips are attached fibers of the internal oblique muscle.

The prominent anterior superior spine provides the lateral attachment of the inguinal ligament and the origin of the sartorius muscle. The anterior inferior spine is separated from the above by a slight concavity from whose surface, and the prominence of the spine, arise the straight head of the rectus femoris muscle and the inferior part of the iliofemoral ligament. From the posterior superior spine to the posterior inferior spine the ilium offers attachment to the upper fibers of the stout sacrotuberous ligament. Below this area, the posterior border of the ilium turns upward and forward and then sweeps downward to form the greater sciatic notch.

The gluteal (lateral) surface of the ala displays the superior, middle and inferior gluteal lines which posteriorly converge upon the greater sciatic notch. Formed by the traction of the intervening fascia, these lines respectively delineate the areas of origin of the gluteus maximus, medius, and minimus muscles.

The medial sacropelvic surface of the ilium presents the smooth slightly depressed anterior iliac fossa, the upper two-thirds of which is covered by the origin of the iliacus muscle. The posterior part of the medial ala surface is roughened. Its superior aspect, the iliac tuberosity, is slightly convex and serves for the attachments of iliolumbar and sacroiliac ligaments. The more inferior and sharply demarcated auricular surface indicates the site of attachment with the corresponding auricular surface of the sacrum to form the slightly moveable diarthrodial sacroiliac joint. Below the anterior part of the auricular surface the body of the ilium is thickened medially to form its contribution to the arcuate line. This thickening also provides a triangular dimension to the body of the ilium which, as the stoutest part of the hip bone, forms the major pillar that transfers the vertical thrust from the hip joint to the vertebral column.

The Ischium

The ischium is the second largest component of the hip bone. Its heavy body provides the posteroinferior two-fifths of the acetabulum and bears a posteromedial projection, the spine of the ischium, that, in conjunction with the sacrospinous ligament, separates the greater from the lesser sciatic notch. This latter aperture give egress to the tendon of the obturator internus muscle. Above and below the depression formed by the lesser sciatic notch arise the superior and inferior gemelli that accompany the obturator tendon to its insertion. The smooth concavity of the notch indicates the interposition of a bursa between the tendon and the bone. Below the level of the spine, the ischium bears the large posteroinferiorly directed sacral tuberosity, with a roughened convexity that serves as an origin for the hamstring muscles, while its lateral edge gives the origin to the quadratus femoris muscle. The medial aspect of the tuberosity receives the sacrotuberous ligament, which converts the greater and lesser sciatic notches into foramina. The narrower remainder of the ischium is abruptly directed forward as the ramus that, with the body, encompasses the posterior half of the obturator foramen. Like the body, the ischial ramus is triangular in its cross section with its sharp internal border giving attachment to the obturator membrane. The anterior end of the ischial ramus fuses with the inferior pubic ramus. The lateral aspect of this conjoined ramus is termed the femoral surface because it faces the femur and serves as an origin for its adductors. The lower margin of the femoral surface of the ischial ramus is the origin for the true adductor magnus because the posterior part of the muscle, which arises from the inferior aspect of the ischial tuberosity, is actually by development and innervation, a hamstring muscle. Where the adductor magnus origin is extended forward on the pubis, it is related inferiorly to the origins of the adductor brevis and gracilis, and superiorly to the bony origin of the obturator externus. The pelvic (inner) surface of the conjoined ramus gives origin to the muscles and fascia of the uorgenital diaphragm.

The Pubis

The pubis is the smallest of the three developmental components of the hip bone, and its body forms only the anteroinferior one-fifth of the acetabulum. In its entirety it is V-shaped, being composed of two prismatic bars of bone with the apex directed toward the pubic symphysis. The upper bar, the superior ramus, which extends ventromedially from the body at the acetabulum to the meeting of its bilateral counterpart at the pubic symphysis, is usually described as having a prismoid lateral part and a flat medial part that had been formerly designated as the body of the pubis. The lateral part has superior, inferior, and dorsal surfaces. On the superior surface is found the iliopectineal line, a lateral continuation of the pectineal line (pectin pubis), which is continuous with the arcuate line of the ilium and thus forms the brim of the lesser pelvis. A roughened expansion of the line, the iliopectineal eminence, may be seen at the junction of the pubis and ilium. Just medial to this point the superior ramus is smooth, indicating the position of the psoas bursa that intervenes between the psoas tendon and the bone. The inferior surface forms the superior boundary of the obturator foramen and is grooved laterally for the passage of the obturator nerve and vessels. Medial to the groove the sharp obturator crest anchors its related fibers of the obturator membrane. The smooth dorsal surface faces the pelvic cavity and its lateral part gives origin to some anterior fibers of the obturator internus muscle.

The medial part of the pubis is flat and quadrilateral in shape with a rough medial surface that, through a fibrocartilagenous pad, unites with its opposite member to form the pubic symphysis. Superiorly the medial part is thickened to form the pubic crest whose lateral projection is termed the pubic tubercle. The tubercle receives the medial attachment of the inguinal ligament and hence the medial insertion of the external abdominal oblique muscle. Just medial to the pubic tubercle and in a line that lies anteroinferior to the pectin, originates the pectineus muscle. To the medial part of the pu-

bic crest are attached the rectus abdominis and pyramidalis muscles; just below this point along the lateral border of the symphysis, the adductor longus arises. The muscular relations of the inferior ramus of the pubis have been discussed in conjunction with those of the inferior ramus of the ischium.

The Acetabulum

The acetabulum (Latin: a wine cup), as its name implies, is a cup-shaped cavity that forms the proximal component of the coxofemoral articulation. Although the articulating surface of the femoral head comprises the greater part of a spheroid, the bearing surface of the acetabulum utilizes only a crescentic part of the cup known as the lunate surface. The central and inferior parts of the cavity show a spoon-shaped depression called the acetabular fossa that is filled with the pulvinar, an extrasynovial pad of fat and vessels. The fossa extends inferiorly and slightly anteriorly through the acetabular rim to produce the acetabular notch that is bridged superficially by the transverse acetabular ligament. The recess of the fossa and the soft pulvinar accommodate the ligamentum teres when the articulating surfaces are in the close-packed position. The opening of the acetabulum is directed laterally inferiorly and slightly anteriorly so that the widest and thickest aspect of the lunate surface is positioned superiorly and slightly anteriorly to transfer the most frequent concentration of forces from the upright body to the head of the femur.

The Proximal Femur

Consistent with its weight-bearing requirements, the femur has the thickest and strongest shaft of all the long bones. It receives the nearly vertical thrusts from the pelvis through its angulated and uniquely configured upper end (Fig. 1–4). This consists of a globular head affixed to a superiorly, anteriorly, and medially directed neck that is distally related to two conspicuous muscular processes, the lateral greater trochanter and the posteromedial lesser trochanter. In contrast to the shallow glenohumeral relation of the freely moveable shoulder joint, the femoral head is deeply and securely engaged in the acetabulum. This provides the stability essential to the load-bearing requirements, but at the cost of a severe limitation in the range of motion. However, this restriction is greatly compensated by the angulation and length of the femoral neck (Fig. 1–4A). This angular relation to the

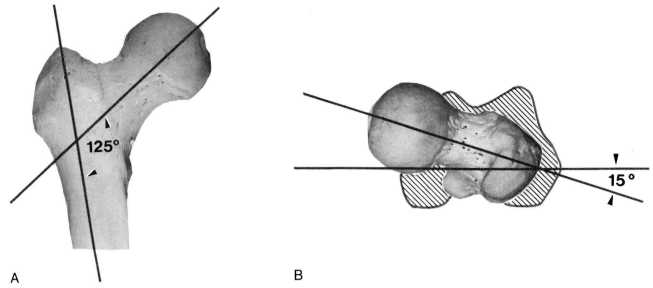

Fɪɢ. **1–4A.** The approximate mean angle of inclination of the adult femoral neck. This value varies in subpopulations, according to age and sex. **B.** The approximate mean of the angle of declination of the femoral neck. It is determined against the intercondylar line of the distal femur shown in shadowed outline. The rotation of this angle is called version, with the anterior rotation being known as anteversion and the posterior rotation termed retroversion.

shaft (the angle of inclination) averages about 125° in the adult.[17] It tends to be increased in the longer femora and in the child and decreased in shorter bones and in the female. By angulation of the neck, the most frequent movements of the thigh, flexion and extension, are converted to a rotation of the head within the acetabulum which, in itself, is virtually unlimited and also maintains a constant amount of bearing surface throughout the range of the actions. Thus the thigh is allowed an extent of flexion only restricted by its contact with the abdomen. Were the head of the femur mounted directly on the shaft, the required depth of the articulation would cause shaft impingement on the acetabular rim after only very limited range of motion. In addition, the length of the angled neck gives a greater leverage for the action of the abductors and a greater space for the bulk of the adductors. The angulation also provides a bone configuration that allows a cranking action of the femur to enhance its rotation. With regard to the ligaments of the joint capsule, the length of the neck permits their distal attachments to be placed much farther from the actual articulation. Thus their length allows for a greater torsional freedom of the capsule before the ligaments are brought up tight.

In addition to the angle of inclination, the neck of the femur is projected obliquely forward with respect to a line joining the condyles of the distal end of the femur. The degree of anterior variance of the neck with respect to this condylar line is known as the version or angle of declination and averages approximately 15° in the adult (Fig. 1–5).

However, the neck angulation and length are not without negative attributes. The downward thrust of the body upon the head and the resistance through the shaft produce displaced parallel lines of force that tend to shear the neck, a risk that is much increased in the demineralized bones of the aged. This detriment is further complicated by the fact that the required distal attachments of the capsule necessitate that the blood supply to the neck and head be closely applied to almost the entire length of the neck and thus share its predisposition to shearing forces.

The head of the femur is entirely intracapsular and its articular surface is more than half a sphere. The surface is entirely covered with articular cartilage except at the *fovea* where it receives the ligamentum teres (Fig. 1–5B).

The expanded base of the neck is delimited anteriorly by the intertrochanteric line and posteriorly by the intertrochanteric crest a prominent traction ridge. The two trochanters form from separate centers of ossification and are essentially traction apophyses. The greater trochanter is quadrilateral in shape and presents a roughened lateral surface. Its anterior lateral surface receives the insertion of the gluteus minimus, whereas its posterolateral surface receives the gluteus medius. An intervening space between these insertions is covered by a bursa to facilitate the motion of the overlying anterior part of the gluteus maximus.

The posterosuperior edge of the greater trochanter (Figs. 1–3, 1–6) is raised to a prominence that overhangs a depression between it and the base of

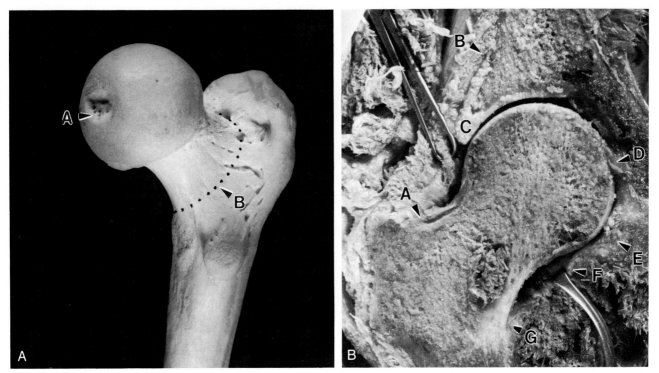

FIG. 1–5A. Posterior oblique view of right femur showing (A) fovea and (B) posterior limit of joint capsule. **B.** Frontal section through hip joint showing (A) lateral superior limit of hip joint capsule with reflected part (retinaculum) that ensheathes the femoral neck. The zona orbicularis is the thickened part of the capsule just above this area. The medial extent of the joint capsule (B) covers the acetabular labrum (C). The attachment of the ligamentum teres (D) lies superior to the fatty pulvinar (E) that fills the acetabular fossa. The transverse acetabular ligament (F) is retracted to the inferior part of the joint capsule to its lateral reflection (G).

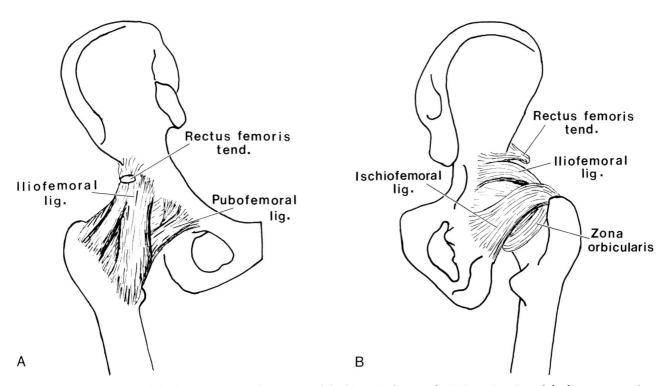

FIG. 1–6A. Anterior view of the ligamentous reinforcements of the hip articular capsule. **B.** Posterior view of the ligamentous reinforcements of the hip articular capsule.

the femoral neck called the trochanteric fossa. The superior edge receives the insertion of the piriformis muscle and the fossa receives the combined tendons of the obturator internus and the gemelli. Just dorsal to the fossa inserts the tendon of the obturator externus and inferior to this the intertrochanteric crest shows a prominence, the quadrate tubercle. To this and the area just below it attaches the tendon of the quadratus femoris muscle.

The lesser trochanter (Figs. 1–3, 1–6) is a rounded posteromedially directed prominence that limits the inferior end of the intertrochanteric crest. It serves as the insertion of the powerful flexor and external rotator of the hip, the iliopsoas muscle. In a line inferior and lateral to the quadrate tubercle, the gluteal tuberosity marks the insertion of the inferior part of the gluteus maximus. At approximately the same level a line or ridge curves inferolaterally from the lesser trochanter, the pectineal line, that receives the insertion of the pectineus muscle. This and the gluteal line converge inferiorly and commence to form a pronounced mid-dorsal ridge, the linea aspera, that descends along the middle third of the femur. The linea aspera shows a medial and lateral lip and receives the insertions of the femoral adductors.

Although some muscular insertions below the linea aspera effect movements of the hip, a detailed discussion of the distal femur is not warranted in an anatomic discourse devoted to the hip joint.

Nonosseous Components of the Hip Articulation

Articular Capsule

The structure of the coxal articular capsule and its reinforcing bands reflects the primary requirements of strength and stability without an appreciable sacrifice of mobility, and its collagenous fibers collectively form one of the strongest ligamentous structures in the body (Fig. 1–6). The entire capsule is quite ample and somewhat slack so that some part of it is relaxed in every position of the limb. Its generalized form is that of a fibrous cylinder, the proximal and distal openings of which are firmly attached to bone. At the pelvis the attachments encircle the acetabulum several millimeters medial and external to its bony rim. Commencing with the fixation of its anterior fibers to the anterior inferior iliac spine and proceeding in a counterclockwise direction, the superior and posterior fibers are bound to the body of the ilium and

are blended with the origin of the reflected tendon of the rectus femoris muscle. Inferiorly, the capsule is attached to the deep aspect of the groove that separates the ischial tuberosity from the corresponding section of the acetabulum from which it continues its attachment to the external surface of the transverse acetabular ligament. Here a partial origin may also be blended with the superior fibers of the obturator membrane. Continuing anteriorly from the acetabular notch the capsular fibers take origin from the superior pubic ramus above the obturator groove and then from the iliopectineal eminence which brings it back to the anterior inferior iliac spine.

At the femoral end of the capsule the anterior attachments are more distal than the posterior. They are bound anterosuperiorly to the union of the neck and the greater trochanter; from there the anterior fibers are fixed to the length of the intertrochanteric line until they reach the medial surface of the femur just anterior to the lesser trochanter. At this point the line of attachment passes posteriorly and then superiorly so that the distal fixation of the posterior capsular fibers follows an oblique line that runs about 15 mm proximal and parallel to the intertrochanteric crest (Fig. 1–5A). It then passes over the neck medial to the trochanteric fossa to attain the anteromedial surface of the greater trochanter.

Some of the distal capsular fibers do not terminate in the bone along the lines of attachment but are reflected medially and passing around the distal margin of the synovial reflection extend under the deep layer of the cervical synovial sheath to achieve a bony fixation closer to the femoral head (Fig. 1–5B). These fibers, collectively termed the retinacula of the capsule, form three fairly distinct bands. Two from the intertrochanteric line are reflected from its superior and inferior parts, respectively, whereas the third is reflected from the middle of the posterior margin of the capsule. The inferior and posterior bands of these retinacular fibers may provide connective tissue support for the cervicocapitular arteries and help them resist the shearing effect of intracapsular cervical fractures.

Thickenings of the capsular fibers along specific lines of stress have produced a number of reinforcing bands that, with respect to the neck, are both longitudinal and circumferential. The three longitudinal bands take their names from their respective origins on the bodies of each of the pelvic bones (Fig. 1–6). With reference to the acetabulum, most of the fibers of these longitudinal ligaments run a spiral clockwise course as they extend distally to their femoral attachments; an arrangement that strongly checks hyperextension through tightening, but progressively relaxes the capsule in hip flexion.

The iliofemoral ligament is the largest, longest, and strongest of the longitudinal capsular bands. Its general appearance is that of a triangle, the apex of which is fixed to the body of the ilium inferior and posterior to the anterior inferior iliac spine, where its most superior fibers blend with those of the reflected origin of the rectus femoris muscle. The fibers descend laterally to their femoral attachments at the anteromedial aspect of the greater trochanter and the entire length of the intertrochanteric line as far inferiorly as the medial femoral surface anterior to the lesser trochanter. The superior fibers run nearly parallel to the superior surface of the neck, but those that attach to the intertrochanteric line show an increasing obliquity toward its inferior end. Frequently there is a visible and palpable division between the upper and lower fibers at the middle of the intertrochanteric line so that the overall configuration of the ligament suggests an inverted "Y" and has been called the "Y" ligament of Bigelow. When the upper fibers are distinct they have been labelled the iliotrochanteric ligament. At the apex of the triangular division between the limbs of the "Y," an artery from the ascending branch of the lateral circumflex artery frequently pierces the capsule as the anterior artery to the neck.

The iliofemoral ligament strongly checks hyperextension of the hip and stoutly splints the anterior capsule against the stress it receives when the vertical thrust of the upright body tries to pivot the pelvis backward upon the femoral heads. This heavy ligament is rarely disrupted in trauma and thus serves as a reliable fulcrum for levering the subluxed femoral head back into the acetabulum.

The pubofemoral ligament is a discrete band of fibers that is shorter and narrower than the other longitudinal capsular ligaments. Its fibers are proximally attached to the iliopectineal eminence and the body of the pubic bone as far inferiorly as the anterior end of the acetabular notch. The fibers of this ligament do not reach the distal attachments of the capsule in themselves, but blend with the more medial and lower fibers of the iliofemoral ligament to transmit their tension to the femur. Thus the pubofemoral ligament assists in limiting hyperextension of the hip in addition to resisting excessive abduction of the femur.

In the variable triangular interval between the pelvic attachments of the ilio- and pubofemoral ligaments, the unreinforced fibers of the anterior capsule may be exposed. Here, in 15% of the cases, an opening permits communication between the synovial cavity of the hip joint and the iliopectineal iliopsoas bursa.

On the posteroinferior surface of the capsule a thick group of fibers forms the strong ischiofemoral ligament. It is proximally attached along the ischial margin of the acetabulum and from the grooved surface between it and the ischial tuberosity and forms a triangular band, the fibers of which pass superolaterally over the posteroinferior aspect of the joint capsule. The most important superior fibers are almost horizontal, but they are joined by the more obliquely spiraling fibers from the lower pelvic attachments and all converge to a fixation on the superior surface of the neck just medial to the trochanteric fossa. Like the other capsular ligaments, the ischiofemoral ligament resists hyperextension of the hip joint.

Some of the deeper fibers of the hip joint capsule are circumferentially disposed forming a garter-like band, the zona orbicularis, located just medial to the distal line of synovial membrane reflexion (Fig. 1–5B). Although it totally encircles the neck external to the outer layer of the synovium, without opening the capsule, it is visible only at the posteroinferior surface of the neck where the fibers of the ischiofemoral ligament fail to attach to the capsular margin.

The Acetabular Labrum and the Transverse Acetabular Ligament

The acetabular labrum is a fibrocartilagenous C-shaped ring that is attached to the bony rim of the acetabulum. It is of variable strength and thickness being stouter in the ilial and ischial sections. A radial cut through the labrum reveals its semitriangular cross section with the internal edge of the base being attached to the inner aspect of the acetabular rim and the articular cartilage. The more extensive external base is fixed to the outer slope of the rim surface as far as the proximal synovial reflexion so that the entire structure is intracapsular, but, being covered by the membrane, it is extrasynovial. The projecting part of the labrum is slightly concave on its inner surface and augments the depth of the acetabulum by 6 to 9 mm. It thus enables the socket to encompass more than half of the spheroidal femoral head so that, even after the capsule is removed, it is still very difficult to extract the head from the acetabulum.

The labrum, like other structures that are largely cartilagenous, may be mostly avascular; the injection of the regional acetabular arteries with a low

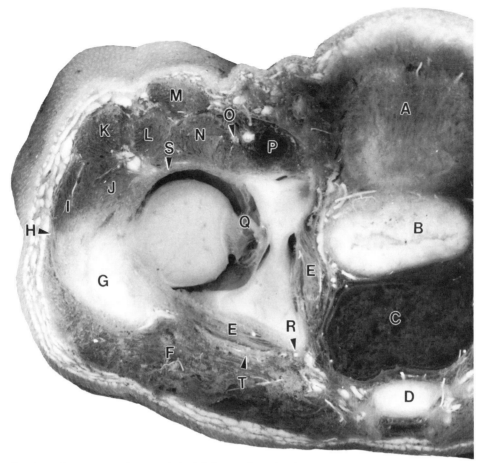

A. Bladder
B. Uterus
C. Rectum (with meconium)
D. Sacrum
E. Obturator internus m.
F. Gluteus maximus m.
G. Greater trochanter
H. Fascia lata
I. Gluteus medius m.
J. Gluteus minimus m.
K. Tensor fasciae latae m.
L. Rectus femoris m.
M. Sartorius m.
N. Iliopsoas m.
O. Femoral nerve (with artery)
P. Femoral vein
Q. Ligamentum teres
R. Internal pudendal artery
S. Hip joint capsule (iliofemoral ligament)
T. Sciatic nerve

Fig. 1–7. Cross-sectional view of the left hemipelvis of a female perinatal cadaver through the level of the hip joint. Especially well shown here is the angulated course of the obturator internus muscle (E), and the early cartilage canal blood supply of the femoral head and acetabulum. Arteries have been injected with white latex.

viscosity medium failed to show evidence of any vessels in the free edge. This suggests that its cellular components derive their nutrients by diffusion from the nearby synovial vessels.

The transverse ligament of the acetabulum is a fibrous completion of the C-shaped ring of the labrum. It contains no chondrocytes and its strength is enhanced by a decussation of fibers as it bridges the acetabular notch. Those that are superficial at its ischial attachment run to the deeper part of the pubic fixation and vice versa. The aperture deep to this ligament gives vascular access to the fatty contents of the acetabular fossa that comprise the pulvinar. This opening also transmits extensions of the synovial membrane that ensheath the ligament to the head and the free surface of the pulvinar.

The ligament of the head of the femur, more commonly called the ligamentum teres (Figs. 1–5, 1–7), extends from the inferior part of the acetabular fossa to the fovea of the head of the femur and is usually about 35 mm in length. It has three proximal attachments; two from the respective ischial and pubic margins of the acetabular notch and a third from the deep inferior fibers of the transverse ligament. The bony fixations usually show some fibers arising external to the notch on the adjacent surfaces of the ischial and pubic bodies, with the posterior (ischial) group being more pronounced. It is flattened on its lateral (capitular) surface and usually presents an elliptical or triangular cross section. As a ligament, the composition is atypical and its function is uncertain. It has a low concentration of fibrous material and it appears slightly redundant so that it may be put under tension only in extreme adduction of the thigh.

The ligamentum teres is completely ensheathed by an extension of the synovial membrane and therefore, like the labrum, is totally intracapsular but extrasynovial. The artery of the ligamentum teres, derived from the posterior branch of the obturator, enters the ligament where its three proximal attachments blend and is present in early fetal life long before it can make any vascular contribution to the osseous tissue of the femoral head (Fig. 1–7).

Undoubtedly the ligament also serves in some capacity to elaborate and distribute synovial fluid through its membranous sheath, a function that is shared by the membrane-covered vascularized tissue of the pulvinar.

Articular Cartilage

As in almost all diarthrodial joints, the articular surfaces of the femoral head and the acetabulum are covered with articular cartilage.

Like a fiber-reinforced plastic, the extracellular matrix of all cartilage is a biphasic system in which collagen fibers hold proteoglycans in a hydroscopic spatial arrangement that binds a relatively large amount of water. However, articular cartilage is a unique form of hyaline cartilage in that the usual random arrangement of the collagen fibers is replaced by a highly organized network that is adapted to load-bearing. The matrix is reinforced by an arrangement of U-shaped fiber bundles, ends of which are anchored into the underlying calcified tissue and the free closed loops are arched into the cartilage toward its bearing surface. These closely packed arcades of Benninghof[2] not only help the cartilage to resist lateral shearing forces, but the collective outer ends of the loops strengthen the outermost aspect of the cartilage by forming a dense layer of collagen fibers that runs mostly parallel to the surface.[3]

The entire tissue is avascular and depends solely on the synovial fluid for its support, but the repeated compression and release experienced through the rolling and sliding of the opposing bearing surfaces has provided an efficient, though labile, system of pumping the fluid-borne nutrients to the deeper chondrocytes. The planes of the loops are not randomly organized, but, as shown by pricking with a round pin, the surface fibers of articular cartilage have consistent patterns of orientation that bear an imperfectly understood relationship to regional stress requirements specific to a particular joint.[4] In the hip articulation, the quantitative distribution of the articular cartilage also reflects the load-bearing characteristics of the joint. A study by Kurrat and Oberlander[13] determined the topographic variations in the relative thickness of the acetabular and femoral cartilage based on systematic sampling according to radial grid projections on the concave and convex surfaces. Their data are graphically indicative that the gradations in cartilage thickness could be arranged in more or less concentric rings receding from the region of maximum loading. This supports what is readily evident in coronal sections of the articulation where the thickest layers of the femoral and acetabular cartilage are seen in apposition at the superior and slightly anterior joint surfaces. When related to an anteroposterior radiogram, the Koch lines of trabecular reinforcement are shown to transmit the loading forces of the femoral shaft and neck directly to that area of the surface where the joint space indicates the cartilage is most ample. Subsequent study of the actual contact pressures by Afore, et al.,[1] has substantiated these observations.

Innervation of the Hip Joint

In accordance to the anatomic generality known as Hilton's Law (the nerve trunks that supply the muscles that move a joint also provide sensory branches to that joint), the nerve supply to the hip joint is rather complex. The classic work of Gardner[6] shows the nerves to be inconsistent in their patterns of distribution because of variant levels and sites of origins from the main trunks or their branches. Nevertheless, when the course and topographic relationship of the nerves effecting hip movement are considered, a conceptual pattern of capsule innervation becomes apparent.

Surprisingly, the innervation to the capsule is rather sparse and with little territorial overlap, a situation that fosters the conclusion that the bulk of sensory spinocerebellar feedback, so necessary and greatly developed with the upright posture, is mediated mostly by neuromuscular and tendinous afferents. Personal dissections have supported Gardner's observations and despite the profusion of variations, a generalized illustration (Fig. 1–8) and verbal description of the hip joint innervation may be presented.

Because both preaxial and postaxial muscles are involved in hip movements, then, per Hilton's Law, nerves from both the anterior and posterior divisions of the lumbosacral plexus will send branches to the joint. The anterior and inferior aspects of the capsule receive sensory nerve fibers from anterior divisions of the lumbar plexus through branches of the femoral and obturator nerves. The femoral branch most frequently supplying fibers to the capsule is the branch to the rectus femoris. This nerve is usually intrapelvic in origin and crosses the joint anteriorly to reach the deep surface of the muscle. It gives one, or more often two, twigs to the capsule.

Frequently, the femoral branch to the pectineus muscle sends fibers to the capsule. These contributions are reciprocal in size to those of the rectus femoris branches.

The inferior aspect of the capsule is innervated

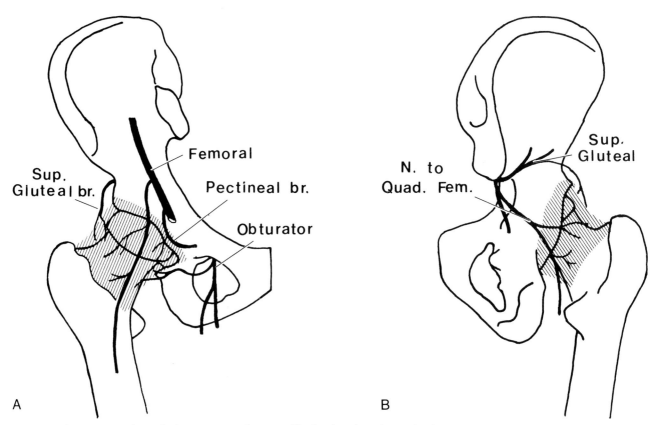

Fig. 1–8. The nerve supply to the hip joint capsule is variable, but based on the work of Gardner and personal observations, a typical arrangement is depicted here. **A.** The anterior part of the capsule is more highly innervated and may receive branches from the quadriceps branch of the femoral nerve, the superior gluteal nerve, a small branch from the pectineal branch, and a substantial branch from the obturator nerve. **B.** The less highly innervated posterior aspect of the capsule receives most of its innervation from a branch of the nerve to the quadratus femoris with a possible small contribution from the superior gluteal.

by a branch from the obturator nerve that tends to be high in origin and separates from the parent nerve in the obturator canal.[6] It then passes posteromedially with the obturator vessels to achieve the medial inferior aspect of the capsule. When accessory femoral or obturator nerves are present they also may contribute fine sensory branches to the joint connective tissue.[10]

The postaxial, posterior division nerves to the joint are sacral plexus branches usually derived from the inferior gluteal nerve and the nerve to the quadratus femoris. The former innervates the superior fibers of the capsule and may accompany the capsular branches of the inferior gluteal artery, whereas the latter, through two or more twigs, supplies the posterior capsule. Occasionally accessory contributions directly from the sciatic nerve have been observed.[21]

Early attempts to relieve the hip pain consequent to degenerative changes focused mainly on the surgical resection of the obturator nerve alone or in combination with a section of the nerve to the quadratus femoris.[15] The results have ranged from good to no improvement, and the permanence of

the relief was always in question. Since the development of more definitive solutions to hip disease, denervation of the joint, as an independent procedure, has been all but abandoned.

Internal Structure of the Proximal Femur

In the growth and remodelling of bone, the deposition of the extracellular matrix is not a random process. Under influences that are not yet clearly understood, the osteoblasts assume a specific polarization and organize the inital collagen formation along lines that are geometrically disposed to provide the greatest resistance to mechanical stress, be it in the form of either tension or compression. The subsequent embedding of these fiber bundles by the precipitation of mineral compounds produces the definitive bone tissue. In compact bone the gross evidences of this osteogenic response to stress are often a general thickening of the cortical shaft to resist compression or the production of asymmetrical ridges (i.e., linea aspera) and protuberances (i.e., lesser trochanter) that are traction apophyses developed in response to tension. In the cancellous bone, the biologic economy of the bone remodeling, through the constant turnover of the osteoblastic-osteoclastic process, eventually achieves a status in which the distribution of the cancellous trabeculae reveals, in the geometric configurations, the definitive stress lines inherent in a specific segment of adult bone.

Nowhere in the skeleton is this stress-related architecture of the trabeculae better demonstrated than in the proximal femur.

As well illustrated in Figures 1–9 and 1–10, the shaft of the femur is a heavy hollow tube of compact bone designed primarily for axial loading, and secondarily, for shear and bend resistance. Just distal to the lesser trochanter, the thickness of the cortex diminishes dramatically so that it is represented only by a relatively thin shell over the external surfaces of the greater trochanter, and neck and head of the femur. However, in common with the epiphyseal regions of other long bones, the thin shell becomes internally reinforced by a system of cancellous trabeculations. An analysis of the frontal sections of a series of femora shows that the arrangement of these trabeculae is remarkably consistent from specimen to specimen. In his classic

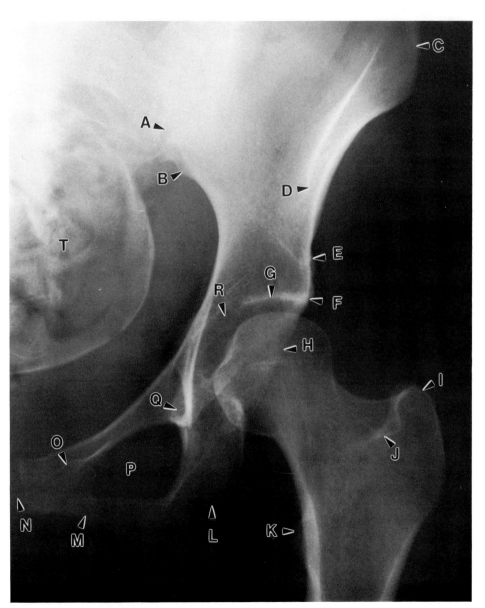

A. Sacroiliac joint
B. Posterior superior iliac spine
C. Iliac tuberosity
D. Anterior superior iliac spine
E. Anterior inferior iliac spine
F. Acetabular crest (margin)
G. Lunate surface of acetabulum
H. Head of femur
I. Greater trochanter
J. Intertrochanteric crest
K. Lesser trochanter
L. Ischial tuberosity
M. Inferior pubis ramus
N. Pubic symphysis
O. Pubic crest
P. Obturator foramen
Q. Kohler's anatomic "teardrop"
R. Acetabular fossa

Fig. 1–9. An anteroposterior x-ray view of the left hip joint of a 18-year-old gravid female. Note the weight-bearing relationships of the acetabulum and femoral head and the consequent alignment of the internal femoral trabeculae.

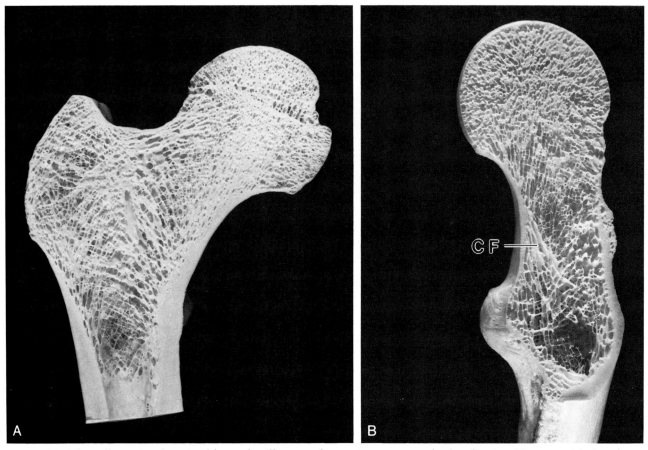

FIG. 1–10A. A frontally sectioned proximal femur that illustrates the consistent pattern of trabeculization. (Compare with the schema in Figure 1–11A.) Note the pattern of medial compression and lateral tension lines. **B.** An oblique cross section of a proximal femur in which the plane of section follows the axis of the femoral neck. Note the convergence of trabeculae that forms the calcar femorale (CF). This aggregate of trabeculae forms a plate-like structure that, because of its "edge effect," is radiologically visible in lateral radiograms of the hip.

work on the mechanical analysis of the moments of force at selected intersecting points in the proximal femur, Koch[12] has demonstrated that the trabeculae are aligned into two major intersecting systems: one to resist tension and the other to resist compression. He assumed a theoretical load on the femoral head and noted ". . . that the trabeculae lie exactly in the paths of the maximum tensile and compressive stresses, and hence these trabeculae carry these stresses in the most economical manner." Koch concluded that there were two major groups of trabeculae. A medial compressive group and a lateral tensile group, each further divided into principal and secondary arrangements (Figs. 1–10, 1–11). The medial compressive group commences on the medial side of the the femoral shaft approximately at the level of the lesser trochanter. Its principal trabeculae course upward nearly parallel to the inferior surface of the neck and terminate in a fan-like arrangement that supports the superior hemisphere of the femoral head. The secondary

compressive trabeculae run immediately lateral to these and gracefully arc toward the greater trochanter. The lateral tensile system begins in the lateral cortex of the femoral shaft and sends its principal members in a curve that runs tangential to the superior surface of the femoral neck to eventually terminate in the inferomedial aspect of the femoral head. Its secondary fibers lie just medial to these and prescribe much tighter curves that terminate in the inferior cortex of the neck. Generally, the trabeculae of the compressive groups tend to be thicker than those of the tensile group. The concentration of trabeculae is least along a "neutral axis" that arises out of the center of the femoral shaft and follows the angulation of the femoral neck in a smooth curve that terminates at the fovea of the head. This axis coincides with the points of intersection of equivalent levels of compressive and tensile trabeculae and shows less bone concentration as some of the antagonistic forces are neutralized at these points. A practical consideration here

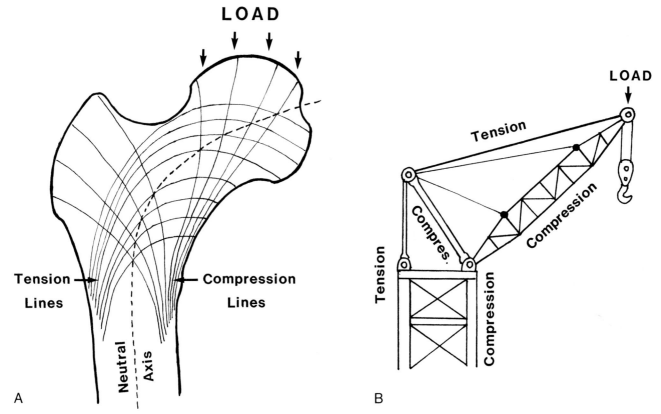

Fig. 1–11A. Schema of the predominant trabecular lines shown in Figure 1–10A. Note the medial trabeculae have a principal compression group that directly supports the load-bearing region of the femoral head and a laterally directed secondary group that is interconnected with the tension trabeculae. The tension trabeculae arise in the lateral femoral shaft and also display a principal lateral group that terminates in the inferior aspect of the head, and a medial secondary group that terminates along the inferior margin of the neck (after Koch). **B.** A gantry crane can be used as the mechanical analogy to the interaction of the compressive and tensile forces in a structure designed to counteract an offset loading, such as in the angulation of the femoral neck.

is that nails or screws driven to align fractures of the femoral neck are best placed close to the cervical cortex because there they gain a better support in the denser concentrations of the trabeculae.

An oblique cross section that follows the axis of the femoral neck reveals a spur-like concentration of trabeculae, the calcar femorale, that converges from the greater trochanter to a point on the posterior cortex of the femoral neck (Fig. 1–10B). The functional significance of this trabecular configuration was not addressed by Koch, but it appears to lend rigidity to the posterior aspect of the femoral neck. The high concentration of trabeculae at the apex of the calcar femorale makes it radiologically visible, particularly in lateral views of the hip joint.

Blood Supply of the Hip Joint

The disruption of the nutritional vascularity to the femoral head that is often consequent to cervi-

cal fractures has directed considerable attention to the sources and collateral relations of the arterial supply to the femur and particularly to that of its proximal region. Although the degree of collateral support provided to the proximal femur by the intramedullary vessels of the shaft is uncertain, their morphologic relationship must be considered in any comprehensive description of the upper femoral blood supply.

The medullary cavity of the femur, from the trochanters to the distal epiphyseal area receives most of its arterial nutrition from one or two nutrient vessels usually derived from the perforating branches of the deep femoral artery (Figs. 1–12, 1–13). According to Laing,[14] the incidence of double or single nutrient arteries to the shaft was about equally distributed in his series of adults and infants examined. He also recorded that whether single or double, these arteries, in most cases penetrated the shaft in the upper half so that the descending intramedullary supply to the distal shaft, like that of the tibia, is more remote from its

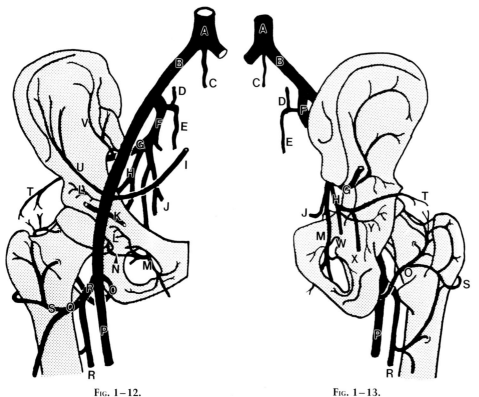

A.   Aorta
B.   Internal iliac a.
C.   Middle sacral a.
D.   Iliolumbar a.
E.   Lateral sacral a.
F.   Hypogastric a.
G.   Superior gluteal a.
H.   Inferior gluteal a.
I.   Inferior epigastric a.
J.   Middle rectal a.
K.   Superficial external puden-
     dal a.
L.   Acetabular branches
M.   Obturator a.
N.   Artery of ligamentum teres
O.   Medial femoral circumflex a.
P.   Femoral a.
Q.   Lateral femoral circumflex a.
R.   Deep femoral a.
S.   Circumflex branch of lateral
     circumflex a.
T.   Capsular branch of superior
     gluteal a.
U.   Deep iliac circumflex a.
V.   Superior gluteal branch to il-
     iac fossa
W.   Internal pudenal a.
X.   Artery to sciatic nerve

Fig. 1–12.   Fig. 1–13.

Fig. 1–12. Anterior view of the major arterial relationships of the right hip. The same labels apply to the posterior aspects shown in Figure 1–13.

Fig. 1–13. Posterior view of the major arterial relationships of the right hip.

source and therefore more precarious in the event of lower shaft fracture. Because the medullary nutrient foramina are located along the linea aspera, the stripping of adductor insertions to the upper half of this line should be done with caution. The ascending intramedullary vessels course upward to reach the intertrochanteric and lower cervical regions where the terminal branches anastomose with those of the more proximal arteries to the femur.[19,22]

The functional significance of these anastomoses has been disputed by Howe and his coworkers,[9] who claim the terminal relationships are too fine to be effective, and the vascular injection studies of Trueta and Harrison[18] have failed to show any anastomoses between the ascending intramedullary terminals and the arterial supply to the head. From a clinical standpoint, then, the intrinsic blood supply to the femoral components above the trochanters depends on branches of the nearby major vessels. These arteries are, in order of importance of their contribution, the medial and lateral femoral circumflexes, the obturator, the superior gluteal, the ascending branch of the first deep femoral perforator, and the inferior gluteal.

Despite some disagreements on relative quantitative aspects, an analysis of the major studies of the vascularity of the upper end of the femur shows that there is a remarkably consistent pattern in the arterial distribution to the femoral head and neck (Fig. 1–14). This is evidently related to the facts that the development and shape of the osseous components and the arrangement of the ligamentous attachments and their synovial reflexions have limited the possible approaches to the sites of vascular access to the bone.

Both of the circumflex vessels supply the trochanteric and cervical regions, but the medial is the major source of nutrition to the head. This artery is usually the first branch of the deep femoral and initially courses downward and medially to curve around the insertion of the iliopsoas, where it gives small nutritional branches to the lesser trochanter. Passing inferior to the obturator externus it then ascends in a superolateral direction along the posterior surface of the femoral neck. During this part of its course it provides two groups of branches to the head. The first of these, the posteroinferior vessel, which may be multiple, leaves the circumflex artery as it clears the posterior border of the obturator

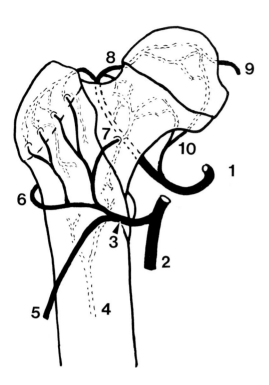

Fig. **1–14.** Typical arterial supply to proximal femur.

1. Medial femoral circumflex a.
2. Deep femoral a.
3. Lateral femoral circumflex a.
4. Ascending branch of internal nutrient a.
5. Muscular branch to quadriceps
6. Circumflex femoral branch
7. Anterior cervical branch
8. Superior branches of medial femoral circumflex a.
9. Artery of ligamentum teres
10. Inferior branches of medial femoral circumflex a.

externus, and enters the distal edge of the joint capsule where it courses upward deep to the synovial reflexion that ensheathes the neck. It subdivides and penetrates several nutrient foramina just distal to the articular rim of the head.

The medial circumflex artery then continues to follow the margin of the attachments of the capsule and usually gives off a cervical branch that penetrates the mid or distal part of the posterior neck surface. After reaching the trochanteric fossa, it gives one or two branches to the greater trochanter and then terminates in two to four larger branches that constitute the posterosuperior group of arteries to the head. After penetrating the capsular margin, these run under the synovium for almost the entire length of the posterosuperior surface of the neck and penetrate a series of nutrient foramina circumferentially arranged around the posterior and superior aspects of the articular rim of the head. Thus, the medial circumflex artery constitutes a vascular ring that follows the posterior femoral attachment of the capsule to encircle nearly two-thirds of the base of the femoral neck.

The lateral femoral circumflex artery also is usually a branch of the first part of the deep femoral artery. Its initial segment is much larger than the medial circumflex because its first major branch supplies the anterior bulk of the quadriceps muscles as far distal as the knee (Fig. 1–15). It continues a nearly horizontal course anterior to the femoral shaft just below the level of the lesser trochanter. The lateral circumflex terminates by wrapping around the lateral infratrochanteric region of the shaft and anastomosing with terminals of the gluteals, posterior branch of the obturator, and ascending branch of the first deep femoral perforator to complete the classical so-called "cruciate anastomoses." With respect to the supply of the upper femur, its anterior ascending branches are most important. The first of these is usually the longest because it serves both the greater trochanter and the neck. This branch, like the medial circumflex, courses along the margin of the joint capsule. However, the anterior capsular margin is more distal than the posterior so that this artery may be seen running along the intertrochanteric line, which is defined by the distal limits of the iliofemoral ligament. Midway in its ascending course this first branch gives rise to a substantial vessel that penetrates the capsule and passes a brief distance under the synovial sheath to penetrate a nutrient foramen in the anterior distal one-third of the neck. The continuation of the main branch then ascends to nutrient foramina in the anterosuperior aspect of the greater trochanter. A small communication with the terminals of the medial circumflex may occur in the trochanteric fossa, thus completing a perivascular ring that almost surrounds the entire distal capsular margin.

The continuation of the lateral circumflex then gives off a variable number of smaller trochanteric branches as it encircles the femoral shaft (Fig. 1–14).

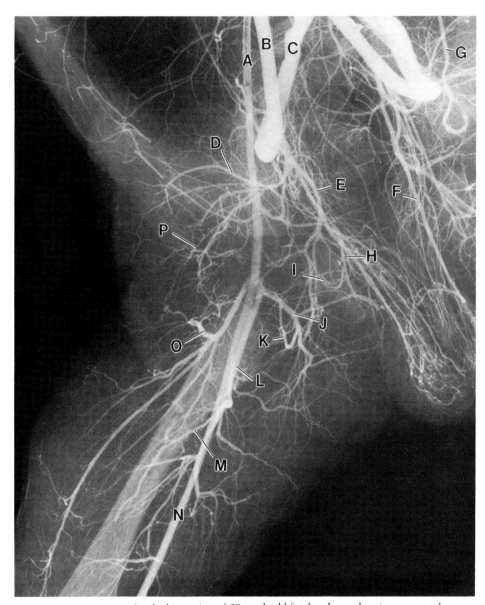

A. External iliac a.
B. Umbilical a.
C. Hypogastric a.
D. Superior gluteal branch
E. Inferior gluteal a.
F. Internal pudendal a. (opposite side)
G. Inferior epigastric a. (opposite side)
H. Obturator a.
I. Posterior branch of obturator to ligamentum teres
J. Medial femoral circumflex a.
K. Medial femoral circumflex branch to hip joint
L. Deep femoral a.
M. Nutrient artery to shaft of femur
N. Femoral a.
O. Lateral femoral circumflex a.
P. Capsular branches of superior gluteal a.

Fig. 1–15. Arteriogram of right hip region of 30-week-old fetal cadaver showing an actual example of the anterior distribution to the hip joint. The acetabulum and the femoral head and cervix are represented by radiolucent cartilage at this stage, but the definitive pattern of circulation has been established.

The artery of the ligamentum teres (foveolar artery) is usually a derivative of the posterior branch of the obturator artery, but origin from the medial circumflex has been noted. It leaves the obturator branch as it passes inferior to the acetabular notch and enters the acetabular fossa deep to the transverse acetabular ligament. Before entering the ligamentum teres it gives off one or more branches to the fossa, which are nutrient to the medial wall of the acetabulum and the tissues that comprise the pulvinar. The artery is incorporated into the ligament, where the deep ischial and pubic attachments of the ligamentum teres blend with its origin from the transverse acetabular ligament. The artery of the ligament may be single or multiple at this point, but it usually elaborates some fine branches within the ligamentous substance before the major vessel(s) enter the head of the femur through nutrient foramina in the fovea.

Several studies have tried to analyse the extent of the collateral support provided to the femoral head by the artery of the ligamentum teres because this is the only capitular supply that is not directly threatened by cervical fracture.[5,19,20,22] All agree that the ligament artery in all but a few cases (110 out 114 of Chandler and Krenscher's series[5]) contributes to the nutrition of the head, but the extent is widely variable. Tucker,[19] who described the presence of an artery entering the head in all ligaments, claimed that in 30% of the cases its size was not sufficient to provide a reliable support should the more distal circulation be interrupted, whereas in the remaining 70% of cases, a variable extent of vascularization might be primarily supplied by the artery of the ligament, ranging from just the proximal foveolar section to the entire head.

Trueta and Harrison[20] have generally substantiated this observation, noting in injected specimens that the injection medium had reached about one-fifth of the head substance in 7 out of 15 specimens; one-half in 1; and as much as two-thirds in the remaining 7.

During the developmental and early childhood periods the artery of the ligamentum teres does not supply any of the chondrous head tissue. According to Wolcott,[22] vessels from the ligament invade the head only after ossification is well underway, and no anastomoses with the distal arterial terminals can be observed until around age 15, when the ossification of the head is nearly complete.

A consistent and immediately recognizable designation for the branches of the circumflex arteries that course along the femoral neck to supply the intrinsic vessels of the proximal neck and head is sadly lacking. Names such as "capsular" and "rectinacular" arteries tend to be confusing. Howe and his associates[9] used the term "capital arteries," and the common label of "ascending cervical branches" at least gives a partial clue to their topographic relations, but their function is still obscure because those of the posterosuperior group supply branches to both the proximal neck and head. Because these arteries are unique in that they run a substantial distance closely applied to the cervical periosteum and are held fairly firmly against the bone by the reflected sheath of synovial membrane, their collective lability and clinical significance in intracapsular fractures should warrant them a consistent and more precise designation. Therefore the label "cervicocapitular arteries" may better indicate the subsynovial branches of the circumflex arteries that are bound around the neck and supply both it and the head.

Most investigations and descriptions of the vascularity of the hip joint fail to even mention the blood supply to the pelvic components of the articulation. This may be understandable when it is considered that although its physiologic significance may be just as great, from the standpoint of

trauma and its surgical implications, its clinical import is far less than that of the proximal femur.

Ribet[18] in 1926, published a remarkable account of the vascular supply to all of the major musculoskeletal articulations. In this much neglected monograph he has provided the first accurate and illustrated description of not only the upper femoral blood supply, but also of the nutritional vessels to the acetabulum. In 1950, Howe and his associates[9] (who were apparently unaware of Ribet's work) compiled an excellent report of the vascularity to the entire coxal articulation, but their description of the acetabular supply was incomplete. By injection studies of the neonatal hip the author has been able to substantiate the observations of Ribet and provide the following account. If the acetabulum is regarded as the face of a clock, then a radially arranged centripetal group of nutrient vessels penetrates the thick supporting acetabular bone from the following sources. From 10 to 2 o'clock a group of penetrating arteries are derived from the inferior branch of the superior gluteal artery. From 2 to 4 o'clock a specific acetabular branch of the femoral artery curves around the acetabular rim. From 4 to 8 o'clock, the posterior branch of the obturator extends nutrient arteries to the inferior acetabular bone, and from 8 to 10 o'clock a branch of the inferior gluteal artery provides nutrient acetabular branches. The obturator branch to the ligamentum teres, as previously noted, sends nutrient branches to the medial acetabular wall through foramina in the acetabular fossa. All of these vessels are schematically depicted in Figure 1–16. What is not shown are the vessels to the medial wall of the acetabulum that penetrate the internal surface of the bodies of the ilium and ischium from iliac branches of the iliolumbar artery. Ribet gave these vessels the collective designation of "cotyloid branches" of their respective source arteries.

All of the above groups of vessels also supply branches to the fibrous sheath, ligaments, and the synovial membrane of the proximal parts of the joint capsule. These may be regarded as the true "capsular" arteries. They anastomose with distal capsular branches from the vascular ring that nearly encircles the distal attachments of the capsule as well as conspicuous contributions from anastomotic connections between a pronounced capsular branch of the inferior (sometimes superior) gluteal artery and ascending trochanteric branches of the lateral femoral circumflex as illustrated in Figures 1–12, 1–13, 1–15.

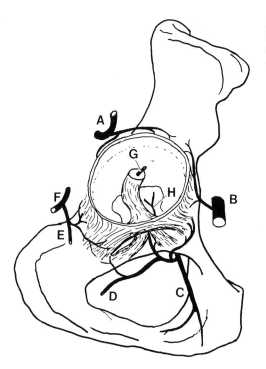

Fɪɢ. **1–16.** Anteroinferior veiw of a right hip bone showing arterial relationships of the acetabulum and proximal connective tissue.

A. Inferior gluteal a.
B. Femoral a.
C. Obturator a.
D. Posterior branch of obturator a.
E. Sciatic branch of inferior gluteal a.
F. Inferior gluteal a.
G. Artery of ligamentum teres
H. Pulvinar a.

Muscle Actions at the Hip

A description of muscles pertaining to a specific joint is usually accomplished by grouping them either topographically or functionally. However, in the case of the hip joint, the muscles are so numerous and complex in their functions and relationships that some consideration of both aspects is warranted. To avoid the prolixity required by a detailed account of each individual muscle, a table grouping the muscles topographically with the essential facts of their innervation and action is presented here (Table 1–1).[7,8,16] This table groups the muscles according to their anatomic compartments and their developmental preaxial and postaxial affinities. The latter categories indicate the original relationship of the muscles to the axis of the limb when it was in its early embryonic and phyletically primative position. With the medial rotation of the limb in subsequent growth, the definitive locations of the muscles do not readily indicate their original relations to the limb axis, but their origins and innervations retain the initial associations. It may be conveniently summarized that those hip muscles originating on the vertebral column and ilium are postaxial and are innervated by the gluteal or femoral nerves (or small individual nerves of equivalent origins from the lumbosacral plexus), whereas the preaxial muscles have origins on the ischium and pubis with innervation from the obturator or sciatic (tibial) nerves (or their small positional equivalents).

The topography of the origins and insertions of the individual hip muscles has been graphically provided in Figures 1–17 and 1–18, so an extensive narrative account of this information is not necessary here. However, during the following discussion of the functional groups of the hip muscles, significant topographic information will be added where appropriate.

Functional Groups of Muscles That Act Across the Hip Joint

The Extensors

The major extensors of the thigh are the gluteus maximus and the ischiocondylar part of the adductor magnus. The gluteus maximus, in its cross-sectional dimension is the largest single muscle of the body. Its extensive origin and double insertion indicate its multiple functions, and the differing actions of the upper and lower fibers have been confirmed electromyographically. The lower fibers insert both in its femoral tendon and the fascia lata of the vastus lateralis and the iliotibial tract, but the extent and effect of the tract insertion have been disputed. The extension effect of the lower gluteus is most active when a powerful thrust, such as in running or climbing, is required. It is also powerful in its correlative action of erecting the spine and pelvis when the body has been bent over at the hips. The superior part of the gluteus is an abductor and lateral rotator of the

TABLE 1–1. *Summation of Segmental Innervation of Muscles Involved with the Hip*

Muscle	Nerve		Segmental Innervation ←—Recorded Range—→ >Essential<		Major Functions at Hip
Postaxial Muscles					
Gluteal Compartment					
Gluteus maximus	Inferior gluteal	L4	L5, S1	S3	Extend, laterally rotate
Tensor fascia latae	Superior gluteal	L4	L4, L5	S1	Flex, abduct, medially rotate
Gluteus medius	Superior gluteal	L4	L4, L5, S1	S2	Abduct, medially rotate
Gluteus minimus	Superior gluteal	L4	L4, L5, S1	S1	Abduct, medially rotate
Piriformis	Nerve to piriformis	L4	S1, S2	S2	Laterally rotate, abduct
Anterior Compartment					
Iliopsoas	Nerves to iliopsoas	L2	L2, L3, L4	L5	Flex, laterally rotate
Rectus femoris	Femoral	L2	L2, L3, L4	L5	Flex
Sartorius	Femoral	L2	L2, L3	L5	Flex, abduct, laterally rotate
Preaxial Muscles					
Medial Compartment					
Obturator externus	Obturator	L2	L3, L4	L5	Laterally rotate
Gracilis	Obturator	L2	L3, L4	L5	Adduct, flex
Pectineus	Femoral or obturator	L2	L2, L3	L4	Flex, adduct, medially rotate
Adductor longus	Obturator	L2	L2, L3	L4	Adduct, flex, medially rotate
Adductor brevis	Obturator	L2	L2, L3	L5	Adduct, flex, medially rotate
Adductor magnus (Pubofemoral part)	Obturator	L2	L3, L4	L5	Adduct, flex, medially rotate
(Ischiocondylar part)	Sciatic (tibial)	L4	L4, L5	S3	Adduct, extend, laterally rotate
Posterior Compartment					
Obturator internus	Nerve to obturator internus	L4	L5, S1, S2	S3	Laterally rotate, extend
Gemellus superior	Nerve to obturator internus	L4	L5, S1, S2	S3	Laterally rotate, extend
Gemellus inferior	Nerve to quadratus femoris	L4	L5, S1	S1	Laterally rotate, extend
Quatratus femoris	Nerve to quadratus femoris	L4	L5, S1	S1	Laterally rotate
Semitendinosus	Sciatic (tibial)	L4	L5, S1	S3	Extend, medially rotate
Semimembranosus	Sciatic (tibial)	L4	L5, S1	S3	Extend, medially rotate
Biceps femoris (Long head)	Sciatic (tibial)	L4	L5, S1	S3	Extend, laterally rotate

thigh and will be discussed in these functional groupings. The posterior (ischiocondylar) part of the adductor magnus is the second most important extensor of the thigh. Whereas the gluteus maximus is most effective in this action when the thigh is in lateral rotation, the adductor magnus is most effective when it is in medial rotation. During extension, the natural adduction of the magnus is neutralized by the synergistic contraction of the gluteus medius. The hamstrings (semimembranosus, semitendinosus, and long head of the biceps) are minor thigh extensors because their function in this capacity is limited to the synergistic concomitant of flexion.

A graphic schema of the thigh extensors is provided in Figure 1–19.

The Flexors

The iliopsoas, pectineus, tensor fasciae latae, and sartorius are the major flexors at the hip. Of these, the iliopsoas is the most powerful. As the combined fibers of the psoas major and the iliacus, the inferior part of this muscle passes over the pelvic brim to course, first anterior and then inferior to the femoral neck. Its insertion in the posteriorly situated lesser trochanter calls for a pulley-like ac-

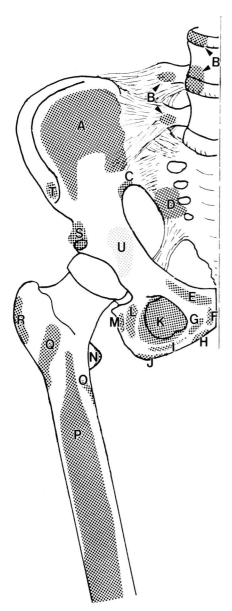

FIG. 1–17. Anterior view of the right hip showing the attachment of regional muscles.

A. Iliacus—origin
B. Psoas—origin
C. Obturator internus—origin
D. Piriformis—origin
E. Pectineus—origin
F. Adductor longus—origin
G. Adductor brevis—origin
H. Gracilis—origin
I. Adductor magnus (pubofemoral)—origin
J. Adductor magnus (ischiocondylar)—origin
K. Obturator externus—origin
L. Quadratus femoris—origin
M. Semimembranosus—origin
N. Iliopsoas—insertion
O. Vastus medialis—origin
P. Vastus intermedius—origin
Q. Vastus lateralis—origin
R. Gluteus minimus—insertion
S. Rectus femoris—origin
T. Sartorius—origin
U. Iliopectineal (psoas) bursa

tion around the contiguous bones. This force actually results in a rotation of the femoral neck, which, because of the neck angulation, is transformed into a flexion of the thigh. When the body is supine and the legs are fixed, the iliopsoas ventroflexes the lumbar spine and flexes the pelvis at the hip joint as in "sit-up" exercises. This function is much emphasized in the running and leaping quadrupeds (e.g., rabbits and kangaroos) whose greatly exaggerated psoas muscles serve to rapidly ventroflex the spine and pelvis and flex the femurs so as to repeatedly and rapidly "cock" the hind limbs for their powerful propulsive extension.

The hip joint actions of the tensor fasciae latae and the sartorius are also primarily that of thigh flexion. This function is also assisted in a lesser degree by the adductors, namely the adductor brevis, adductor longus, and the anterior (pubofemoral) part of the adductor magnus. The flexion contribution of these muscles is proportional to the degree in which pelvic origins of the fibers are positioned anterior to the axis of the femur in extension. The anterior fibers of the deeper gluteals (medius and minimus) may also provide minor assistance in thigh flexion. Although the rectus femoris is primarily an extensor at the knee joint, its pelvic origins provide for some flexion at the hip. Its effectiveness in this role is diminished by flexion at the knee and increased with flexion of the thigh. This last functional aspect probably results from the fibers of the reflected (acetabular) part of its dual tendon of origin being brought more into line with

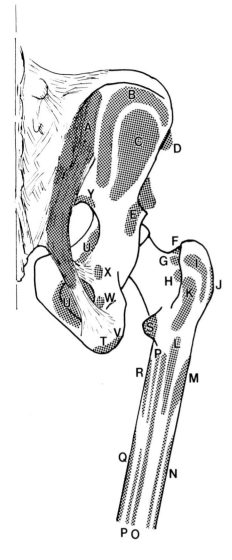

Fɪɢ. 1–18. Posterior view of right hip showing attachments of regional muscles.

A. Gluteus maximus—origin
B. Gluteus medius—origin
C. Gluteus minimus—origin
D. Tensor fasciae latae—origin
E. Rectus femoris (reflected and straight heads)—origin
F. Piriformis—insertion
G. Obturator internus (with gemelli)—insertion
H. Obturator exturnus—insertion
I. Gluteus minimus—insertion
J. Gluteus medius—insertion
K. Quadratus femoris—insertion
L. Gluteus maximus—insertion
M. Vastus lateralis—origin
N. Vastus intermedius—origin
O. Adductor magnus—insertion
P. Adductors brevis and longus-insertion
Q. Vastus medialis—origin
R. Pectineus—insertion
S. Iliopsoas—insertion
T. Semitendinosus—origin
U. Obturator internus—origin
V. Biceps femoris—origin
W. Gamellus inferior—origin
X. Gamellus superior—origin
Y. Piriformis—origin

the major direction of the muscle contraction during flexion. Another anterior femoral muscle, the sartorius, assists in flexion at the hip. Like the rectus it is a two-joint muscle with a greater effect on knee joint action and a more complex relationship with lateral rotation of the thigh. However, with its pelvic origin being superior to that of the rectus, it possesses a greater mechanical advantage in the earlier stages of thigh flexion. The topographic relations of the hip flexion are depicted in Figure 1–20.

The Abductors

The principal abductors of the thigh are the gluteus medius and minimus. Both of these muscles have an extensive origin from the external surface of the ala of the ilium and they insert respectively on the posterior and anterior edges of the greater trochanter. By their position relative to the hip joint, it is self evident that their combined contraction elevates the trochanter and thus abducts the thigh. However, a less obvious but extremely important function of these muscles is their ability to pull down on the wing of the ilium when their respective leg is bearing weight and firmly grounded. By using the entire pelvis as a lever with the fulcrum being the ipsilateral femoral head, these two glutei hold the opposite side of the pelvis in a level position as the contralateral leg is raised off the ground for its forward non-weight-bearing swing in the stride cycle. Because of the fan-like extensive origins of these two gluteal muscles, their more anterior and posterior fibers also give minor contributions to thigh rotation, flexion, and extension. The shortening of the leg in the supine postion, that is pathognomonic of femoral neck fractures, is

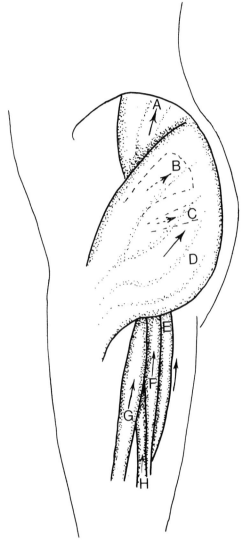

FIG. 1–19. Extensors of the thigh.

A. Gluteus medius (dorsal fibers)
B. Gluteus minimus (dorsal fibers)
C. Piriformis
D. Gluteus maximus
E. Ischiocondylar part of adductor magnus
F. Semitendinosus
G. Biceps femoris
H. Semimembranosus

caused, to a great part, by the contraction of these deep gluteal muscles.

Thigh abduction is also assisted by the tensor fasciae latae, the sartorius, and the superior fibers of the gluteus maximus. In addition, when the thigh is flexed, the small, deep lateral rotators may be recruited in this action.

The abductors of the thigh are shown in Figure 1–21.

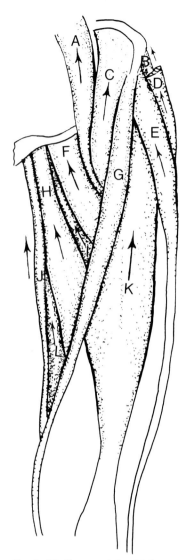

FIG. 1–20. Flexors of the thigh.

A. Psoas
B. Gluteus minimus
C. Iliacus
D. Gluteus medius
E. Tensor fasciae latae
F. Pectineus
G. Sartorius
H. Adductor longus
I. Adductor brevis
J. Gracilis
K. Rectus femoris
L. Adductor magnus

The Adductors

The chief adductors of the thigh are the pectineus, and the adductors longus, brevis, and magnus. All of these, with the exception of the posterior fibers of the magnus, arise on the pubis, which, being more medially placed than the ischium and

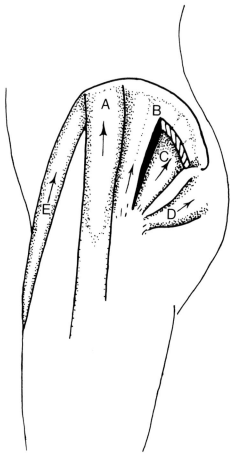

FIG. 1–21. Abductors of the thigh.

A. Tensor fasciae latae
B. Gluteus medius
C. Gluteus mimimus
D. Piriformis
E. Sartorius

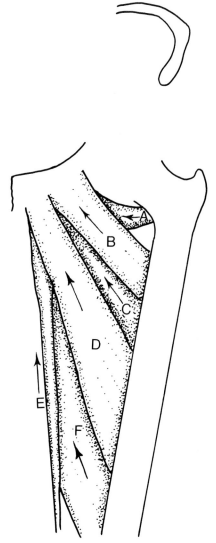

FIG. 1–22. Anterior adductors of the thigh.

A. Obturator externus
B. Pectineus
C. Adductor brevis
D. Adductor longus
E. Gracilis
F. Adductor magnus

ilium, establishes a good mechanical advantage for this action. The pectineus originates on the superior pubic ramus and forms a large part of the floor of the femoral triangle. The interval between its superolateral border and the iliopsoas gives passage to the medial circumflex artery that is the major source of vascularity to the femoral head and neck. Developmentally, the pectineus received contributions from both preaxial and postaxial precursors that account for its frequent ambiguous innervation from both femoral and obturator nerves. From a closely grouped origin, the adductors longus and brevis, and the pubofemoral part of the magnus, fan out to insert on the greater part of the linea aspera with the fibers of the first two muscles attaching medially to those of the magnus. In addition to strong adduction, they also contribute to flexion (v.s.), and rotation (v.i.). Adduction of the thigh also

receives considerable assistance from the gracilis and the inferior fibers of the gluteus maximus. Although adduction of the thigh is one of the primary functions of the gracilis, its size and postion do not allow it to be a major contributor in this respect, for its surgical relocation for reconstructive procedures in the perineum is not followed by any appreciable loss of adductive power.

The obturator externus, iliopsoas, and the collective hamstrings all provide minor contributions to adduction. Electromyography shows that the abductors must be recruited to counteract this ten-

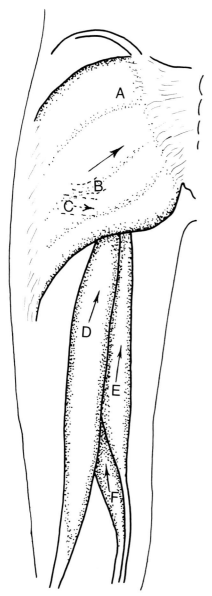

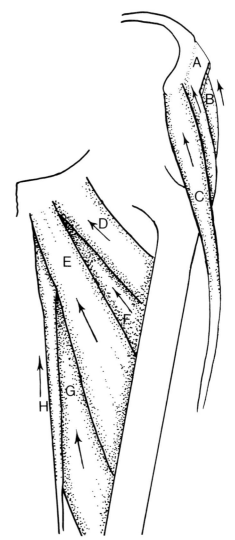

Fig. **1–24.** Medial rotators of the thigh.

A. Gluteus medius
B. Gluteus minimus
C. Tensor fasciae latae
D. Pectineus
E. Adductor longus
F. Adductor brevis
G. Adductor magnus
H. Gracilis

Fig. **1–23.** Posterior adductors of the thigh.

A. Gluteus maximus
B. Obturator externus
C. Quadratus femoris
D. Biceps (long head)
E. Semitendinosus
F. Semimembranosus

dency when they are involved in their other primary functions. The topographic relations of the thigh adductors are shown in Figures 1–22 and 1–23.

The Rotators

Medial (Internal) *Rotation.* The primary contributors to this action are the gluteus medius and

minimus, the tensor fasciae latae, the pectineus, the adductors longus and brevis, and the pubofemoral part of the magnus. The anterior fibers of the deep gluteals and the tensor fasciae latae combine to pull the greater trochanter and the overlying lateral fascia lata forward, and hence pivot the hip joint medially in an obvious mechanical relationship. The rotative actions of the adductor group, however, have not been so obvious. An agreement that they contributed to rotation of the thigh has been universal, however, there has been much confusion regarding the direction in which they pro-

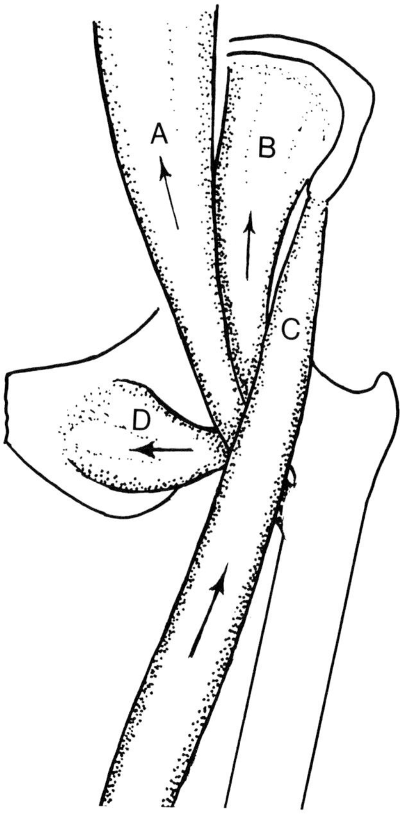

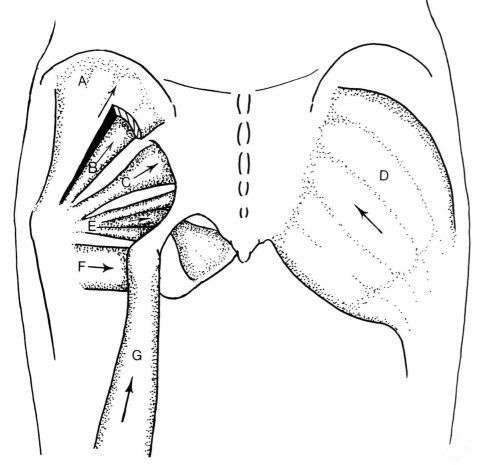

Fig. 1–25. Anterior lateral rotators of the thigh.

A. Psoas
B. Iliacus
C. Sartorius
D. Obturator externus

Fig. 1–26. Posterior lateral rotators of the thigh.

A. Gluteus medius
B. Gluteus minimus
C. Piriformis
D. Gluteus maximus
E. Obturator internus and ga-
melli
F. Quadratus femoris
G. Biceps

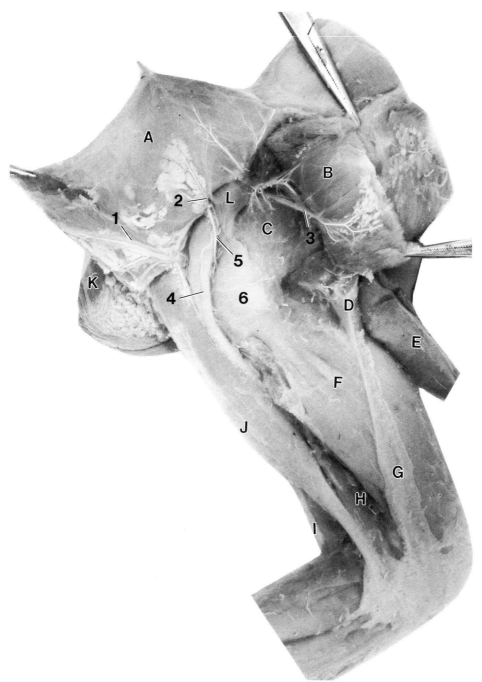

A. Gluteus maximus m.
B. Gluteus medius m.
C. Gluteus minimus m.
D. Tensor fasciae latae m.
E. Reflected skin
F. Vastus lateralis m.
G. Iliotibial tract
H. Short head, biceps femoris m.
I. Semitendinosus m.
J. Long head, biceps femoris m.
K. Levator ani m.

1. Posterior femoral cutaneous nerve and concurrent branch of inferior gluteal artery
2. Inferior gluteal nerve and artery
3. Superior gluteal nerve and artery
4. Sciatic nerve
5. Artery to sciatic nerve
6. Trochanteric bursa

Fɪɢ. 1–27. Dissection of the gluteal region of a perinatal cadaver that well shows the relationships of the major vessels and nerves to the hip joint. The thigh is in the flexed position that is the normal attitude of the newborn and quadrupeds. Note that the perineum extends below the pelvic outlet in the infant. The muscles are labeled with letters; nerves and neurovascular bundles are designated with numbers.

duced the rotational force. The popular anatomic texts, up to and including Hollinshead's classics, have all listed the adductor group as lateral rotators, but the electromyographic evidence has shown them to be medial rotators. The source of this error probably lay in the superficial analysis of the directions of force in relation to the femoral

axis of rotation. With the exception of the ischiocondylar part of the magnus, the adductors insert on a prominence on the posterior aspect of the femur. A cross-sectional image of this arrangement coupled with the hasty assumption that the axis of femoral rotation somewhat parallels the axis of the femoral shaft would immediately suggest that the

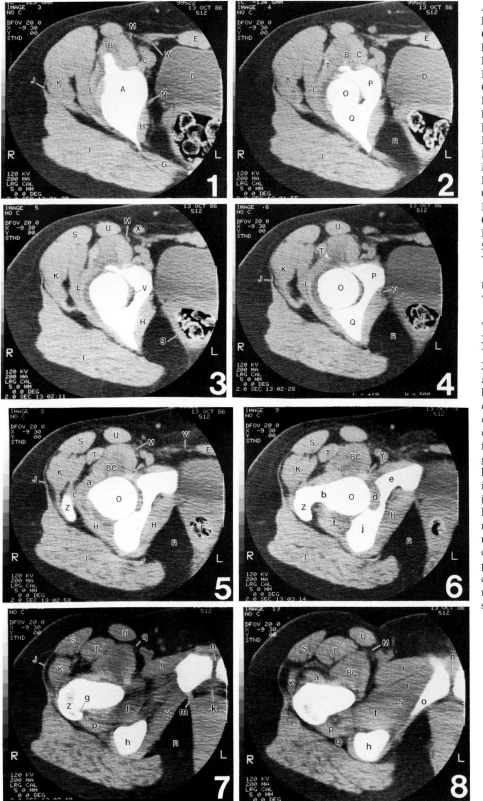

A. Body of ilium
B. Iliacus m.
C. Psoas m.
D. Bladder
E. Rectus abdominis m.
F. Rectum
G. Coccygeus m.
H. Obturator internus m.
I. Gluteus maximus m.
J. Fascia lata
K. Gluteus medius m.
L. Gluteus minimus m.
M. Femoral nerve
N. Obturator nerve and vessels
O. Femoral head
P. Body of pubis
Q. Body of ischium
R. Ischiorectal fossa
S. Tensor fasciae latae m.
T. Rectus femoris tendon (calcified)
U. Sartorius m.
V. Ligamentum teres

W. Inguinal ligament
X. Inguinal lymph node
Y. Femoral artery and vein
Z. Greater trochanter
a. Vastus intermedius m.
b. Femoral neck
c. Obturator canal
d. Acetabular notch
e. Body of ischium
f. Obturator externus
g. Trochanteric fossa
h. Ischial tuberosity
i. Pectineus m.
j. Body of ischium
k. Retropubic space
m. Pubococcygeus m.
n. Pubic symphysis
o. Inferior pubic ramus
p. Inferior gemellus
q. Sciatic nerve
r. Adductor longus m.
s. Adductor brevis m.

FIGS. 1–28.1 TO 1–28.8. Sequential cross-sectional views of a normal hip joint provided by CT scanning. The first image sections the base of the ilium at the level of the anterior inferior iliac spine, and the last sections the femur through the level of the junction of the inferior aspect of the neck and the femoral shaft. The same legend is applicable to all eight images. Note the calcification of the tendon of the rectus femoris.

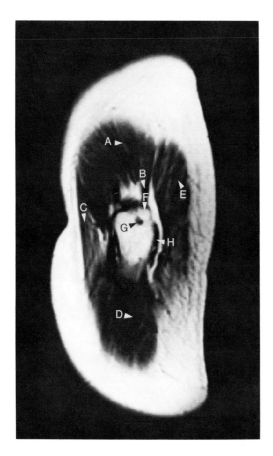

Fig. 1–29. Sagittal MRI views of the hip region of an adult female.

A. Gluteus medius m.
B. Gluteus minimus m.
C. Tensor fasciae latae m.
D. Vastus lateralis m.
E. Gluteus maximus m.
F. Greater trochanter
G. Trochanteric fossa
H. Obturator externus m.

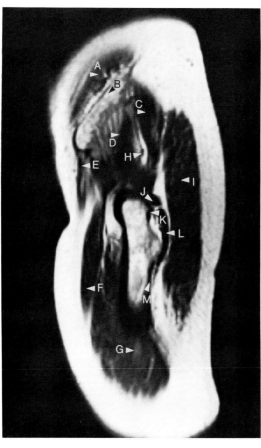

Fig. 1–30. Sagittal MRI views of the hip region of an adult female.

A. Internal oblique m.
B. Iliac crest
C. Gluteus medius m.
D. Gluteus minimus m.
E. Sartorius m.
F. Rectus femoris m.
G. Vastus lateralis m.
H. Superior gluteal artery
I. Gluteus maximus m.
J. Piriformis m.
K. Obturator internus m.
L. Obturator externus m.
M. Quadratus femoris m.

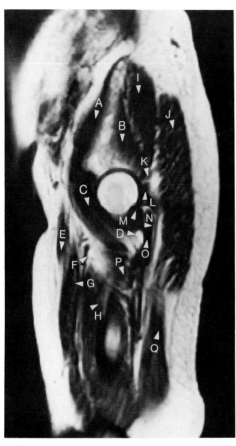

Fig. **1–31.** Sagittal MRI views of the hip region of an adult female.

A. Iliacus m.
B. Gluteus minimus m.
C. Iliopsoas m.
D. Lesser trochanter
E. Sartorius m.
F. Femoral artery and nerve
G. Rectus femoris m.
H. Vastus lateralis m.
I. Gluteus medius m.
J. Gluteus maximus m.
K. Piriformis m.
L. Obturator internus and gamelli mm.
M. Obturator externus m.
N. Sciatic nerve
O. Quadratus femoris m.
P. Pectineus m.
Q. Biceps femoris m.

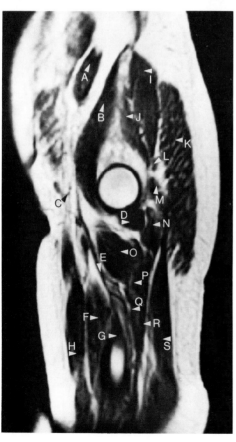

Fig. **1–32.** Sagittal MRI views of the hip region of an adult female.

A. Sigmoid colon
B. Psoas m.
C. Inguinal ligament
D. Obturator externus m.
E. Deep femoral artery
F. Vastus intermedius m.
G. Vastus medialis m.
H. Rectus femoris m.
I. Gluteus medius m.
J. Gluteus minimus m.
K. Gluteus maximus m.
L. Piriformis m.
M. Obturator internus and gemelli mm.
N. Quadratus femoris m.
O. Pectineus m.
P. Adductor brevis m.
Q. Adductor longus m.
R. Adductor magnus m.
S. Semimembranosus m.

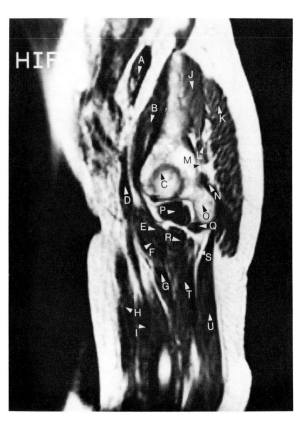

Fɪɢ. **1–33.** Sagittal MRI views of the hip region of an adult female.

A. Sigmoid colon
B. Psoas m.
C. Acetabulum
D. Rectus femoris m.
E. Pectineus m.
F. Adductor brevis m.
G. Adductor longus m.
H. Rectus femoris m.
I. Vastus medialis m.
J. Gluteus medius m.
K. Gluteus maximus m.
L. Piriformis m.
M. Sciatic nerve
N. Obturator internus and gemelli mm.
O. Ischial tuberosity
P. Obturator internus m.
Q. Quadratus femoris m.
R. Adductor minimus m.
S. Semimembranosus tendon
T. Adductor magnus m.
U. Semitendinosus m.

adductors laterally rotate the femur. However, the true axis of thigh rotation is described by a line dropped from the fovea of the femoral head to the adductor tubercle of the medial condyle. Thus almost all of the femur, and particularly its upper parts lies lateral to this line. With the bulk of the adductor fibers arising on the anterior parts of the pelvis, the direction of the fibers from origin to insertion describes a line that lies considerably anterior to this axis of rotation. Thus, the vectors of adductor contraction literally "crank" the upper femur medially around the true rotational axis as substantiated by electromyography. Because their ischiadic origin lies medial to their femoral insertions, the semimembranosus, semitendinosus, and the long head of the biceps femoris also tend to adduct the thigh when engaged in their major functions of thigh extension and leg flexion. This action is compensated by synergistic contraction of the abductors.

The positional relationships of the thigh medial rotators are shown in Figure 1–24.

Lateral (External) ***Rotation.*** The lateral rotators of the thigh are the most numerous functional group and some of the included smaller muscles have a complex ontogenetic and phyletic history. The gluteus maximus, piriformis, quadratus femoris, and the obturators externus and internus are the major contributors to this action. With the ex-

ception of the obturator externus, all of these muscles are best visualized from a posterior anatomic approach. When the inferior gluteal fibers, which are its stronger lateral rotators, are elevated from their insertion, the deeper lateral rotators are readily exposed. The posterior fibers of the gluteus medius and minimus, which both contribute some accessory effort to this action, may be dissected in the superior part of the subgluteal region. Inferior to this, the triangular piriformis passes laterally out of the pelvis through the greater sciatic foramen to insert on the superior aspect of the greater trochanter. By mechanical relationship to the hip joint, the piriformis should laterally rotate, and, depending on thigh position, should assist in abduction and extension. However, its size seems to preclude any effective degree of contribution in these respects. The phyletic relationships of the piriformis and its nerve supply indicate that this muscle represents a migration of the most posterior fibers of the original gluteus medius, and its disproportionate number of nerve spindles may indicate that it serves more as a proprioceptive sensor than an effector of limb motion. From a topographic sense, however, the piriformis serves as a central anatomic landmark in the subgluteal region. Through the interval between the piriformis and the gluteus medius superiorly, and a corresponding space between the piriformis and the superior gamellus inferiorly, the

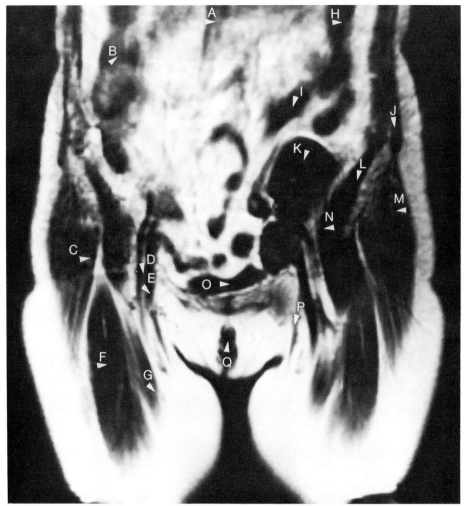

A. Aorta
B. Ascending colon
C. Tensor fasciae latae m.
D. Femoral artery
E. Femoral vein
F. Rectus femoris m.
G. Vastus medialis m.
H. Descending colon
I. Sigmoid colon
J. External oblique m.
K. Sigmoid colon
L. Iliacus m.
M. Gluteus maximus m.
N. Psoas m.
O. Bladder
P. Saphenous vein
Q. Vulva

Fɪɢ. 1–34. Frontal MRI views of the pelvis and hip regions of the same adult female.

major nerves and vessels leave the pelvis and enter the posterior limb compartments. In the medial part of the superior piriformic recess the superior gluteal nerve and arterial complex exit to supply the deep gluteal muscles and the tensor fasciae latae. Through the medial part of the inferior piriform interval passes the inferior gluteal nerve and artery, and the internal pudendal nerve and artery; the latter structures loop around the sacrospinous process to enter the perineum. In the more lateral part of this interval, the massive sciatic nerve, the posterior femoral cutaneous nerve (lesser sciatic), the nerves to the quadratus femoris and inferior gemellus, and to the obturator internus and superior gemellus pass out of the pelvis to enter the posterior compartment of the thigh. In about 85% of the observed cases, the combined tibial and peroneal components of the sciatic nerve pass inferior to the piriformis. The balance of instances shows either one or both components of the nerve splitting the fibers of the piriformis. Inferior to the piri-

formis are found the fibers of the superior and inferior gemelli flanking the tendon of the obturator internus to form with it a combined insertion into the trochanteric fossa. The obturator internus arises from almost the entire internal aspects of the pubic and ischiadic bones where it lines the anterolateral walls of the lesser pelvis. Its fibers converge posteriorly toward the lesser sciatic foramen to take a greater than 90° turn around a bursa-protected groove and then travel anterolaterally to reach the greater trochanter. The pulley-like arrangement of this muscle may be appreciated in the photograph of the cross-section of the newborn pelvis shown in Figure 1–7. The two gemelli originate on either side of the groove that passes the extrapelvic part of the obturator internus. Like the piriformis, these small muscles ostensibly assist in lateral femoral rotation, but also like the piriformis, they are probably more functional in a proprioceptive capacity. The heavy quadrilateral quadratus femoris that lies inferior to the above muscles is of sufficient size to provide a sub-

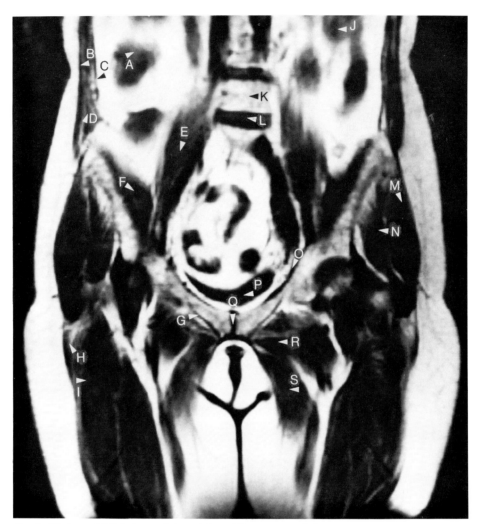

Fᴵɢ. 1–35. Frontal MRI views of the pelvis and hip regions of the same adult female.

A. Ascending colon
B. External oblique m.
C. Transversus abdominis m.
D. Internal oblique m.
E. Psoas m.
F. Iliacus m.
G. Lacunar ligament
H. Gluteus maximus m.
I. Rectus femoris m.
J. Descending colon
K. L₃ vertebral body
L. L₃₋₄ disc
M. Gluteus maximus m.
N. Gluteus medius m.
O. Obturator internus m.
P. Bladder
Q. Pubic symphysis
R. Pectineus m.
S. Adductor longus m.

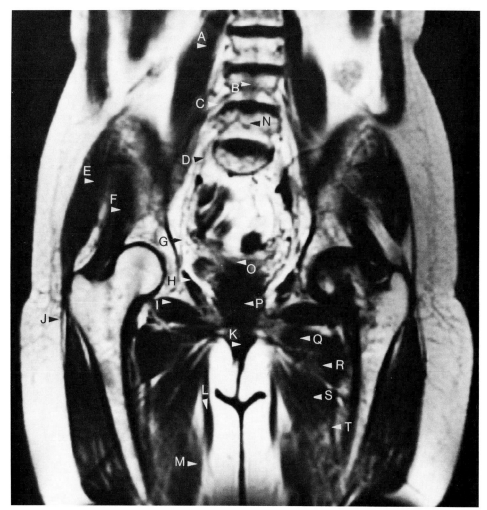

Fig. 1–36 Frontal MRI views of the pelvis and hip regions of the same adult female.

A. Psoas m.
B. Dura in spinal cord
C. L₃ spinal nerve
D. Lumbosacral trunk
E. Gluteus maximus m.
F. Gluteus medius m.
G. Obturator nerve
H. Obturator internus m.
I. Obturator externus m.
J. Iliotibial tract

K. Vagina
L. Gracilis m.
M. Adductor magnus m.
N. L₄ vertebral body
O. Uterus
P. Bladder
Q. Pectineus m.
R. Adductor brevis m.
S. Adductor longus m.
T. Femoral artery

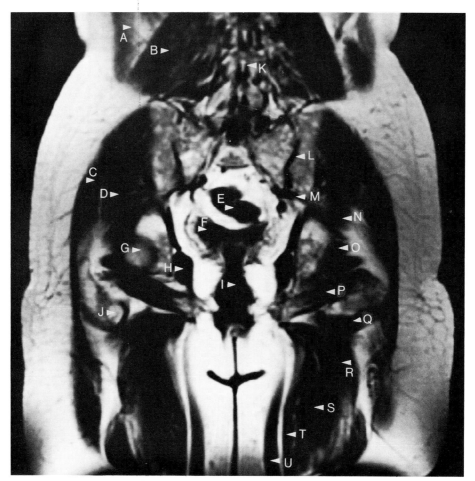

FIG. 1-37. Frontal MRI views of the pelvis and hip regions of the same adult female.

A. Transversus abdominis m.
B. Quadratus lumborum m.
C. Gluteus maximus m.
D. Gluteus medius and minimus mm.
E. Rectum
F. Uterus
G. Femoral head
H. Obturator internus m.
I. Vaginal fornix
J. Lesser trochanter
K. Spine of L$_4$ vertebra

L. Sacroiliac joint
M. Superior gluteal artery
N. Piriformis m.
O. Obturator internus and gamelli mm.
P. Obturator externus m.
Q. Quadratus femoris m.
R. Adductor magnus m.
S. Semitendinosus m.
T. Semimembranosus m.
U. Biceps femoris m.

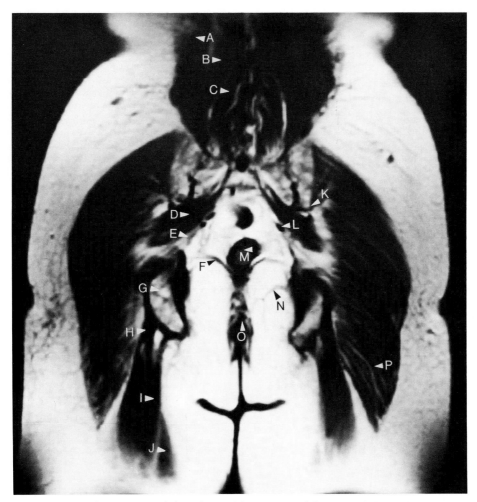

FIG. 1–38. Frontal MRI views of the pelvis and hip regions of the same adult female.

A. Erector spinae m.
B. Semispinalis m.
C. Multifidus m.
D. Piriformis m.
E. Sciatic nerve
F. Pelvic diaphragm
G. Ischial tuberosity
H. Biceps femoris m.
I. Semimembranosus m.
J. Semitendinosus m.
K. Superior gluteal vessels
L. Inferior gluteal vessels
M. Rectum
N. Inferior rectal vessel
O. Anus
P. Gluteus maximus m.

stantial contribution to the lateral rotation of the thigh. The sartorius, iliopsoas, and the long head of the biceps femoris also provide assistance in this function.

With the thigh in the flexed position, the lateral rotators arising from the pelvis act as thigh abductors, and from an evolutionary standpoint this was evidently their primary function. In the quadruped, the normal anatomic position of the thigh is that of flexion. A similar situation prevails in the human newborn (which is actually a quadruped in its thigh-pelvis relationships) for the first few months of life. A photograph of the exposed subgluteal region in a newborn cadaver (Fig. 1–27), well illustrates this intitial flexed status of the thigh and indicates the primative abductor function of the deep lateral rotators. It also illustrates the relationships of the nerves and vessels to the landmark piriformis muscle, and the intimate relationship of these structures to the posterior aspect of the hip joint capsule.

The general topographic relations of these rotators of the thigh are graphically shown in Figures 1–25 and 1–26.

The large aggregate of muscle that surrounds and moves the hip shows an intricate arrangement that may be visually appreciated in the CT cross-sectional views of the joint (Figs. 1–28.1 to 1–28.8). The same area is depicted in Figures 1–29 to 1–33, a series of sagittal MRI views that progresses from lateral to medial. Figures 1–34 to 1–38 show the frontal MRI view. The series progresses from anterior to posterior.

References

1. AFOKE NYP, BYERS PD, HUTTON WC: Contact pressures in the human hip joint. J Bone Joint Surg, 69B:536–541, 1987.
2. BENNINGHOFF A: Spaltlinen am knocken. Anat Aug, 60:189–206, 1925.
3. BENNINGHOFF A: Form und bau dev gelenknorpel in ihren beziehungen zur funktion. Z Zellforsch Mikrosk Anat, 2:782–862, 1925.
4. BULLOUGH P, GOODFELLOW J: The significance of the fine structure of cartilage. J Bone Joint Surg, 50B:852–857, 1968.
5. CHANDLER SB, KREUSCHER PH: A study of the blood supply of the ligamentum teres and its relations to the circulation of the head of the femur. J Bone Joint Surg, 14:834–846, 1932.
6. GARDNER E: The innervation of the hip joint. Anat Rec, 101:353–371, 1948.
7. HOLLINSHEAD WH: Anatomy for Surgeons, Vol 3. New York, Harper and Row, 1971.
8. HORWITZ MT: The anatomy of (A) the lumbosacral nerve plexus—its relation to variations of vertebral segmentation, and (B) the posterior sacral nerve plexus. Anat Rec, 74:91–107, 1939.
9. HOWE WW, LACEY T, SCHWARTZ, RP: A study of the gross anatomy of the arteries supplying the proximal of the femur and the acetabulum. J Bone Joint Surg, 32A:856–866, 1950.
10. KAPLAN EB: Resection of the obturator nerve for relief of pain in arthritis of the hip joint. J Bone Joint Surg, 30A:213–218, 1948.
11. KEISER, RA: Obturator nervectomy for coxalgia: an anatomic study of the obturator and accessory obturator nerves. J Bone Joint Surg, 31A:815–819, 1949.
12. KOCH JC: The laws of bone architecture. Am J Anat, 21:177–298, 1917.
13. KURRAT HJ, OBERLANDER W: The thickness of cartilage in the hip joint. J Anat, 126:145–155, 1978.
14. LAING PG: The blood supply of the femoral shaft: anatomical study. J Bone Joint Surg, 35B:462–466, 1953.
15. OBLETZ BE, LOCKIE LM, MILCH E, HYMAN I: Early effects of partial sensory denervation of the hip for relief of pain in chronic arthritis. J Bone Joint Surg, 31A:805–816, 1949.
16. PATERSON AM: The origin and distribution of nerves to the lower limb. J Anat Physiol, 28:84–102, 1893.
17. PICK JW, STACK JK, ANSON BJ: Measurements on the human femur: lengths, diameters and angles. Northwest Med School, 15:281–291, 1941.
18. RIBET M: Les Artères Osteo-Articulaires. Alger, Imprimerie Moderne, 1926.
19. TUCKER FR: Arterial supply to the femoral head and its clinical importance. J Bone Joint Surg, 31B:82–93, 1949.
20. TRUETA J, HARRISON MHM: The normal vascular anatomy of the femoral head of the adult man. J Bone Joint Surg, 35B:442–461, 1953.
21. WERTHHEIMER LG: The sensory nerves of the hip joint. J Bone and Joint Surg, 34A:447–485, 1952.
22. WOLCOTT WE: The evolution of the circulation in the developing femoral head and neck. Surg Gynecol Obstet, 77:61–68, 1943.

CHAPTER TWO

Basic Science Aspects of Cemented Total Hip Arthroplasty

WILLIAM J. HOZACK

Introduction

The success of total hip replacement depends on three critical factors—patient selection, prosthesis selection, and surgical technique. Probably the most important single determinant of a good surgical result is proper patient selection. Improper patient selection can overwhelm the most advanced prosthetic design and the most expert technical surgeon.

Given proper patient selection, however, close attention to the details of prosthesis selection and surgical technique can virtually guarantee consistent, reliable, and enduring results. Yet this guarantee is not absolute. As Charnley has noted "neither surgeons nor engineers will ever make an artificial hip joint which will last thirty years and at some time in that period enable the patient to play football."[29] Extensive basic research and clinical experimentation has outlined the many factors that can influence the outcome and success of total hip replacement. The following chapter attempts to review many of these factors.

Because a total hip replacement is a mechanical device consisting of three parts—metal, polyethylene, and cement—it is not surprising that the major long-term problem with total hip replacement is mechanical failure of one or all of the parts. The forms of failure include fatigue fractures of the metal stem, wear and fracture of the high density polyethylene cup, and loosening of the cement grout.

This chapter examines many of the theoretical and practical means by which a successful result may be achieved. Both experimental and clinical evidence is examined. In most areas consensus exists; in others, debate continues to rage.

Mechanical Failures

Polyethylene Failure

Although polyethylene failure can occur because of fracture[64,105,135,144] or external wear,[155,159] the most common mode of failure of the polyethylene is through internal wear at the metal-plastic interface (Fig. 2–1). Considering that the load borne by the acetabulum ranges between 3 and 5 times body weight, depending upon activity, it is not surprising that some wear does occur. The actual extent of this polyethylene wear and its significance is not clear. A finite element analysis by Bartel[8] suggested that the polyethylene in the cup is protected from large stresses and large variations in stress by the high conformity of the head-cup surfaces. He predicted, however, that the thickness of the polyethylene should be maximized to reduce contact stresses that can lead to surface damage. Minimum plastic thickness of 6 mm was recommended (especially in the low conformity total knee arthroplasty).[7] Furthermore, Bartel's model predicted higher contact stresses with the 22-mm head as compared to a 28-mm head. However, no long-term data exists to suggest that there is more wear with the 22-mm internal diameter cups. Rather, Charnley found in his Teflon cups that the smaller head size produced less volumetric wear debris than did 41-mm heads.[27]

However, Charnley noted that the linear distance penetrated into the cup was greater with the 22-mm head.[27] In 1978, Griffith and Charnley performed a thorough radiographic evaluation of socket wear in 491 total hip replacements at an average of 8.3 years postoperatively.[61] The mean cup wear was 0.59 mm, which corresponded to 0.07 mm per year. Only 4% had wear greater than 1.5 mm. Wear was not correlated with weight in this study (and in most others). However, heavy wear was more common in younger patients. In 1985,

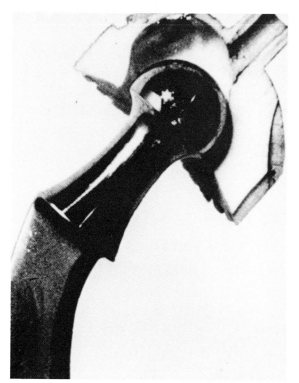

Fig. 2–1. Internal wear is dramatically visualized in the early teflon cups.

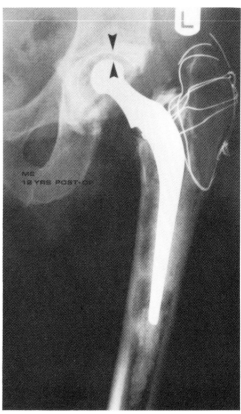

Fig. 2–2. Wear of the polyethylene acetabular component as indicated by the arrows may be responsible for the calcar and endosteal resorption visualized around the femoral component. (From Rothman RH, Hozack WJ: Complications of Total Hip Arthroplasty. Philadelphia, WB Saunders, 1988.)

Wrobleski reported on 22 retrieved acetabular cups.[157] The rate of wear was 0.19 mm per year (ranging from 0.17 mm to 0.52 mm). He felt that mechanical impingement of the neck onto the socket would occur after 0.4 to 0.56 mm of wear and that this wear could lead to late dislocations and loosening. Support for this statement has been provided by Coventry[36] who found that patients with late dislocations had a greater range of motion, implying that prosthetic neck-cup impingement was instrumental in these dislocations. Internal polyethylene wear would certainly aggravate this tendency toward late impingement and dislocation.

Rose[131] felt that the major long term problem from polyethylene wear would not be mechanical impingement secondary to dimensional changes within the cup but rather would be the adverse tissue reaction to the polyethylene debris created by wear. In his study on a total joint simulator, he found that a major contributing factor to the variable wear rates encountered was the variable molecular weights of the plastic. The true wear rate of the polyethylene as measured by volume of debris ranged from 0.3 to 10.2 mg per year. This accounted for only 3 to 30% of the dimensional change in the cup, the remainder being caused by creep. Furthermore, he felt that none of the true wear rates were large enough to cause mechanical

dysfunction. The biologic effect of wear debris may be the more important concern because it may be responsible for calcar resorption and possibly even component loosening (Fig. 2–2).[155] If the noncemented total hip components do solve the long-term problem of component fixation, wear of the polyethylene may become a prominent future concern.[43] For this reason, research into alternatives to ultra-high molecular weight polyethylene (such as ceramics) is warranted.

Metal Failure

Metal failure as a cause of a failure of a total hip replacement is rare. However, the range of incidence in studies is surprisingly variable—from 0.23% to 11%.[58] Fortunately for current orthopaedic practice, the causes of premature metal failure are well recognized and therefore, for the most part, entirely avoidable.

Metallurgic defects that act as crack initiation points[59,99] can be responsible for early metal failure or at least contributory, however this type of problem has been properly addressed by quality control in the manufacturing process. The actual metals themselves (primarily cobalt-chromium or titanium alloys) have fatigue strengths and endurance limits that far exceed predicted in vivo stress levels. However the addition of porous ingrowth surfaces and modular head-neck attachments has created new areas of weakening or stress concentration that may predispose to fracture.[98,122] Iatrogenic stress risers, such as wire nicks and accidental drill bit scoring, must be avoided.[25]

The most common underlying cause for metal failure is related to a combination of poor cement technique and unfavorable patient characteristics. The largest series reported was by Wroblewski, who reviewed 120 cases of fracture of the femoral component.[156] He found a significant linear relationship between patient weight and the time of fracture. The active, young, heavy male is at greatest risk of fatigue failure of the metal.

Most studies have found that a varus position of the femoral component predisposes to earlier failure.[25,30,32,128] This is most likely related to the inadequate cement mantle support proximally that occurs with the varus position. With poor proximal support and good distal fixation, prosthetic toggle will occur and lead eventually to fatigue failure.

Galante[58] has provided a useful classification of femoral stem fractures:

Cantilever bending. This includes problems with varus positioning of the femoral component, failure to remove the weak cancellous bone in the proximal-medial calcar area, calcar resorption, and good distal fixation (Fig. 2–3).[25,30,32]

Overstress. Included here are the heavy, active, youthful patients (Fig. 2–4).[30,128]

Stress concentration. Stress risers come in numerous forms—nicks, metallurgic defects, serrations, sharp edges, and "porous ingrowth" coatings (Fig. 2–5).

Most likely, a combination of several of these factors is needed before a femoral component fracture could occur. Careful attention to proper cement technique, the use of stronger alloys, proper patient selection, and avoidance of iatrogenic stress risers will keep this problem to a minimum.

Cement Failure

Clinical experience has shown that aseptic loosening of cement is, as Charnley wrote, "the central and most serious problem with which we are faced in total hip replacement at the present moment."[31] Early clinical reviews identified the femoral side as

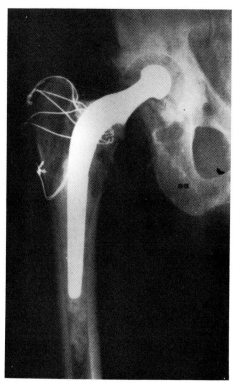

FIG. 2–3. Fracture of the femoral component in its midportion was most likely related to the combination of varus component position and inadequate proximal cement and bony support for the component. (From Rothman RH, Hozack WJ: Complications of Total Hip Arthroplasty. Philadelphia, WB Saunders, 1988.)

an immediate problem.[9,19,116] Consequently, much early basic research examined methods to improve durability of the femoral component. However, later studies with longer followup showed that aseptic loosening of the acetabular component was equally problematic.[31,84,141,142] Clearly the literature implicates polymethylmethacrylate (PMMA) as the weakest component of the implant chain. The degree to which the surgeon adheres to the principles of proper patient selection, prosthesis selection, and surgical techniques that protect this weak link will ultimately determine the long term success of conventional total hip replacement.

Wiltse, in 1957,[150] evaluated methyl methacylate for possible surgical application. He concluded that "although at the present time, no uses in orthopaedic surgery can be recommended unequivocally, it is believed that it may find a place following more research on the basic material." Since then the general physical properties of polymethylmethacrylate (PMMA) have been reviewed extensively. PMMA has 50 to 75% of the compressive strength, 25% of the tensile strength, and less than 50% of the fatigue strength of cortical bone.[133] PMMA is brittle—it undergoes relatively little deformation before fracture. Finally it has 10% of the stiffness of

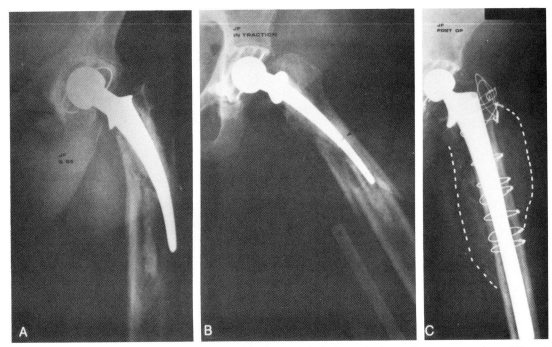

Fɪɢ. 2−4. **A.** This patient suffered a comminuted fracture of the femoral shaft about the femoral component after a fall. **B.** The patient was initially placed in traction, and a radiograph revealed a femoral component fracture as well (arrow). **C.** An early revision was undertaken in this patient, and a satisfactory result was obtained with a combination of a long-stem noncemented prosthesis, multiple cerclage wires, and extensive bone grafting using allograft bone (dotted line). This was a heavy, active, youthful patient who suffered a fall while dancing. (From Rothman RH, Hozack WJ: Complications of Total Hip Arthroplasty. Philadelphia, WB Saunders, 1988.)

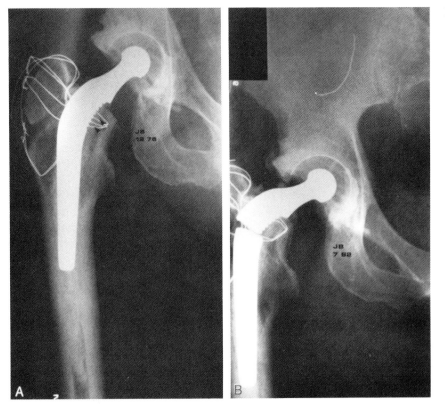

Fɪɢ. 2−5. **A.** An old version of the Charnley component had a serrated proximal medial face. Note also that this component was placed varus. **B.** The patient suffered a fracture of the femoral component through these medial stress risers. The excessive weight of the patient and the varus position of the femoral component probably contributed to this fracture. (From Rothman RH, Hozack WJ: Complications of Total Hip Arthroplasty. Philadelphia, WB Saunders, 1988.)

cortical bone. Placed as a mechanical grout between two stronger and stiffer materials—a metal femoral component and cortical bone—it would seem doomed to failure. Furthermore, as shown by Pilliar,[118] the endurance limit of cement is very close to physiologic stress levels.

However numerous clinical studies have shown that cement can be used successfully and reliably when proper attention is paid to its preparation and delivery.[68,77] Because cement is the weak link in the system, the present solutions are to avoid the cement, strengthen the cement, or protect the cement.

Avoid the Cement

Noncemented total hip replacement is currently a popular alternative to the traditional cemented arthroplasty. Whether, in the long run, it will be a better and more durable alternative remains to be seen (Fig. 2–6). The specifics of noncemented total hip replacement are discussed elsewhere in this book.

Strengthen the Cement

Preparation Techniques. Porosity of the cement has long been recognized as a primary source of mechanical weakness for the cement. Haas[63] found porosity to range from 1 to 10% of the cement volume with hand mixing. Vigorous hand mixing causes highest porosity. The pores are weak points through which the cement can fracture under physiologic stress. Cement porosity can develop through several mechanisms:

1. Entrapment of air during mixing.
2. Release of absorbed air during polymerization.
3. Air entrapment during delivery into the femur, especially with a cement gun.
4. Monomer evaporation, especially with thick cement mantles.

Reduction of cement porosity would seem an ideal method of enhancing the cement fatigue life and thereby reducing longterm prosthetic loosening rates. However a dissenting opinion was voiced by Rimnac, et al., in 1986.[126] They argued that surface irregularities, which are inevitably present at the cement-bone interface because of the interdigitation of the cement with the trabecular bone, overwhelmingly control the material properties of the cement. Using fracture toughness tests, stress concentration at these surface imperfections resulted

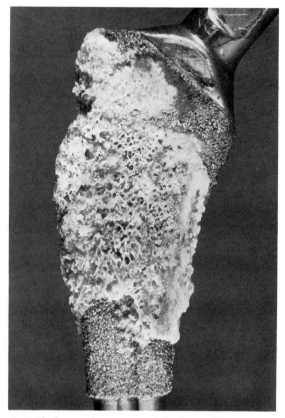

Fɪɢ. **2–6.** If adequate bony ingrowth is obtained in noncemented total hip replacement, as evidenced by this picture, the problems associated with cemented total hip arthroplasty may be avoided.

in early crack propagation, regardless of the underlying cement porosity. On the other hand, Davies, et al.,[45] argue that it is the structural properties of the cement that are most important. They tested trabecular bone/PMMA composite specimens and notched PMMA specimens (Table 2–1). In the centrifuged specimens with lower porosity they found a significantly higher fatigue strength. Furthermore, although fracture occurred at the notch in 13 of 15 of the centrifuged, low porosity specimens, 11 of 15 uncentrifuged specimens broke at a void. In the four that did break at the notch, a void was also present there. From this study they concluded "that porosity reduction of the cement would be a clinical advantage."

This porosity reduction can be achieved through several methods. Slow hand mixing (1 beat per second) has been shown to entrap less air than more rapid beating.[63,57] Air entrapment in the femoral canal at the site of a distal plug can be avoided by using a vent-opening tool. A small hole in the plug allows air to escape distally during pressurization with the cement gun. Avoiding excessively thick cement mantles would seem prudent in view of the findings of Meyer, et al.[101] Cement mantles 10 mm thick developed maximal setting temperatures

TABLE 2–1. *Effect of Centrifugation on Cement Strength*

Preparation	Maximum Initial Tensile Stress	Weibull Fatigue Life (Mean)	Confidence of Significant Difference
Trabecular bone/PMMA component			
Centrifuged	15MPa	9121 (n = 7)	>99%
Uncentrifuged	15MPa	1593 (n = 7)	
Notched specimen			
Centrifuged	15MPa	47,652 (n = 7)	>99%
Uncentrifuged	15MPa	3,229 (n = 7)	

Table 2–1. Centrifugation and cement strength. Centrifugation of the cement significantly increases the fatigue life of the trabecular bone/PMMA composites, and specifically notched specimens. The trabecular bone/cement composites were used to simulate the clinical situation when cement is pressurized within the femoral canal. This examines the fatigue life of the centrifuged versus uncentrifuged bone cement in the presence of surface irregularities. Even in the presence of grossly notched specimens the centrifuged cement displayed an increased fatigue life. (From Davies JP, et al.: The effect of centrifugation on the fatigue life of bone cement in the presence of surface irregularities. Clin Orthop, 229:156, 1988.)

(T_{max}) of 107° C as compared to mantles 3 mm thick that developed maximal setting temperatures of 60° C. Aside from the possible thermal effects of this thick cement mantle, one must also consider the deleterious effect of monomer evaporation at these higher temperatures. Noble, et al.,[107] also found a significant influence of mantle thickness upon cement porosity, with porosity being the least in cement mantles less than 2.5 mm thick. Finally, in an attempt to avoid air adsorption in the prepolymerized powder, evacuated powder mixing has been attempted by Noble, et al.[109]

Clinically, centrifugation and vacuum mixing of cement are the two most useful means of reducing cement porosity. Saha and Pal[133] subjected bone cement mixtures to ultrasonic vibration and found a 10 to 15% increase in ultimate compressive strength and energy absorption capacity. Burke, et al.,[16] found that machined, centrifuged specimens were significantly stronger, with static increases in ultimate tensile strength of 24% and in fatigue life of 136%. Furthermore, overall strength was more consistent with the centrifuged specimens. Not all cements respond to centrifugation with porosity reduction. Jasty, et al.,[75] found no reduction in porosity with centrifugation of Palacos R, Palacos with gentamicin, CMW, and LVC cements. Both Jasty[75] and Davies[44] found Simplex P to respond most favorably to centrifugation with the largest reduction in porosity and the greatest increase in fatigue strength. Simplex P is therefore recommended as the cement of choice if centrifugation is used. Centrifugation should be performed for 60 to 120 seconds depending upon the cement brand, cement temperature, room temperature, and centrifuge speed.

Vacuum mixing of cement has been recommended by several authors.[3,49,83,151] Similar increases in static and fatigue strength have been noted. This mixing technique uses an operating room vacuum at 550 mm Hg for 60 to 90 seconds.

Three studies have compared the two techniques. Noble[108] found that centrifugation reduced porosity by 45%, removed large pores, and left uniformly small pores behind. Vacuum mixing reduced porosity by 70% but created more variability of pore size with large pores still visible on x-ray (Fig. 2–7). Tensile strength of the cement was raised 15 to 30% by centrifugation and 10 to 20% by vacuum mixing. Davies[46] found that centrifugation was preferable because it created more consistent and uniform specimens as compared to vacuum mixing. Schreurs'[138] study found just the opposite. Unfortunately these studies are difficult to compare because of major differences in the technical aspects of cement preparation and testing.

Although centrifugation and vacuum mixing seem useful and both can be applied clinically with ease, one must remember that no clinical followup yet exists to support their use. However, porosity reduction would seem a reasonable and laudable goal.

Cement Mantle. Specific characteristics of the cement mantle are important for the longevity of the total hip arthroplasty (Fig. 2–8). A smooth, even cement mantle would appear most desirable because it obviates any local stress concentration caused by a thinner cement mantle. As demonstrated by Oh[110,112] an eccentric cement results in local areas of higher strain that could lead to cement fracture and component loosening. In that same study Oh[112] found that as the cement mantle

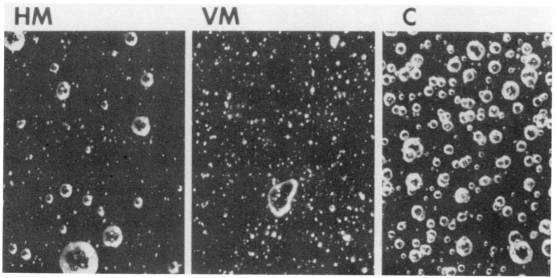

F**IG.** **2–7.** A visual representation of the effects of hand mixing vs. vacuum mixing vs. centrifugation. Vacuum mixing reduces the overall number of pores within the cement, whereas centrifugation merely reduces the overall average size of the pores present. (From Noble PC: Innovations in cementing techniques in total hip replacement. 54th Meet Am Acad Orthop Surg, Jan 1987.)

increased in thickness from 2 mm to 5 mm, the amount of strain in the cement decreased. However, because of various constraints (e.g., acetabular size and the need for an adequate thickness of poly-

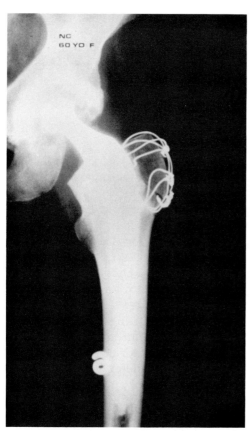

F**IG.** **2–8.** Cement technique, as demonstrated in this postoperative x-ray, virtually guarantees a long lasting and successful clinical result.

ethylene) his recommendation was for a concentric 3-mm cement mantle. Obtaining this type of even cement mantle in the acetabulum is difficult because of the irregular anatomy and because "bottoming out" of the cup against the subchondral bone tends to occur during cup placement. For this reason the use of PMMA pods on the cup was introduced.[112,113] These pods will come up against the subchondral bone, in theory insuring the proper cement mantle thickness. Hopefully no stress concentration effect of the pods will occur.

The characteristics of the cement mantle are equally important for the femoral side. Lindberg[91] and Beckenbaugh[9] each found that an inadequate (less than 1 mm) and uneven cement mantle resulted in increased rates of loosening. Varus positioning of the femoral component has been shown in several studies to be associated with higher loosening rates,[9,71,116,124,142,] which is directly related to the inadequate cement mantle associated with the varus position. A 2- to 3-mm, even, circumferential cement mantle is ideal. Currently, experience is being obtained with the use of component centralizing devices.[109] These devices control the position of the tip of the femoral component within the canal, thus ensuring an even mantle. They are formed of PMMA and fuse chemically with the cement mantle, thereby avoiding any stress concentration effects (Fig. 2–9). Excessively thick cement mantles should be avoided. The thermal effects of a thick cement mantle will cause bone necrosis[63,10] and can also lead to monomer evaporation. Monomer evaporation creates voids within the cement mantle, thus weakening it. Furthermore, an exces-

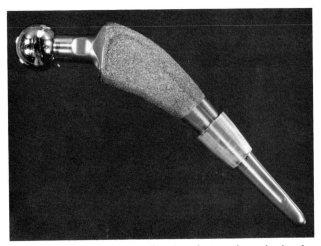

Fɪɢ. 2–9. Component centralization devices formed of polymethylmethacrylate can aid in the creation of an even cement mantle. One particular type is shown in this picture.

sively thick cement mantle (5 mm or more) implies improper selection of a small femoral component.

The distal cement mantle should extend 2 cm past the prosthetic tip. This distance can easily be ensured with the use of a distal cement plug (Fig. 2–10). A finite element analysis by Shinner[140] comparing 1-, 2-, and 3-cm long canal plugs found that a 2-cm plug was most effective in allowing a more even stress distribution in that area, thus eliminating the stress concentration at the distal tip of the femoral component. No effects of the plugs were seen on proximal stress distribution. Clinical support for distal cement mantles has been provided by Beckenbaugh[9] and by Ianotti.[74] Becken-

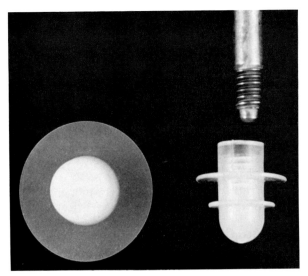

Fɪɢ. 2–10. Distal cement plugs can be made of various materials, including plastic, as demonstrated in this figure. Not only does this guarantee an adequate distal cement mantle but it also aids dramatically in improving pressurization of the cement during cement delivery.

baugh found that the distance that the cement extended past the prosthetic tip was inversely proportional to the incidence of femoral loosening (p < .001). Ianotti found that failure to place cement past the tip of the prosthesis again was associated with a higher incidence of femoral bone-cement demarcation. A mechanical study by Savino[137] also confirmed the beneficial effect of a distal cement plug.

Delivery Techniques

Lamination and blood entrapment can seriously weaken the cement mantle. Gruen, et al.,[62] found a drop in tensile strength to only 46% of normal when lamination occurred. Blood entrapment in the lamination caused a more significant drop down to only 23% of clean unlaminated cement. Black and Greenwald[11] noted a decrease in shear strength of 63 to 78% when additional acrylic cement was added to an already polymerizing cement mass. The weakness was created in the added cement because of a significant increase in porosity. Lee, et al.,[88] found that "specimens deliberately prepared to preserve laminations showed large variations in strength and it was possible to see that failure most often began at laminations in the cement." Furthermore, although they found that admixture of 2 ml of blood to the cement during mixing did not affect strength, "certain specimens failed completely at laminations caused by a blood-cement interface."[88]

Clinically it is important to avoid blood admixtures and lamination. Smooth, rapid, and careful injection of cement with a cement gun is the best method of creating a homogenous cement mantle. Thorough cleansing of the bone with water lavage and the use of thrombin-soaked gelfoam (in the acetabulum) and sponges (in the femur) can reduce the bleeding during cement delivery. Should large doses of cement be necessary, as in revision surgery, all the cement should be mixed simultaneously to avoid the need for adding additional cement to an already polymerizing cement mantle.[11] Finally, should recementing to old cement be undertaken during revision surgery, the need for a clean, dry interface cannot be over emphasized.[11]

Additives. Barium sulfate (BaSO₄), used for radiographic contrast, is a common additive to cement. Combs[33] found no significant reduction in shear strength of the cement until the barium sulfate was increased to 60% by weight. Two other authors[56,149] have found no weakening effect of up to 10% BaSo₄. On the other hand Haas[63] found a 10%

reduction in tensile and fatigue strength when 10% $BaSo_4$ was included in the powder.

Antibiotics are added to cement for their local bacteriocidal effects, especially in revision surgery, but also in primary joint arthroplasty. Marks, et al.,[97] found a slight but insignificant loss of compressive and tensile strength by adding 2 gm or less of powdered gentamicin, oxacillin, or cefazolin to 40 gm of polymer. They did find that liquid antibiotics interfered with the early phases of cement polymerization and caused a weakening of the cement. Hughes, et al.,[73] found no significant change in breaking stress and modulus of Simplex P or CMW cements until at least 8 gm of antibiotic was added. On the other hand, Moran[104] found a significant drop in shear strength with the addition of 0.5, 1.0, and 2.0 gm of gentamicin powder to 40 gm of Palacos. They ascribed these findings to crack propagation from defects created by the larger size of the gentamicin particles. Lautenschlager[87] found that the addition of 4.5 gm of powdered gentamicin to 40 gm of cement reduced compression strength to a level below that recommended as the minimum by the American Society for Testing of Materials (ASTM). Bargar[6] noted a 13% drop in flexural strength after adding 1.2 gm of tobramycin to 40 gm of Simplex P. These conflicting results most likely result from the sensitivity of cement strength to the mode of preparation, conditions of polymerization, and parameters of mechanical testing, all of which vary considerably between laboratories. One further study also demonstrated that in vitro tests may not reflect in vivo actuality. Weinstein[147] found that Prostaphlin added to cement resulted in increased tensile strength in vitro but reduced tensile strength in vivo. Clinically, the durability of antibiotic-impregnated cement has been confirmed in several studies.[14,20,158]

Thus it appears that powdered antibiotics added to the polymer powder do cause some drop in mechanical strength of the cement but this drop is not significant if the dosage of antibiotic is kept below 2 gm per 40 gm of powder. Furthermore, the antibiotic powder must contain fine granules (a mortar and pestle may be necessary for some antibiotics), and it must be thoroughly and completely mixed and integrated with the powdered polymer prior to adding the liquid monomer. This will avoid creating large clumps of antibiotic powder that act as crack initiation points.

Although $BaSo_4$ and antibiotics are additives not designed to enhance the mechanical properties of the cement, several other additives have been studied specifically for this reason. These include metal wire reinforcement,[143] bone particles,[92] and various fibers such as carbon,[118,132,134] steel,[54] Aramid,[154] and graphite.[80] Metal wire reinforcement of cement has been shown to improve the maximum tensile strength of the PMMA, but this technique is not practical for total hip replacement because of the narrow canal of the femur.[143] In an attempt to induce bone ingrowth into cement while maintaining the mechanical properties of the cement, Liu[92] studied bone-particle-impregnated cement. They found a tenfold improvement of crack propagation velocity and a 50% increase in modulus but also noted a 30% decrease in ultimate tensile strength and a 21% drop in impact strength. Furthermore, the cement viscosity was increased.

This problem of increased viscosity has been the limiting factor for most cement additives. Carbon fiber reinforced cement has enhanced tensile (increased up to 60%), compressive, shear, and fatigue strengths (increased 25 to 50%).[118,132,134] This is true also for steel, Aramid, and glass fiber reinforced cements. Yet research has failed to find a clinical use because of the poor intrusion characteristics of these materials. Unfortunately graphite reinforced low viscosity cement has demonstrated significantly less fracture toughness than plain PMMA.[80] One other criticism of stainless steel fiber reinforcement has been the potential for corrosion after implantation.[54]

These fiber additives raise the elastic modulus of the cement composite from 30 to 100%. As Crowninshield[37] has pointed out, this rise in modulus could actually be detrimental because it causes more weight-bearing stress to be shared by the cement. This does not necessarily lead to early cement failure if the fatigue strength of the cement is also raised proportionately. However, as noted by Crowninshield this increase in elastic modulus might raise the tensile stresses transferred to the cement to such an extent that the fiber reinforced cement might actually show reduced endurance as compared to plain PMMA.

New Cements. There are numerous different bone cements available today, including Simplex P, Palacos, CMW, AKZ, Zimmer Regular, and LVC. The mechanical and handling properties of each of these cements is highly variable within one brand and between brands, depending on mixing and delivery conditions as well as in vitro testing parameters.[82] Several studies have compared the cements but no definitive statement can be made about which cement is "the best." On the other hand, there is no doubt that there is room for improvement, and possibly a need for change. Most investigations have been directed toward increasing the strength of the cement (see previous section) but this has not been clinically successful except with centrifugation or vacuum mixing, which increases the structural fatigue strength of PMMA without affecting its modulus.

The possibility that modulus and ductility of cement may be more important than tensile or fatigue strength has lead Weightman, et al.,[146] to develop a new cement called polyethylmethylmethacrylate. This new cement has one-half the modulus and ultimate tensile strength of CMW but has 5 to 10 times the ductility and toughness and 30 to 40 times the fatigue resistance. In theory this new cement could allow controlled subsidence of the femoral component and therefore proximal load transfer without cement fracture. If proximal load transfer is clinically important, then this new cement might be a definite improvement.

Low viscosity cement (LVC) was introduced as a means of increasing the penetration of acrylic into the interstices of the cancellous bone, thereby enhancing the mechanical interdigitation, increasing the area for load transfer, and reducing the local bone-cement interface stresses. However, several reports question the mechanical strength of LVC[44,60,130] and one clinical study demonstrated the LVC did not improve prosthetic fixation.[103] One possible explanation for the lack of improvement in fixation in spite of better intrusion has been put forward by Rey, et al.[125] In this comparative study of intrusion characteristics of LVC, Simplex P, and Palacos cement in a bovine cancellous bone model, they found that the cement intrusion obtained for all three cements was greater in depth than the remaining cancellous bone bed after femoral preparation for cement delivery during total hip replacement. Therefore, the additional penetration possible with LVC was not clinically important (Table 2–2).

Table 2–2. **Cement Intrusion with Different Cements**

| | Cement intrusion depth (mm) | |
	20 PSI	40 PSI
LVC	8	12
Simplex	2.2	4.2
Palacos	1.4	2.4
Chilled Simplex	5.8	8.2
17° C Simplex	6.3	10.8
26° C Simplex	2.2	4.2

Table 2–2. Cement intrusion depth was measured using various types of cements. Note that the intrusion depth with the low viscosity cement is significantly greater than would be possible clinically. More than adequate penetration can be obtained using Simplex-P cement. Chilling the Simplex-P cement allows delivery into the bone with the cement in a more viscous state. (From Ray RM, et al.: A study of intrusion characteristics of low viscosity cement, Simplex-P, and Palacos cements in a bovine cancellous bone marrow. Clin Orthop, 215:272, 1987.)

Protect the Cement

Specific consideration of the cement-prosthesis interface, the cement-bone interface, and specific details of component design can protect the cement and therefore enhance the longevity of a total hip replacement.

Cement-Prosthesis Interface. The interface between the prosthesis and the cement is a frequent area of failure in total hip arthroplasty (Fig. 2–11). Amstutz[4] identified a radiolucent line at the proximal-lateral portion of the stem-cement interface in 10% of 454 cases, Beckenbaugh[9] noted the same finding in 24% and Carlson[18] in 36%. Stauffer[141] noted radiographic evidence of failure of the stem-cement interface in 56 out of 69 femoral components. These findings tended to occur early—Paterson[117] noted that 97% of these radiolucent lines were already visible after 2 years. The ability to maintain the mechanical bond between the cement and the prosthesis can directly influence the durability of the arthroplasty; poor bonding at the interface creates uneven stresses proximally, whereas failure of the interface creates high distal cement stresses. Most of the early total hip arthroplasties used a smooth-surfaced stem. However, as shown by Welsh,[148] the mechanical interlock of cement with the prosthesis is poor, only

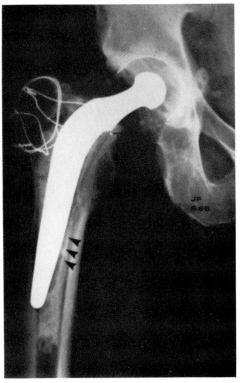

Fig. 2–11. Failure of the cement prosthesis interface is dramatically demonstrated in this radiograph. (From Rothman RH, Hozack WJ: Complications of Total Hip Arthroplasty. Philadelphia, WB Saunders, 1989.)

one-third the strength of the cement itself. The problem of improving the carrying and fatigue properties of the stem-cement interface has been addressed in two different manners: first, by enhancing the mechanical interlock through textured, irregular, or porous surfacing techniques and, second, by creating a chemical bond through the use of a polymethylmethacrylate precoat.

Gross mechanical interlock can be improved by placing recesses, grooves, or undercuts onto the femoral component but these techniques may subject the cement to localized stress concentration (Fig. 2–12). Porous coated surfaces dramatically and significantly improve the fatigue resistance of the cement-prosthesis interface. Welsh[148] noted a fourfold increase in push-out strength comparing porous Vitallium mesh to a smooth-surfaced Vitallium. Manley and Stein[95] and Bundy[15] also showed improved fatigue properties of the stem-cement interface in a porous coated prosthesis. The findings of Cook are shown in Figure 2–13.

An alternative method of enhancing the stem-cement interface strength is through the use of a PMMA precoat. As has been shown by Raab,[120,121] Lane,[85] Price,[119] and Ahmed,[1] the chemical bonding that occurs between the cement and the precoat is significantly stronger with a higher fatigue resistance than the cement itself. A study by Davies[47] found that the porous titanium mesh coating interface was significantly stronger than the PMMA precoat interface. However both interfaces were significantly increased in strength over controls (smooth stem) (Table 2–3). Because of the need to enhance proximal loading to avoid calcar atrophy and the advisability of making prosthetic extraction feasible, most of these surfaces should be confined to the proximal one-third of the femoral component.

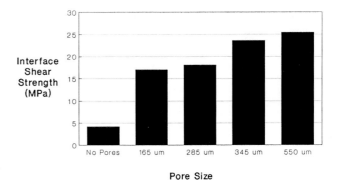

FIG. 2–13. The effect of pore size on cement-prosthesis interfacial strength. A significant increase in shear strength was noted for all pore sizes as compared to a prosthesis with no pores. The larger two pore sizes (345 microns and 550 microns) also were statistically significantly stronger in shear strength as compared to the smaller two pore sizes (165 microns and 285 microns). (From Cook SD, et al.: Optimum pore size for bone cement fixation. Clin Orthop 223:296, 1987.)

The acetabular prosthesis-cement interface does not fail as frequently but the same principles apply. In a comprehensive study by Oh,[112] increased torsional resistance of the prosthesis-cement interface was created in cups having surface irregularities as opposed to smooth-surfaced cups (Fig. 2–14). The effect of porous surfaces or PMMA precoating has not been examined directly but can be inferred from studies on the femoral component-cement interface.

Surgical technique is critical. Fornasier and Cameron[55] and Cook[34] noted that any interposition of blood between the cement and stem or any motion during the setting of the cement significantly compromises the mechanical integrity of that interface. This important point has previously been noted by DeLee and Charnley[48] regarding the acetabular component. They felt that a potential technical pitfall was to use the acetabular holder too long, the result being macromotion of the cup during setting of the cement (caused by patient respiration and inadvertent movement of the surgeon's hands.) They recommended using a small diameter acetabular

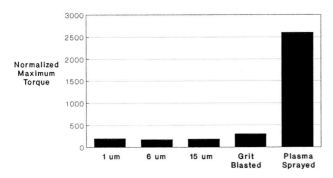

FIG. 2–12. Cement-prosthesis interfacial strength. The strength of the metal-bone cement interface (as measured by normalized maximum torque) increases dramatically as one goes from a smooth nonporous surface to a plasma sprayed porous surface. (From Bundy KJ, et al.: The effect of surface preparation on metal/bone cement interfacial strength. J Biomed Mater Res 21:773, 1987.)

TABLE 2–3. *Cement Prosthesis Interfacial Strength*

Specimen	n	Cycles to Failure
Uncoated	15	9,486 +/− 24,790
Precoated	15	224,251 +/− 299,193
Porous coated	7	No failure

Table 2–3. The cement prosthesis interfacial strength. Both the precoated prosthesis and the porous coated prosthesis have significantly increased cement prosthesis bonds as compared to uncoated specimens. The porous coat used in this experiment was titanium mesh, and no failure could be elicited using the porous coat to enhance the cement/prosthesis bond. (From Davies JP, et al.: Fatigue strength of cement/metal interfaces. Trans Orthop Res Soc, 34:367, 1988.)

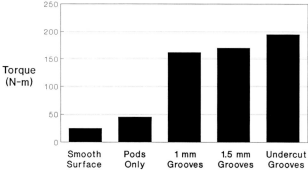

FIG. 2–14. The effect of pod and groove design on fixation strength of the acetabular component. The use of surface irregularities, including small pods and grooves in the acetabular component, significantly increased the ability of the cement-prosthesis interface to resist torque. (From Oh I, et al.: Acetabular cup groove and pod design and its effect on cement fixation in total hip arthroplasty. Clin Orthop 189:308, 1984.)

pusher that would allow angulatory movements between the pusher and the socket without translating any motion to the underlying prosthesis-cement or cement-bone interfaces (Fig. 2–15).

Cement-Bone Interface. Numerous studies have documented high rates of failure at the cement-bone interface (Fig. 2–16). At ten years of followup Johnston[77] and Salvati[136] reported radiographic loosening of the acetabular component of between 8 and 11%, and of the femoral component of 9%. Stauffer[141] noted a significantly higher rate of radiographic loosening of the femoral component (30%). Sutherland[142] found acetabular migration in 17% and femoral migration in 20%. Radiographic evidence of loosening is even higher in younger patients as shown by Chandler[23] and Dorr.[50] To reduce this unacceptably high rate of radiographic failure specific attention must be paid to methods of enhancing the cement-bone interface strength.

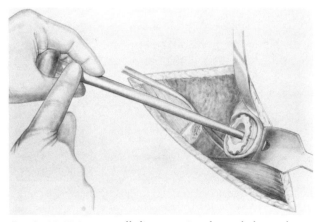

FIG. 2–15. Using a small diameter tipped acetabular pusher to hold the cup in place while the cement is setting, any inadvertent motion by the hand of the surgeon will not be translated into motion of the cup.

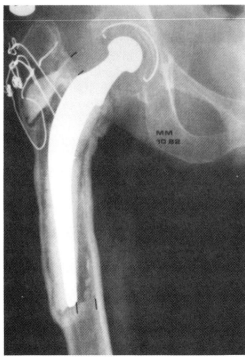

FIG. 2–16. Failure of the cement-bone interface occurred in this total hip arthroplasty. (From Rothman RH, Hozack WJ: Complications of Total Hip Arthroplasty. Philadelphia, WB Saunders, 1989.)

Failure to achieve a good mechanical interlock between the acrylic and the bone allows micromotion to occur at this interface and ultimately leads to loosening and failure. Close adherence to the fine points of surgical technique can significantly reduce this problem.[35]

Adequate operative exposure is essential for adequate surgical technique. It was partially for this reason that Charnley advocated trochanteric osteotomy.[52] Failure to properly expose the acetabulum or femur inhibits adequate visualization of the bony surfaces and can greatly impair the quality of the surgical technique.

Proper preparation of the bony surfaces requires close attention to numerous small details (Fig. 2–17). The bony surfaces should be as clean and as dry as possible prior to cement insertion. Pulsatile water lavage is an effective means of removing blood and debris from the interstices of the trabecular bone.[102,81] Sponge packing of the acetabulum and femoral canal during cement mixing is helpful for hemostasis. Thrombin-soaked gelfoam also provides effective control of bleeding in the acetabulum. Failure to adhere to these specific techniques will result in interposition of blood between the cement and bone[102] with resultant weakening of the mechanical bond.

On the acetabular side a good mechanical inter-

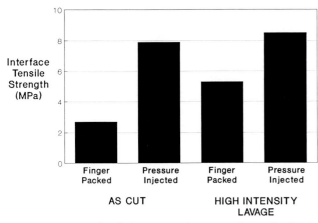

Fig. 2–17. Strength of the cement-bone interface. The bone-cement interface tensile strength was significantly increased by pressure-injecting the cement as opposed to finger-packing, and by using high intensity lavage as a means of preparing the bony surface to receive the cement. (From Krause WR: Strength of the cement-bone interface. Clin Orthop 163:290, 1982.)

Table 2–4. *Effect of Anchoring Holes on Acetabular Fixation*

Specimen Type	Hole Diameter (cm)	Hole Depth (cm)	Mean Maximum Torque
3 large holes	1.2	0.8	121
3 small holes	0.85	0.8	84
6 small holes	0.85	0.8	157

Table 2–4. Acetabular bone/cement interface strength. In terms of maximum torque resistance, the most effective means of obtaining bone/cement fixation in the acetabulum is by multiple small anchoring holes. An additional advantage of the smaller and shallower anchoring holes is that they are easy to make and are less likely to penetrate through the acetabulum. (From Oh I: A comprehensive analysis of the factors affecting replacement arthroplasty. Trans 11th Meet Hip Soc, p. 129, 1983.)

lock with cancellous bone could be obtained but this is not advisable because subchondral bone retention is important for reduction of cement stresses.[22] An alternative method of enhancing the ability of the cement-bone interface to resist torsional loads has been investigated by Oh.[112] He recommended creating multiple small "anchoring" holes drilled through the retained subchondral bone (Fig. 2–18). In this fashion the torsional rigidity of the interface is significantly increased (Table 2–4).

On the femoral side, the surgeon should concentrate heavily on mechanical preparation of the cement-bone interface. Curettage of the weak cancellous bone proximal-medially and thorough debridement of the femoral canal with a plastic bone brush are effective means of cleansing the endosteal bone. Beckenbaugh[9] found that an inability to obtain a good cement column proximal-medially was associated with a statistically significant increase in the incidence of femoral component loosening. Only by careful curettage can this problem be avoided. Miller[102] noted that blood clots and debris could not be debrided ade-

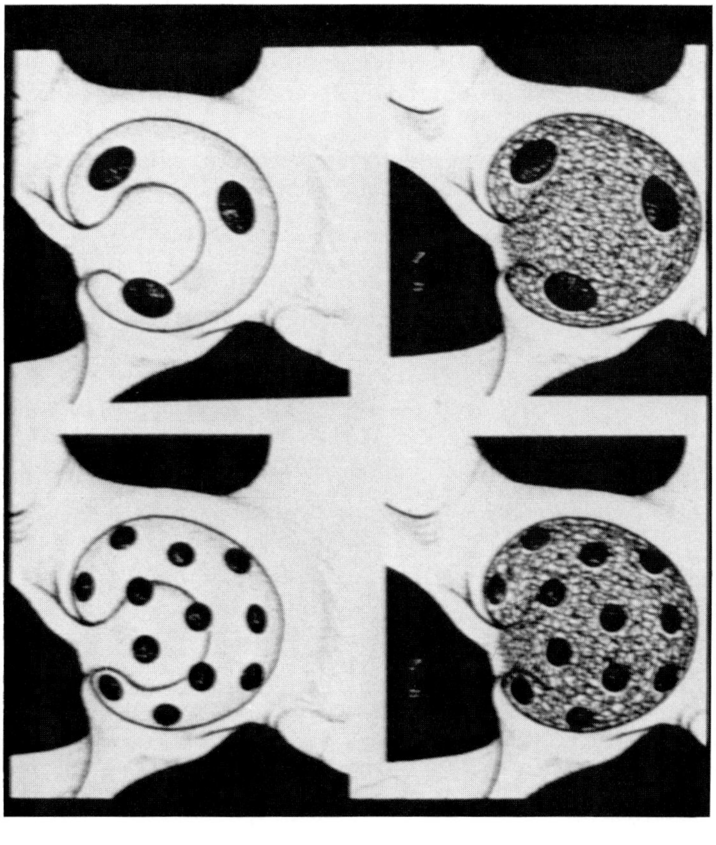

Fig. 2–18. Diagrammatic representation of acetabular preparation techniques that might enhance cup fixation. Subchondral bone has been sacrificed in the upper two figures and multiple small holes have been created on the right as compared to three larger fixation holes as demonstrated on the left. In this experiment the best fixation was obtained by preserving subchondral bone and by using multiple small fixation holes. (From Oh HI: A comprehensive analysis of the factors affecting acetabular cup fixation and design in total hip replacement arthroplasty. Trans 11th Meet Hip Soc, p 129, 1983.)

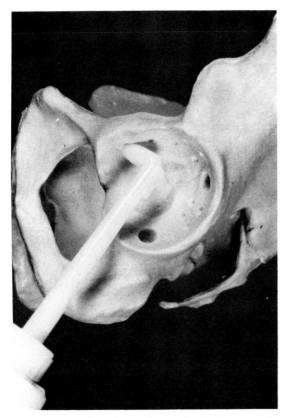

FIG. 2–19. Using the right angle nozzle, the larger anchoring holes can be injected with cement and pressurized in a more controlled and satisfactory fashion.

quately from the femoral canal with pulsatile lavage alone. They found that this problem could easily be overcome through the use of an intramedullary bone brush. Proper use of this brush enhances the radiographic appearance of the bone-cement interface.

Pressurization of the cement is critical because it increases the intrusion pressure and cement penetration into the bone interstices, resulting in better component fixation. As demonstrated by Oh,[112] the use of a special acetabular cement compressor significantly increased the intrusion of cement into the bone. However, care has to be taken to prevent cement extrusion through the fovea; excessive cement in this direction could injure neurovascular structures. Specific injection of the anchoring holes using a right-angled cement nozzle prior to inserting the bolus of cement also will improve fixation (Fig. 2–19).

Innovations on the femoral side include pressurizing against a distal cement plug and using a special cement injection system (Fig. 2–20). The intrusion pressures are greatly increased with the use of a distal plug[94,110] and a femoral cement compactor system has been shown to be superior to finger-packing for cement intrusion (Fig. 2–21).[81,110,111] Clinical support for these two techniques has been provided by Harris.[68,67]

Prosthetic design considerations can influence the degree of pressurization obtained. The use of a flange for the acetabular cup has been advocated. Oh[114] showed that a continuous 2.5-mm flange acted as a restrictor for cement extrusion resulting in significantly higher cement intrusion depths and pressures as compared to nonflanged or partially flanged cups (Fig. 2–22). Larger flexible flanges can also greatly enhance cement pressurization,[139] but improper trimming of the flange may compromise proper component positioning, which is critical to implant stability. Bourne[13] outlined an additional method of enhancing femoral cement pressuriza-

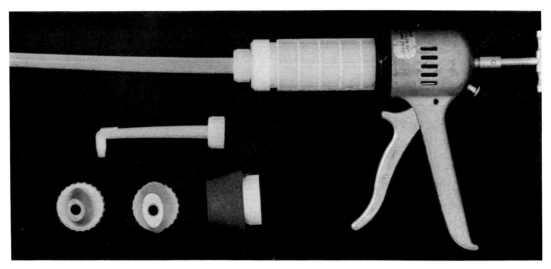

FIG. 2–20. Femoral cement delivery system. The gun and the long plastic tube are used to deliver the cement in a retrograde fashion into the femoral canal. The malleable plastic nozzles (lower left) are used to occlude the proximal opening of the femoral canal and pressurize the cement after it has been delivered into the distal canal. The right-angled nozzle is used on the acetabular side. Using this cement delivery system, controlled delivery and excellent pressurization of the cement can reliably and repeatably be obtained.

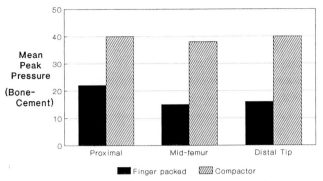

Fig. 2–21. Comparison of cement pressurization techniques. A special femoral cement compactor system was consistently more effective than finger-packing in achieving higher mean bone cement pressures. (From Oh I, et al.: The femoral cement compactor. J Bone Surg 65A:1335, 1983.)

tion (Fig. 2–23). In studying the role of different femoral stem sizes and shapes, this study found that a larger stem significantly increased cement intrusion pressures distally as compared to a smaller femoral component.

Component Design

Acetabulum

On the acetabular side, cement can be protected from excessive stress by either using more cement or thicker polyethylene components. However excessively thick cement mantles are poor mechanical structures and acetabular anatomic size often prevents the surgeon from using the thicker components. Therefore metal-backing of the acetabular component is the primary method of stress-shielding the acetabular cement.

The metal backing, having a relatively high modulus, will bear most of the stresses during loading

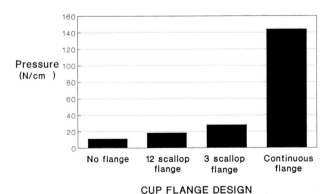

CUP FLANGE DESIGN

Fig. 2–22. Cup flange designs and cemented intrusion pressure. Continuous unbroken flanges on the acetabular cups resulted in significantly higher pressures for cement intrusion. (From Oh I, et al.: Total hip acetabular cup flange design and its effect on cemented fixation. Clin Orthop 195:304, 1985.)

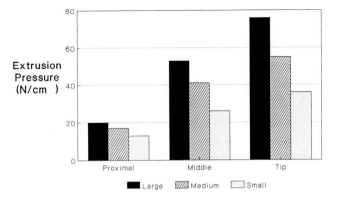

Component Size and Location

Fig. 2–23. The effect of component size on cement pressurization. Better pressurization of the cement was obtained as the components were increased in size. This effect was particularly evident in the distal tip area. (From Bourne RB, et al.: Femoral cement pressurization during total hip arthroplasty. Clin Orthop 183:12, 1984.)

of the hip thus protecting the underlying cement. Finite element analyses by Carter[21] and Crowninshield[41] lend support to this statement. One further advantage of metal-backing of the cup is that stresses are presented to the pelvis in a more physiologic fashion. The metal-backed cup serves to transfer loads directly to the walls of the ilium and spares the underlying weak cancellous bone. This does not occur to any appreciable extent without metal backing.

Clinical support for the use of a metal-backed acetabular component has been provided by Harris[66,70] and Mattingly.[100] In patients whose average age was less than 45, a significantly lower rate of acetabular loosening was present at 6 to 7.5 years of followup as compared to rates in series with non-metal-backed acetabuli. When Harris[69] extended his followup to 11.3 years, the loosening rate of the cup was 12.5%, which is half that experienced by Charnley at 12 to 15 years of followup. This is especially significant because the patients in Harris' series were much younger (average age 41) and, by inference, more active than the patients in Charnley's series.

As has been shown by Carter[22] and Crowninshield,[41] retention of subchondral bone during preparation of the acetabulum is essential in sparing the underlying weak cancellous bone from excessive stresses. However, retention of subchondral bone is not always possible because of anatomic constraints. Furthermore, Carter[22] found that the subchondral bone will not completely protect the cement from high stresses. Only the metal-backed acetabular component is effective in this manner. One additional advantage of the metal-backed acetabular component is its ability to act as a substitute for subchondral bone. Carter[21] and Crowninshield[41] each demonstrated mathematically that a metal-backed cup protects the underlying trabecular bone from excessive stresses should the subchondral bone be absent. Crowninshield took his analysis one step further in his stress analysis of reconstruction of acetabular protrusion[40] where he showed that stress levels in the underlying bone *and* cement were best reduced by an anatomically placed metal-backed acetabular component.

Femur

A dramatic change in the distribution of stress in the femur occurs after insertion of a total hip prosthesis (Fig. 2–24). Oh and Harris[115] found that proximal calcar stress was drastically reduced with a concomitant rise in distal bone stresses. Clinically, according to Wolf's Law, proximal calcar resorption and distal bony hypertrophy occurs. To prevent this problem a collar was added to the femoral component, thus providing direct transfer of stress from the prosthesis to the calcar area. A secondary benefit was obtained because the proximal cement stresses also were reduced. In a finite element analysis by Crowninshield,[39] stresses in the proximal-medial femur were increased to within 40 to 50% of normal and proximal cement stresses were reduced by 60 to 70% with a properly functioning collar. These findings were echoed by Lewis,[90] who also found that proximal cement stress was reduced to low levels by a functioning collar.

In spite of these finite element studies, calcar atrophy appears to spare no prosthetic design. One study by Rand[123] compared the collarless Charnley prosthesis to the collared T-28 prosthesis and found no difference in the degree of calcar atrophy. Furthermore, it seems that the proximal bony remodeling tends to stabilize early and not progress with time.[141] Several authors have suggested that unloading of the calcar by the femoral component may play only a minor part in causing calcar atrophy. Bocco[12] and Johnson and Crowninshield[77] emphasized how acetabular polyethylene debris actually may play a more important role. Improved medial cement techniques[12] and valgus orientation to the femoral component[72] also seem to reduce calcar atrophy.

A study by Lanyon[86] demonstrated that resorption of the proximal medial femur may not be caused only by a loss of calcar loading but rather to total reorganization of proximal bone strains. Using a collar to load only medially may not sufficiently influence these major changes in strain patterns. In addition, a larger stiff stem can negate the effectiveness of a collar altogether; Lewis[90] found that they could obtain only up to 30% of normal calcar stresses with a large-collared cobalt-chromium prosthesis.

The real technical problem in using a collared prosthesis is in insuring intimate calcar-collar contact. As demonstrated by Markolf[92] this may be dif-

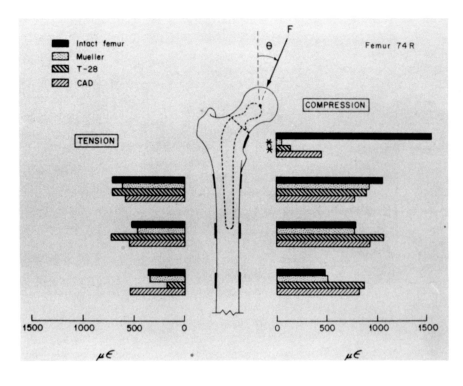

Fig. 2–24. After insertion of a femoral component the distribution of compression forces is essentially reversed as compared to the normal intact femur. Particularly significant is the sparing of compression forces on the proximal medial cortex. (From Oh I, Harris WH: Proximal strain distribution in the loaded femur. J Bone Joint Surg 68A:75, 1978.)

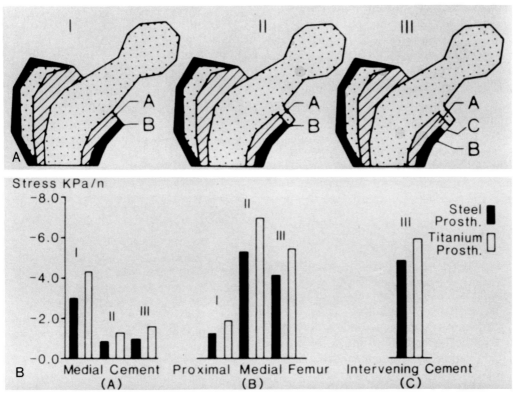

Fig. 2–25. The effect of a femoral component collar on proximal stresses. **A.** Diagrammatic representation of three different situations. I. Collarless cemented femoral component. II. Collared cemented component with perfect apposition of the collar to the proximal medial femoral cortex. III. Collared cemented femoral component with imperfect apposition of the collar to the proximal medial femoral cortex and interposition of some proximal cement. **B.** Comparing the collarless to the collared prosthesis the proximal medial cement stresses are significantly reduced using the collared prosthesis and the proximal medial femoral cortical stresses are increased. However, should any intervening cement come to lie between the collar and the femoral cortex, this would be subject to excessively high forces. (From Crowninshield LD: An analysis of collar function and the use of titanium in femoral prostheses. Clin Orthop 158:271, 1981.)

ficult if not impossible to achieve. If the collar is supported by both bone and cement, then the intervening cement stresses will be exceedingly high (Fig. 2–25).[39] Because protecting the cement is a goal of total hip replacement, the situation is less than ideal. In most cases, it is likely that at least 1 to 2 mm of bone necrosis will occur after calcar molding with reamers. Even if it does not initially, the inability to create a stress level higher than 30% normal[90] will likely cause calcar atrophy to occur eventually. Thus, in spite of intimate initial contact the collared prosthesis will ultimately act as one without a collar. A study by Kareh and Harrigan[79] compared stresses in the cement mantle from finite element analyses to experimental data and found that the finite element analyses that assumed no collar-calcar contact were more representative of the experimental values.

One potential advantage of a collar is to allow the surgeon to place the final prosthetic component in exactly the same position as the trial component. On the down side, however, a badly designed collar can compromise component removal, espe-

cially if the collar is circumferential, or it may force the surgeon to place the component in a varus attitude to achieve calcar-collar contact, especially if the collar is too short. Thus the need for a collared femoral component is still an unsettled issue.

In general, two types of stem materials are available for use—cobalt chromium alloys (CoCr) and titanium alloys. Although micrograin cobalt chromium alloys have a higher tensile strength and fatigue strength than titanium alloys, these differences are inconsequential because both materials have enough strength to function satisfactorily as a total hip prosthesis. As far as the cement is concerned the important materials difference between the two types of metals is in modulus; titanium alloy has a significantly lower modulus than cobalt chromium alloy. Because of this lower modulus, titanium stems increase the proximal cement stresses by 40% as compared to the cobalt chromium stems.[39] Lewis quantified this to be approximately 10% of failure stress. On the other hand, Lewis[90] found that maximum cement stresses were present distally with all prosthetic designs (Fig.

2–26), and that cobalt chromium stems were responsible for the highest distal cement stresses (up to 40% of failure stress and 80% of fatigue limit). Therefore as stated by Crowninshield,[39] "if fracture of the cement about the distal tip of the prosthesis . . . is a concern, then titanium implants may be a logical choice. However, if proximal loosening of femoral components . . . is a critical problem, then titanium due to increased proximal cement stresses would be a poor choice." These theoretical differences may have no clinical value however. One variable that is often ignored when discussing modulus differences between titanium and cobalt chromium alloys is component size. As the femoral components get larger, they become stiffer. With the larger stems now in use, differences in modulus may be overwhelmed by the structural stiffness. This may offer a partial explanation for the finding of Burke and Davis[17] and Kareh, et al.,[79] in testing high modulus versus low modulus stems. They found no significant advantage could be demonstrated between the two different alloys for proximal femoral bone strains or cement mantle strains.

Stem geometry critically affects cement integrity. Several design features are well established (Fig. 2–27). When one examines results of Suther-

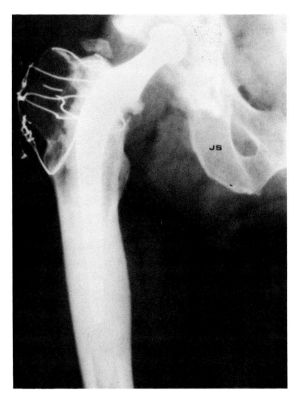

FIG. 2–26. Distal cortical hypertrophy as demonstrated in this x-ray suggests that distal stresses are large. These stresses are being shared by the femoral component, the bone, and the cement.

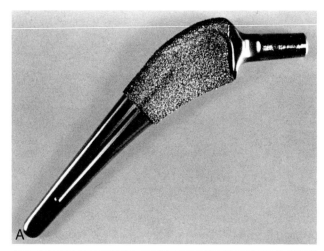

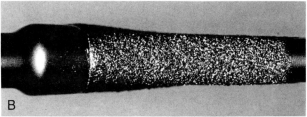

FIG. 2–27. Design features of the cemented femoral component. **A.** Features that may be beneficial include: 1. Straight stem design. 2. Bulky proximal and middle third to prevent stem fractures. 3. The Cobra flange proximolaterally to enhance cement pressurization. 4. Porous coating to enhance the cement-prosthesis bond. 5. Stem tapering to allow for controlled settling. **B.** A broad medial face with smooth rounded corners provides an even load to the cement without stress risers. In addition a thicker lateral than medial cross section places more of the cement under compression, the mode in which cement is most strong.

land's review of curved-stem Mueller prostheses[142] with numerous reports of good long-term results with the straight-stemmed Charnley prosthesis, the value of a straight stem cannot be denied.

A broad medial face with smooth rounded edges provides an even load to the cement without stress risers. Stem designs that are thicker laterally than medially place more cement under compression— the mode in which the cement is most strong. A finite element analysis by Crowninshield in 1980[38] clearly emphasizes the importance of these design features (Fig. 2–28).

As the stem length is increased the cement stresses fall. However, the proper length is unknown. In general, the component should extend into the isthmic area of the femur to reduce the tendency of the femoral component to toggle within the canal. Stem-neck angle is another unsettled issue (Fig. 2–29). The choice of angle can affect the joint contact forces, the torque force on the femoral component, and the efficiency and func-

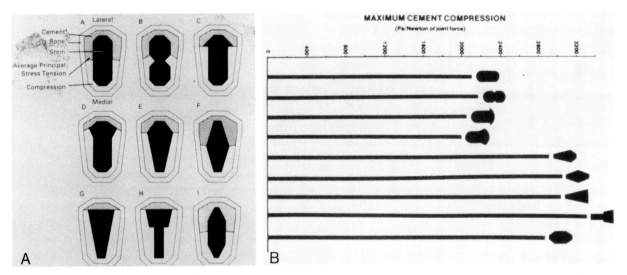

Fig. 2–28. A. Demonstration of the distribution of compressive vs. tensile forces within the cement using various femoral cross sectional designs. Those stems with a wider dimension laterally resulted in larger regions of the cement being under compression—a favorable situation for cement durability. **B.** Those designs with a smoother medial face created less maximum cement compressive force as compared to those designed with sharper medial faces. (From Crowninshield RD, Cohen A: The effect of femoral stem cross-sectional geometry on cement stresses in total hip reconstruction. Clin Orthop 146:71, 1980.)

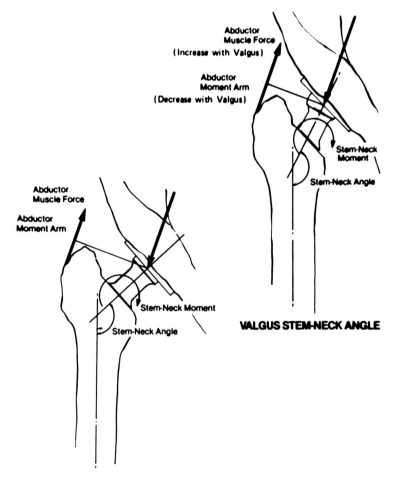

Fig. 2–29. The effect of changes in the stem-neck angle on forces about the hip. An increase in the valgus of the stem-neck angle causes the abductor muscles to work at decreased moment arm. These muscles would therefore need to work harder to sustain normal ambulation. Prostheses of this design are more likely to result in persistent postoperative limp. In addition, this increased abductor muscle force will translate into a higher resultant force in the acetabulum and may predispose to early acetabular loosening.

tion of the abductor muscles. Johnston[76] showed that valgus neck-stem angles reduce the torque on the femoral component and thus reduce the femoral component stresses. Theoretically, this will reduce the risk of loosening. On the other hand the abductor muscles will have to pull harder because of the reduced moment arm and therefore acetabular joint contact forces will be increased. This may adversely affect the longevity of the acetabular component. Johnston, et al.,[76] suggest that the ideal shaft-prosthetic neck angle is 130°. Offset of the prosthesis, that is, the distance from the femoral component to the center rotation of the hip, is an important consideration for stability and leg length and has been discussed previously in this chapter. Finally, tapering of the femoral component may be beneficial because it allows for a more gradual transfer of stresses from the femoral component to the cement. The clinical significance of this is unknown. An additional claimed advantage of a tapered component is that it may allow the prosthesis to settle into a position of stability with time.[22]

Stability and Dislocation

Dislocation of a total hip replacement is a worrisome problem that can usually be prevented. Factors that have an important influence on hip stability include: (1) patient position, (2) component position, (3) soft tissue balance. Because the surgeon can exert only partial control over patient activities in the form of recommendations (Figs. 2–30 and 2–31), careful decision-making with respect to the other two factors is critical.

Charnley[27] recommended a cup position of 45° of abduction and neutral version with the femoral component also in neutral version. Harris[65] recommends a cup position of 30° of abduction and 20° of anteversion. Lewinnek[89] suggested a "safe range" of cup anteversion to be 15 ± 10°, and cup abduction to be 40 ± 10°, with a dislocation rate of 1.5% inside this range and 6.1% outside. Excessive cup anteversion causes anterior instability in extension and external rotation especially with smaller head sizes and anterior surgical approaches (Fig. 2–32). Any cup retroversion can cause posterior instability in flexion, especially with posterior surgical approaches. The same holds true for the femoral component. Excessive anteversion of the cup and femoral component was the most common positional error noted in the study by Ali Khan.[2] Dorr[51] recommends using the anterior acetabular rim as a guide with the cup being 15° anteverted if its anterior edge is aligned with the bony anterior rim. Excessive cup abduction causes instability in adduction (Fig. 2–33) whereas an excessively horizontal

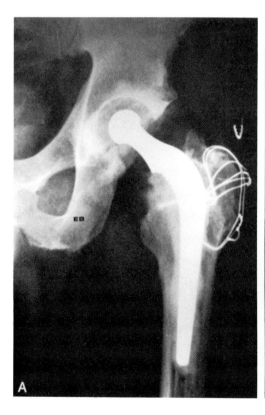
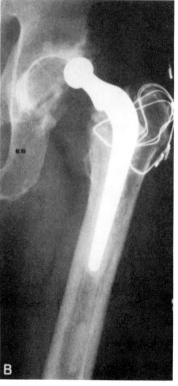

Fig. 2–30. A. A technically satisfactory total hip replacement is seen here with good orientation of the cup, no evidence of wear, and restoration of Shenton's line. B. In spite of this the patient had three episodes of subluxation and one episode of dislocation, shown here. This patient refused to discipline himself regarding body positioning. (From Rothman RH, Hozack WJ: Complications of Total Hip Arthroplasty. Philadelphia, WB Saunders, 1988.)

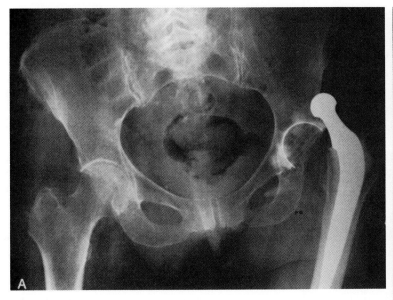
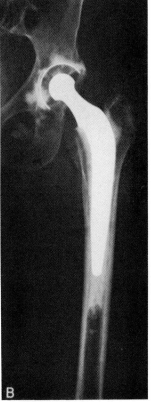

FIG. 2–31. **A.** This patient experienced two episodes of dislocation, each time after reaching forward to trim her toenails. **B.** After the patient was educated about the correct joint precautions, she experienced excellent function of this total hip replacement. (From Rothman RH, Hozack WJ: Complications of Total Hip Arthroplasty. Philadelphia, WB Saunders, 1989.)

cup does not present any problems with instability. Therefore, one should err on the side of the cup being more horizontal.

Head size has been considered an important factor in hip stability. Charnley[27] himself thought that the 22-mm head was inherently unstable and therefore emphasized the need for trochanteric transplantation. Several head sizes are currently popular—22, 26, 28, and 32 mm. Aside from stability, the choice of head size can influence wear, loosening rates, and range of motion. Polyethylene wear has been discussed previously in this chapter.

Charnley chose the 22-mm head in an effort to reduce the frictional torque experienced at the acetabular bone-cement interface.[27] Charnley demonstrated a 50% increase in frictional torque when going from a 22.5-mm femoral head to a 50-mm head. Ma and Amstutz[93] showed an increase in frictional torque proportional to the increase in head size, which was most dramatic at higher loads. In this study they also found that a thicker polyethylene component could reduce this increase in torque. Metal backing of the cup also reduces the degree of frictional torque transferred to the cement-bone interface.[21,41]

On the other hand, torque created by the frictional resistance between the head and socket may not be enough by itself to cause component loosening especially when one considers the amount of stress placed on the cement-bone interface by body weight. Andersson, et al.,[5] measured strengths of bone-cement interfaces in cadaveric specimens and found that the static failure strength of the bond at the cup-cement or cement-bone interface was much higher than any frictional moment acting on the two surfaces.

However, there are three clinical studies that confirm the beneficial influence of the 22-mm head on cup loosening. Ritter, in 1983,[127] compared 67 Mueller and 84 Charnley total hip arthroplasties. At 7 years, the acetabular loosening rate in the Mueller 32-mm prosthesis was 15%, whereas in the Charnley 22-mm prostheses loosening was present in only 4%. This was a statistically significant difference. A later study by Ritter[129] (1987) reconfirmed these findings. Morrey[106] compared 4576 22-mm and 487 32-mm femoral head designs. For the 22-mm heads, the 10 year probability of acetabular revision was 0.7%; for the 32-mm heads, it was 3.5%.

One additional important consideration for choosing a head size is in small or dysplastic acetabuli where the 22-mm head as compared to a 32-mm head allows the surgeon to preserve more bone stock and to allow adequate polyethylene thickness (Fig. 2–34).

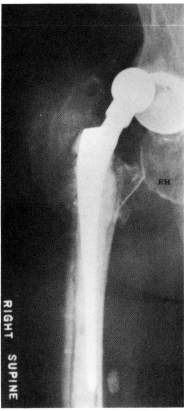

Fig. 2–32. This patient suffered an anterior dislocation of the hip secondary to an excessively anteverted acetabular cup. (From Rothman RH, Hozack WJ: Complications of Total Hip Arthroplasty. Philadelphia, WB Saunders, 1989.)

Range of motion can be influenced by head size. Johnston and Smidt, in 1970,[78] demonstrated that 120° of flexion, 20° of abduction, and 20° of external rotation in the hip was necessary for most common

activities of daily living. A study by Woolson, et al.,[153] found that total hip replacement gave adequate abduction and external rotation but the mean flexion range was only 94°. However, this motion is adequate for most patients, allowing them to pick up objects off the floor, dress, and go up stairs. A study by Chandler, et al.,[24] of 22-, 28- and 32-mm heads in a cadaveric pelvis showed that all head sizes provided at least 100° of flexion (120° at 30° of abduction), 80° of external rotation, and 30° of abduction. All head sizes, therefore, provide a functional hip range of motion especially if flexion is accompanied by abduction and external rotation. Certainly the 32-mm head allows for a greater impingement free range of motion and therefore should enhance stability. However, no clinical evidence exists to indicate a higher incidence of dislocation when the heads are small.[51,53,152]

The explanation is that head size plays a relatively minor role in stability. A variety of other component design variables are equally important. These include socket-rim design, head-neck diameter ratio, neck length, and neck offset. An extended posterior wall as suggested by Charnley[28] will significantly enhance stability for all head sizes (Fig. 2–35). A head-neck diameter ratio of two or more is important to allow for more prosthetic motion before impingement.[4] For example, a design change in the 22-mm Charnley prosthesis from a 12.5-mm neck to a 10-mm neck resulted in an average increase in motion before impingement of 18° (Fig. 2–36).[157]

Neck length and neck offset are two important factors relating to the third cause of hip instabil-

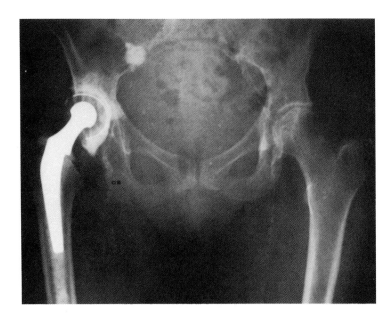

Fig. 2-33. An excessively vertical acetabular cup was responsible for multiple episodes of dislocation in this patient. (From Rothman RH, Hozack WJ: Complications of Total Hip Arthroplasty. Philadelphia, WB Saunders, 1989.)

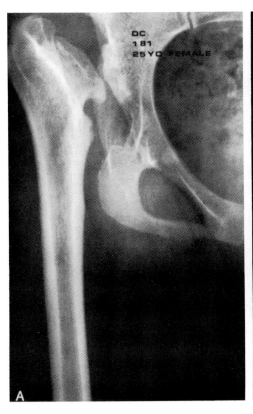
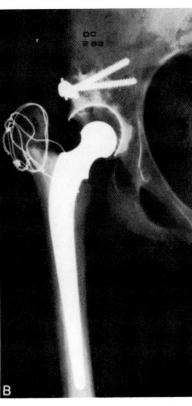

FIG. 2–34. Small femoral components and the 22-mm head size were essential in this patient in order to reconstruct the hip joint. **A.** Preoperative x-ray. **B.** Postoperative x-ray.

ity—soft tissue imbalance. Soft tissue tension about a total hip replacement must be correctly balanced at the time of surgery or dislocation is likely to occur.

Component position can influence soft tissue tension. On the acetabular side, superior placement of the cup makes it more difficult to obtain ade-

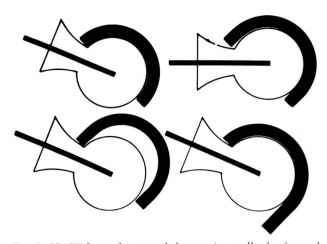

FIG. 2–35. Without the extended posterior wall, the femoral head can dislocate from the acetabular component when the neck impinges on the acetabular component (bottom left). With the extended posterior wall (bottom right) no such subluxation or dislocation occurs. (From Charnley J: The rationale of low friction arthroplasty. Proc 1st Meet Hip Soc, p 92, 1973.)

quate soft tissue tension (as determined by "toggle" of the femoral head within the cup on a simple pull test intraoperatively). Excessive medial deepening of the acetabulum with reaming will result in premature bony impingement with hip motion and lead to dislocation. On the femoral side, an excessively aggressive femoral neck cut will have the same effect as a superior cup placement. Excessive valgus placement of the femoral component decreases the distance from the greater trochanter to the femoral head and thereby results in earlier bony impingement.[53] Thus, the relationship between stability and soft tissue tension is complex. Traditionally, one can restore soft tissue tension through variations in neck length. Modular systems now available give a wide range of choices. The advantage of a modular neck length is demonstrated in this 65-year-old female patient with degenerative arthritis who underwent a right total hip replacement (Fig. 2–37). At surgery she had a 22-mm acetabular cup inserted and a femoral component with a short neck. Intraoperatively she appeared to have a stable hip with no toggle and equal leg lengths by examination (this patient was supine for surgery). In the recovery room however the hip was found to be dislocated. She was relocated in the recovery room but a repeat x-ray revealed what appeared to be inadequate soft tissue tension. The head seemed

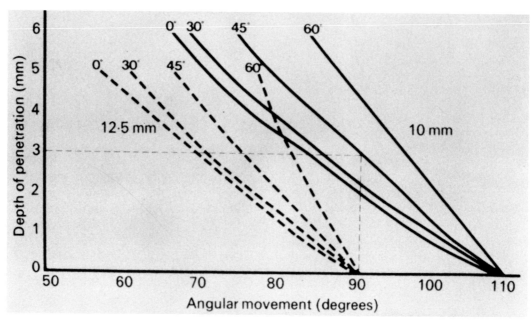

FIG. 2–36. By modifying the neck design in the Charnley 22-mm prosthesis, an increase in range of motion before impingement is obtained. As shown by the dotted lines in this chart, and assuming a 45° angle of wear, a total of 3 mm of plastic wear could occur before the angle of movement before impingement would be reduced to 90° using the 10-mm neck diameter. With the larger 12.5-mm neck diameter this degree of wear only would allow approximately 75° of motion before impingement would occur. (From Wrobleski BM: Direction and rate of socket wear in Charnley low-friction arthroplasty. J Bone Joint Surg 67B:157, 1985.)

to be out of the cup. She was returned immediately to the operating room where re-examination revealed excessive tissue toggling. Had a modular system not been used, she would have needed a revision of either the femoral or acetabular compo-

nent. With the modular system we merely had to pop off the short neck and reimplant a longer neck. Currently, she has a stable hip with equal leg lengths.

The problem with adjusting only the neck length

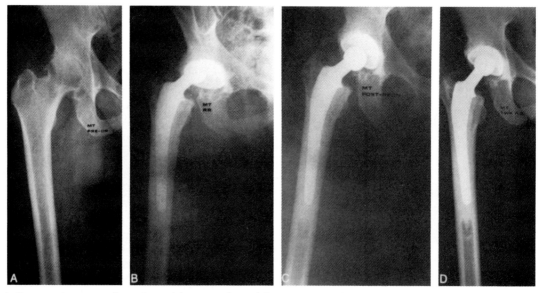

FIG. 2–37. **A.** Preoperative x-ray of a patient with uncomplicated degenerative arthritis of the hip. **B.** Recovery room x-ray showing a dislocation in spite of a horizontally oriented acetabular cup. **C.** The patient's hip was relocated without difficulty in the recovery room. The post reduction x-ray, however, reveals that the femoral component is not well seated within the acetabular cup. This suggests that adequate soft tissue tension has not been restored. **D.** The patient was taken immediately back to the operating room and a longer-neck femoral head was attached to the femoral stem. Adequate soft tissue tension was restored and the patient's hip was made stable. (From Rothman RH, Hozack WJ: Complications of Total Hip Arthroplasty. Philadelphia, WB Saunders, 1989.)

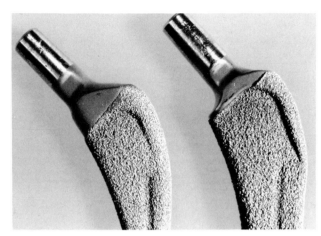

Fig. 2–38. A lateral offset component (left) pushes the femur away from the pelvis, thus increasing soft tissue tension without leg lengthening and also reduces bony impingement at the extremes of motion as compared to the standard offset prosthesis (right).

as a means of creating adequate soft tissue tension and thus stability is that excessive leg lengthening may occur. Leg length inequality is bothersome to the patient and a source of embarrassment for the surgeon. Furthermore, it is possible, although unproven, that leg length inequality can aggravate and even cause low back pain and possibly even prosthetic loosening.[145] The challenge of hip arthroplasty is to re-establish proper soft tissue tension and stability without excessively lengthening the extremity. The ability to adjust neck offset with a modular system can allow the surgeon to adjust to the anatomical variations of patient's bony architecture about the hip. A lateral offset prosthesis (Fig. 2–38) not only tightens the soft tissues without leg lengthening but also significantly reduces bony impingement at extremes of position. This particular design adds 6 mm of increased tissue ten-

TABLE 2–5A. *Standard Offset Prosthesis with 28 mm Head*

Stem	Neck Length (mm)		
	−6	0	+6
10 mm	33	37	41
16 mm	36	40	44

TABLE 2–5B. *Lateral Offset Prosthesis with 28 mm Head*

Stem	Neck Length (mm)		
	−6	0	+6
10 mm	39	43	47
16 mm	42	46	50

Table 2–5B. The numbers represent the degree of increasing offset (and therefore increased soft tissue tension) with the lateral offset as compared to standard offset prosthesis.

sion without increasing leg length (Tables 2–5A,B). In a patient with a varus angle to the femoral neck whose femur is located relatively far away from the pelvis as demonstrated by the broad shape to Shenton's line (Fig. 2–39) a lateral offset prosthesis is necessary not only to create stability and equal leg lengths but also to recreate the normal anatomical configuration to the pelvis.

Another particular advantage of increased femoral offset is that it enhances the mechanical advantage of the abductor muscles and should reduce postoperative limp. Although it can be argued that a larger offset will increase the moment arm that tends to twist or bend loose the femoral component, the increased efficiency of the abductor muscles (that is, reduced force needed for ambulation) should partially or completely negate the effect of increased femoral component distance from the pelvis.[42,79] Furthermore, because of the decreased abductor force required the joint reactive force will be lower and, in theory, this will reduce acetabular component loosening.[42]

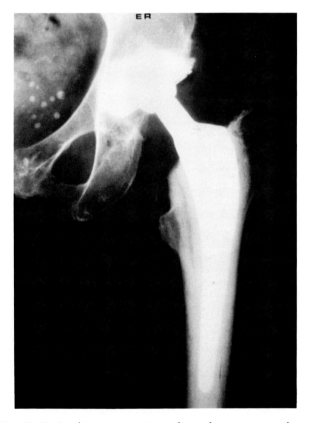

Fig. 2–39. In this postoperative radiograph one can see how Shenton's line has actually been widened with the lateral offset prosthesis. The lateral offset prosthesis was absolutely necessary in this patient in order to restore stability at surgery without leg lengthening.

Conclusion

Total hip replacement surgery must be based on science in order for it to be successful. As outlined in this chapter, a great deal of scientific data is available to us and if the surgeon pays close attention to the details of patient selection, prostheses selection, and surgical technique, consistent and enduring results can readily be achieved. Hopefully, as time passes, continued research will overcome all of the unsolved problems of cemented total hip arthroplasty—the problems of fixation, durability, and wear, for example. Until that time however, total hip replacement surgery will continue to be an art form that only some can truly master.

References

1. AHMED AM, et al.: Metal/cement interface strength in cemented stem fixation. J Orthop Res 2:105, 1984.
2. ALI KHAN M, et al.: Dislocation following total hip replacement. J Bone Joint Surg, 63B:214, 1981.
3. ALKIRE MJ, et al.: High vacuum as a method of reducing porosity of polymethacrylate. Orthopaedics, 10:1553, 1987.
4. AMSTUTZ HC, MARKOLF KL: Design features in total hip replacement. Bioengineering and Arthritis of the Hip. Chapter 7:111, 1974.
5. ANDERSSON, GBJ, et al.: Loosening of the cemented acctabular cup in total hip replacement. J Bone Joint Surg, 54B:590, 1972.
6. BARGAR WL, et al.: The addition of tobramycin to contrast bone cement: effect on flexural strength. J Arthroplasty, 1:165, 1986.
7. BARTEL DL, et al.: The effect of conformity and plastic thickness on contact stresses in metal-backed plastic implants. J Biomech Eng, 107:193, 1985.
8. BARTEL DL, et al.: The effect of conformity, thickness, and material on stresses in ultra-high molecular weight components for joint replacement. J Bone Joint Surg, 68A:1041, 1986.
9. BECKENBAUGH RD, ILSTRUP DM: Total hip arthroplasty: a review of three hundred and thirty-three cases with long follow-up. J Bone Joint Surg, 60A:306, 1978.
10. BERMNA AT, et al.: Thermally induced bone necrosis in rabbits. Clin Orthop, 186:284, 1984.
11. BLACK JD, GREENWALD AB: Structural weakness of layered acrylic bone cement. Clin Orthop, 171:94, 1982.
12. BOCCO F, et al.: Changes in the calcar femoris in relation to cement technology in total hip replacement. Clin Orthop, 128:287, 1977.
13. BOURNE RB, et al.: Femoral cement pressurization during total hip arthroplasty. Clin Orthop, 183:12, 1984.
14. BUCHOLZ HW, et al.: Management of deep infection of total hip replacement. J Bone Joint Surg, 63B:342, 1981.
15. BUNDY KJ, PENN RW: The effect of surface preparation on metal/bone cement interfacial strength. J Biomed Mat Res 21:773, 1987.
16. BURKE DW, et al.: Centrifugation as a method improving tensile and fatigue properties of acrylic bone cement. J Bone Joint Surg, 66A:1265, 1984.
17. BURKE DW, et al.: Stem modulus in total hip design. Proc 10th Annu Meet Soc Biomat, p. 320, 1984.
18. CARLSSON AS, GENTZ CF: Mechanical loosening of the femoral head prosthesis in the Charnley total hip arthroplasty. Clin Orthop, 147:262, 1980.
19. CARLSSON AS: 351 Total hip replacements according to Charnley. Acta Orthop Scand, 52:339, 1981.
20. CARLSSON AS, et al.: Radiographic loosening after revision with gentamicin-containing cement for deep infection in total hip arthroplasties. Clin Orthop, 194:271, 1985.
21. CARTER DR: Finite-element analysis of a metal-backed acetabular component. Proc 11th Meet Hip Soc, p. 216, 1983.
22. CARTER DR, et al.: Peri-acetabular stress distributions after joint replacement with subchondral bone retention. Acta Orthop Scand, 54:29, 1983.
23. CHANDLER HP et al.: Total hip replacement in patients younger than thirty years old. J Bone Joint Surg, 63A:1426, 1981.
24. CHANDLER DR, et al.: Prosthetic hip range of motion and impingement. Clin Orthop, 166:284, 1982.
25. CHAO EYS, COVENTRY MB: Fracture of the femoral component after total hip replacement. J Bone Joint Surg, 63A:1078, 1981.
26. CHARNLEY J: A biomechanical analysis of the use of cement to anchor the femoral head prosthesis. J Bone Joint Surg, 47B:354, 1965.
27. CHARNLEY J: Total hip replacement by low-friction arthroplasty. Clin Orthop, 72:7, 1970.
28. CHARNLEY J: The rationale of low frictional arthroplasty. Proc 1st Meet Hip Soc, p. 92, 1973.
29. CHARNLEY J: Arthroplasty of the hip: a new operation. Lancet, p. 1129, 1961.
30. CHARNLEY J: Fracture of femoral prostheses in total hip replacement. Clin Orthop, 111:105, 1975.
31. CHARNLEY J: Long-term results of low-friction arthroplasty. Proc 10th Meet Hip Soc, p. 42, 1982.
32. COLLIS DK: Femoral stem failure in total hip replacement. J Bone Joint Surg, 59A:1033, 1977.
33. COMBS SP, GREENWALD AS: The effects of barium sulfate on the polymerization temperature and shear strength of surgical Simplex P. Clin Orthop, 145:287, 1979.
34. COOK SD, et al.: Optimum pore size for bone cement fixation. Clin Orthop, 223:296, 1987.
35. CORNELL CN, RANAWAT CS: The impact of modern cement techniques on acetabular fixation in cemented total hip replacement. J Arthroplasty, 1:197, 1986.
36. COVENTRY MB: Late dislocation in patients with Charnley total hip arthroplasty. J Bone Joint Surg, 67A:832, 1985.
37. CROWNINSHIELD RD, et al.: An analysis of femoral component stem design in total hip arthroplasty. J Bone Joint Surg, 62A:68, 1980.
38. CROWNINSHIELD RD, et al.: The effect of femoral stem cross-sectional geometry on cement stresses in total hip reconstruction. Clin Orthop, 146:71, 1980.
39. CROWNINSHIELD RD, et al.: An analysis of collar function and the use of titanium in femoral prostheses. Clin Orthop, 158:270, 1981.
40. CROWNINSHIELD RD, et al.: A stress analysis of acetabular reconstruction in protusio acetabuli. J Bone Joint Surg, 65A:495, 1983.
41. CROWNINSHIELD RD, et al.: Analytical support for acetabular component metal backing. Proc 11th Meet Hip Society, p. 207, 1983.
42. DAVEY JR, et al.: Femoral component offset: its effect on strain in the cement, bone and prosthesis. Trans Orthop Res Soc, 34:528, 1988.

43. Davidson JA, Schwartz G: Wear, creep, and frictional heat of femoral implant articulating surfaces and the effect on long-term performance. J Biomed Mater Res, 21:261, 1987.
44. Davies JP, et al.: Comparison of the mechanical properties of Simplex P, Zimmer Regular, and LVC bone cements. J Biomed Mater Res, 21:719, 1987.
45. Davies JF, et al.: The effect of centrifugation on the fatigue life of bone cement in the presence of surface irregularities. Clin Orthop, 229:156, 1988.
46. Davies JP, et al.: Comparison of centrifuged and vacuum mixed Simplex P. Trans Orthop Res Soc, 34:221, 1988.
47. Davies JP, et al.: Fatigue strength of cement-metal interfaces: comparison of porous, precoated and smooth specimens. Trans Orthop Res Soc, 34:367, 1988.
48. DeLee JG, Charnley J: Radiologic demarcation of cemented sockets in total hip replacement. Clin Orthop, 121:20, 1976.
49. Demarest VA, et al.: Vacuum mixing of acrylic bone cement. Proc 9th Annu Meet Soc Biomater, p. 37, 1983.
50. Dorr LD, et al.: Total hip arthroplasties in patients less than forty-five years old. J Bone Joint Surg, 65A:474, 1983.
51. Dorr LD, et al.: Classification and treatment of dislocation of total hip arthroplasty. Clin Orthop, 173:151, 1983.
52. Eftekar N: Charnley "low friction torque" arthroplasty. Clin Orthop, 81:93, 1971.
53. Fackler CD, Foss R: Dislocation in total hip arthroplasties. Clin Orthop, 151:169, 1980.
54. Fishbane BM, Pond RB: Stainless steel fiber reinforcement of polymethylmethacrylate. Clin Orthop, 128:194, 1977.
55. Fornasier VL, Cameron HU: The femoral stem/cement interface in total hip replacement. Clin Orthop, 116:248, 1976.
56. Freitag TA, et al.: Fracture characteristics of acrylic bone cements. J Biomed Mater Res, 10:805, 1976.
57. Fumich RM, Gibbons DF: Rate of mixing and the strength of methylmethacrylate bone cements. Orthop Rev, 8:41, 1979.
58. Galante JO: Causes of fractures of the femoral component in total hip replacement. J Bone Joint Surg, 62A:670, 1980.
59. Galante JO, et al.: Failed femoral stems in total hip prostheses. J Bone Joint Surg, 57A:230, 1977.
60. Gates EI, et al.: Comparative fatigue behavior of different bone cements. Clin Orthop, 189:294, 1984.
61. Griffith MJ, et al.: Socket wear in Charnley low friction arthroplasty of the hip. Clin Orthop, 137:37, 1978.
62. Gruen TA, et al.: Effects of laminations and blood entrapment on the strength of acrylic bone cement. Clin Orthop, 119:250, 1976.
63. Haas SS, et al.: A characterization of polymethyl methacrylate bone cement. J Bone Joint Surg, 57A:380, 1975.
64. Harley JM, Boston DA: Acetabular cup failure after total hip replacement. J Bone Joint Surg, 67B:222, 1985.
65. Harris WH: Loosening. Proc 8th Meet Hip Soc, p. 162, 1978.
66. Harris WH: Advances in total hip arthroplasty: the metal-backed acetabular component. Clin Orthop, 183:4, 1984.
67. Harris WH, et al.: Femoral component loosening using contemporary techniques of femoral cement fixation. J Bone Joint Surg, 64A:1063, 1982.
68. Harris WH, McGann WA: Loosening of the femoral component after use of the medullary—plug cementing technique. J Bone Joint Surg, 68A:1064, 1986.
69. Harris WH, Penenberg B: Further follow-up on socket fixation using metal-backed acetabular components for total hip replacement. J Bone Joint Surg, 67A:1140, 1987.
70. Harris WH, White RE: Socket fixation using a metal-backed acetabular component for total hip replacement. J Bone Joint Surg, 64A:745, 1982.
71. Hierton C, et al.: Factors associated with early loosening of cemented total hip prostheses. Acta Orthop Scand, 54:168, 1983.
72. Hierton C, et al.: Factors associated with calcar resorption in cemented total hip prostheses. Acta Orthop Scand, 54:584, 1983.
73. Hughes S, et al.: The physical properties of antibiotics in bone cement. J Bone Joint Surg, 61B:379, 1979.
74. Ianotti JP, et al.: Aseptic loosening after total hip arthroplasty. J Arthroplasty, 1:99, 1986.
75. Jasty M, et al.: Porosity measurement in commercial bone cement preparation and the effect of centrifugation on porosity reduction. Trans Orthop Res Soc, 31:239, 1985.
76. Johnston RC, et al.: Reconstruction of the hip: a mathematical approach to determine optimum geometric relationships. J Bone Joint Surg, 61A:639, 1979.
77. Johnston RC, Crowninshield RD: Roentgenologic results of total hip arthroplasty. Clin Orthop, 181:92, 1983.
78. Johnston RC, Smidt GL: Hip motion measurements for selected activities of daily living. Clin Orthop, 72:205, 1970.
79. Kareh J, et al.: The effect of markedly varying head offset cement modulus, and stem modulus on the stress transfer around total hip replacement prostheses. Trans Orthop Res Soc, 34:528, 1988.
80. Knoell A, et al.: Graphite fiber reinforced bone cement. Ann Biomed Eng, 3:225, 1975.
81. Krause WR, et al.: Strength of the cement-bone interface. Clin Orthop, 163:290, 1982.
82. Krause W, Mathis RS: Fatigue properties of acrylic bone cements: review of the literature. J Biomed Mater Res, 22:37, 1988.
83. Kummer FJ: Improved mixing of bone cement. Trans Orthop Res Soc, 31:327, 1985.
84. Lachiewicz PF, Rosenstein BD: Long-term results of Harris total hip replacement. J Arthroplasty, 1:229, 1986.
85. Lane T, et al.: PMMA bone precoating—a new technique to optimize the bone-cement interface. Trans Orthop Res Soc, 28:247, 1982.
86. Lanyon LE, et al.: In vivo strain measurements from bone and prostheses following total hip replacement. J Bone Joint Surg, 63A:989, 1981.
87. Lautenschlaeger EP, et al.: Mechanical properties of bone cement containing large doses of antibiotic powders. J Biomed Mater Res, 10:929, 1976.
88. Lee AJC, et al.: Some properties of polymethylmethacrylate with reference to its use in orthopaedic surgery. Clin Orthop, 95:281, 1973.
89. Lewinnek GE, et al.: Dislocation after total hip replacement arthroplasties. J Bone Joint Surg, 60A:217, 1978.
90. Lewis JL, et al.: The influence of prosthetic stem stiffness and of a calcar collar on stresses in the proximal end of the femur with a cemented femoral component. J Bone Joint Surg, 66A:280, 1984.
91. Lindberg HO, Carlsson AS: Mechanical loosening of the femoral component in total hip replacement, Brunswik design. Acta Orthop Scand, 54:557, 1983.
92. Liu YK, et al.: Bone-particle-impregnated bone cement. J Biomed Mater Res, 21:247, 1987.
93. Ma SM, et al.: Frictional torque in surface and conventional acetabular cup in total hip replacement. J Bone Joint Surg, 54B:590, 1972.
94. Mallory TH: A plastic intermedullary plug for total hip arthroplasty. Clin Orthop, 155:37, 1981.
95. Manley MT, et al.: The load carrying and fatigue properties

of the stem-cement interface with smooth and porous coated femoral components. J Biomed Mater Res, 19:563, 1985.

96. MARKOLF KL, et al.: The effect of calcar contact on femoral component micromovement. J Bone Joint Surg, 62A:135, 1980.
97. MARKS KE, et al.: Antibiotic-impregnated acrylic bone cement. J Bone Joint Surg, 58A:358, 1976.
98. MARMOR L, et al.: Stem fractures of extra-heavy cobra femoral hip prostheses. Clin Orthop 190:148, 1984.
99. MARTENS M, et al.: Factors in the mechanical failure of the femoral component in total hip prosthesis. Acta Orthop Scand, 45:693, 1974.
100. MATTINGLY DA, et al.: Aseptic loosening in metal-backed acetabular components for total hip replacement. J Bone Joint Surg, 67A:387, 1985.
101. MEYER PR, et al.: On the setting properties of acrylic bone cement. J Bone Joint Surg, 55A:149, 1973.
102. MILLER J, et al.: Pathophysiology of loosening of femoral components in total hip arthroplasty. Proc 6th Meet Hip Soc, p. 64, 1978.
103. MJOBERG B, et al.: Low—versus high—viscosity bone cement. Acta Orthop Scand, 58:106, 1987.
104. MORAN JM, et al.: Effect of gentamicin on shear and interface strengths of bone cement. Clin Orthop, 141:96, 1979.
105. MORELAND JR, JINNAH R: Fracture of a Charnley acetabular component from polyethylene wear. Clin Orthop, 207:94, 1986.
106. MORREY BF, ILSTRUP D: Size of the femoral head and acetabular revision in total hip-replacement arthroplasty. J Bone Joint Surg, 71A:50, 1989.
107. NOBLE PC, et al.: The distribution of porosity in acrylic bone cement. Trans Orthop Res Soc, 31:242, 1985.
108. NOBLE PC, et al.: Innovations in acrylic bone cement. Proc 53rd Annu Meet Am Acad Orthop Surg, 1986.
109. NOBLE PC, et al.: Innovations in cementing technique in total hip replacement. Proc 54th Annu Meet Am Acad Orthop Surg, 1987.
110. OH I, et al.: Improved fixation of the femoral component after total hip replacement using a methacrylate intramedullary plug. J Bone Joint Surg, 60A:608, 1978.
111. OH I, et al.: The femoral cement compactor. J Bone Joint Surg, 65A:1335, 1983.
112. OH I: A comprehensive analysis of the factors affecting acetabular cup fixation and design in total hip replacement arthroplasty. Trans 11th Meet Hip Soc, p. 129, 1983.
113. OH I, et al: Acetabular cup groove and pod design and its effect on cement fixation in total hip arthroplasty. Clin Orthop, 189:308, 1984.
114. OH I, et al.: Total hip acetabular cup flange design and its effect on cemented fixation. Clin Orthop, 195:304, 1985.
115. OH I, HARRIS WH: Proximal strain distribution in the loaded femur. J Bone Joint Surg, 60A:75, 1978.
116. OLSSON SS, et al.: Clinical and radiological long-term results after Charnley-Muller total hip replacement. Acta Orthop Scand, 52:531, 1981.
117. PATERSON M, et al.: Loosening of the femoral component after total hip replacement. J Bone Joint Surg, 68:392, 1986.
118. PILLIAR RM, et al.: Carbon-fiber-reinforced bone cement in orthopaedic surgery. J Biomed Mater Res, 10:893, 1976.
119. PRICE H, et al.: PMMA precoating. A study of the effects of pre- and post-coating treatment on bone cement adhesion. Trans Orthop Res Soc, 31:91, 1985.
120. RAAB S, et al.: PMMA precoated implants—interface optimization. Trans Orthop Res Soc, 26:251, 1980.
121. RAAB S, et al.: Thin film PMMA precoating for improved

implant bone-cement fixation. J Biomed Mater Res, 16:679, 1982.
122. RAND JA, CHAO EY: Femoral implant neck fracture following total hip arthroplasty. Clin Orthop, 221:255, 1987.
123. RAND JA, ILSTRUP DM: Comparison of Charnley and T-28 total hip arthroplasty. Clin Orthop, 180:201, 1983.
124. REIKERAS O: Ten-year follow-up of Muller hip replacement. Acta Orthop Scand, 53:919, 1982.
125. REY RM, et al.: A study of intrusion characteristics of low viscosity cement, Simplex-P, and Palacos cements in a bovine cancellous bone model. Clin Orthop, 215:272, 1987.
126. RIMNAC CM, et al.: The effect of centrifugation on the fracture properties of acrylic bone cements. J Bone Joint Surg, 68A:281, 1986.
127. RITTER MA, et al.: Correlation of prosthetic femoral head size and/or design with longevity of total hip arthroplasty. Clin Orthop, 176:252, 1983.
128. RITTER MA, CAMPBELL ED: An evaluation of Trapezoidal-28 femoral stem fractures. Clin Orthop, 212:237, 1986.
129. RITTER MA, CAMPBELL ED: Longterm comparison of the Charnley, Muller and Trapezoidal-28 total hip prostheses. J Arthroplasty, 2:299, 1987.
130. ROBINSON RP, et al.: Mechanical properties of poly (methyl methacrylate) bone cements. J Biomed Mater Res, 15:203, 1981.
131. ROSE RM, et al.: On the true wear rate of ultra high-molecular-weight polyethylene in the total hip prostheses. J Bone Joint Surg, 62A:537, 1980.
132. SAHA S, PAL S: Strain-rate dependence of the compressive properties of normal and carbon-fiber-reinforced bone cement. J Biomed Mater Res, 17:1041, 1983.
133. SAHA S, PAL S: Mechanical properties of bone cement: a review. J Biomed Mater Res, 18:435, 1984.
134. SAHA S, PAL S: Mechanical characterization of commercially made carbon-fiber-reinforced polymethylmethacrylate. J Biomed Mater Res, 20:817, 1986.
135. SALVATI EA, et al.: Fracture of polyethylene acetabular cups. J Bone Joint Surg, 61A:1239, 1979.
136. SALVATI EA, et al.: A ten-year follow-up study of our first one hundred consecutive Charnley total hip replacements. J Bone Joint Surg, 63A:753, 1981.
137. SAVINO AW: The influence of femoral stem thickness and implantation technique on the strength of the bone cement bond. Acta Orthop Scand, 53:23, 1982.
138. SCHREURS BW, et al: Effects of preparation techniques on the porosity of acrylic cements. Acta Orthop Scand, 59:403, 1988.
139. SHELLEY P, WROBLEWSKI BM: Socket design and cement pressurization in the Charnley low-friction arthroplasty. J Bone Joint Surg, 70B:358, 1988.
140. SKINNER HB, et al.: Stress changes in bone secondary to the use of a femoral canal plug with cemented hip replacement. Clin Orthop, 166:277, 1982.
141. STAUFFER RN: Ten-year follow-up study of total hip replacement. J Bone Joint Surg, 64A:983, 1982.
142. SUTHERLAND CJ, et al.: A ten-year follow-up of one hundred consecutive Muller curved-stem total hip-replacement arthroplasties. J Bone Joint Surg, 64A:970, 1982.
143. TAITSMAN JP, SAHA S: Tensile strength of wire-reinforced bone cement and twisted stainless steel wire. J Bone Joint Surg, 59A:419, 1977.
144. THIRUPATHI RG, HUSTED C: Failure of polyethylene acetabular cups. Clin Orthop, 179:209, 1983.
145. TURULA KB, et al.: Leg length inequity after total hip arthroplasty. Clin Orthop, 202:163, 1986.
146. WEIGHTMAN B, et al.: The mechanical properties of cement

and loosening of the femoral component of hip replacements. J Bone Joint Surg, 69B:558, 1987.

147. WEINSTEIN AM, et al.: The effect of high pressure insertion and antibiotic inclusions upon the mechanical properties of polymethylmethacrylate. Clin Orthop, 121:67, 1976.

148. WELSH P, et al.: Surgical implants. The role of surface porosity in fixation to bone and acrylic. J Bone Joint Surg, 53A:963, 1972.

149. WILDE AH, GREENWALD AS: Shear strength of self-curing acrylic cement. Clin Orthop, 106:126, 1975.

150. WILTSE LL, et al.: Experimental studies regarding the possible use of self-curing acrylic in orthopaedic surgery. J Bone Joint Surg, 39A:961, 1957.

151. WIXSON RL, et al.: Vacuum mixing of methylmethacrylate bone cement. Trans Orthop Res Soc, 31:327, 1985.

152. WOO RYG, MORREY BF: Dislocation after total hip arthroplasty. J Bone Joint Surg, 64A:1295, 1982.

153. WOOLSON ST, et al.: Time-related improvement in the range of motion of the hip after total replacement. J Bone Joint Surg, 67A:1251, 1985.

154. WRIGHT TM, TRENT PS: Mechanical properties of Aramid fiber reinforced acrylic bone cement. J Mater Sci, 14:503, 1979.

155. WROBLEWSKI BM: Wear of high-density polyethylene on bone and cartilage. J Bone Joint Surg, 61B:498, 1979.

156. WROBLEWSKI BM: Fractured stem in total hip replacement. Acta Orthop Scand, 53:279, 1982.

157. WROBLEWSKI BM: Direction and rate of socket wear in Charnley low-friction arthroplasty. J Bone Joint Surg, 67B:757, 1985.

158. WROBLEWSKI BM: One-stage revision of infected cemented total hip arthroplasty. Clin Orthop, 211:103, 1988.

159. WROBLEWSKI BM, et al.: External wear of the polyethylene socket in cement total hip arthroplasty. J Bone Joint Surg, 69B:61, 1987.

CHAPTER THREE

Surgical Approaches

RICHARD A. BALDERSTON

Introduction

Over the last three decades consideration of the various surgical approaches to the hip joint has been stimulated by three major developments in hip surgery. The first is total hip arthroplasty, the goal of which is to insert prosthetic components into a satisfactorily prepared bony bed.[9,20,37] In the process minimal trauma should occur to the muscular, tendinous, ligamentous, and fascial structures that must be retracted or incised to complete the operation. The second major impetus for development of surgical approaches comes from the treatment of complex acetabular and pelvic fractures. With the means to both obtain and maintain an anatomic reduction, and thus restore function to a maximal level, the requirement of early motion and muscle function necessitated review of the surgical approach possibilities that would minimize loss of abductor function. The third major area of surgical endeavor comes from the field of musculoskeletal tumor surgery around the hip joint. For any given tumor at the level of the acetabulum or proximal femur, the surgical approach must respect the planes of dissection necessary for tumor control and consider subsequent muscle function after the tumor surgery. Because of differences in size, configuration, and microscopic indications of tumor aggressiveness, no set formula exists to surgically remove each particular neoplasm. This set of unique pathologic characteristics in each case dictates a fresh consideration of the various surgical approach possibilities before treatment is rendered.

Historically, the surgical approaches that are reviewed in this chapter have developed in accordance with a particular pathologic entity to be considered. The hip surgeons of the early twentieth century were interested in the treatment of septic arthritis as well as the eradication of tuberculosis infection from the hip joint.[1,12,15] Their surgical approaches to the hip reflected their desire to obtain drainage of the hip joint as well as to carry out surgical debridement of dead bone and soft tissue. With the arrival of the mold arthroplasty, and subsequently the proximal femoral endoprosthesis, the surgical approaches were modified to reflect completely different goals of the surgical procedure.[2] No longer was a functionally limited hip expected after hip surgery for infection. In a significant number of cases both Vitallium mold arthroplasty and endoprosthetic replacement were able to provide a patient with a functionally normal hip. Thus, the consideration of the abductor mechanism as well as the other soft tissue structures violated in a surgical approach became more important. With the advent of total hip replacement as devised by Charnley, the role of the surgical approach has become even more vital.[9]

Decision Making and Choice of Surgical Approach

The following sections detailing the anterior, lateral, posterior, and medial approaches to the hip demonstrate a large number of possibilities to initiate exposure of the hip joint. Many factors should be considered by the surgeon before any operation is begun. The surgeon must first consider patient position on the operating table. The patient may be placed in a straight supine position or may have the operated side elevated by a towel or rolled blanket. The pelvis can be elevated to 45° with the use of a bean bag, or the patient can be placed in the straight lateral position with the use of abdominal and lumbar supports. Whatever position is chosen, it is extremely important that the surgeon remains aware of the position of the pelvis at all times during the surgery.

A number of patient considerations enter into the surgeon's consideration for operative approach. Patients who have large bulk may require more extensive exposure. Often, patients with well developed musculature may require a surgical approach that is more extensile of muscle planes to allow adequate exposure. Patients who have an increased size because of subcutaneous adipose tissue may only require a longer incision to allow the same exposure in a deeper surgical site. Patients who are in precarious health and who may be subject to poor wound healing because of nutritional considerations may require an approach that requires less in the way of soft tissue and bony healing. In patients with neuromuscular disease and when muscle function is partly absent around the hip, an approach must be chosen that does not require those particular muscles for subsequent stability of the hip joint. Patients who have had cerebrovascular accidents often posture with the hip in flexion, adduction, and internal rotation; the choice of a posterior approach that would violate the supporting structures posteriorly might increase the risk of dislocation of an endoprosthesis or total hip replacement. In patients who might require treatment for myositis with radiation, consideration should be given to an operative approach that does not require the bony healing of a trochanteric osteotomy.

Patients who have had previous surgery on the affected hip present a number of problems. The previous incision may not have incorporated the approach that the revision surgeon would like to use. Additional incisions about the hip put the skin at increased risk for necrosis. Incisions more anterior to a previous incision are said to be more at risk than those incisions posterior to a previous incision. Whenever possible our attempt has been to incorporate the old incision with extensions superiorly and inferiorly in an anterior or posterior direction that would allow approach of the fascia through a routine incision. Consideration must also be given to the effect of the previous surgery on the bony anatomy that awaits the surgeon after the soft tissue dissection. In general, a more extensile exposure must be planned in a revision situation.

Consideration must also be given to the limitations of the operating room support personnel. The experience of the anesthesia team with the supine and lateral positions of the patient must be considered. The anesthesia department's experience with spinal anesthesia in both the supine and lateral positions is critical. In addition, the availability of surgical assistance to accomplish any approach is important. The surgeon must have the critical retractors necessary to maintain exposure as well as the necessary assistance to accomplish this retraction.

At this point the surgeon must judge the extent of exposure required to accomplish the surgical goal. For instance, with total hip replacement, the selection of the prosthesis is critical to the determination of the surgical approach that may be required. In patients with whom methylmethacrylate is used to anchor an acetabular component, exposure must be adequate so that the methylmethacrylate can be contained and removed once the acetabular component is in position.[9] Components that do not require methylmethacrylate may require slightly less definition of the surrounding soft tissues.[19] The surgeon must be able to judge whether the hip joint is stable after the given surgery and that the patient's leg length discrepancy has been minimized as much as possible.

The final and most important consideration in the choice of surgical approach to the hip is the surgeon's experience. Many surgeons have advocated a particular approach for a wide variety of surgical interventions about the hip joint, and claimed excellent results both in the short and long term. With increasing experience with a given exposure, the surgeon develops respect for the soft tissues and understands the limits to which the exposure can practically be accomplished.

Surgical Anatomy

The critical structures that should be considered before any surgical approach are the surface landmarks and critical blood vessels, nerves, and muscles that will be encountered during the surgical approach.

Surface Landmarks

The critical bony prominences that the surgeon must be able to palpate include the anterior superior iliac spine, posterior superior iliac spine, iliac crest, and greater trochanter (see Fig. 1–1). For most hip operations the ankle and knee are draped freely so that the surgeon can readily ascertain the position of the tibia in space with the knee flexed 90°. This information will assist the surgeon in assessing femoral neck anteversion at the time of prosthetic implantation. Also, palpation of the lumbar spine and sacrum is easier with the patient in the lateral decubitus position.

The surgeon must keep in mind that the relationships between the greater trochanter, anterior superior iliac spine, posterior superior iliac spine, and iliac crest may be altered significantly with the various diseased states. In patients with severe degenerative joint disease where the femoral head is partially destroyed, the femur may migrate one or two centimeters superiorly. This situation may also occur with femoral neck fractures, so the surgeon should take these factors into account when planning his incision. Also, acetabular and pelvic fractures as well as previous surgery about the greater trochanter will alter these relationships.

Key Muscular and Fascial Relationships About the Hip

Beneath the skin and subcutaneous adipose tissue along the lateral aspect of the thigh lies the fascia lata. At this level the gluteus maximus arises from the posterior gluteal line of the ilium as well as the iliac crest that lies superior to it (see Figs. 1–19, 1–23). The fibers of the gluteus maximus muscle proceed distally and anteriorly and end in an extremely broad aponeurosis that inserts into the fascia lata and femur at the level just distal to the trochanters. The tensor fascia femoris arises from the anterior aspect of the iliac crest at the level of the anterior superior spine (see Fig. 1–21). Its fibers run distally to insert into the iliotibial tract anterior to the aponeurosis of the gluteus maximus tendon. At the level of the iliac crest the deep investing fascia between these two muscles forms a cover for the gluteus medius muscle.

Perhaps the most critical muscle in any lateral approach to the hip is the gluteus medius (see Figs. 1–19, 1–21). It arises from the entire outer surface of the ilium from the iliac crest to the anterior and posterior gluteal lines. The muscle is shaped like a fan and converges into a strong flattened tendon that inserts obliquely along the lateral surface of the greater trochanter. It must be remembered that the point of insertion of the gluteus medius is not a single point but actually a broad attachment along the outer surface of the greater trochanter. It must also be remembered that when one is palpating the medial surface of the greater trochanter the insertion of the gluteus medius is entirely superficial to this area. The superior gluteal nerve innervates both the gluteus medius and tensor fascia lata (see Fig. 1–27).

The gluteus minimus lies deep to the gluteus medius (see Fig. 1–21). This muscle is also fan shaped and arises from the outer surface of the ilium caudal to the anterior and posterior gluteal lines. This muscle is much smaller in bulk than the medius and converges to a much smaller tendon that has an insertion along the anterior and medial aspect of the greater trochanter. In addition

the gluteus medius inserts directly onto the capsule of the hip joint. This muscle may be thin posteriorly and is often mistaken for capsule and left behind when the surgeon intends to retract both gluteus medius and minimus muscles in a posterolateral approach to the hip.

The most superior of the external rotators is the piriformis muscle, which lies parallel to the posterior margin of the gluteus medius (see Fig. 1–21). After arising from the pelvis it becomes a long rounded tendon that inserts into the superior border of the greater trochanter. The obturator internus arises from inside the pelvis in a broad expansion that includes the superior and inferior rami of the pubis as well as the ischium. At the level of the lesser sciatic notch just inferior to the sacrospinous ligament the bands converge and proceed to their insertion on the greater trochanter. Because it lies outside the pelvis the obturator internus muscle is flanked on its superior and inferior side by the gemellae. These two small muscles arise from the ischium and insert onto the posteromedial surface of the greater trochanter. The quadratus femoris is the most inferior external rotator and arises from the tuberosity of the ischium. The insertion of the quadratus femoris is more posterior than that of the other external rotators; the insertion proceeds distally from the intertrochanteric crest, and at this level of the femur there is a close relationship with the branches of the medial femoral circumflex artery.

Vascular Relationships About the Hip

The primary vasculature to the hip is from the medial and lateral femoral circumflex vessels that are branches of the profunda femoris artery (see Fig. 1–12, 1–13). These two vessels encircle the intertrochanteric region of the femur. The lateral femoral circumflex arises from the profunda femoris and proceeds in a lateral direction anterior to the femur. The medial femoral circumflex arises at the same level as the preceding artery but procedes medially and posteriorly until the medial border of the femur is reached, and then proceeds laterally to give branches that form anastomotic network around the proximal femur. When making a lateral approach to the hip, a large branch of the lateral femoral circumflex vessel is encountered at the junction of the gluteus medius muscle with the anterior border of the greater trochanter at the level of the femur. The femoral artery lies directly anterior to the hip joint.

Both the inferior and superior gluteal arteries leave the pelvis at the level of the greater sciatic notch (see Figs. 1–12, 1–13). The superior gluteal vessel accompanies the superior gluteal nerve and lies between the superior aspect of the notch and the piriformis muscle. This artery is most commonly at risk with posterior procedures that involve dissection about the greater sciatic notch. The inferior gluteal artery accompanies the inferior gluteal nerve and arises from the greater sciatic notch inferior to the piriformis tendon and is much less commonly injured.

Another vessel that is frequently encountered during hip surgery is the lateral or posterior branch of the obturator artery as it appears beneath the transverse acetabular ligament and enters the acetabular fossa (see Fig. 1–16). A small branch is given off to the ligamentum teres and enters the head of the femur. With reaming of the acetabulum, the surgeon must control bleeding from this vessel.

Peripheral Nerves About the Hip

The femoral nerve lies lateral to the femoral artery as they emerge from the inguinal canal. This nerve is most at risk with anterior approaches to the hip; although with extensive retraction during an anterolateral or direct lateral approach or in cases of revision surgery with extensive scarring, this nerve is at risk for neuropraxia and in rare cases neuroptmesis secondary to retraction or surgical dissection. The superior gluteal nerve is accompanied by the superior gluteal artery as it leaves the greater sciatic notch superior to the piriformis muscle. This nerve proceeds between the gluteus medius and gluteus minimus muscle in an anterior direction. Branches of this nerve may lie 2 centimeters above the level of the greater trochanter and dissection posteriorly at this level may denervate the anterior aspect of the gluteus medius, gluteus minimus, and the entire tensor fascia muscle.

The sciatic nerve classically passes anterior to the piriformis tendon (see Fig. 1–27). The nerve then proceeds, under cover of the gluteus maximus muscle, in a position posterior to the rest of the external rotators. The common peroneal portion of the sciatic nerve may lie posterior to the piriformis muscle or rarely the entire sciatic nerve may lie posterior to the piriformis muscle. Great care must be taken with any posterior or posterolateral approach to the hip or pelvis to know the position of the sciatic nerve at all times during the execution of the operation.

Application of Neuromuscular Anatomy for Surgical Exposure

Four peripheral nerves innervate major muscle groups that have action across the hip joint: the femoral, superior gluteal, sciatic, and obturator. The nerves, muscles, and principal actions are listed in Table 3–1. The femoral nerve supplies the rectus femoris division of the quadriceps mechanism as well as the sartorius; these muscles act primarily as flexors of the hip. The superior gluteal nerve supplies the primary abductors of the hip, which are the gluteus medius, gluteus minimus, and tensor fascia lata. The sciatic nerve supplies primarily extensors of the hip including the biceps femoris, semitendinosis, and semimembranosus, as well as the posterior portion of the adductor magnus. The obturator nerve supplies the adductors longus, brevis, and magnus, as well as the gracilis and obturator externis; these muscles function primarily as adductors of the hip. The inferior gluteal nerve innervates the gluteus maximus, which is the primary extensor of the hip joint. The nerve to the obturator internis, nerve to the quadratus femoris, and nerve to the piriformis complete the innervation of the musculature of the hip and supply the small external rotators, which in addition to their external rotation activity, can act as extensors.

For any operation about the hip one guiding principle is that the musculature should be traumatized to the least extent possible. Direct injury to the muscles through retraction, loss of continuity of either insertion or origin or direct sectioning of the muscle is to be avoided, if possible. Great care must also be taken to respect the integrity of the peripheral nerves that supply these same muscles. Surgical exposures of the hip joint can be classified according to their relationship to the plane of exposure with each of these muscle groups. The anterior approach proceeds between the nerve territories of the femoral nerve and the superior gluteal nerve; thus theoretically, the muscles within the extensor and abductor groups are traumatized to a minimal extent. The lateral approaches as a group are the most diverse, but all of them stay posterior to the tensor fascia lata muscle. The superficial muscular layer split is either between the gluteus maximus and tensor fascia or extends into the gluteus maxi-

TABLE 3–1.

Group	Nerve	Divisions of Lumbosacral Plexus	Muscles	Principal Action
I	Femoral	Dorsal L-2 L-3 L-4	Iliopsoas Pectineus Sartorius Rectus femoris	Flexion
II	Superior gluteal	Dorsal L-4, L-5 S-1	Gluteus medius Gluteus minimus Tensor fasciae latae	Abduction
III	Sciatic	Ventral L-4 L-5 S-1 S-2 S-3	Biceps femoris Semitendinosus Semimembranosus Adductor magnus	Extension
IV	Inferior gluteal	L-5, S-1, S-2	Gluteus maximus	Extension
V	Nerve to piriformis	S-1, S-2	Piriformis	External Rotation
VI	Nerve to obturator internus	L-5, S-1, S-2	Obturator internus Superior gemellus	External Rotation
VII	Nerve to quadratus femoris	L-4, L-5, S-1	Quadratus femoris Inferior gemellus	External Rotation
VIII	Obturator	Ventral L-2 L-3 L-4	Adductor longus Adductor brevis Adductor magnus Gracilis Obturator externus	Adduction

mus muscle in a posterolateral direction. Once the abductor mechanism is encountered there are multiple approaches for mobilization of the gluteus medius, minimus, and greater trochanter. Posterolateral approaches remain posterior to the muscles of the superior gluteal nerve. The tensor fascia lata, gluteus medius, and gluteus minimus are retracted anteriorly. The gluteus maximus is split in a more posterior direction and the muscle group of external rotators including the obturator, internus, superior and inferior gemelli, and quadratus femoris as well as the piriformis are retracted posteriorly. The seldom used medial approach uses a plane through the muscles of the obturator nerve.

Anterior Approaches to the Hip

The utility of the anterior approach to the hip was greatest during the period when cup arthroplasty was the most common procedure for degenerative arthritis.[2] The plane of exposure is between the muscles of the flexor and abductor groups supplied by the femoral and superior gluteal nerves respectively. Superficially, the dissection proceeds between the tensor fascia lata and the sartorius muscle; deeper dissection separates the gluteus medius from the rectus femoris muscle, which then leads to the hip capsule.

The most common indications for the anterior approach today include intra-articular hip fusions and pelvic osteotomies. Biopsies of the hip or anterior pelvis, as well as internal fixation of anterior pelvic fractures can be performed through this approach. This technique may also be appropriate in patients who require endoprosthetic replacement in the presence of severe hip flexion contractures or for those who require total hip replacement.

Unfortunately, many limitations and complications may be encountered. The principal limitation of the exposure is an inability to mobilize the femur in an extensile manner. Although the exposure of the anterior acetabulum is often adequate, consideration of the posterior wall of the acetabulum is limited. With dissection along the anterior femur distally, the quadriceps mechanism and the lateral femoral cutaneous nerve provide a barrier for further exposure of the femur.

Great care must be taken during the approach to ligate the ascending branch of the lateral circumflex artery that travels between the abductor and flexor muscle planes. In addition, the lateral femoral cutaneous nerve crosses the plane of dissection two finger breadths below the anterior superior iliac spine and care should be taken that this structure is not ligated, but gently retracted.

Smith-Peterson first reported on this approach to the hip in 1917 in the American Journal of Ortho-

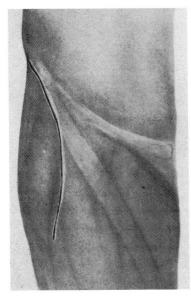
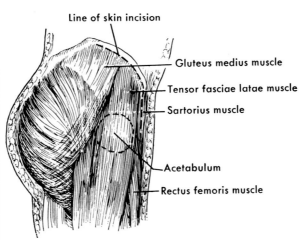

Line of skin incision

Gluteus medius muscle

Tensor fasciae latae muscle

Sartorius muscle

Acetabulum

Rectus femoris muscle

Fig. 3–1. The anterior iliofemoral approach to the hip by Smith-Peterson. **Left.** Anterior view of the skin incision. **Right.** Lateral view of the skin incision. Depending on the operation to be performed, the direction of the distal limb of the incision may be altered. (From Crenshaw AM: Campbell's Operative Orthopaedics. St. Louis, Mosby, 1963.)

paedic Surgery.[46] The patient is placed in the supine position on the operating table. Incision is begun at the middle of the iliac crest and carried anteriorly to the iliac spine and then distally and laterally for a distance of 10 cm along the lateral aspect of the femoral shaft (Figs. 3–1, 3–2, 3–3). After division of the superficial fascia, the interval between the tensor fascia lata and the sartorius is sought. This interval is more easily discernable in the distal aspect of the wound where the deep fascia is not as thick and the muscle bellies themselves are more easily identified. The deep fascia is then split superiorly to the anterior superior spine and dissection is begun on the ilium to free the origins of the tensor fascia lata, gluteus medius, and gluteus minimus musculature. Because this step is carried out with a Cobb elevator, the muscles are packed to limit bleeding. With the tensor

fascia retracted laterally, the interval between the rectus and the gluteus medius can be palpated bluntly. At this step the ascending branch of the lateral femoral circumflex artery, which usually lies 4 to 5 cm distal to the hip joint, is ligated. At all times care must be taken that the lateral femoral cutaneous nerve is gently retracted medially.

At this point if tissues are contracted an osteotomy may be performed of the anterior superior iliac spine to allow retraction of the sartorius medially. In addition, more posterior dissection may be performed of the gluteus medius and minimus muscle to allow a broader exposure of the distal deeper structures. At this point the rectus femoris muscle itself is identified as it lies anterior to the hip capsule. The origin of the direct head of the rectus from the anterior inferior iliac spine as well as the

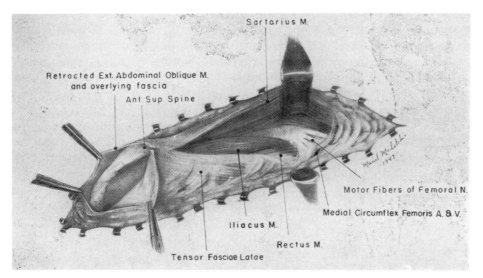

Sartorius M.

Retracted Ext. Abdominal Oblique M. and overlying fascia

Ant Sup Spine

Motor Fibers of Femoral N.

Medial Circumflex Femoris A. & V.

Iliacus M.

Rectus M.

Tensor Fasciae Latae

Fig. 3–2. Anterior iliofemoral approach to the hip by Smith-Peterson. The superficial aspect of the dissection has been developed, exposing the iliacus with overlying motor fibers of the femoral nerve. Superiorly, the muscular periosteal attachments have been reflected from the medial and lateral surfaces of the ilium. (From Crenshaw AM: Campbell's Operative Orthopaedics, St. Louis, Mosby, 1963.)

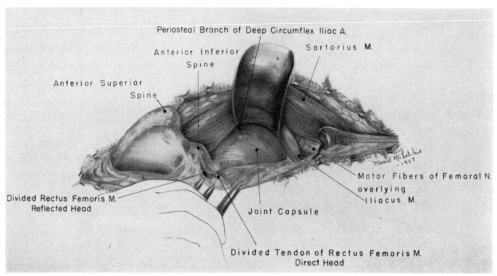

Periosteal Branch of Deep Circumflex Iliac A.

Anterior Inferior
Spine

Sartorius M.

Anterior Superior
Spine

Divided Rectus Femoris M.
Reflected Head

Motor Fibers of Femoral N.
overlying
Iliacus M.

Joint Capsule

Divided Tendon of Rectus Femoris M.
Direct Head

Fig. 3-3. Anterior iliofemoral approach to the hip by Smith-Peterson. The capsule of the hip joint has been exposed with retraction of the rectus, femoris, and iliacus muscles. Bleeding is usually encountered from the periosteal branch of the deep circumflex iliac artery. The surgeon should be ready to bove this vessel when encountered. (From Crenshaw AM: Campbell's Operative Orthopaedics. St. Louis, Mosby, 1963.)

reflected head from the superior acetabulum and hip capsule are divided and retracted medially.

The hip capsule is now easily exposed along its entire anterolateral aspect. At this point a capsulectomy can be performed if required or a T-shaped incision may be made in the capsule with a transverse incision perpendicular to the femoral neck at the level of the acetabular margin. A central incision may then be made to the femoral neck and extending distally to the intertrochanteric line. Gentle external rotation and adduction will place tension on the ligamentum teres, which may then be divided with a curved knife or scissors. Further external rotation and adduction, as well as slight flexion, will allow dislocation of the femoral head.

The approach may be extended at this point to include a subperiosteal dissection along the inner aspect of the pelvis. Osteotomy of the anterior superior iliac spine allows the sartorius to be retracted medially and using a Cobb elevator with blunt dissection, the muscles of the abdominal obliques, as well as the iliacus are dissected from the iliac crest and inner surface of the ilium. Utilizing this technique, the anterior acetabular wall can be easily exposed.

In 1955 Luck reported the variation on this approach that allowed a more extensive exposure of the proximal femur.[32] The same intermuscular planes are utilized; however he advocated division of the tensor fascia lata across the distal third of its belly and consideration of division of the gluteus medius and minimus from the greater trochanter or trochanteric osteotomy for increased exposure of the lateral femoral neck (Fig. 3-4).

The patient is placed in the supine position and a skin incision is made between the mid point of the anterior superior spine and the symphysis pubis and is carried laterally to an end joint just lateral to the greater trochanter. After dissection of the subcutaneous tissue, the fascia lata is identified and at a point distal to the greater trochanter is divided transversely to permit identification of the tensor fascia muscle. The branch of the superior gluteal nerve to the tensor fascia lata enters that muscle in its proximal half from the posterior aspect. Therefore, the muscle is divided as far distally in the wound as possible to prevent injury to this feeder nerve. The gluteus medius and tensor fascia can be retracted laterally without significantly taking down the origin of this abductor muscle group. The rectus femoris is identified and can usually be retracted although the origins from the anterior inferior spine and from the acetabulum may be divided. The anterior fibers of the gluteus medius and gluteus minimus may be dissected from the greater trochanter or a trochanteric osteotomy may be performed depending on the exposure necessary. The greater trochanteric fragment can then be transplanted distally at the time of closure. Again, great care must be taken to control bleeding from the ascending branch of the lateral femoral circumflex and to preserve function of the lateral femoral cutaneous nerve.

Closure of anterior approaches to the hip is facilitated by flexion of the thigh on the pelvis. The tensor fascia in the case of the Luck approach is closed with interrupted sutures and the fascia lata is closed with interrupted figure-8 sutures.

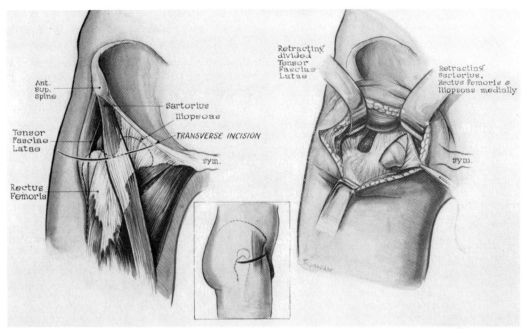

Fig. 3–4. The transverse anterior approach to the hip by Luck. A transverse incision is made over the anterior aspect of the hip followed by division of the tensor fascia lata across the distal third of its muscle belly. The sartorius rectus femoris and iliopsoas are retracted medially while the remaining abductors are retracted laterally. (From Luck VC: A transverse anterior approach to the hip. J Bone Joint Surg, 37A:534, 1955.)

Numerous variations have been reported on these two approaches to gain increased exposure and more versatility. Cubbins, Callahan, et al.,[13] described a distal posterior extension of the Smith Peterson incision that allowed a more distal transverse incision across the fascia lata. Sutherland and Rowe[47] recommended extensive bony osteotomies to preserve the tendinous attachments of the origins of the rectus and sartorius as well as the insertions of the gluteus medius and minimus. Fahey[15] recommended an oblique excision running from anteromedial to posterolateral to decrease scarring along the iliac crest.

Lateral Approaches to the Hip

Lateral approaches to the hip are defined as dissections that proceed within the group of muscles innervated by the superior gluteal nerve. Approaches in this group have in common that the tensor fascia lata remains intact and retracted anteriorly. Because the innervation of the nerve is superior and posterior, the muscle is not denervated unless extensive dissection is required to remove the origin of the tensor from the iliac wing.

The multiple variations of the lateral approach are among the most commonly performed as the initial step for a wide variety of hip procedures. Ol-

lier,[12] in the late nineteenth century, described an approach to the hip that used trochanteric osteotomy. Watson-Jones[51] in 1936 described an anterolateral approach to the hip leaving the trochanter intact. Variations on these two approaches have been described by numerous authors. The indications for lateral approach to the hip are most commonly total hip replacement, but also include endoprosthetic replacement, open reduction, internal fixation of fractures, and biopsies of the proximal femur.

The limitations of the lateral approaches in general include inadequate exposure of the ilium unless anterior or posterior exposures are added. Generally, an excellent exposure of the distal femur is possible with incision of the vastus lateralis muscle. The most common complication with these approaches includes injury to the abductor mechanism. These exposures require either sectioning of the anterior fibers of the gluteus medius as suggested in the Watson-Jones approach, elevation of the gluteus medius origin that is recommended in the approaches of McFarland and Osborne[35] and McLauchlin[37] and Hardinge,[19] or elevation of the greater trochanter as recommended by Ollier,[12] Charnley,[9] and Harris.[20,21] Thus, at the level of the insertion of the abductor muscles, it is possible to lose continuity of either the muscle fibers themselves or of the greater trochanter from the rest of the proximal femur. Great attention must be placed on the closure of these incisions once the total hip replacement or other intraarticular procedure is carried out. The method of trochanteric reattachment and the execution of that step are often as important as the technique required for the hip replacement itself.

The technique of the anterolateral approach according to Watson-Jones[51] begins with the patient in the supine position. The incision is made from a point 2.5 cm distal and lateral to the anterior superior spine and curved distally and posteriorly over the lateral aspect of the greater trochanter and down the lateral aspect of the femoral shaft to 6 cm distal to the base of the trochanter. At this point the deep investing fascia of the thigh is visualized. Beginning in the distal aspect of the incision the iliotibial band is split at a level below the greater trochanter. Blunt tipped scissors are used to carry the incision of the iliotibial band proximally to the inferior border of the tensor fascia lata. Blunt dissection at this level can be used to facilitate the exposure of the interval between the tensor fascia lata and the gluteus medius. The anterior border of the greater trochanter can be palpated and thus the anterior border of the gluteus medius is directly visualized. The transverse branch of the lateral femoral circumflex artery is then ligated at the junction of the greater trochanter with the anterior surface of the gluteus medius. The hip is maintained in 45° of flexion to facilitate relaxation of the anterolateral musculature. The hip capsule lies directly within this field, the gluteus medius is retracted posteriorly and, to increase exposure, the anterior fibers may be sectioned at their insertion on the greater trochanter, as suggested by Mueller.[41] The vastus lateralis may be elevated from the proximal femur and retracted distally and medially. The gluteus medius insertion may also be elevated with a piece of greater trochanter to allow bone to bone healing should more exposure of the lateral femoral neck be necessary.

Ollier[12] described an approach that used the trochanteric osteotomy to elevate the gluteus medius and minimus and to expose the lateral aspect of the hip joint as shown in Figure 3–5. Simply using the U-shaped incision does not allow exposure of the proximal femur but numerous variations have been described that allow a third limb of the incision to be created that proceeds distally along the lateral femur. The technique includes an incision at the anterior superior iliac spine that passes distally to the greater trochanter and then continues proximally in a posterior direction to end half way between the trochanter and the posterior superior iliac spine. The dissection is carried medially to the

greater trochanter where the interval between the tensor fascia lata and the gluteus medius is identified. The anterior and lateral aspects of the greater trochanter are defined and then separated with an osteotome to remove enblock the trochanter with the insertions of the gluteal muscles as well as the piriformis, gemelli, and obturator internus muscles. As the trochanter is elevated, the fibers of the gluteus maximus are separated in a longitudinal direction. The capsular branch of the medial femoral circumflex artery is present at the posterior border of the greater trochanteric fragment and is controlled by cautery.

Charnley's[9] lateral approach to the hip also is based on the interval between the gluteus medius and tensor fascia muscles. With a trochanteric osteotomy the fibers of the gluteus medius and minimus are kept intact and their length may be readjusted depending on the level of the trochanteric reattachment. Thus trochanteric osteotomy has the theoretical advantage that the mechanics of the hip joint may actually be improved after surgery by increasing the abductor moment arm. However, with any approach that requires trochanteric osteotomy there is the possible complication of trochanteric fibrous union, nonunion, or frank migration with complete loss of abductor function.

Charnley's approach begins with the patient in the supine position with a bump placed under the sacrum to allow posterior displacement of adipose tissue. The hip is flexed 45° and the greater trochanter is palpated. A point is chosen one-third of the distance between the anterior and posterior borders of the trochanter. The incision from this point proceeds 10 cm distally along the shaft of the femur and superiorly curves slightly posteriorly for a distance of 8 cm. The deep fascia is then identified and incision is made in the lateral fascia at the level of the mid trochanter and extended distally and then proximally over the greater trochanter (Fig. 3–6A). This maneuver is facilitated with the hip in slight abduction. The incision in the fascia is then curved posteriorly at 45° until the gluteus maximus muscle is encountered and is then split bluntly into the posterior aspect of the wound. The trochanteric bursa is then incised and the trochanteric notch is palpated posteriorly. Attention is then turned to the vastus lateralis where the adipose tissue is swept superiorly along the anterior aspect of the femur to expose the anterior margin of the gluteus medius (Fig. 3–6B). A retractor is placed anteriorly to elevate the tensor fascia lata and rectus femoris origins (Fig. 3–6C). The reflected head of the rectus as it inserts onto the anterior acetabulum and onto the hip capsule is then

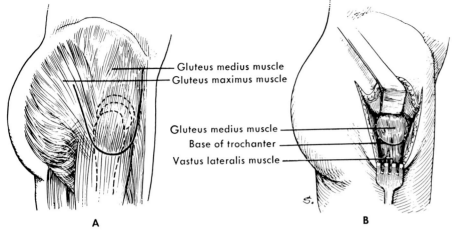

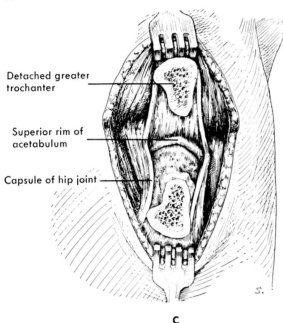

Gluteus medius muscle
Gluteus maximus muscle

Gluteus medius muscle
Base of trochanter
Vastus lateralis muscle

A

B

Detached greater
trochanter

Superior rim of
acetabulum

Capsule of hip joint

C

FIG. 3–5. The Ollier lateral U approach to the hip. **A.** Relation of skin incision to deep structures. **B.** Incision has been made and skin flap has been retracted. **C.** Greater trochanter has been osteotomized and retracted superiorly along with its muscle attachments. Joint capsule has been incised both anteriorly and posteriorly to expose the femoral neck and hip joint. (From Crenshaw AM: Campbell's Operative Orthopaedics. St. Louis, Mosby, 1963.)

sectioned allowing for complete exposure of the anterior capsule. Once anterior capsulectomy has been performed, the superior bony neck of the femur is palpated. Trochanteric osteotomy is performed with an osteotome or Gigli saw and is kept intracapsular to allow retraction of not only the gluteus medius and minimus muscles but also the entire lateral and superior capsule (Fig. 3–6D). Once the posterior capsule has been cut after elevation of the greater trochanter the hip may be dislocated and total hip replacement can then be accomplished (Fig. 3–6E).

The most critical aspect of this approach includes reattachment of the greater trochanter. The bony bed on the proximal femur must be preserved and it is also critical that the trochanteric fragment be approximated so that a maximal surface area exists for healing between the femur and greater trochanter. If distal advancement is possible, then the

vastus lateralis must be elevated from the proximal femur so that muscle fibers do not interpose between the healing bony fragments.

In 1967 Harris[20] described a lateral approach for the hip that allows for extensive mobilization of the proximal femur with dislocation in both an anterior and a posterior direction. The patient is placed with the hip elevated roughly 60° from the scapula to the sacrum using a long roll, sandbags, or a blanket. An incision is made 5 cm posterior and slightly proximal to the anterior superior spine and is curved distally and posteriorly to the posterior superior corner of the greater trochanter and then is extended longitudinally for 8 cm. The iliotibial band is divided beginning distally in the line with the skin incision (Fig. 3–7A). The insertion of the gluteus maximus tendon on the gluteal tuberosity is palpated and the incision continues one finger breadth anterior to this insertion. The

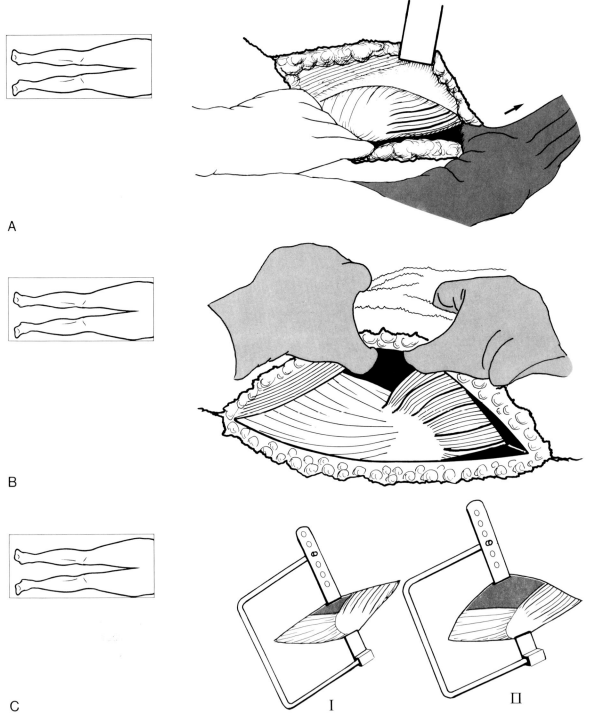

Fig. 3–6. A. Incision to the deep fascia-proximal extension. Access in the headward direction is completed by splitting the muscle fibers of the gluteus maximus with the thumb. **B.** Exposure of the gluteus medius. To complete the blunt stripping of the anterior margin of the gluteus medius both thumbs are now inserted under the anterior edge of the deep fascia as in the diagram. **C.** Initial retraction. Figure I shows how restricted the exposure of the front of the neck of the femur can be if incision in the fascia is straight and centered over the trochanter. Figure II shows how the curved incision in the fascia lata, convex anteriorly centered anterior to the trochanter makes for easy access to the front of the neck of the femur.

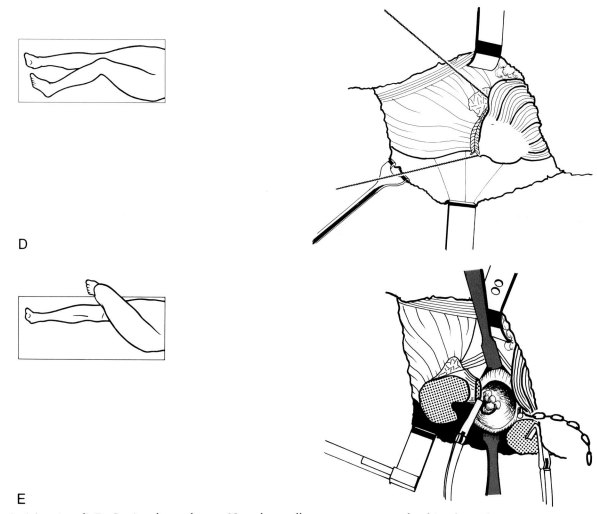

D

E

Fɪɢ. 3–6 *(continued)*. **D.** Cutting the trochanter. Note the small retractor to protect the skin edges. The surgeon must operate the Gigli saw slowly and watch the advance of the anterior and posterior ends alternatively at each traction stroke. The Gigli saw must emerge through the middle of the vastus lateralis ridge. **E.** Hohman retractors. The anterior and posterior lips of the acetabulum are exposed with Hohman retractors, which take a purchase on bone and reveal the acetabulum. (From Charnley J: Low Friction Arthroplasty of the Hip: Theory and Practice. New York, Springer-Verlag, 1979.)

incision in the fascia lata proceeds proximally in line with the skin incision thus exposing the gluteus medius. The fascia lata is incised posteriorly to obtain wide exposure of the external rotators (Fig. 3–7B). A periosteal elevator is now placed along the anterior capsule to the acetabulum and utilizing a blunt retractor, the iliotibial band and tensor fascia lata are retracted anteriorly. Attention is then turned to the femur where the origin of the vastus lateralis is reflected distally using sharp dissection and the abductor muscles are isolated by placing an instrument between the abductors and the superior surface of the joint capsule (Fig. 3–7C). Osteotomy is performed with a Gigli saw and with the greater trochanter and gluteus medius and minimus elevated the entire superior aspect of the joint capsule is visualized. With internal rotation of the hip the external rotators are visualized and incised

at their insertion on the proximal femur (Fig. 3–7D). At this point a complete anterior, superior, and posterior capsulectomy may be performed under direct vision. With anterior dislocation of the femoral head utilizing extension, adduction, and external rotation, the anterior femur may be well visualized. Adduction, flexion, and internal rotation will dislocate the femoral head posteriorly allowing excellent visualization of the entire acetabulum (Fig. 3–7E,F).

In 1954 McFarland and Osborne[35] made the observation that the gluteus medius muscle and vastus lateralis muscles are in functional continuity through a thick periosteum that covers the greater trochanter. They were able to sharply incise the trochanteric fascia such that the greater trochanter could be separated in a sagittal manner from the overlying gluteus medius-vastus lateralis complex.

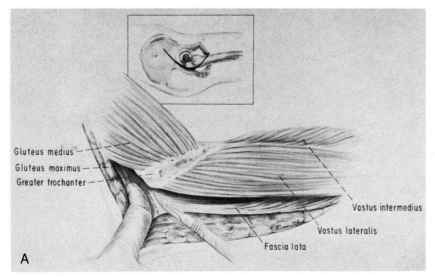

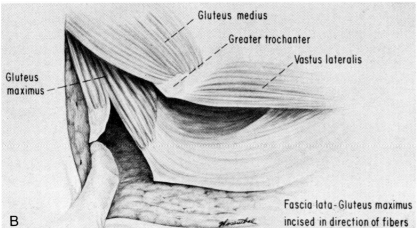

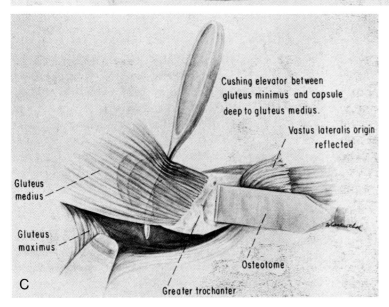

Fig. 3-7. The lateral approach of Harris. A. The insert shows the relationship of the lateral incision to the anterior superior iliac spine and posterior border of the greater trochanter. A parallel U-shaped incision is made in the fascia lata to expose the vastus lateralis and gluteus medius. Exposure of the short external rotator muscles in the posterior portion of the hip capsule remains restricted by that portion of the fascia lata posterior to the incision. B. Once the fascia has been incised, the area posterior to the greater trochanter becomes available to inspect the posterior portion of the capsule's short external rotators and also provide space for posterior dislocation of the femoral head if necessary. C. The direction of the osteotomy of the greater trochanter is defined by passing an elevator from anterior to posterior deep to the gluteus medius and minimus, along the superior aspect of the capsule.

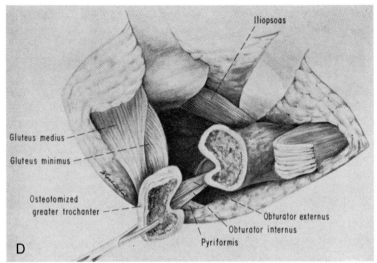

D

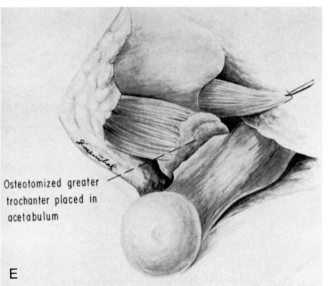

E

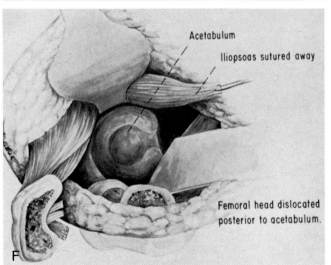

F

Fig. 3–7 *(continued)*. **D.** After osteotomy the greater trochanter is reflected superiorly putting the short external rotators on stretch. After they have been divided, the posterior portion of the capsule can be incised at the posterior rim of the acetabulum under direct vision. **E.** The femoral head is brought into full view by anterior dislocation of the hip in extension, adduction, and external rotation. **F.** Wide exposure of the acetabulum is thus achieved by posterior dislocation of the femoral head into the space provided by incision of the gluteus maximus. (From Harris WH: A new lateral approach to the hip joint. J Bone Joint Surg, 49A:891, 1967.)

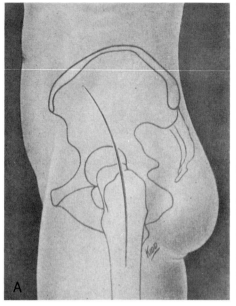

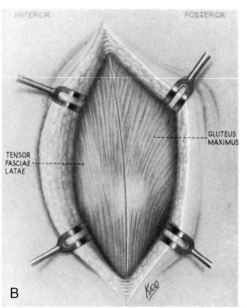

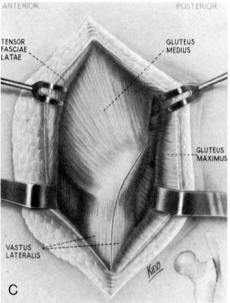

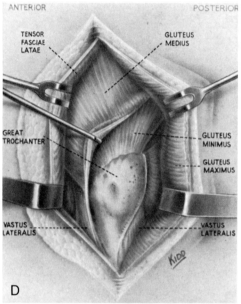

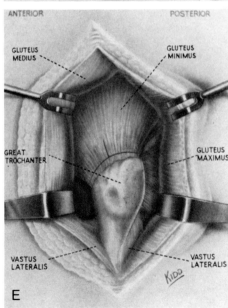

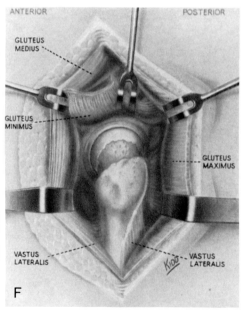

FIG. 3-8. The lateral approach to the hip of McFarland and Osborne. A. The skin incision. B. Incision of the fascia lata between the tensor fascia lata and the gluteus maximus. C. Incision at the posterior margin of the gluteus medius and vastus lateralis, showing the line at which loosening of periosteum of the trochanter begins. D. Anterior displacement of the gluteus medius and vastus lateralis in continuity. E. Gluteus minimus revealed with a line for the division of its tendon. F. Hip joint revealed with neck and upper shaft of the femur. (From McFarland B, Osborne, G: Approach to the hip: a suggested improvement on Kocher's method. J Bone Joint Surg 36: 364, 1954.)

Their approach involved a midline incision centered over the greater trochanter (Fig. 3–8A). The gluteal fascia and iliotibial band are divided in a straight mid lateral line parallel to the skin incision over the mid portion of the trochanter (Fig. 3–8B). The gluteus maximus may then be retracted posteriorly and the tensor fascia retracted anteriorly. The gluteus medius is bluntly dissected from the piriformis and gluteus minimus tendons. At the posterior border of the gluteus medius, where it joins the posterior edge of the greater trochanter, an incision is made down to bone through the periosteum and fascia obliquely (Fig. 3–8C). The incision is carried distally along the anterior greater trochanter to the trochanteric ridge and continued in the substance of the vastus lateralis for approximately 5 cm. From this incision down to bone the vastus lateralis and gluteus medius are elevated subperiosteally from

the greater trochanter and lateral femur. Great care is taken that the continuity between the gluteus medius and the vastus lateralis is maintained (Fig. 3–8D). The entire muscle mass is then retracted anteriorly exposing the gluteus minimus, which is then sectioned to expose the hip capsule. A capsulotomy or capsulectomy may be performed as indicated (Fig. 3–8E,F).

At the time of closure, the gluteus minimus and capsule are sutured as one structure with hip in abduction and slight extension. In this position the gluteus medius and vastus lateralis can be returned to their original position.

Two variations of this approach have been described. McLauchlin[37] used a similar skin incision and fascial incision with exposure of the greater trochanter, gluteus medius, and vastus lateralis (Fig. 3–9A). The gluteus medius is split in the line

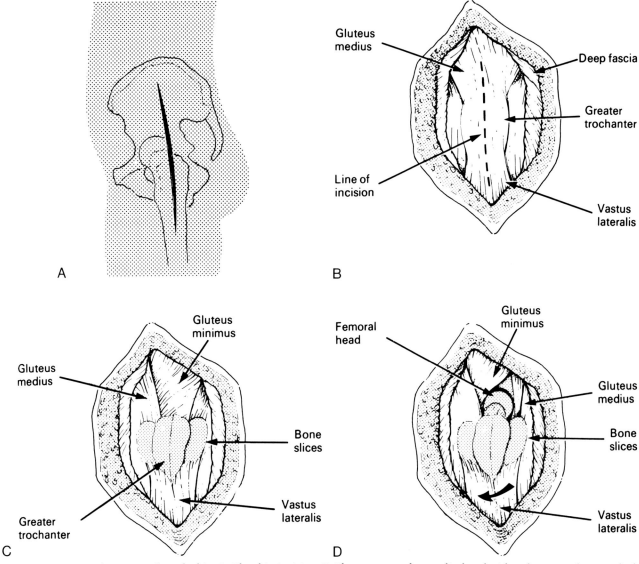

Fig. 3–9. The Stracathro approach to the hip. **A.** The skin incision. **B.** The greater trochanter displayed with a gluteus medius attached proximally and vastus lateralis distally. **C.** Slices of the trochanter with gluteus medius attached proximally and vastus lateralis distally. Retraction reveals the gluteus minimus. **D.** The hip is dislocated anteriorly with flexion in lateral rotation. (From McLauchlin J: The Stracathro approach to the hip. J Bone Joint Surg, 66B:30–31, 1984.)

of its fibers and an osteotome is used to elevate two rectangular slices of greater trochanter, one anterior and one posterior (Fig. 3–9B). Both slices of greater trochanter have gluteus medius attached proximally and vastus lateralis attached distally forming two separate bands with a continuum of muscle and fascia. The anterior band is retracted anteriorly and the posterior band is retracted posteriorly to reveal the gluteus minimus, which is usually detached from the greater trochanter (Fig. 3–9C). A capsulectomy may be performed with dislocation of the hip anteriorly with flexion and external rotation (Fig. 3–9D). At the time of closure the trochanteric slices are wired to one another and, because the continuity of the gluteus medius and vastus lateralis has not been interrupted, union is said to occur without difficulty.

Hardinge[19] described a variation of the McFarland approach. Instead of taking the entire gluteus medius muscle, a split is developed in the gluteus medius superior to the greater trochanter. The posterior fibers are not elevated from the greater trochanter but the anterior vastus lateralis in continuum with the anterior and superior fibers of the gluteus medius are elevated sharply from the greater trochanter and femoral neck. A cuff of gluteus medius tendon is left at the insertion on the greater trochanter to allow ease of reattachment (Fig. 3–10).

Posterolateral Approaches to the Hip

The definition of posterior lateral approach to the hip includes a dissection plan that is posterior to the muscles of the adductor mechanism innervated by the superior gluteal nerve. Langenbeck[28] and Kocher[12] are traditionally credited with the first description of this approach and subsequent modifications have been advanced by numerous authors. The advantage of the technique is that the abductor mechanism is not disturbed because the origin, the insertion, and the muscle bellies of the gluteus medius or minimus are not disturbed.

The common indications for the posterior approach are total hip replacement, endoprostheses of the proximal femur, open reduction of posterior hip dislocations, posterior joint arthrotomy for sepsis, and the open reduction and fixation of posterior acetabular fractures.

The limitations of the posterior approach include the necessity for using the lateral decubitus position. The ability to determine the exact position of the pelvis is limited compared to approaches that

allow the patient to be in the supine position. The patient's body is less intrinsically stable so that more supports are required to maintain a true lateral of the torso as well as the pelvis. In the lateral position it is more difficult to maintain equalization of leg length with total hip arthroplasty. The unaffected limb is placed in slight flexion for stability and thus leg lengths cannot be checked during the operation.

One possible complication of the posterior approach is injury to the sciatic nerve, which is directly in the field, as compared to the lateral and anterior approaches. Usually a cuff of external rotators is placed over the sciatic nerve after the external rotators have been sectioned from the proximal femur. Great care must be taken that the sciatic nerve is not injured during surgery through the posterior approach.

Most of the posterolateral skin incisions follow the line of the femur distally from the greater trochanter for a variable distance of 4 to 10 cm. Above the level of the greater trochanter the Gibson[17] approach recommends a 30 to 45° limb that proceeds to a point just anterior to the posterior superior iliac spine (Fig. 3–11A). The classic Kocher-Langenbeck incision has its proximal limb in a direction to a point at, or just inferior to, the posterior superior iliac spine. The Moore[38] approach includes an incision that begins 10 cm distal to the posterior iliac spine and extends laterally parallel to the fibers of the gluteus maximus to the posterior margin of the greater trochanter and then extends distally parallel to the femoral shaft. Once the subcutaneous tissue has been divided, the gluteus maximus is exposed. The gluteus maximus musculature is then split bluntly at the level of the hip joint and the fascia lata is then split distally down the femur (Fig. 3–11B).

With hip flexion and internal rotation the anterior gluteus maximus can be retracted anteriorly with the rest of the fascia lata. Retraction of the posterior aspect of the gluteus maximus exposes the sciatic nerve and external rotators as well as the posterior border of the gluteus medius. At this point, Gibson's approach recommends dividing the gluteus medius and minimus muscles at their insertion but leaving the insertion of the external rotators (Fig. 3–11C). With retraction of these muscles anteriorly the joint capsule is now exposed and a capsulotomy may be performed, followed by dislocation by flexing and externally rotating the thigh.

The more common technique after blunt dissection of the gluteus maximus has been described by

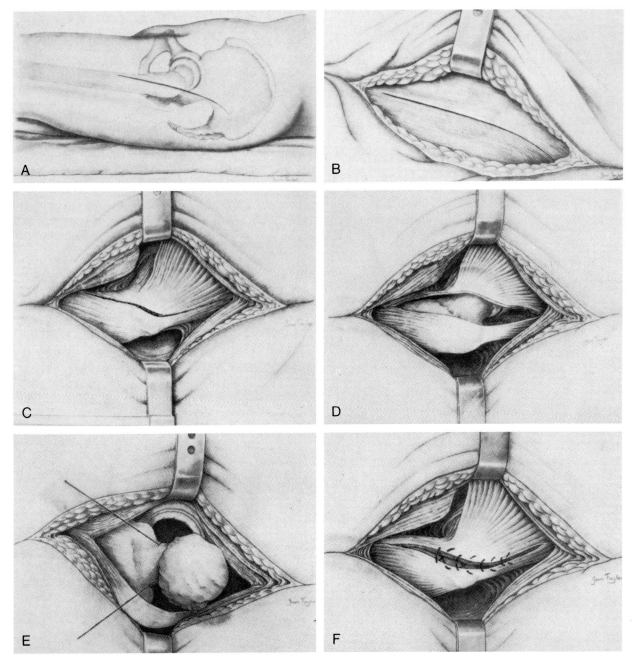

Fɪɢ. 3–10. The direct lateral approach to the hip by Hardinge. **A.** The skin incision is parallel to the femur distally curving posteriorly with the greater trochanter at its midpoint. **B.** Incision of the fascia lata in line with the skin incision. **C.** Incision of the tendon of the gluteus medius leaves a cuff of tendon attached to the greater trochanter to facilitate closure and early function. **D.** Adduction of the thigh causes the anterior half of the gluteus medius to swing forward to reveal the gluteus minimus. **E.** The neck of the femur can be divided with a Gigli saw because the axis of the neck and shaft of the femur are anterior to the apex of the trochanter and the main mass of the gluteus medius is undisturbed. **F.** Closure of the gluteus medius tendon allows early mobilization with partial weight-bearing. (From Hardinge K: The direct lateral approach to the hip. J Bone Joint Surg, 64B:17, 1982.)

Osborne[44] and Moore.[38] Instead of sectioning the gluteus medius and minimus, the external rotators along with the piriformis tendon, superior and inferior gemella, and obturator internus are dissected sharply from their insertion on the posterior femur (Fig. 3–12A,B). The superior half of the quadratus femoris may also have to be incised if exposure is necessary. Great care must be taken that the branches of the medial femoral circumflex artery are cauterized at the superior border of the quadratus femoris muscle. The piriformis tendon may be tagged at this point for future reattachment at the

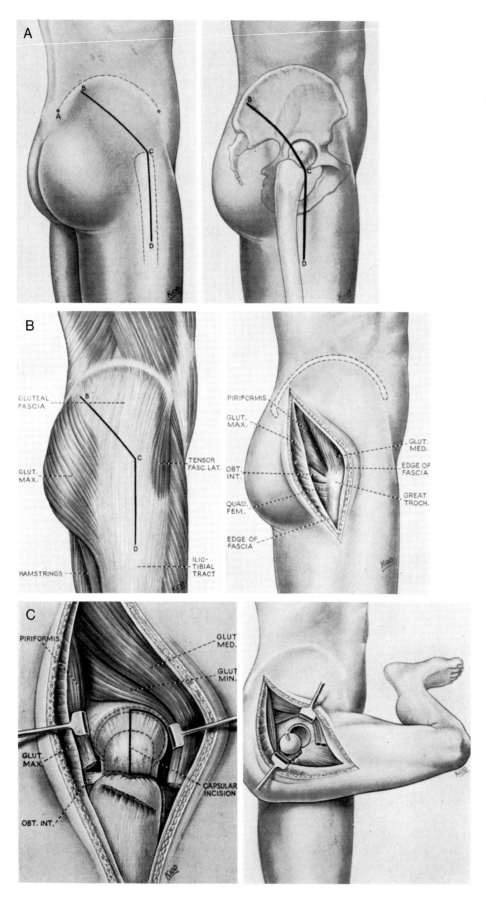

FIG. 3–11. The Gibson posterior exposure of the hip joint. **A.** The skin incision is made along the shaft of the femur to the tip of the greater trochanter and then posteriorly to a point just anterior to the posterior superior iliac spine. **B.** The gluteal fascia is divided in the same line as the skin incision and the whole mass of gluteus maximus with its aponeurotic prolongation is retracted posteriorly, exposing the short external rotators attached to the greater trochanter. **C.** The capsule of the hip joint is incised and reflected anteriorly by detaching it from the margin of the acetabulum and base of the neck. Dislocation is accomplished by flexion, adduction, and external rotation of the limb. (From Gibson A: Posterior exposure of the hip. J Bone Joint Surg, 32:183, 1950.)

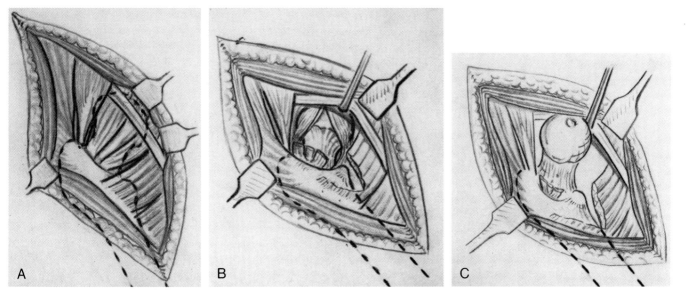

Fig. 3–12. The Moore posterior approach to the hip joint. A. Retraction of the gluteus maximus and tensor fascia reveal the external rotators and gluteus medius lying just posterior to the hip joint. B. After sectioning of the short external rotators the sciatic nerve is retracted medially and the hip capsule is opened with a T-shaped incision. C. Dislocation of the hip is carried out with internal rotation. Occasionally the gluteus maximus insertion must be incised to allow adequate room for dislocation. (Moore AT: The self-locking metal hip prosthesis. J Bone Joint Surg, 39A:811, 1957.)

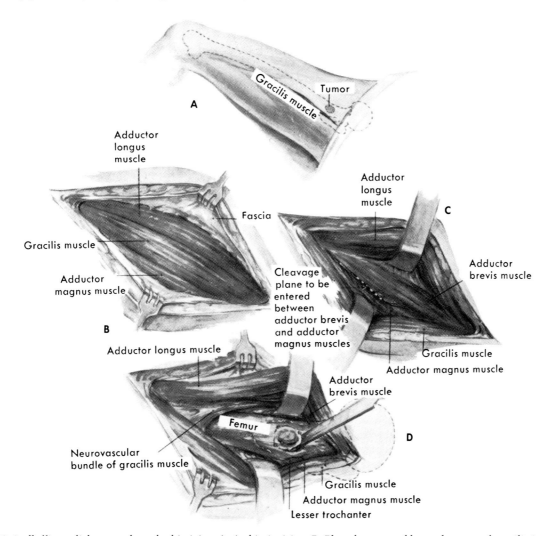

Fig. 3–13. Ludloff's medial approach to the hip joint. A. A skin incision. B. Plane between adductor longus and gracilis is to be developed. C. Adductor longus has been retracted anteriorly and the gracilis and adductor magnus posteriorly. D. Lesser trochanter has been exposed. (From Crenshaw AM: Campbell's Operative Orthopaedics. St. Louis, Mosby, 1963.)

end of the surgery. The most common position of the sciatic nerve is that it passes anterior to the piriformis muscle but posterior to the rest of the external rotators. Thus, with retraction of the external rotators, these muscles can be wrapped posteriorly around the sciatic nerve to protect it. A retractor is then placed between the gluteus minimus and the hip capsule and the entire lateral and posterior aspects of the hip capsule are visualized. Capsulectomy, or more commonly a T-shaped posterior capsulotomy, may be performed as indicated. Should greater exposure be required, a trochanteric osteotomy may be added to this approach to facilitate more anterior exposure. Dislocation of the hip is performed with flexion, internal rotation and adduction (Fig. 3–12C).

Henry[23] has described a variation on the posterior approach that includes a posterior dissection of the sciatic nerve.

Medial Approaches to the Hip

The medial approach to the hip was first described by Ludoff[33] in 1913 and was designed primarily to treat congenital dysplasia of the hip in the pediatric age group. The other possible indications for this approach include release of the psoas tendon, obturator neurectomies, biopsies of the medial femur and lesser trochanter, and adduction contracture releases of the hip. The greatest limitation of this approach is the inability of the surgeon to obtain an extensile exposure.

The technique requires the patient to be placed supine with the hip flexed, abducted and externally rotated. A longitudinal incision is made along the medial aspect of the thigh beginning 2 to 3 cm distal from the pubic tubercle at the lateral margin of the adductor longus muscle (Fig. 3–13). The intermuscular plane between the gracilis and adductor longus is then palpated and dissected bluntly. The adductor longus and subsequently the adductor brevis are retracted anteriorly, whereas the adductor magnus and gracilis are retracted posteriorly. The gracilis muscle is innervated by the anterior division of the obturator nerve, which runs just posterior to the adductor brevis muscle. Great care must be taken that this neurovascular bundle is not avulsed from the gracilis muscle as the interval is deepened. The innervation of the adductor magnus is from the posterior division of the obturator nerve as well as the tibial portion of the sciatic nerve. Between the adductor brevis and the adductor magnus the lesser trochanter and medial hip capsule is palpated.

References

1. ALLISON N: Arthrotomy of the hip. Surg Gynecol Obstet, 47:375, 1928.
2. AUFRANC OE: Constructive Surgery of the Hip. St. Louis, Mosby, 1962.
3. BANKS SW, LAUFMAN H: An Atlas of Surgical Exposures of the Extremities. Philadelphia, Saunders, 1968.
4. BOST FC, SCHOTTSTAEDT ER, LARSEN LJ: Surgical approaches to the hip joint. Am Acad Orthop Surg Lect, 11:131, 1954.
5. BOYD HB: Anatomic disarticulation of the hip. Surg Gynecol Obstet, 84:346, 1947.
6. BRACKETT E: A study of the different approaches to the hip joint, with special reference to the operations for curved trochanteric osteotomy and for arthrodesis. Boston Med Surg J, 166:235, 1912.
7. BURWELL, HN, SCOTT D: A lateral intermuscular approach to the hip joint. J Bone Joint Surg, 36B:104, 1954.
8. CAPENER N: The approach to the hip joint (editorial), J Bone Joint Surg 32-B:147, 1950.
9. CHARNLEY J: Low Friction Arthroplasty of the Hip: Theory and Practice. New York, Springer-Verlag, 1979.
10. COLONNA PC: The trochanteric reconstruction operation for ununited fractures of the upper end of the femur. J Bone Joint Surg, 42B:5, 1960.
11. COX HT: The cleavage lines of the skin. Br J Surg, 24:234, 1942.
12. CRENSHAW AM: Campbell's Operative Orthopaedics. St. Louis, Mosby, 1963.
13. CUBBINS WR, CALLAHAN JJ, SCUDERI CS: Fractures of the neck of the femur, open operation and pathologic observations: new incisions and new director for use of simplified flange. Surg Gynecol Obstet 68:87, 1939.
14. ETIENNE E, LAPEYRIE M, CAMPO A: The route of internal access to the hip joint. Int. Abstr. Surg., 84:276, 1947.
15. FAHEY JJ: Surgical approaches to bone and joints. Surg Clin North Am 29:65, 1949.
16. DE FRENELLE D: La voie d'acces anterieure de l'articulation de la hanche (Anterior "U" iliofemoral incision). Par Chirurg 16:1, 1924.
17. GIBSON A: Posterior exposure of the hip joint. J Bone Joint Surg, 32-B:183, 1950.
18. GIBSON A: Vitallium cup arthroplasty of the hip joint. J Bone Joint Surg, 31-A:861, 1949.
19. HARDINGE K: The direct lateral approach to the hip. J Bone Joint Surg, 64B:17, 1982.
20. HARRIS WH: A new lateral approach to the hip joint. J Bone Joint Surg, 49A:891, 1967.
21. HARRIS WH: Extensive exposure of the hip joint. Clin Orthop, 91:58, 1973.
22. HARTY M, JOYCE JJ: Surgical approaches to hip and femur. J Bone Joint Surg, 45A:175, 1963.
23. HENRY AK: Extensile Exposure. Edinburgh, Livingstone, 1966.
24. HOROWITZ T: The posterolateral approach in the surgical management of basilar neck, intertrochanteric and subtrochanteric fractures of the femur. Surg Gynecol Obstet, 95:45, 1952.
25. IYER KM: A new posterior approach to the hip joint. Injury 13:76, 1981.
26. JERGESEN F, ABBOTT LC.: A comprehensive exposure of the hip joint. J Bone Joint Surg, 37-A:798, 1955.
27. KAPLAN EB: The blood vessels of the gluteal region. Bull Hosp Joint Dis, 7:165, 1946.
28. VON LANGENBECK B: Ueber die Schussverletzungen des Huftgelenks. Arch Klin Chir, 16:263, 1874.

29. LETOURNEL E, JUDET R: Fractures of the Acetabulum. New York, Springer-Verlag, pp. 242–243, 1981.

30. LIPSCOMB PR: A comparison of the Gibson posterolateral and Smith-Petersen iliofemoral approaches to the hip for Vitallium mold arthroplasty. Am J Surg, 87:4, 1954.

31. LUCK JV: An approach for hip construction: broad visualization without osteotomy of the greater trochanter. Clin Orthop, 91:70, 1973.

32. LUCK VC: A transverse anterior approach to the hip. J Bone Joint Surg, 37A:534, 1955.

33. LUDLOFF K: The open reduction of the congenital hip dislocation and anterior incision. Am J Orthop Surg, 10:438, 1913.

34. MARCY GH, FLETCHER RS: Modification of the posterolateral approach to the hip for insertion of femoral-head prosthesis. J Bone Joint Surg, 36-A:142, 1954.

35. McFARLAND B, OSBORNE G: Approach to the hip: a suggested improvement on Kocher's method. J Bone Joint Surg, 36-B:364, 1954.

36. McGEE GK: Development of total prosthetic replacement of the hip. Clin Orthop, 72:85, 1970.

37. McLAUCHLAN J: The Stracathro approach to the hip. J Bone Joint Surg, 66B:30–31, 1984.

38. MOORE AT: The self-locking metal hip prosthesis. J Bone Joint Surg, 39A:811, 1957.

39. MOORE AT: The Moore self-locking Vitallium prosthesis in fresh femoral neck fractures. Am Acad Orthop Surg Lect, 16:309, 1959.

40. MOSLEY HF: An Atlas of Musculoskeletal Exposures. Philadelphia, Lippincott, 1955.

41. MÜLLER ME: Total hip prosthesis. Clin Orthop, 72:46, 1970.

42. NICOLA T: Atlas of Orthopaedic Exposures. Baltimore, Williams & Wilkins, 1966.

43. OBER FR: Posterior arthrotomy of the hip joint. JAMA 83:1500, 1924.

44. OSBORNE RP: The approach to the hip-joint: a critical review and a suggested new route. Br J Surg, 18:49, 1930–1931.

45. SMITH-PETERSEN MN: A new supra-articular subperiosteal approach to the hip joint. Am J Orthop Surg, 15:592, 1917.

46. SMITH-PETERSEN MN: Approach to and exposure of the hip joint for mold arthroplasty. J Bone Joint Surg, 31A:40, 1949.

47. SUTHERLAND R, ROWE MJ Jr.: Simplified surgical approach to the hip. Arch Surg, 48:144, 1944.

48. THOMPSON JEM: The Jan Zahradnicek surgical approach to the problem of congenital hip dislocation. Clin Orthop, 8:237, 1956.

49. TRONZO RG: Surgery of the hip joint. New York, Springer-Verlag, 1984.

50. VOSMER AM, VAN LINGE B: Surgical exposure of the lesser trochanter and the medial proximal part of the femur. Acta Orthop Scand, 47:214, 1976.

51. WATSON-JONES R: Fractures of the neck of the femur, Br J Surg, 23:787, 1935–1936.

52. ZAZEPEN S, GAMIDOV E: Tumors of the lesser trochanter and their operative management. Am Dig Foreign Orthop Lit Fourth quarter, p. 191, 1972.

PART II

Pediatrics

CHAPTER FOUR

Congenital Dislocation of the Hip

WILLIAM McCLUSKEY
WILLIAM P. BUNNELL

Introduction

Idiopathic congenital dislocation of the hip (CDH) at birth represents a spectrum of clinical and radiographic pathologic conditions ranging from acetabular dysplasia to a frank, irreducible dislocation. The essential thrust of modern management of CDH has been early diagnosis through neonatal screening and effective treatment with avoidance of iatrogenic complications such as ischemic necrosis of the femoral head. Unfortunately, neonatal screening and early orthotic treatment have not solved all the problems related to CDH. Dislocations still are diagnosed late, either because they were missed on the infantile examinations or because they are true late dislocations of a preluxation hip. Complications such as avascular necrosis and physeal arrests still occur, although with a decreased incidence. The goal of management of CDH should be a hip that will function normally for that patient's lifetime. This means achieving a concentric reduction and avoiding secondary deformities. It is these secondary deformities, either of the femoral head or of persisting acetabular dysplasia, even if relatively mild, that may predispose to early degenerative joint disease.

Terminology

There are three types of dislocated hips identified in neonates. The *idiopathic dislocated hip* (Fig. 4–1A–C) occurs at or near the time of birth, has no secondary adaptive changes, and usually reduces easily with orthotic treatment. The *neuromuscular dislocated hip* often reduces easily but, because of muscle imbalance, redislocates easily. With a *teratologic dislocation* (Fig. 4–1D), secondary soft tissue and bony changes are already present at birth. This type of dislocation often cannot be reduced by an Ortolani maneuver.

The word "dysplasia" refers to abnormal growth or development about the hip. This could be a primary acetabular dysplasia intrinsic to the developing cartilaginous anlage of the acetabulum. The defect also could be a secondary adaptive response to the abnormal position and pressures of the dislocated femoral head. The working definition of acetabular dysplasia is radiographic. There is a greater than normal slope of the superior osseous portion of the acetabulum. This radiographic description, however, does not indicate whether the unossified cartilaginous model is deformed. The term "dysplasia" does not indicate instability or necessarily an intrinsic abnormality. In some cases, however, it may indicate a "preluxation" state, which would predispose the hip to dislocate at a later date. Persistence of this increased slope into adulthood also may predispose the hip to early degenerative joint disease.

The term "dysplasia" often is used to describe the delayed or irregular ossification of the ossific nucleus of the femoral head in subluxated or dislocated hips. Again, dysplasia does not indicate any degree of instability and does not define any pathologic process other than the ossification asymmetry.

In a newborn with a dislocated hip, the femoral head is completely displaced from the acetabulum. If it can be reduced, an active reduction is required. An irreducible dislocated hip often is referred to as an "Ortolani-negative hip" because this maneuver fails to reduce the hip. When the femoral head is in the acetabulum with the hip at rest but can be completely displaced with a provocative maneuver, it is termed "dislocatable." When the leg is released, the femoral head usually reduces spontaneously. The "subluxatable" hip is reduced at rest, but with a provocative maneuver, the femoral head can be displaced significantly, although not completely, from the acetabulum. This is the most difficult condition to detect clinically. It often is referred to as an "unstable hip;" however, this is a vague term that does not indicate the degree of in-

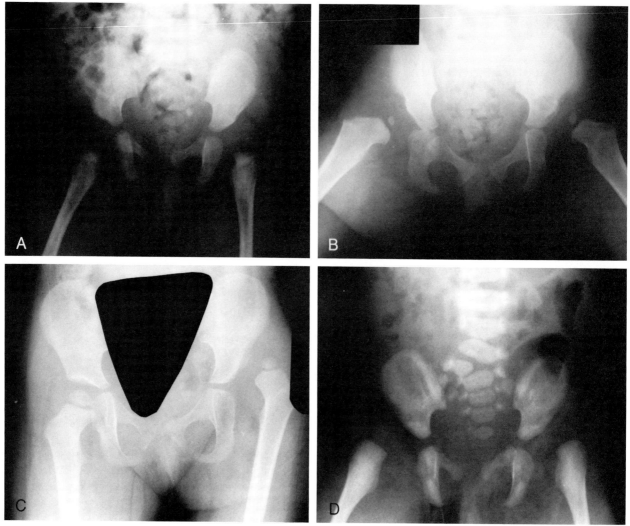

FIG. 4-1. Four examples of dislocated hips. **A.** Newborn with hip displaced laterally, without superior migration, on the left. **B.** Older infant with bilateral dislocations, dysplastic acetabula, and delayed appearance of the femoral ossific nuclei. **C.** Older child with a displaced left hip with established acetabular dysplasia. **D.** Newborn with bilateral teratologic dislocations. Note the spine and sacral abnormalities.

stability. By definition, clinically apparent CDH must have some degree of laxity or instability.

Two useful categories are used in retrospective studies. The "intermediate hip" was defined by Ramsey and associates[88] to denote an irreducible dislocation that reduces spontaneously after the passage of time in a Pavlik harness. Another term has been used to describe the hip that has been diagnosed at an advanced age. The term applied exhibits the bias of the user in regard to the cause of the dislocation. It is called a "late dislocation"[15,45] or a "missed dislocation."[44,45,73] The term "failed infantile CDH"[122] has been used to describe those juvenile unstable hips that had been treated in infancy but had inadequate followup. Some are dislocated, although most are subluxated or show evidence of avascular necrosis.

Incidence

Figures based on recent studies of the prevalence of newborn hip instability show that the condition occurs in 5.9 to 21.8 of every 1000 infants. A mean figure of 11.7 of every 1000 infants is acceptable, with subluxatable hips occurring in 9.2 of every 1000 infants, dislocatable hips occurring in 1.2 of every 1000 infants, and dislocated hips occurring in 1.3 of every 1000 infants.[64] Roughly 1 of every 85 newborns will have an instability. Seventy-five percent of neonatal CDH is unilateral. The left hip is involved in 60% of cases, the right hip in 20%, and both hips in 20%. In most series, the infant female-to-male ratio ranges between 4:1 and 8:1. Dislocation is distinctly uncommon in blacks. All of the dislocations show a tendency to be laterally and superiorly displaced. The literature is divided on whether the neonatal hip is predominantly anteriorly or posteriorly unstable. Theoretically, capsular laxity with femoral anteversion and hip extension should combine to subluxate the head anteriorly. The provocative tests for instability are biased toward detecting the posteriorly unstable hip, even though there may be a global instability caused by capsular laxity. The late dislocated or persistently displaced hip is displaced predominantly posteriorly, and neonatal splinting (in a Pavlik harness with femoral external rotation) provides a position of stability for posterior dislocations.

Breech presentation is associated with 20% of all dislocations. The risk group identified consists of first-born girls with a breech presentation. In an Alfred I. duPont Institute study of 25,000 newborns,[64] this group showed a true dislocation in 1 out of every 35 births. Other associations are also noted. Twenty percent of children with torticollis and 1.5% of children with metatarsus adductus also have an abnormal hip.

Natural History

The natural history of the unreduced congenitally dislocated hip is largely anecdotal, with few series being reported.[20,71,115] Minimal disability is reported, especially when the dislocation is bilateral. In Wedge and Wasylenko's series of 42 dislocated hips in patients 16 to 86 years old,[115] some functional impairment was seen in every patient, although 40% were pain free. Only 1 of the 18 patients in Crawford and Slovek's study had hip pain.[20] Most patients had an unstable Trendelenburg gait. Those with only a unilateral dislocation had a more severe disability, with a hip adduction contracture, a short leg, and ipsilateral genu valgum with a high incidence of gonarthrosis. Only 13 of the 42 dislocated hips developed osteoarthritis, and 10 of these were rated poor. (Only 19 of the total group of 42 hips were poor.) The development of osteoarthritis was more common in those with a well developed false acetabulum.[115] The incidence of disability from back pain was the same as that in the general population. It is unclear at what age a completely dislocated hip becomes symptomatic enough to present a functional disability beyond the baseline mechanical disadvantage. The demands placed on the hip influence the age of onset of symptoms. There are reports of asymptomatic unilateral dislocated hips with a contralateral sub-

luxated hip that had disabling osteoarthritis. Wedge and Wasylenko reported that although only 25% of dislocated hips showed degenerative changes; subluxated hips showed osteoarthritis more frequently.[115]

A subluxated femoral head is associated with dysplasia of the acetabulum. This is a clinical observation, with causality being momentarily irrelevant. Acetabular dysplasia and hip subluxation have been blamed for 20 to 48% of the incidence of adult coxarthrosis.[19,40,102,120] The mean age for the appearance of significant degenerative changes is 55 years. Many patients with coxarthrosis and dysplasia have dysplasia in the opposite asymptomatic hip.[102] Given this population, we must identify uniquely three entities, so that their natural histories may be followed. These are: Group 1—primary acetabular dysplasia without subluxation; Group 2—acetabular dysplasia with a subluxated hip, and Group 3—dysplasia (Group 1) with subluxation secondary to coxarthrosis and not directly related to the dysplasia. Groups 2 and 3 cannot be distinguished radiographically with certainty, so that the contribution of Group 1 to the problem is probably underestimated.

Wiberg,[120] Cooperman and coworkers,[19] and Stulberg and Harris[102] looked at the association between coxarthrosis and dysplasia, with and without subluxation. Wiberg[120] showed that the age of onset of radiographic and clinical degenerative disease correlated with the severity of the dysplasia, as measured by a decrease in the center-edge (CE) angle. The subluxated hips were the most dysplastic and had the lowest CE angles, and all had onset of degeneration by the age of 42 years. Cooperman and colleagues[19] reported on hips without subluxation but with CE angles less than 20°. Although only 4 of 32 hips had significant arthritis in the fourth and fifth decades, only 2 hips had no significant arthritis at the final followup in the seventh and eighth decades. It would appear that dysplasia alone, especially in women, predisposes to coxarthrosis. The severity of the dysplasia, however, did not correlate directly with the rate of arthritic progression.

Wedge and Wasylenko[115] define three peaks in the onset of complaints: at skeletal maturity, after pregnancy, and at menopause, depending on the severity of subluxation. The mean age was 35 years in female patients and 55 years in male patients. Initially, the symptoms were postexertional aching and fatigue. Clinical symptoms precede radiographic changes by approximately 5 years and significant radiographic signs of coxarthrosis by 10 to

15 years. Although only 42% of subluxated hips and 41% of dislocated hips were rated as good in Wedge and Wasylenko's series, the subluxation group was younger and had a more rapid worsening of symptoms.

It is important to compare the results of reduction of CDH with the expected natural history. Long-term followup studies (greater than 40 years) are lacking, and those available utilized techniques of reduction from 40 years ago. Severin[95] reported on 448 hips reduced in children greater than 1 year old. All initially were termed "successful," although on followup all had radiographic abnormalities. Ponseti[84] reviewed patients treated between 1940 and 1968 and found only 3 with complaints of pain (2 had residual subluxation and 3 had deformed femoral heads). The only generalization to be made is that there is a poor correlation between the clinical examination at maturity and the eventual outcome. The Severin grade radiographically at maturity (a measure of femoral head deformity, subluxation, and arthritis) had the closest correlation with the eventual outcome.

Because the expected incidence of persisting dislocation in an unscreened population is about 1 per every 1000 infants (1.5 to 1.7 per 1000[6]), all abnormally lax hips diagnosed at neonatal screening are not destined to be adult dislocated hips. The incidence of lax hips on neonatal examination is from 10 to 20 times greater than expected (28.7 per 1000[21]). When discussing the natural history of lax hips, part of the difficulty is the reliability of the diagnosis. Interobserver reliability in the clinical diagnosis of dislocated or dislocatable hips, by provocative tests such as the Ortolani and Barlow maneuvers in the neonatal period, is good among experienced examiners and on repeat examination by the same observer. Barlow[6] found a spontaneous recovery rate of 58% in the first week and 88% within 2 months in those patients with dislocated or dislocatable hips. Tredwell and Bell[110] and Fredensborg and Nilsson[30] also found a spontaneous recovery rate of 80 to 90%. Because approximately 5 to 10 of every 1000 infants are diagnosed as having lax hips at birth, the 10% persistent instability rate correlates well with expected numbers. The natural history of the labrum and acetabular index is discussed later in the chapter.

For subluxatable hips, however, the clinical diagnosis is unreliable, with interobserver reliability approaching random occurrence. If a subluxatable hip cannot be diagnosed with certainty, its natural history cannot be followed. With the advent of ultrasonography, the asymptomatic dysplastic hip and the subluxatable hip have been identified and can be quantified, but a natural history has not been reported yet. Gross and associates[34] have reported that in their series of patients suspected of having subluxatable hips and left untreated, no patient progressed to a late diagnosed acetabular dysplasia (increased acetabular index and frank subluxation at a later date). The subluxatable hip in CDH appeared to be a normal variant with no predisposition to acetabular dysplasia and dislocation.

To be successful, neonatal hip screening should show some effect on the natural history of the unstable hip. If neonatal screening is foolproof and the neonatal unstable hip is the same disease process as the late diagnosed hip (diagnosed after 1 year of age), the screening program should eliminate the late diagnosis of CDH. The early studies of Finlay and colleagues[27] and Palmen[80] eliminated the late diagnosis of CDH. Paterson[81] reported a decrease in the incidence of CDH diagnosed in children older than 18 months from 1.2 per every 1000 children to 0.2 per every 1000 children with screening. Lehmann and Street[61] reported a decrease in late diagnosis (over 1 month old) from 1.4 per every 1000 children to 0.3 per every 1000 children for senior staff diagnoses and 0.8 per every 1000 children for resident diagnoses. In Tredwell and Bell's study,[110] only one case of CDH was missed in 32,000 infants screened.

Some studies have reported an increased incidence in the late diagnosis of CDH. In one Norwegian study,[10] the incidence of "missed" CDH was 2 per every 1000 infants. Barlow[5] reported a late diagnosis rate of 0.18 per every 1000 infants, and MacKenzie and Wilson[65] cited a rate of 1.11 per every 1000 infants despite screening. (See Table 4–1 for missed and incidence rates.) In these studies, the late or missed dislocation rate approximated the dislocation rate expected in unscreened populations. Barlow's[6] concept of the natural history of an unstable hip consists of the following: (1) All hips at risk can be diagnosed clinically at birth. (2) There is no "preluxation hip" (a hip with a normal clinical examination that will subluxate progressively because of acetabular dysplasia). And (3), approximately 12% of unstable hips at birth will persist without treatment. If one assumes that Barlow's concept is correct, either these results are due to poor or ineffective (ineffective in technique or frequency in the first year of life) screening examinations in which clinical signs that are present are missed, or they are a result of ineffective treatment that allows diagnosed lax hips to proceed to dislocation.

The natural history of acetabular dysplasia ("preluxation hip") as a cause of late dislocation is pre-

TABLE 4–1. *Incidence of Early and Late Diagnosis of CDH*

Author(s)	Location	Population Size	Number Unstable Per 1000 Births*	Number Diagnosed Late Per 1000 Births†
von Rosen (1960)[112]	Sweden	31,200	2.18	0
Palmen (1961)[80]	Sweden	12,394	5.6	0
Barlow (1962)[6]	England	9,289	14.9	0
Barlow (1966)[5]	England	19,625	18.2	0.18
Finlay et al (1967)[27]	England	14,594	4.1	0.07
von Rosen (1968)[113]	Sweden	24,000	1.7	0.04
Hiertonn and James (1968)[43]	Sweden	11,868	19.0	0.42
Mitchell (1972)[73]	Scotland	31,961	7.1	0.13
Wilkinson (1972)[121]	England	6,272	5.9	1.3
Williamson (1972)[124]	Ireland	~300,000	2.6	0.63
Bjerkreim and Van Der Hagen (1974)[10]	Norway	NR	7.0	2.0
Artz (1975)[3]	USA	23,408	13.3	0.3
Fredensborg and Nilsson (1976)[30]	Sweden	58,759	9.3	0.07
Paterson (1976)[81]	Australia	7,409	5.5	0.26
Dunn (1976)[25]	England	23,002	19.3	0.44
Jones (1977)[48]	England	29,366	2.6	0.58
Noble et al (1978)[77]	England	25,921	10.4	0.15
Ponseti (1978)[84]	USA	51,359	1.4	0.07
Galasko et al (1980)[32]	England	11,980	14.9	0.83
Monk and Dowd (1980)[74]	England	25,263	11.0	0.16
Lehmann and Street (1981)[61]	Canada	16,045	6.0	0.3
MacKenzie and Wilson (1981)[65]	Scotland	53,033	28.4	1.11
Tredwell and Bell (1981)[110]	Canada	32,480	9.8	0.03
McKinnon et al (1984)[70]	USA	15,149	9.7	0.13
Heikkila (1984)[41]	Finland	151,924	6.8	0.85
Bialik et al (1986)[9]	Israel	12,891	5.9	2.8

NR = not reported.

*The exact definition of instability is not uniform in the literature. See reference for details.

†A uniform definition of "late" diagnosis could not be applied to the data in the literature. "Late" implies a diagnosis beyond 1 month of age in some reports and in other reports is applied only to those over 1 year old. See reference for details.

dominantly anecdotal. It is presumed that the hip is reduced at birth, but because of the dysplastic, shallow acetabulum, there is a progressive subluxation. With activity and weight-bearing, the hip should progress to frank dislocation. Some late-diagnosed CDH has been blamed on acetabular dysplasia, yet this natural history has not been well documented radiographically. Of 10 late-diagnosed cases reviewed by Ilfeld and Westin,[45] only 1 case with a dislocated right hip found at 6 months of age had neonatal radiographs that were not misinterpreted. These showed a normal hip without evidence of acetabular dysplasia. Davies and Walker,[24] however, followed radiographically 10 children with normal neonatal examinations who were believed to be at risk (neonatal hip click, breech presentation, positive family history). All 10 hips showed signs of developing acetabular dysplasia, with an increased acetabular index but without subluxation. Four of these hips progressed to frank

dislocation. Because acetabular dysplasia in its earliest phases is not clinically apparent, and established dysplasia with dislocation or subluxation cannot be classified with certainty to be primary or secondary in origin, this question cannot be answered without a mass radiographic or ultrasound screening program testing children from birth through walking age.

The natural history can be summarized as follows: (1) The disease CDH is present from the perinatal period, although it may not be clinically apparent on the neonatal examination. (2) About 10% of dislocatable and dislocated hips will have persisting dislocation unless treated. (3) Subluxatable hips are probably a variation of normal, without predisposition to acetabular dysplasia or dislocation (unless other environmental factors intervene). And (4), it is unclear whether some late dislocations may be caused by a primary acetabular dysplasia. If this mechanism does occur, the incidence is certainly less than the rate required to account for all the late-diagnosed hips (up to 10% of all CDH[45]).

Etiology of CDH

Most congenital dislocations occur during the perinatal period. The predisposition to proceed to a frank dislocation is caused by interaction between environmental and genetic factors. The genetic factor has been demonstrated in studies dealing with racial predilection, twin studies, and family studies. Racial studies suggest a genetic linkage, although cultural patterns probably also contribute to interracial differences (for example, swaddling an infant to a cradle board). Twin studies have shown that in monozygotic twins, the incidence of CDH (in the second twin) is 34% to 50%. If this were strictly a result of the mechanical factor of restricting two fetuses in the same uterus, dizygotic twins should show a similar risk. Although the risk is greater than that expected in singletons, it is only 3%, much less than the concordance rate seen in monozygotic twins.

Familial studies also show an increased risk within families, with the incidence of CDH in siblings ranging from 2.2% to 14%. The female sex preference among siblings is still preserved, although the risk is slightly higher if the proband is male. The risk for the total population is 2 per every 1000 children, whereas that for first-born female is 1 per every 150 children and that for breech presentation is 1 per every 15 children. If one sibling has CDH, the risk is about 6 per every 100 children. If one parent has CDH, the risk is 12 per every 100 children (6% for male children and 17% for female children). If one parent and one sibling are affected, the risk increases to 36 per every 100 children.[125]

The mechanism of the genetic contribution to CDH has two components. There is a primary acetabular dysplasia with a presumed polygenic inheritance, and joint laxity with a polygenic or monogenic autosomal dominant inheritance. Primary acetabular dysplasia in childhood is difficult to define precisely. The radiographic measurement of the acetabular index has a broad normal range, with a measurement greater than 30° generally considered abnormal. Graf[33] has better defined the dysplastic acetabulum with ultrasound. Patients with radiographically increased acetabular indices have two different soft tissue anatomies on ultrasound. Some have a well developed cartilaginous labrum with delayed or immature ossification. The second group has a defective, inadequate labrum that is

dysplastic. It is the second group that appears to be at greater risk of dislocation. Wynne-Davies[126] and Czeizel and associates[22] have noted that parents of children with CDH have more shallow acetabula than normal. Wynne-Davies[126] divided the dislocated hips into "joint laxity type" and "acetabular dysplasia type," suggesting that the late-diagnosed CDH corresponded to the latter type. Czeizel and colleagues[22] found that the age at diagnosis in the two proposed types did not differ, suggesting that neonatal and late-diagnosed CDH are not distinct entities. The extent to which acetabular dysplasia is influenced by joint laxity in childhood is unknown, although there appears to be an association in Czeizel and coworkers' study. At a more practical level, in cases of unilateral dislocated hips in which the opposite acetabulum is dysplastic, this bilateral process correlates with a poor response to treatment of the dislocated hip.

Joint laxity has three proposed components: a physiologic (hormonal) laxity, an exaggerated physiologic laxity, and a familial, autosomal dominant joint laxity based on connective tissue structure. All of the components are presumed to be genetically controlled. The hormonally induced laxity is temporary and has a female predominance. It is assumed that once out of the maternal environment, the laxity would disappear. This theory would account well for the spontaneous resolution of joint laxity seen in the first postpartum weeks. The familial joint laxity, however, is persistent and affects both sexes.

The three hormones responsible for relaxation, directly or indirectly, are estrogen, progesterone, and relaxin. Human and animal studies have shown that an estrogen-primed uterus will produce relaxin in response to progesterone. The relaxation is not confined to the pelvic ligaments—hip capsule laxity also can be seen in female animal models. In fact, Wilkinson[123] used estrogen- and progesterone-conditioned animals and lateral rotation splinting (breech posture with knees extended) to produce posterior hip dislocations in adult female rabbits.

Because relaxin and estrogen production is more prominent in the female fetus, because relaxin affects ligament laxity more in females than in males, and because "femaleness" is a genetic trait, it would appear that a definite genetic link had been found. Episodes of familial CDH could be a result of an inherited defect of hepatic estrogen metabolism (accounting somewhat for Navajo and South Tyrol racial predilections). Andren and Borglin[2] found increased urinary estrone and 17 beta-estradiol in patients with CDH. Thieme and associates[105] found increased blood hormone levels in CDH patients. Most other studies do not confirm any statistically significant differences.[1] Whatever the details may be, the hormonal environment is established to produce a temporary laxity in the late second to third trimester, when mechanical forces are coming into play.

Persistent joint laxity (benign hypermobility syndrome) in children was initially described in 1920.[63] Although familial laxity as a part of a generalized collagen disorder is known (Ehlers-Danlos syndrome, Marfan's syndrome, homocystinuria), it also can be seen as an isolated phenomenon. It occurs in male and female children and has an autosomal dominant inheritance pattern. Although the degree of joint laxity is difficult to quantitate precisely, it has been shown that exaggerated generalized laxity is seen in 5 to 7% of normal schoolchildren.[16,47] In patients with CDH, 75% of the male children had a generalized laxity, and 33% of the female children had this laxity. Of 100 consecutive patients with familial hypermobility, 6 had a history of treated CDH.[28] In addition to simple joint laxity, a more severe laxity with multiple dislocated joints exists but is rare.

Jensen and colleagues[46] looked at the collagen content of umbilical cords of children with radiographically confirmed CDH. Total content was reduced and the Type 3 to Type 1 ratio was higher than normal, similar to ratios seen in osteogenesis imperfecta or Type 4 Ehlers-Danlos syndrome. In normal fetal development, there is a redistribution of collagen types that appears to be delayed in association with CDH. The results have not been confirmed by others. It is clear clinically, however, that boys with unilateral and especially bilateral dislocations do not respond well to treatment and may represent a forme fruste of a collagen disorder.

Mechanical and environmental factors exert influence in the last trimester and the early postnatal period. The clinical observations regarding breech presentation, left hip predominance, and the "molded baby syndrome" suggest a role for mechanical factors working to restrict space for the fetus and fetal motion. In teratologic dislocations, the fetal motion is restricted by the neuromuscular deficit, which makes these mechanical factors the more important cause of dislocation. Much of the data on the role of abnormal fetal positioning comes from work with arthrogryposis and the myelodysplasias.

In normal fetal development,[122] the initial fetal posture is one of a "frank" breech presentation, with hips flexed, knees extended, and thighs rotated slightly laterally. At 26 to 32 weeks, the nor-

mal folding of the fetus should occur as knee flexor and hip external rotation power increases. If the folding mechanism does not occur, the legs are held in the extended breech position, which prevents spontaneous cephalic version from occurring. The final position is one of hip flexion, thigh medial rotation, knee flexion, and often a calcaneus foot position. The persisting fetal malposition, which causes an arrest in development at the first or second stage and thus causes the breech presentation, is also responsible for hip dislocation.

The malposition may be caused by maternal anatomic factors. Sixty percent of the patients with CDH are firstborns, which means their mothers had relatively tight uterine and abdominal muscles. There is also an association with oligohydramnios and twinning. With restricted space available in the uterus, normal fetal movement (kicking) and limb folding are inhibited. The arrest also may be caused by a physiologic delay, such as a delay in neurologic development; however, there is no direct evidence for this in CDH.

Of the two types of breech presentation (Fig. 4–2), frank breech presentation with extended knees and medially rotated thighs (Stage 1 arrest) is uncommon. In this mechanism, the child is born with dislocated or hyperextended knees. The medial rotation of the hip theoretically confers some stability to the hip, producing a hip dislocation in only about 17% of cases.[122]

As explained by Wilkinson,[122] the more common position is one of incomplete knee flexion with the hip flexed and the thigh laterally (externally) rotated. Full flexion of the hip will direct the subluxation forces posteriorly when the thigh is laterally rotated. These abnormal pressures would retard the

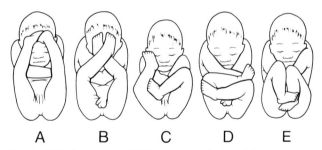

FIG. 4–2. Birth postures. **A.** Hips are acutely flexed, knees are extended, and thighs are internally rotated. **B.** Hips are acutely flexed, knees are extended, and thighs are externally rotated. **C,D.** Incomplete folding; knees are flexed and thighs are externally rotated. **E.** Hips are fully flexed, normal posture. Positions A, B, C, and D account for 65% of breech births and 80% of all congenital hip dislocations. (Adapted from Wilkinson JA: A post-natal survey for congenital displacement of the hip. J Bone Joint Surg 54B:40–49, 1972. *In* Tonnis D: Congenital Dysplasia and Dislocation of the Hip in Children and Adults. New York, Springer-Verlag, 1987.)

growth of the femoral head and would stretch the posterior capsule. The dislocation forces are further enhanced by an adduction moment on the flexed thigh. Many breech presentations tend to lie with the left thigh held against the maternal sacrum. This could help account for the left side predominance of CDH (55% had CDH on the left side, 20% had CDH on the right side, and 25% had bilateral CDH). The molded baby syndrome with torticollis, plagiocephaly, and metatarsus adductus would be further manifestations of the fetal malposition. Wilkinson successfuly produced hip dislocations in a rabbit model using rotational positioning and hormone-induced laxity.[128]

Salter and colleagues[92] also have shown in a pig model that forced hip extension can promote hip dislocation. Prenatally, the hip cannot be extended in the uterus. However, extension, especially in combination with hip adduction postnatally, is the position assumed by a swaddled infant or one wrapped to a cradle board. A child with hips flexed and abducted, as seen in an unbound infant in the prone position, is the more physiologic position. It is unclear whether the extended position promoted acetabular dysplasia; however, the flexed and abducted position seems to promote normal acetabular development. The contribution of weight-bearing to problems caused by the extended hip is also unclear, although theoretically, by increasing the forces across the hip, it should promote dislocation.

Pathologic Anatomy of CDH

Although several etiologic factors are suspected of contributing to dislocation of the hip, the typical congenital dislocation is essentially idiopathic. This is convenient because it distinguishes the idiopathic form from the teratogenic form, which usually has a more severely distorted anatomy. The time of onset of the dislocation or the predisposing factors influence the degree of laxity and the severity of the pathologic changes. In the typical congenital dislocation, the predisposing factors are active in the last trimester, with the dislocation occurring either prior to birth or in the first postpartum months. The anatomic changes are subtle and reversible. In the teratologic hip, the pathologic condition is usually more severe. Dislocation takes place early in fetal life, which allows time for adaptive changes in both the femur and the acetabulum by the time birth occurs. The abnormal muscles also are a more significant deforming force than in idiopathic CDH.

Normal development of the hip and acetabulum shows a progressive series of changes after approximately 8 weeks, when the hip joint forms by cleavage. Early in fetal life, the acetabulum is a deep cavity that totally encloses the femoral head. In the normal hip, the bony acetabulum progressively provides less coverage, with superior coverage being provided more by the fibrocartilaginous labrum. At birth, the true acetabular depth is small but thereafter increases as the labrum ossifies. During fetal development, the acetabulum becomes progressively more anteverted, until it reaches approximately 10° at birth. During the first half of fetal life, the femur is retroverted to a variable degree. By birth, the femur is anteverted an average of 35°, decreasing to approximately 12° at maturity. Whether the femur is anteverted or retroverted at birth depends on the torsional forces on the hip prenatally. The fully flexed cephalic presentation of the infant holds the hips in internal rotation during the last trimester. The internal rotation force on the flexed hip acts to place an anteversion force on the hip. In the lateral rotation breech posture, the thighs are externally rotated and locked in this position for the last trimester. With flexion, there is a retroverting force on the hip. Wilkinson[122] has shown that these children have retroverted femoral heads as predicted. If the posterior capsule fails to act as a restraining force, these lateral breech hips will dislocate but will not be as retroverted. It is significant that some stable hips may be retroverted, because although both anteverted and retroverted hips are neonatally less stable in forced extension, the anteverted hip is more stable in internal rotation, and the retroverted hip is more unstable in internal rotation.

The subluxatable hip (Fig. 4–3A,B) is essentially normal. Ponseti,[83,84] Stanisavljevic and Mitchell,[100] and Ogden[79] have seen minimal changes. The acetabulum may be mildly elliptical in shape. The femoral neck is anteverted, but the femoral head is normal. There may be some contracture of the anterior capsule. There will be some posterior capsular laxity or redundancy. The labrum may show delayed ossification. If the head is eccentric, it can be concentrically reduced easily by flexion and abduction.

With a more pronounced subluxation and with chronicity (Fig. 4–3C), the anatomic changes become worse. The femoral neck shows increased anteversion, and the head loses its sphericity, usually with some posteromedial or posteroinferior flattening. The posterior capsule is further distended and lax, with increasing contracture of the anterior capsule. As the head subluxates, the fibrocartilaginous

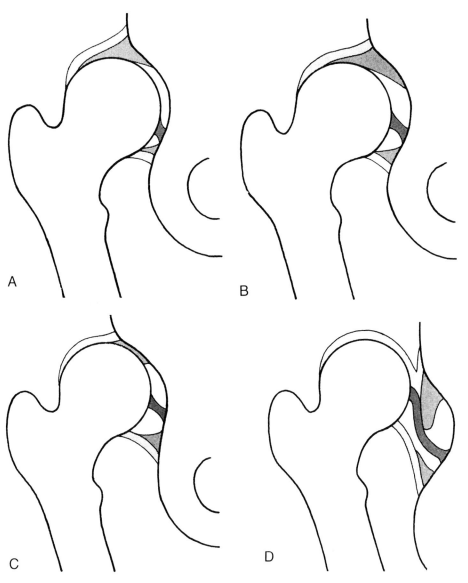

Fɪɢ. 4–3. **A.** Normal hip. **B.** Subluxatable hip. There is little deformity. The labrum is distorted posterosuperiorly. **C.** Subluxated hip. The labrum and the acetabulum are more deformed. The femoral head is subluxated, with the inferior capsule and transverse acetabular ligament distorted. **D.** Dislocated hip. The femoral head has dislocated out of the acetabulum. The labrum is inverted and hypertrophied, and the acetabulum is shallow. (From Tonnis D: Congenital Dysplasia and Dislocation of the Hip in Children and Adults. New York, Springer-Verlag, 1987.)

labrum is everted superiorly. The margin between the labrum and the hyaline cartilage of the acetabulum becomes the site for hypertrophy of the fibrocartilage to form the "inverted limbus." The "inverted limbus" is probably not an acute, inverting process caused by attempts at early reduction by abduction before proper length is regained, as some have suggested. Although on a rare occasion this mechanism may apply, in the majority of cases the inversion is the result of a slow process of plastic deformation of the labral fibrocartilage and remodeling of the superolateral acetabular margin (pseudolimbus). In the subluxated hip, the limbus does not obstruct reduction, although when the hip is reduced, there is some incongruity not seen in the less severely affected hip.

The normal development of the acetabulum depends on the normal femoral head being contained within it as a stimulus for growth. With the head subluxated, the acetabulum is shallow. The posteriorly displaced femoral head erodes the posterior acetabular margin, forming an elliptical, relatively more retroverted acetabulum. Anteriorly, because of adduction contractures, the lesser trochanter and femoral metaphysis are held apposed to the anterior acetabular rim, causing erosion and a relative anterior acetabular deficiency. In general, the more severe the subluxation and the more chronic the process, the more advanced the secondary femoral and acetabular changes.

In the completely dislocated hip (Fig. 4–3D), the pathology covers a broad spectrum of severity. Although more severe than the subluxated hip, the nonteratologic dislocated hip at birth usually has few or no irreversible changes. Most of the secondary changes occur with chronicity. There is posterior capsular redundancy and anterior capsular contracture. Initially, there is no muscle contracture. Later, adduction or flexion contracture is common. The head tends to be more aspheric, with posteromedial flattening. Femoral anteversion may be severe (greater than 90°) and often is accompanied by valgus deformity of the femoral neck. This, however, is not always seen, as demonstrated by Ogden,[79] who found that the dislocated head in a false acetabulum showed only 20° of anteversion.

The femoral head is usually small and shows a delay in ossification of the nucleus. As the head migrates more superiorly, the labrum is further everted, and the discrete limbus develops by deformation and hypertrophy. The ligamentum capitis femoris (ligamentum teres) elongates and hypertrophies. The inferior margin of the acetabulum is pulled superiorly across the inferior quadrant of the acetabulum. This structure includes the fibrocartilaginous transverse acetabular ligament. The entrance to the acetabulum is then restricted superiorly by the limbus and inferiorly by the capsule and transverse acetabular ligament. The acetabular depth itself is occupied by the pulvinar, a fibrofatty tissue. The entrance to the acetabulum may be compromised further by a superiorly displaced iliopsoas tendon indenting the anteroinferior capsule.

Many of the secondary acetabular changes seen in the subluxated hip are now more prominent. The anterior acetabulum is further eroded, and the posterior acetabulum is more deficient. The superolateral acetabular margin has remodeled, with the acetabulum assuming a shallow, elongated form. Often, the acetabulum may appear slightly anteverted because of the severity of the anterior acetabular deformity. With time, the ligamentum teres may attenuate, or it may hypertrophy and even erode a notch in the femoral head.

The false acetabulum is a structure of variable anatomic distinction. The capsule and labrum are everted by the dislocated head and pushed against the ilium. Then secondary osseous remodeling of the ilium and secondary metaplasia of the fibrocartilaginous labrum occurs, forming what is, at times, a very well defined anatomic structure.

As the psoas shifts superiorly, so, too, do the vascular structures. The medial circumflex artery has been reported to shift superiorly to a space between the psoas and the pubic ramus, where it is vulnerable to injury. The posteroinferior branches also may be at risk. Both may be difficult to dissect from the surrounding soft tissue.

To a variable extent, these pathologic changes can interfere with obtaining a concentric reduction by closed manipulation. Acetabular dysplasia and femoral anteversion do not impede reduction but influence the stability of the reduction. The soft tissues may impede reduction in the older child. The pulvinar and ligamentum teres and some capsular adhesions are soft obstructions that usually do not cause failure of reduction. Tightness of the iliopsoas muscle may impede reduction, but this could be stretched by traction. Assuming a dislocated Ortolani-negative hip has been converted into an Ortolani-positive hip, with the head being brought down to the level of the triradiate cartilage, those structures that may keep the hip seated laterally are the limbus and the inferior capsular structures (transverse acetabular ligament).

The inverted limbus and pseudolimbus (hyaline hypertrophy) superiorly and the transverse acetabular ligament inferiorly form a constriction (or hourglass deformity) at the introitus to the depths of the acetabulum. The iliopsoas also may contribute to the narrowing of the hourglass. The presence of these deformities does not make incision of the transverse ligament or limbusectomy imperative to achieve concentric reduction. If by closed reduction the head can be brought to the level of the triradiate cartilage, so that despite slight lateral displacement the head points centrally and is inferior to the limbus, the head is said to be "docked." After being held in this "docked" position for 2 to 4 months, the femoral head in the young child seats itself with a full concentric reduction, with either the limbus everting or the pseudolimbus remodeling. Arthrographically, the medial dye pool has resolved (Fig. 4–4). This occurrence requires the following vague criteria to be met: the child must be young enough that the limbus will remodel (through either persisting plasticity or growth potential in the acetabulum) and young enough that the inferior capsular structures are elastic enough to stretch and allow the head to be brought initially inferior to the limbus. The age limit appears to be approximately 3 to 4 years of age, although failures occur even well before that age. The main risk is avascular necrosis.

Once the head has been reduced, what becomes of the secondary adaptive changes seen in the femur and acetabulum? The femur has a natural reduction in anteversion until maturity. There is no evidence that this process is accelerated when an abnormally anteverted hip is held reduced. There is evidence that the acetabulum will remodel.[38,39,62,83] The greatest growth rate and the greatest potential for remodeling of the acetabulum are in the first 2 months of life, with significant remodeling possible to about 12 months. If the hip in

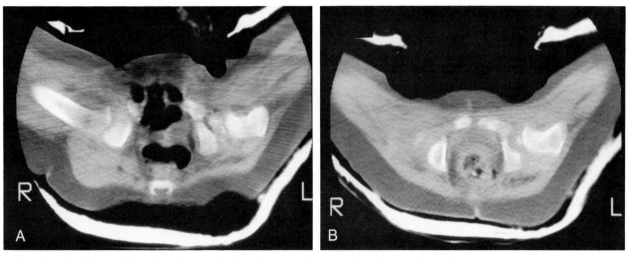

Fig. 4–4. A. Left dislocated hip after closed reduction. Computed tomography shows a "docked" hip, with slight lateral displacement of the femoral head. **B.** Two months later, the femoral head is completely reduced.

a young child with a dysplastic acetabulum is held in concentric reduction, there will be a progressive decrease in the acetabular index, continuing until the age of 8 years. Most of the remodeling occurs within the first 1 to 2 years after reduction. Although some investigators[90] believe that the remodeling potential past 18 months of age is insufficient to produce a normal-appearing hip, many others have stated that a reduction by the age of 4.5 to 5 years may allow for sufficient remodeling to achieve a normal hip. Even for those who advocated a higher age limit, the percentage of failure was higher in those hips reduced when older than 2 years and in those with avascular necrosis or persisting subluxation. In Lindstrom and coworkers' study,[62] 49.2% of the patients achieved an acetabular index less than 20° (normal) within 8 years of reduction. Staheli and associates[98] report that a limbusectomy does not affect acetabular development.

Diagnosis of CDH

The diagnosis of CDH neonatally is a clinical determination based on instability. Radiographs at birth are not indicated. A successful screening program relies on several examinations and as many modalities of examination as needed. The hip should be examined at birth (within 24 hours) and then at about 6 weeks of age, 3 months of age, 6 months of age, and around walking age. Radiographs become useful at approximately 6 to 12 weeks after birth, although teratologic dislocations and other early dislocations will be apparent earlier. Indications for imaging examination are clinical instability, limited abduction, or shortening of the leg. Imaging of all at-risk patients (female infants with breech presentation) does not appear necessary, although there are many reports of patients at risk without instability or other classic signs of dislocation but with radiographically very abnormal hips. Imaging is indicated in patients with persisting metatarsus adductus. If any neonatal imaging examination is equivocal, it should be repeated, with a radiograph obtained again at approximately 3 months or an ultrasound examination performed again in approximately 1 month. Followup of the older child is done most effectively with radiographs. If the hip is reduced, most of the pathologic condition is clinically silent and is apparent only on radiograph.

Who should screen for CDH is essentially a moot issue. The necessity for repeat examinations during the first year of life places the responsibility on the pediatricians who provide well-baby care. If only a single neonatal examination was needed, an experienced orthopedist could be used to provide good results, as in Barlow's initial work. Certainly, from Lehmann and Street's study,[61] it is clear that in screening there is a learning curve, with older, more experienced examiners, whether pediatricians or orthopedists, missing fewer abnormalities than residents and those with less training.

Examination of the Normal Child

The normal range of motion of the infant is different from that of the adult. Hass and colleagues[35] reported normal motion to be an average internal rotation of 62.9° (range, 35 to 100°), average external rotation of 89.1° (range, 45 to 110°), average abduction in flexion of 76.4° (range, 50 to 90°), and average flexion contracture of 27.9° (range, 10 to 75°). The normal range is influenced by the prenatal posture, with hip flexion and usually hip external rotation. About 50% of the children will show 90° of abduction, with most normal hips having greater than 60° of abduction. As the child grows, the hip abduction naturally decreases, so that by approximately 9 months, abduction is limited to approximately 60° from a birth value of 90°. At birth, abduction less than 60° is abnormal, and if less than 50°, it is almost certainly pathologic.

Stanisavljevic[99] reported on his hip-knee-hip triad, which he described as follows: In the normal infant who is 1 to 4 days old and did not have a breech presentation, hip extension is the most difficult position to achieve, followed by knee extension and hip abduction. If the hip abduction is the most difficult position to achieve, presumably be-

cause of iliopsoas overpull, the triad is abnormal, and there is a risk of subluxation.

Examination of the Hip for Instability

The diagnosis of CDH in the newborn is based on the clinical examination. The most reliable methods are those described by Barlow[6] (or variations of that method). For any of these tests, the infant must be lying quietly supine on a firm surface with the diaper removed and the pelvis stabilized.

The Ortolani examination (Fig. 4–5A–C) attempts to demonstrate a dislocation by the movement of the hip as the femoral head is reduced into the acetabulum. With one hand holding the pelvis, the examiner flexes the hip 90° and flexes the knee 90° or more, with the thumb of the examining hand on the medial aspect of the thigh and the index and

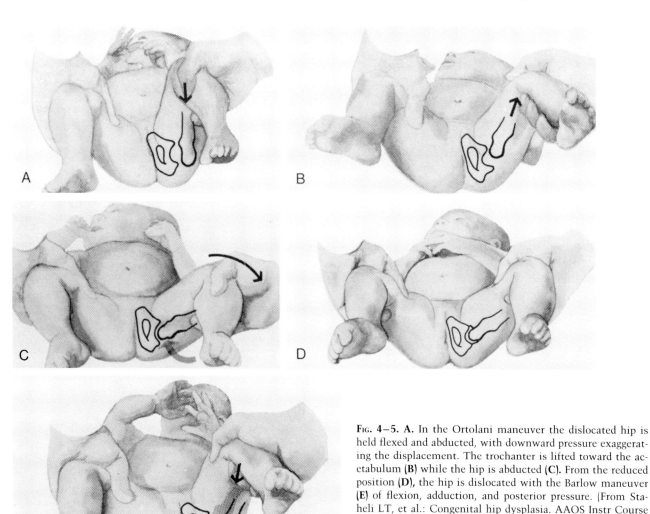

Fig. 4–5. **A.** In the Ortolani maneuver the dislocated hip is held flexed and abducted, with downward pressure exaggerating the displacement. The trochanter is lifted toward the acetabulum (**B**) while the hip is abducted (**C**). From the reduced position (**D**), the hip is dislocated with the Barlow maneuver (**E**) of flexion, adduction, and posterior pressure. (From Staheli LT, et al.: Congenital hip dysplasia. AAOS Instr Course Lect 33:350–363, 1984.)

middle fingers over the greater trochanter. The hip is gently abducted while the trochanter is lifted toward the acetabulum. If the maneuver is successful and the hip is reduced, there will be a proprioceptive sensation of the hip moving into the acetabulum. This may or may not be associated with a jerk, click, or snap. By adducting the thigh and applying pressure with the thumb medially, the hip then can be displaced again.

The positive Ortolani sign is reliable at birth as long as the examiner does not require a "jerk sign" to demonstrate dislocation. The originally described "jerk of reduction" is most common in late infancy, peaking at approximately 3 months of age. Ortolani believed it was not present at less than 3 months of age. In young children, there is usually only a sensation of movement and reduction. Many sharp palpable and audible clicks about the hip are ligamentous and myofascial in origin. After 3 months of age, the incidence of Ortolani-positive examination decreases as the secondary contractures progress. In the neonate, the extent of hip abduction is not helpful, because a reducible or irreducible hip (Ortolani-positive or -negative) can have full and symmetric hip abduction because of the capsular laxity.

The Barlow examination (or its variations by Palmen[80] and Coleman[18]) is a provocative test for dislocation. It is the Barlow maneuver that identifies the subluxatable neonatal hip, so that complete dislocation most often will not be demonstrated (Fig. 4–5D,E). The examiner again uses one hand to stabilize the pelvis, placing the fingers on the sacrum and the thumb on the symphysis pubis. The thumb of the examining hand is placed on the medial thigh, exerting pressure laterally with the hip flexed to 90°. The thigh can be held in slight abduction, adduction, or adduction with internal rotation, with some gentle pressure exerted posteriorly to dislocate the hip. In many cases, posterior pressure is not needed to dislocate the hip, because it is unstable in flexion and adduction alone.

The proprioceptive sensation produced by the Barlow test is one of movement of the femoral head posteriorly or laterally. A thumb over the groin or fingers placed posteriorly can be used to help locate the femoral head with respect to the acetabulum. The femoral head may be felt to dislocate completely from the acetabulum. Usually, the femoral head reduces spontaneously when the pressure is released, although when the capsule is lax, the head may remain in the dislocated position. The subluxatable hip allows displacement of the femoral head to the acetabular rim.

In some cases, the completely dislocated hip is neither Barlow- nor Ortolani-positive. The irreducible dislocated hip may show some movement in its dislocated position. If the hip is held as for an Ortolani maneuver, flexed 90° and abducted approximately 60°, and the thigh is alternately flexed and extended about 40°, the reduced hip will be felt to rotate in a fixed position in the acetabulum. The dislocated hip will be felt to displace up and down. The dislocated hip may demonstrate apparent femoral shortening, with uneven knee heights and asymmetric thigh folds (Allis test). The greater trochanter of the flexed hip may be felt to displace toward the examining table or may be felt to lie above Nelaton's line (a line drawn from the ischial tuberosity to the anterosuperior iliac spine). Ludloff's sign also may confirm the dislocation. The normal infant with a maximally flexed and abducted hip cannot extend the knee. The dislocated hip will displace in the soft tissues and allow the knee to extend.

The classic signs of limited abduction, thigh fold asymmetry, and femoral shortening usually are absent or not useful. Fifty percent of newborns show thigh asymmetry. Femoral shortening is reliable when present but unreliable in bilateral dislocations and in neonates with hip dislocations that show lateralization and no proximal migration. Limitation of abduction becomes more prominent as contractures progress. Although instability is common in infants younger than 1 month old (100%), limitation of abduction was reported in only 7% of the infants.[18] By 3 months of age, instability was reduced to 29%, and by 6 months of age, it was reduced to 15%, although limitation of abduction was a more common sign, increasing to 86% by 6 months of age. By 6 months of age, the dislocated hip has become stable in its position of dislocation. In fact, persistence of instability is believed to correlate with a poorer prognosis.

The pathoanatomy of CDH has an effect on signs seen clinically. The most common neonatal dislocations are Grade 1 or 2, which are lateral and minimally superiorly displaced. The reduction will be a subtle event without a jerk or clunk. Even in older children, the limbus or the other pathologic conditions that may obstruct reduction will make the reduction indistinct. A shallow acetabulum also may make the sensation of reduction muffled. The distinct clunk of reduction appears to be present in older children whose soft tissues offer more resistance to reduction and in those who do not have any obstructions to reduction. Occasionally, the child's voluntary muscle action is sufficient to stabilize a hip that is either reduced or dislocated and to obscure the pathologic process on clinical examination. Often, the Ortolani-negative hip becomes Ortolani-positive when guarding is abolished by anesthesia.

Other signs also can be seen. Although anterior thigh fold asymmetry is common and benign, gluteal fold asymmetry with apparent leg-length inequality and pelvic obliquity have been associated with abduction contracture and acetabular dysplasia. The buttock also may appear flattened with dislocation. The dislocated hip may be found to lie externally rotated and slightly flexed and abducted. In the neonatal period, the child may show signs of fetal molding, which would suggest a breech position. Plagiocephaly, metatarsus adductus (Fig. 4–6), calcaneovalgus foot deformity, torticollis, and scoliosis have been reported to be associated with CDH. If the newborn's legs are folded onto the chest, as allowed by contractures, the legs may be found to lie in an extended or breech position.

After walking age, there is usually a limp. If the dislocation is bilateral, the perineum will be wide and the trochanters prominent. About 20% of children with CDH do not walk before 18 months of age (in the normal population, only 5% of the children do not walk before 18 months of age). The gait may be waddling, with a marked lumbar lordosis. The Trendelenburg sign is usually positive in the older child.

Obviously, the physical examination and history must exclude other diagnoses. Infantile coxa vara will not be distinguishable clinically. Hip dislocation caused by trauma, sepsis, collagen disorders, and neurologic defects should be suggested clinically. Exstrophy of the bladder, prune belly syndrome, and skeletal dysplasias such as Larsen's syndrome also should not be overlooked.

Imaging Techniques in CDH

The radiographic changes seen with CDH are those that show displacement and secondary osseous changes. Because the femoral capital epiphysis is not ossified at birth, displacement must be measured indirectly. By 6 months after birth, 79% of normal hips have started to ossify, and by 7 months after birth, 90% of normal hips have a radiographically apparent ossification center. The dysplastic hip has delayed ossification, with the asymmetry of ossification being apparent. Before ossification of the nucleus, Hilgenreiner's measurements can be used (Fig. 4–7). Even in the neonate, however, these measurement can be inaccurate, especially the acetabular index, because the superior border of the acetabulum is indistinct. Perkin's line (P) is a variation on the "d" index of Hilgenreiner and is subject to the same limitations.

The classic radiographic changes are (1) a break in Shenton's line, (2) an increased acetabular index, (3) a shortened "h" and lengthened "d" in Hilgenreiner's method, (4) an ossific nucleus or medial metaphyseal beak lateral to Perkin's line, and (5) a displaced hip on von Rosen's view. Near birth, when the dislocation is often only a slight lateral displacement without superior migration, and before secondary bone changes have occurred, these signs may be absent. Shenton's line may not be broken. The acetabular index may be difficult to determine, although asymmetry of the acetabular index may be apparent. Using the published normal values for the acetabular index and Hilgenreiner's "h" and "d" indices is misleading because pelvic positioning may alter the radiographic topology. Side-to-side rotation may make one hip appear uncovered or have an abnormally high acetabular index. Anteroposterior pelvic rotation or tilt can alter the acetabular index so that the measurement is unreliable. This is especially true in newborns with hip flexion contractures, in whom extending the thighs to be parallel with x-ray plate causes an anterior pelvic tilt.

Positioning the patient can be difficult. Holding the hips extended and neutral, a position that should demonstrate the pathologic condition of the hip at its worst, can rotate the pelvis. The child can reduce the hip at times by contracting the pelvic muscles. This may occur when an infant is placed on a cold x-ray plate. If the child is allowed to lie

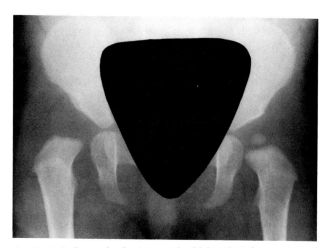

Fig. 4–6. Radiograph of a 12-month-old female infant evaluated for persisting metatarsus adductus. The hip examination was normal, without limitation of motion or instability. The appearance of the right femoral capital ossific nucleus is delayed, and acetabular dysplasia is evident.

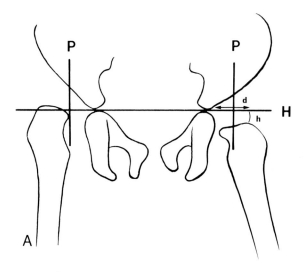

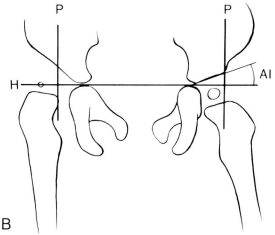

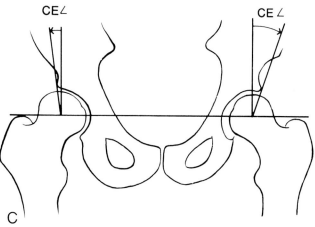

FIG. 4–7. Radiographic evaluation of CDH. **A.** Hilgenreiner's line (H) and Perkin's line (P). In the normal hip, the medial femoral metaphysis is medial to Perkin's line. (d = Hilgenreiner's d index [ischiofemoral distance]; h = Hilgenreiner's h index [trochanteric height].) **B.** The acetabular index (AI) is the angle between Hilgenreiner's line (H) and the slope of the acetabulum. **C.** The center-edge (CE) angle is the angle between a line drawn through the center of the femoral head to the lateral edge of the acetabulum and a line drawn perpendicular to Hilgenreiner's line (H). (From Staheli LT, et al.: Congenital hip dysplasia. AAOS Instr Course Lect 33:350–363, 1984.)

naturally, with hips slightly flexed and externally rotated, the anatomic landmarks for Hilgenreiner's measurements are obliterated. A full frog-leg position in flexion and abduction may reduce a hip (essentially a radiograph of a hip reduced by an Ortolani maneuver). The von Rosen view of abduction and internal rotation of the hip (in the dislocated hip, the metaphysis points above the triradiate cartilage) also may demonstrate a reduced hip.

Although a positive radiograph is helpful in the neonatal period, a normal radiograph cannot prevail over an abnormal clinical examination. As secondary changes become more established, the femur will have a more noticeable proximal migration, a false acetabulum may be noted, and Shenton's line will be broken. This occurs beginning at approximately 6 weeks of age, with the radiograph providing fairly consistent information from approximately 3 months of age. Several national and regional radiographic screening programs have advocated a single radiograph of the hips and pelvis at 3 months of age.

For the neonatal period, ultrasound examination of the hip recently has been shown to be accurate and informative, its drawback being its limited availability. Ultrasound has provided the ability to visualize cartilaginous structures such as the labrum, medial and superior acetabulum, and triradiate cartilage and their relationship to the femoral head. Ultrasound cannot penetrate bone, so that an ossified femoral head would inhibit visualization of the medial acetabulum, making information about the depth of reduction unavailable. As long as the ossific nucleus is less than 10 mm in diameter, the triradiate cartilage will be visualized. The ossific nucleus is usually not large enough to interfere until approximately 1 year of age.

The technique can be either real-time in two planes (coronal and transverse, in hip flexion and extension) as described by Harcke and Grissom[37] (Figs. 4–8 to 4–10) or can be a single-plane B-scan technique as described by Graf.[33] Using the B-scan method, Graf identified several sonographic stages of development based on the configurations of the

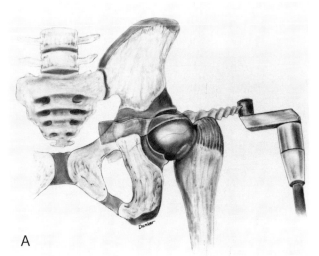

A

Fɪɢ. 4–8. Transverse view of hip in neutral position. **A.** The transducer is placed lateral to the hip, with the sector perpendicular to the long axis of the body and the axis of the femur. **B.** Sonogram of normal hip shows the femoral head (curved arrow) positioned against the bony acetabulum. The triradiate cartilage (open arrow) is open, allowing sound transmission into the acoustic shadow behind the ilium (straight closed arrow). **C.** Sonogram of dislocated hip, with femoral head (curved arrow) resting against the bony ilium (open arrow), without apparent acetabular landmarks. (A = anterior; L = lateral; P = posterior.) (A, from Harcke HT, et al.: Examination of the hip with real-time ultrasound. J Ultrasound Med 3:131–137, 1984; B and C, from Harcke HT, Grissom LE: Sonographic evaluation of the infant hip. Semin Ultrasound, CT, MR 7:331–338, 1986.)

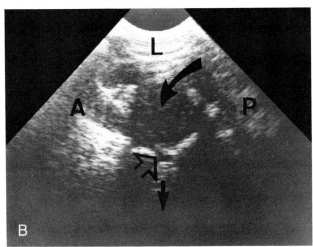

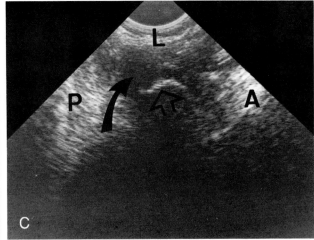

osseous and cartilaginous portions of the acetabular roof (a sonographic acetabular index corrected for the sufficiency of superior and lateral labral coverage of the femoral head). The radiographically dysplastic hip with an increased acetabular index showed delayed ossification of the advancing bony acetabular roof. Most hips in these children under 3 months of age fit the criteria for physiologic immaturity (Graf type 2a) and resolved spontaneously. However, a lower-risk group with persisting osseous deficiency and labral structural insufficiency (Graf type 2b) was identified. This delayed ossification (Graf type 2) could progress to decentration (Graf type 3), with the labrum being superiorly deformed by a subluxating head, or could progress to dislocation (Graf type 4). In 2000 newborns, Szoke and colleagues[104] found 48% normal, 50.4% physiologically immature, 1.5% dysplastic (Graf type 2b), 0.3% type 3, and 0.15% type 4.

In Harcke and Grissom's series,[37] no frank dislocations were missed. Detection of subluxation had a 1.8% false negative rate and a 2.4% false positive

rate. Boal and Schwentker[11] had no false positive or false negative results. Graf,[33] Harcke and Grissom,[37] Dahlstrom and associates,[23] and Boal and Schwentker[11] agree, however, that ultrasound is sensitive, detecting abnormalities in hips that were normal radiographically and clinically. In Dahlstrom and coworkers' series,[23] 63% of all clinically unstable hips referred for examination were found to be normal, and 11% of the clinically normal hips were unstable and 9% were dislocatable. The data correlating clinical stability examinations to sonographic abnormalities are incomplete.

Presently, ultrasound is indicated for screening purposes because it is an imaging method that does not use ionizing radiation. It can detect dislocation and subluxation. With real-time sonography, laxity can be assessed by visualizing subluxation on provocative manipulation. Reduction of the hip can be demonstrated, as well as the stability of the reduction with respect to the position of the hip in flexion and abduction. The patient can be examined in a Pavlik harness, in which reduction can be assured

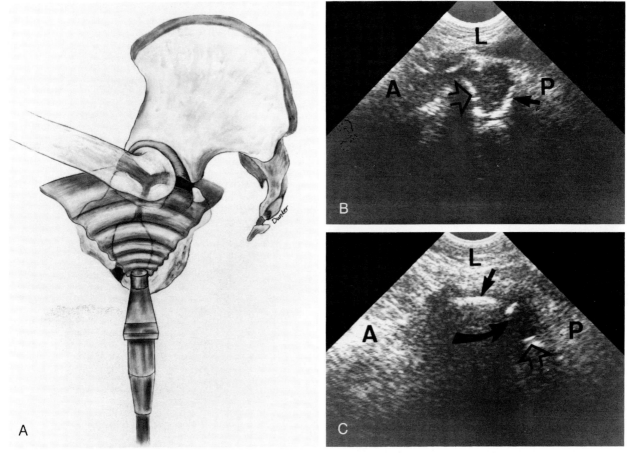

FIG. 4–9. Transverse view of hip in flexed position. **A.** The transducer is placed laterally, with the sector perpendicular to the long axis of the body but parallel to the long axis of the flexed femoral shaft. **B.** Sonogram of a normal hip. The sonolucent cartilaginous femoral head is bounded by the femoral metaphysis anteriorly (open arrow) and the back of the acetabulum posteriorly (closed arrow), making a U- or V-shaped configuration. **C.** Sonogram of a dislocated hip. The femoral shaft (straight closed arrow) and femoral head with an ossific nucleus (curved arrow) are lateral to bone (open arrow), without acetabular landmarks. (A = anterior; L = lateral; P = posterior.) (A, from Harcke HT, et al: Examination of the hip with real-time ultrasound. J Ultrasound Med 3:131–137, 1984. B and C, from Harcke HT, Grissom LE: Sonographic evaluation of the infant hip. Semin Ultrasound, CT, MR 7:331–338, 1986.)

and the hip position can be adjusted under direct visualization. This also can be done for the casted hip, but with more difficulty. Acetabular anatomy can be seen well. One can assess the depth and configuration of the bony acetabulum, as well as the anatomy of the cartilaginous labrum, as noted previously. The ossification of the ossific nucleus also can be followed sonographically.

Computed tomography (CT) has limited but uniquely useful indications. Foremost, it has the ability to confirm radiographically reduction of the hip of a child in a spica cast when the lack of an ossific nucleus and the thickness of the plaster make routine radiographic visualization difficult. CT scans also can be useful in assessing the degree of femoral anteversion, and they are good for providing information regarding acetabular anatomy, especially in assessing anterior coverage versus posterior deficiency. The indications for magnetic resonance imaging (MRI) are not clear yet, although

this imaging modality has been useful in assessing ischemic disorders of the femoral head.

Arthrography is a useful modality, although indications vary among clinicians. The primary use is to assess concentricity of reduction. Incidental information relates to extent of hip laxity, stability of reduction, and, if there is not concentric reduction, information on the anatomy preventing reduction. Anatomy is especially important in the patient with a failed open reduction or a redislocation after an apparently adequate closed reduction.

The study can be performed by an anterior approach or a medial approach, using a 20-gauge short spinal needle. A small amount of dilute contrast material is used (usually less than 2 ml), so that the contrast material will not obscure the femoral head. If too much contrast material is used, an iatrogenic increase in the medial dye pool will be produced. This can be avoided if the syringe is disconnected after injection and some dye is allowed to

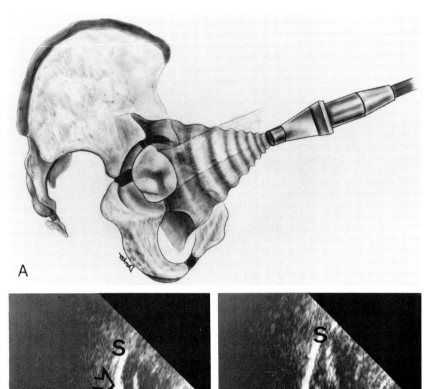

FIG. 4–10. Coronal view of hip in flexed position. **A.** The transducer is placed laterally, with the sector in a coronal plane, parallel to the long axis of the body and perpendicular to the long axis of the flexed femoral shaft. This is the plane used by Graf. **B.** Sonogram of a normal hip. The femoral head (curved arrow) is in the acetabulum (straight closed arrow). Superior to the head is the ilium (open arrow), with the gluteal muscle (+) overlying the head and labrum. **C.** A posteriorly dislocated femoral head (curved arrow) rests against the posterior acetabular margin where the bony ilium meets the posterior limb of the triradiate cartilage (open arrow). (L = lateral; S = superior.) (A, from Harcke HT, et al: Examination of the hip with real-time ultrasound. J Ultrasound Med 3:131–137, 1984. B and C, from Harcke HT, Grissom LE: Sonographic evaluation of the infant hip. Semin Ultrasound, CT, MR 7:331–338, 1986.)

escape, releasing the back pressure. The hip can be examined dynamically under fluoroscopy, with final radiographs taken in extension-neutral rotation, extension-abduction, abduction-internal rotation, and flexion-abduction.

Arthrographic anatomy and pathologic conditions are discussed in the treatment section as needed, in instances in which the indications for arthrography can be demonstrated.

Treatment

Overview

The object of treatment is to obtain a concentric reduction of the femoral head into the acetabulum and to maintain that position until the hip is stabilized in the reduced position. Stabilization means the reversal of the pathologic secondary changes of capsular laxity, femoral anteversion, and acetabular dysplasia. The younger the child is at the time of reduction, the fewer the secondary changes and the faster the return to normal anatomy. The greatest remodeling potential is within the first year of life. When older than 18 months of age, even after achieving a concentric closed reduction, an increasing number of hips require secondary acetabular or femoral procedures for residual dysplasia or subluxation.

Acetabular Dysplasia Without Instability

The patient with an abnormally high acetabular index (greater than 30°) appears to be at risk for progressive dysplasia. The defect in ossification appears to be defined better with sonography than with radiography. The dysplastic hip should be splinted in abduction, as with a Pavlik harness or with an Atlanta abduction brace in the older child. The most improvement occurs in the acetabular index within the first 6 months of life. If dysplasia persists or is noted in a walking-age child, an abduction brace is suggested and is usually worn half time. Failure of the dysplasia to resolve may indicate the need for a pelvic osteotomy at a later date. The duration of splinting may be prolonged by slow progress in remodeling and may span 1 or more years.

Dislocatable and Subluxatable Hip

The neonatal dislocatable hip usually has no secondary deformity or contracture. Treatment involves early orthosis wear, keeping the hips flexed and abducted, as with a Pavlik harness. Many dislocatable hips will resolve spontaneously in the first weeks of life. The orthosis acts as a positioning device, with resolution occurring over 6 to 12 weeks. Because these hips are radiographically normal, progress is monitored by clinical examination or sonogram. Often, weaning from the device starts at 8 weeks, and removal occurs by 12 weeks.

Treatment should start in the immediate neonatal period. Some advocate waiting for the first 7 days, initiating treatment only on those with persistent instability. At one time, it was argued that treatment of CDH should be delayed for as long as 1 year, because the risk of avascular necrosis was too high. Waiting 7 or 14 days is a compromise, because 60% of neonatally unstable hips can be spared treatment. The incidence of avascular necrosis with the Pavlik harness is low,[51,53] because these children have no secondary deformity or adduction contractures. It can be argued that any risk of iatrogenic avascular necrosis in treatment of what may be a benign, spontaneously resolving condition is unacceptable. However, until those dislocatable hips at risk not to resolve are distinguished from those that will resolve, gentle, careful orthotic use is indicated and, as shown by Kalamchi and associates,[51,53] has a very low risk.

Subluxatable hips are controversial, with some observers maintaining that the hips are normal. With the diagnosis being so qualitative and interobserver reliability being so poor, can we be sure on a single examination that today's subluxatable hip was not yesterday's dislocated or dislocatable hip? If sonographic instability or radiographic abnormality can be demonstrated, orthotic treatment is indicated, as it is for the dislocatable hip. If radiographically and sonographically normal, these children can be observed, with repeat sonograms obtained at 6 weeks or radiographs obtained at 3 months. If reliable sonography is not available, treatment with an orthosis, as for a dislocatable hip, is indicated.

Occasionally, a child younger than 1 year old will present with a hip that is unstable but not dislocated. This may be residual deformity from previous CDH. Although the child is too old for a Pavlik harness, an abduction brace is indicated. This brace, initially worn full time, will allow standing and should provide stability and stimulate acetabular remodeling. Bracing may be needed for a year or more, with residual deformity requiring surgical correction.

Dislocated Hip

The dislocated hip can be reducible (Ortolani-positive) or irreducible (Ortolani-negative). Rarely is a nonteratogenic dislocation irreducible prior to 6 months of age. Usually, the secondary changes in the femur or acetabulum are severe enough to make a reduction unstable only after the age of 3 months.

Are there indications not to reduce a dislocated irreducible hip? Many authors suggest that bilateral dislocations in children older than 5 to 7 years of age and unilateral dislocations in children older than 8 to 10 years of age should be left unreduced. Coleman[18] believes that reduction should be attempted for unilateral dislocation at any age. Although incongruity between the acetabulum and femur may be severe, in unilateral cases a Colonna arthroplasty with femoral shortening may be more desirable than the alternative of leaving the hip dislocated.

There are relative contraindications, depending on your viewpoint. Although it is accepted that the hip in the neonatal period is the least difficult to reduce, the unossified femoral head is at relative risk of ischemic damage.[106] Some suggest that attempts at reducing an Ortolani-negative hip should be delayed until 9 to 12 months of age, after the ossific nucleus has appeared. The secondary adaptive changes that occur by that time are minimal and should resolve after reduction. Refinement in the methods of closed reduction have reduced this complication.

An attempt at closed reduction is indicated in all patients less than 18 months of age. The femoral head is gently repositioned, giving either a concentric reduction or an eccentric (docked) reduction. The slight residual displacement is caused by a socket narrowed by labral or capsular obstruction. If the docked position is maintained for 6 to 8 weeks, the head often will medialize as the limbus remodels or everts, producing a concentric reduction (see Fig. 4–4).

For the nonteratogenic dislocated hip, Tonnis[106] believes that there are relative contraindications to attempting closed reduction. He recommends routine arthrography on all children. The group at risk for ischemic necrosis[107] are those with high dislocations, an inverted labrum with a narrow introitus (an hourglass configuration with a width less than 18 mm), and persistent lateral displacement of greater than 3 mm on attempted reduction. This risk is compounded in the older child (greater than 1 year of age) and in the absence of an ossific nucleus. In this case, he recommends a primary open reduction.

Many believe that closed reduction is the initial treatment of choice up to 3 years of age. Arzimanoglu[4] reported successful closed reductions in 3- to 11-year-old children after soft tissue release and prolonged traction. Until 3 years of age, the rate of avascular necrosis is acceptably low and the rate of remodeling is high enough to justify closed reduction only, followed by observation. Harris and colleagues[38,39] thought that a closed reduction by age 4.5 years was compatible with a normal outcome by age 8 years. In Zionts and MacEwen's series,[127] two-thirds of patients 1 to 3 years old subsequently required femoral or pelvic osteotomies for residual deformity in order to stabilize the reduction.

Although most concede that open reduction is almost always indicated after 36 months of age,[94] the 18 to 36 months age period is still controversial.[8,127] Hall[36] and Salter and Dubos[90] believe that acetabular remodeling potential after 18 months is inadequate to assure normal acetabular formation. Early pelvic osteotomy after open or closed reduction after 18 months of age manages both acetabular dysplasia and mild femoral anteversion. One also could argue that the incidence of avascular necrosis following closed reduction after 18 months of age is too high. If the secondary changes can be corrected and avascular necrosis can be avoided by open reduction (Berkeley and associates[8] had no avascular necrosis in their patients), closed reduction may be contraindicated after 18 months of age. Tonnis[106] supports this with his observation that the rate of avascular necrosis in open reduction alone was 8.4%, whereas the rate was 28% in open reduction after failed closed reduction. We believe that closed reduction should be attempted as a primary, initial method up to 3 years of age. The closed reduction should be done with gentleness and an appreciation of soft tissue tensions.

Closed Reduction

In the infant, generally before the age of 6 months, concentric reduction can be achieved with simple positioning. As the child becomes older and develops shortening and contractures, skin traction may be required prior to reduction. After reduction, the hip is held in either a cast or an orthosis, such as the Pavlik harness. The manipulation for reduction is the same as that for performing an Ortolani maneuver, in which the flexed hip is abducted while the thigh is lifted forward. The hip should remain reduced while the thigh remains flexed and abducted, without pressure on the legs. If the capsule is very lax, excessive flexion may dislocate the head inferiorly, with excessive abduction dislocating the head anteriorly. The knees are usually flexed. A reduced hip may be dislocated by extending the knees if the hamstrings are tight. Positioning is important, because the force must be enough to maintain reduction without producing avascular necrosis.

Initially, reduced hips were held in a Lorenz frog-leg position of 90° of flexion and 70° of abduction; however, the incidence of avascular necrosis was high. Excessive abduction (greater than 45°) was believed to contribute to avascular necrosis[31,91] by compressing the posterosuperior branch of the medial circumflex artery in the intraepiphyseal groove and between the iliopsoas and adductors. These complications can be avoided by flexing the hip to greater that 90°, and limiting abduction to the safe zone of Ramsey[1] (Fig. 4–11). Abduction is only for positioning the head stably in the acetabulum. The femur should not be abducted to create tension in a tight adductor muscle (bowstringed) to secure the reduction by force across the joint, because this increases the risk of avascular necrosis. In the newborn, there is often no adductor contracture, so that effortless abduction may be 90°. Although such full abduction is of less risk in neonates, avascular necrosis still may occur. Flexion will tend to center the head toward the triradiate cartilage. Most failures of reduction are caused by inadequate flexion, not inadequate abduction.

Pavlik Harness

In general, in the child younger than 6 months of age, the hip will reduce easily with the Ortolani

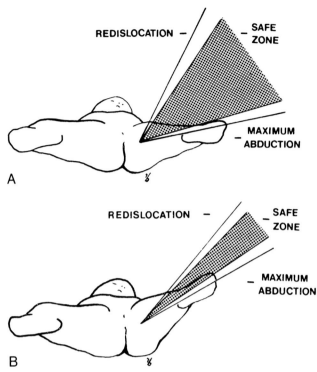

Fɪɢ. **4–11.** **A.** The safe zone of Ramsey is the arc of abduction that is shaded. The zone is bounded by the angle of adduction at which dislocation occurs, and in maximal abduction by the patient's comfort and ease of abduction. **B.** In a patient with an adduction contracture, the safe zone is narrow. Abduction is limited, and the angle of comfortable abduction is close to the angle of dislocation. (From Ramsey PL, et al.: Congenital dislocation of the hip. J Bone Joint Surg 58A:1000–1004, 1976.)

maneuver, and the hip can be held in a reduced position by a Pavlik harness. The position is comfortable and safe, allowing motion within the zone of reduction but maintaining reduction without forced abduction. The Pavlik harness (Fig. 4–12) has an abdominal strap, two shoulder straps, and two leg stirrups. The harness is applied with the legs flexed to 100° and the thighs abducted freely under the weight of the legs. Flexion up to 120° may be needed for reduction.[76, 88]

Once the hip flexion is set by adjusting the anterior strap, the hip is reduced by an Ortolani maneuver with gentle abduction. The hip is then adducted with a Barlow maneuver to redislocate the hip. The posterior strap is adjusted to prevent the thigh from adducting enough to enter the zone of dislocation. The posterior strap had originally been used to hold the hip in maximal abduction (Lorenz), but the incidence of avascular necrosis was high. With present use of the harness, the thigh experiences no forced abduction. The posterior strap serves as a check rein to adduction. In general, it is loose enough to allow the knees to be adducted to within 5 cm of the midline. The hip is allowed free motion

within the safe zone of Ramsey. The hip and knee are not allowed to extend in the device. If there are adduction contractures, the posterior strap should not be tightened to stretch the adductors. The weight of the thighs in flexion will slowly increase abduction. When the child sleeps prone in the harness, gentle abduction is encouraged. At times, if the safe zone is narrow, keeping the hip from reducing, adductor tenotomies may be useful. However, at this point, many prefer to use traction.

Once the harness is applied, reduction should be confirmed by radiography or sonography. The most common error is inadequate flexion, pointing the femoral head toward the superior acetabulum and not toward the triradiate cartilage. The infant remains in the harness full time, because the harness allows for diaper changes and feeding with relative ease. The device can be removed for bathing once the hip stabilizes. As anatomic deformity progresses after 3 months of age, the reduction tends to be more unstable. If the head is slightly laterally displaced or is not pointing centrally, tightening the posterior strap is not the solution.

Adduction contracture usually resolves within 2 weeks. Persisting contracture does not demand tenotomy. It may mean that the hip is not reduced, usually associated with inadequate flexion at the hip. Initially, the harness is left on full time and is examined in a few days to check for harness positioning and complications. The infant is then examined at weekly intervals for stability (clinical or sonographic) until the hip is reduced and stabilized. The average treatment time is 3.6 months for infants who start to wear the harness when they are younger than 1 month of age, 7 months for those who start at 1 to 3 months of age, and 9.3 months for those who start at 3 to 6 months of age. A good estimate of the time required is two times the age of the child when the device is applied.[88] When the hip is stable, the harness is weaned off by gradually increasing the time out of the brace by 4 to 6 hours per day after 2 to 3 weeks. Before weaning, the hip should be stable clinically, reduced radiographically or sonographically, and have a stable or improving acetabular index.

The harness can be used effectively and safely after 6 months of age; however, it cannot be used once the child starts to walk. At walking age, the child often must be placed in another orthosis, such as an Atlanta abduction brace. For persisting dysplasia, the abduction brace also is used after discontinuation of the Pavlik harness.

Kalamchi and MacFarlane[53] observed the constraints of the concept of the safe zone and reported no avascular necrosis in 122 patients 6 to 9 months

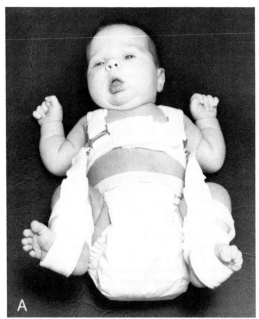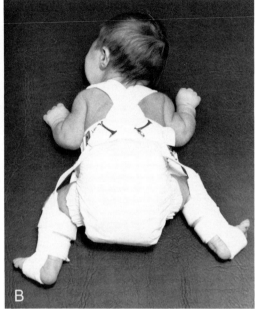

Fɪɢ. **4–12.** The Pavlik harness. **A.** Front view. The harness holds the hips and knees flexed. There is ample room to change the diaper without manipulating the harness. **B.** Back view. The prone child fully abducts her legs. The posterior straps are seen to be slack. The ankles are not being forced into a dorsiflexed position.

of age, with a success rate of 88% in treatment of the dislocated hips. In Bradley and coworkers' group of patients,[14] in whom treatment was initiated at less than 6 weeks of age, 5% needed subsequent surgery, with approximately 1.2% having avascular necrosis. Treatment failure is often caused by lack of recognition that the hip was not reduced initially.

If the hip cannot be reduced with an Ortolani maneuver and the child is younger than 6 months old, a Pavlik harness can be tried. With the hip held flexed, irritability and adductor contracture will resolve, and the hip may reduce spontaneously. This trial is only for 2 weeks. No abduction force is applied to the hip. The hip that responds to this treatment has been termed an "intermediate" hip.

If the hip in the harness does not reduce or if the child is older than 6 months of age, a period of skin traction is indicated. Traction continues until the hip becomes Ortolani-positive or until the ossific nucleus has been brought to a level opposite the triradiate cartilage as seen on radiograph. Occasionally, a very lax hip cannot be held reduced by a harness, with the hip dislocating anteriorly, posteriorly, or inferiorly, depending on position. This hip may be held reduced in skin traction. For the dislocated hip, traction is followed by reduction under anesthesia and spica-cast immobilization.

Traction has been used in several different ways. Morel[75] placed a child in longitudinal traction (4 to 10 kg) with the hips and knees extended. Gradu-

ally, the thighs were abducted and internally rotated, with the femoral head being positioned into the acetabulum without a discrete Ortolani-type maneuver. This position is then held casted. This procedure was successful in approximately 66% of the patients up to 6 years of age and had a low incidence of avascular necrosis. If there was no reduction after 6 weeks of traction, open reduction was indicated. All of the patients required subsequent pelvic osteotomy.

Bryant's traction has been used, which consists of the knees extended and the hips flexed to 90°, with gradual abduction of the thighs. The Southampton method[122] applies 0.5 to 1.5 kg of weight to each leg, enough to raise the buttocks from the bed. After 10 days of traction in 10° of abduction, the thighs are abducted 10° per day for 10 days until the hips are abducted 80°. Young children may require 4 weeks of traction and older ones 6 to 8 weeks of traction. The Bryant's overhead position is not suggested for children older than 4 years of age, because peripheral circulation may be inadequate. In fact, some suggest that the extended knee in children older than 2 years may impair popliteal artery blood flow. As little as 10° of knee flexion will prevent this. At the end of traction, 15% of the hips were reduced and stable, 83% were reducible but required casting or open reduction for stabilization, and 2% were still irreducible. Avascular necrosis was minimal.

We recommend a modified split-Russell skin

traction (Fig. 4–13). The hips are flexed approximately 30 to 45°, the thighs are abducted 20°, and the knees are allowed to flex slightly to relax the hamstrings and popliteal neurovascular bundle. Elastic bandages are used to hold nonadhesive foam strips to the sides of the legs. They extend from groin to malleoli and end in spreaders to protect skin and circulation at the ankle. The elastic bandage is rewrapped frequently, with care being taken to avoid neurovascular compromise due to constriction. The traction is removed routinely to allow feeding, washing, and some free time for play. The traction is otherwise essentially continual (day and night) for 2 to 3 weeks. The weight starts at about 0.5 to 1.0 kg per leg and is increased gradually in increments of 0.5 kg to a maximum of 2.5 kg per leg (usually no more than a total of one third of the patient's body weight). Some patients need countertraction with a diaper-like padded restraint (preferred) or by placing the bed in a head-down (Trendelenburg) position. The hips are periodically assessed clinically and radiographically to determine the laxity of the hip and its reducibility. Traction continues (1) until the hip is reduced spontaneously, (2) until the hip has been converted to a reducible (Ortolani-positive) hip without forceful reduction, or (3) until the femoral head has been pulled distally enough to lie below the level of the acetabulum, allowing a safe reduction. If radiographs show only minimal or no distal migration in traction, an adductor tenotomy or an adductor and psoas tenotomy may be performed, and the patient is then returned for further traction.

Skeletal traction may be considered if more longitudinal force is needed to pull the hip distally. Skin integrity limits the amount of weight applied in skin traction. A large threaded Steinmann pin in

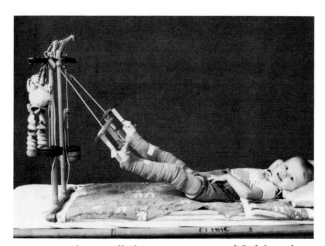

Fig. 4–13. Split-Russell skin traction, as modified for a home traction program.

the distal femoral metaphysis, avoiding the growth plate, can be used. This method was previously popular in heavier, older (greater than 18 months old) children or in children with a high-riding dislocation. The trend now has moved away from skeletal traction with its risks of growth plate injury, pin cut out, pin tract infection, and fracture (of femur or pin). The increased distraction forces possible with heavy skeletal traction, pulling the hip to station +2, may lead to increased pressure on the reduced femoral head when the traction is released, leading to an increased incidence of avascular necrosis. (The Gage stations are 0 if the head is only slightly superior, +1 if it is at the level of the opposite reduced hip, and +2 if it is pulled more distally than the normal hip.) In many cases in older children, open or closed reduction with diaphyseal femoral shortening has been advocated as superior to closed reduction after traction.

Skin traction prior to closed reduction has been shown to decrease the incidence of avascular necrosis and to minimize the severity of that which does occur, presumably by stretching the tight soft tissues. Although Gage and Winter[31] showed less avascular necrosis correlated with more distal traction stations (4.5% at station +2, 21.2% at station +1, and 41.4% at station 0), it appears that duration of traction may be more significant, with 21 days or more giving the best results. Even with traction, however, the older child (greater than 1 year old) is at a greater risk of avascular necrosis. Interestingly enough, 14% of the avascular necrosis in Weiner and associates' study[116] occurred in children younger than 3 months old, which suggests that the cartilaginous femoral head prior to ossification is at risk of avascular necrosis. Despite this risk, we believe that an infant less than 3 months of age with an irreducible hip should be placed in traction, because the risk of avascular necrosis is offset by the potential good of obtaining a reduction early while remodeling is active. If a reduction cannot be achieved by traction, the child can be left free until open reduction is done at a slightly older age (6 months or older). Home traction appears to be as effective and safe as hospital traction, with a similar incidence of avascular necrosis.[114]

Once traction has been successful, the dislocated hip is gently reduced or repositioned under general anesthesia, with full muscle relaxation. An Ortolani-like maneuver is used, with the child supine on the table and the pelvis stabilized. The flexed hip is adducted with gentle longitudinal traction. The femoral head is guided to the acetabulum, with pressure lifting the greater trochanter anteriorly by the thigh being abducted to 50 to 60°. All maneuvers are done gently, with the reduction being a repositioning of the head in the acetabulum. If adductor tightness blocks reduction (it should not after traction) or limits abduction, a subcutaneous adductor tenotomy is indicated.

The hip is positioned within the safe zone. With the hip reduced and flexed, the thigh is allowed to fall freely into abduction. This is the maximum safe abduction. The thigh is then adducted back toward the midline until the hip dislocates. The hip is then positioned reduced midway in the safe zone, rarely exceeding 60° of abduction. When reduction is achieved, with hip and knee flexed, one is unable to extend the knee fully without redislocating the hip. If the safe zone is found to be narrow (abduction limited), the thigh should not be forcibly abducted to stabilize the reduction under pressure. An adductor tenotomy should be performed. If the safe zone is still less than 25°, with the hip still dislocated in moderate abduction, a redislocation in

the cast is likely. The child can be returned to traction with increasing abduction, or open reduction may be considered.

Although clinical signs may suggest reduction, the hips should be imaged to confirm reduction. In the operating room, arthrography with image intensification is helpful. It is especially useful if the ossific nucleus is small. Routine radiographs are adequate when the head is better developed. Arthrography is useful to confirm reduction or to explain why reduction has not occurred (Fig. 4–14). A successful reduction[87] will show an intact Shenton's line, medial dye pooling of 2 mm or less, and no soft tissue interposition. The medial joint space, as measured from the acetabular cortex to the beak of the medial metaphysis of the femur, should show less than 2 mm of discrepancy when compared with the normal hip. If one accepts "docking" as an adequate reduction, up to 5 mm of lateralization or 7 mm of medial dye pooling can be

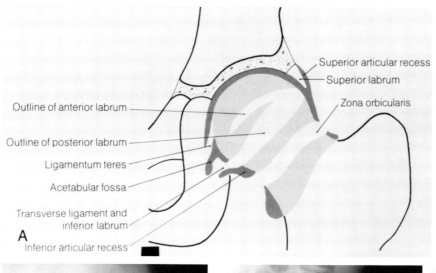

Outline of anterior labrum
Outline of posterior labrum
Ligamentum teres
Acetabular fossa
Transverse ligament and inferior labrum
Inferior articular recess

Superior articular recess
Superior labrum
Zona orbicularis

A

FIG. 4–14. **A.** Schematic drawing of an arthrogram of a normal hip. **B.** Arthrogram of a normal hip. The superior labrum (arrow) is outlined sharply. There is no medial dye pooling. **C.** The hip is dislocated, with a narrowed introitus. The acetabulum is shallow, and the limbus (arrow) is apparent superiorly, obstructing the reduction. **D.** On attempted reduction, the femoral head is still laterally displaced. The rounded, inverted limbus is seen superior to the head (arrow). (A, from Tönnis D: Congenital Dysplasia and Dislocation of the Hip in Children and Adults. New York, Springer-Verlag, 1987.)

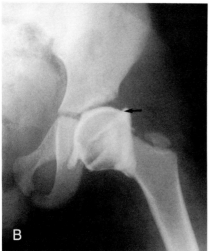
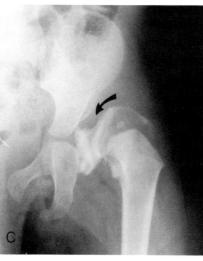
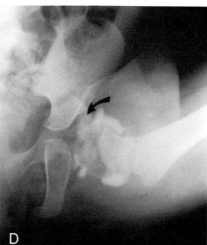

allowed. In this case, some soft tissue interposition is expected. Once casted, the hips are best visualized by computed tomography.

The cast is applied with the hips flexed about 100°, abduction in the safe zone, and the knees flexed 45°. The cast extends from the nipple line to the malleoli. The cast must be well molded over the trochanters to maintain the reduction. Shoulder straps are applied to hold the cast proximally. Four cast problems that may lead to a redislocation are:

1. Downward migration of the heavy cast, which extends the hips (prevented by shoulder straps).
2. Lack of posterior or posterolateral support of the trochanters and buttocks, allowing the buttocks to fall out of the back of the cast, with adduction of the thighs.
3. Initially allowing the knees to kick free and extend.
4. Poor cast placement because of looseness or pulling the hips into extension as the plaster is wrapped about the inguinal crease.

The child should be comfortable. If the child is crying within the first 6 to 12 hours after cast application, the cast should be removed. Impending avascular necrosis is an important cause of pain in the immediate postreduction period. Cast immobilization is for 6 to 9 months. Casts are changed at 2 to 3 months, and gentle clinical evaluation is performed under anesthesia. If arthrography had shown slight lateralization of the initial reduction, it is repeated at 6 to 8 weeks. Renshaw[89] and Race and Herring[87] have demonstrated that reduction of the lateralized hip is not a dependable event. If the hip has not centralized, open reduction is indicated. If the hip stabilizes, at 4 to 6 months the knees can be cut free to allow extension. If residual subluxation of the hip exists when the cast is removed, an abduction brace can be used for an additional 6 to 12 months. The brace is removed for bathing and is weaned off slowly as the hip stabilizes. Persisting subluxation of the head in a neutral weight-bearing position often requires surgical femoral or pelvic stabilization.

Occasionally, in the older child, excessive anteversion may require casting of the hip in internal rotation for stability. This is rare if the child is less than 12 months old. Excessive rotation to maintain reduction is an indication for open reduction.

Open Reduction

The absolute indication for open reduction is failure to achieve a concentric reduction by closed means. This is an Ortolani-negative hip for which traction is unsuccessful, a hip that on reduction under anesthesia has a narrow (less than 25°) safe zone despite adductor tenotomy, a hip that cannot be docked at least under the labrum (as with an hourglass constriction), or one that remains slightly lateral after 6 weeks in a docked position. In general, previous failed closed reductions place the hip at risk for another attempt. Most other indications for open reduction in children younger than 3 years old are relative, depending on the surgeon's perception of the risks of redislocation and avascular necrosis and the age-related potential for acetabular recovery. Although closed reduction after 3 years of age is possible, open reduction is indicated most frequently, often with femoral shortening or other extra-articular procedures.

Open reduction as an isolated procedure has one goal: to allow as complete a concentric reduction as permitted by the deformity of the femoral head. Secondary procedures addressing stabilization of the reduction are a separate issue and are performed at the time of the open reduction or at a later date. Combining open reduction with intertrochanteric osteotomy or pelvic osteotomy increases the difficulty of surgery and may increase the risk of avascular necrosis and redislocation.[57,85] Femoral diaphyseal shortening as a combined procedure has appeared to have fewer complications.

The open reduction can be done through a medial or an anterolateral approach. The medial approach is reserved for children younger than 18 months of age when the child is small and the hip is not teratogenic, high riding, or stiff. The medial approach of Ferguson[26] allows psoas and adductor tenotomy and reduction, but superior capsulorrhaphy is not possible. This approach allows plication of the redundant capsule. There is a high incidence of avascular necrosis (as much as 67%),[54,117] redislocation, persistent instability, and need for secondary procedures. Careful casting is required, with positioning in 10° of flexion, 30° of abduction, and 20° of internal rotation.

The more common procedure is by an anterior approach. An oblique ilioinguinal incision is used. In exposing the hip capsule, the psoas tendon but not the muscle is sectioned. The adductor also can be tenotomized through a separate incision, as needed. This soft tissue release allows the femoral head to be reduced under less pressure and, with the psoas tenotomy, allows for better visualization of the crucial inferior capsular contracture. In opening the capsule, the metaphyseal vessels on the femoral neck are avoided. The ligamentum teres is excised from the femoral head and is traced proximally to define the true acetabulum. The fibrofatty pulvinar is excised gently with a pituitary rongeur, with care being taken not to damage the articular cartilage. With the acetabulum visualized, the inferior capsular contracture must be released to create an inferior pocket in which to drop the head. This involves the sectioning of the transverse acetabular ligament with scissors, usually guided by palpation.

The infolded labrum then can be seen superiorly. A blunt elevator or rongeur is used to elevate and evert the labrum over the reduced femoral head. This may be facilitated by two or three radial cuts in the labrum. Although some advocate excising the limbus, or at least cannot document arrest of the triradiate cartilage or acetabular dysplasia secondary to excision, we recommend eversion of the limbus, with excision only as a last resort. The head is then deeply and concentrically reduced, and the capsule is plicated to remove the superior and posterior redundancy.

Occasionally, the hip will not reduce because of tight soft tissues, as will be seen in older children without traction. In children older than 3 years of age, skeletal traction has been avoided because of stiffness, a 54% incidence of avascular necrosis, and a 31% incidence of redislocation.[94] Femoral shortening has been advocated as an alternative, with a redislocation rate of 8% and an avascular necrosis rate of 8% or less.[18] This is usually a subtrochanteric shortening osteotomy, removing approximately 2 cm of the diaphysis. A higher incidence of avascular necrosis has been reported for varus intertrochanteric osteotomies performed for the same purpose.

The patient is casted with the hips flexed 20°, abducted 20°, and internally rotated as required by the femoral version. The reduction is confirmed radiographically in the cast. Casting is continued for 6 to 8 weeks, followed by mobilization. Longer casting is unnecessary, resulting only in more stiffness. Residual subluxation can be managed by positioning in an abduction brace.

Apparent redislocation after open reduction is most often caused by failure to concentrically reduce the hip at the time of surgery.[93] Occasionally, the incompletely reduced hip is not recognized, and a pelvic osteotomy is used to gain lateral coverage of the head. A pelvic osteotomy is a means of stabilizing a concentric reduction, not a means of gaining reduction. When improperly performed in these circumstances, the pelvic osteotomy carries a high risk of posterior dislocation and avascular necrosis. Occasionally, the anterior capsular repair is too tight and drives the head posteriorly into lax residual posterior redundancy. Infection, inadequate casting, and capsular dehiscence also are seen as causes of failure (Fig. 4–15).

For many children, if femoral shortening is not planned, preoperative traction for 3 weeks is indicated. In children having a repeat open reduction after a previous failed attempt, the fibrosis of the

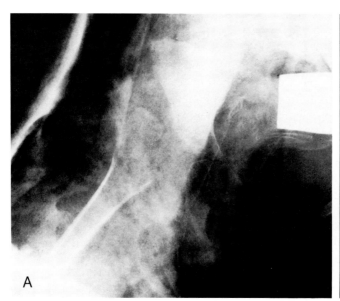
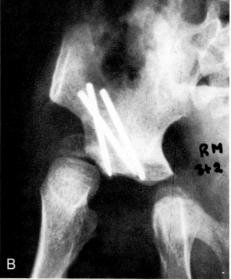

Fɪɢ. 4–15. **A.** Radiograph, in postoperative cast, of open reduction of right hip with capsular dehiscence. **B.** Inadequately reduced right hip with a simultaneous Salter innominate osteotomy. Dislocation is apparent postoperatively.

capsule and soft tissues is tight and will not stretch with traction. Preoperatively, these children should be allowed to be free to work out their stiffness, with traction being used only as an adjunct to increase hip range of motion. [13]

Secondary Procedures

If a concentric reduction is achieved by open or closed methods before 1 year of age, secondary procedures on the femur or acetabulum usually are not necessary. There is adequate acetabular remodeling potential remaining, and anteversion should not cause significant instability. In Zionts and MacEwen's series of patients between 1 and 3 years of age,[127] 62% of the hips reduced by open procedure and 66% of those reduced by closed procedure received secondary procedures for persisting subluxation. In Westin's group,[118] 30% of those hips reduced prior to 3 years of age and 48% of those reduced after age 3 required a subsequent acetabuloplasty.

Secondary procedures are indicated to correct persisting instability or subluxation caused by the adaptive changes in the femur or acetabulum and occasionally are indicated to overcome adaptive shortening of the soft tissues about the hip. The surgery should be directed at the most deformed component. As a rule, extra-articular procedures produce less stiffness than intra-articular procedures. The greater the number of open procedures, the greater the stiffness and the potential for complications.

For any of the reconstructive procedures, the primary prerequisite is that the hip be concentrically reduced. Because the surgery is performed for residual subluxation, this appears to be a contradiction. If a femoral head is radiographically and concentrically reduced and stable in a position of abduction and internal rotation, the prerequisite is considered fulfilled.

The femoral osteotomies have several indications. If excessive internal rotation (greater than 60°) is needed after reduction to center the head, a derotation osteotomy is indicated. If the proximal femur is deformed by anteversion or valgus angulation of the femoral neck and the subluxated head can be centralized by abduction and internal rotation, a varus derotation osteotomy may be indicated. The results of this procedure have been reliable in children younger than 4 years of age. The desired response, an improvement in the acetabular index, occurs most rapidly in the first 6 months af-

ter the head is concentrically and stably reduced (whether it be after a primary closed reduction or a reconstructive procedure, regardless of age). Kasser and associates[55] reported an average decrease of 10° in the index over the first 2 years postoperatively.

Although it is apparent that a valgus anteverted femur is a less stable mechanical configuration than one corrected to more a varus and less anteverted position, there is no indication that hip development is improved by routinely doing a varus derotation osteotomy on a normal, undeformed proximal femur. Occasionally, a shortening osteotomy of an undeformed femur is required for reduction to overcome limitations posed by tight soft tissues.

A purely rotational osteotomy can be done at the subtrochanteric or supracondylar area. Varus derotation osteotomies may be intertrochanteric or subtrochanteric, with varying degrees of rigidity of fixation. In young children, the varus angle is reduced to 110°, and in older children greater than 7 years of age, it is reduced to no less than 125°. In the young child, the femur often will remodel rapidly back to a more valgus position, which may require a pelvic procedure for stabilization. Both Kasser and colleagues[55] and Jones[49] demonstrated remodeling of the proximal femur back to a more valgus position after varus osteotomy. In no instance did this recurrent valgus deformity contribute to treatment failure, although in one case we have seen a hip progressively subluxate as it remodeled back to a valgus position. Ten to fifteen degrees of anteversion should remain postoperatively.

Some of the more severe valgus deformities are associated with avascular necrosis, with damage to the growth plate of the greater trochanter or lateral plate of the femoral head. Some have advocated femoral osteotomies as the best approach, because the varus position does not increase pressure on the femoral head the way a pelvic osteotomy may. However, care must be taken not to use an extreme varus position, because the potential for the femur to remodel into valgus is limited by the growth disturbance. In fact, some reports suggest that intertrochanteric osteotomies themselves have a higher risk of avascular necrosis than subtrochanteric osteotomies.

Other problems associated with femoral osteotomies include the limp often seen postoperatively, especially in older children. The limp may be a persistent problem, resistant to physical therapy. Less-than-good results are seen in those hips that are congruously incongruent, in which the osteotomy forces the hip into an incongruously incongruent configuration. If the head is grossly unstable, an excessive derotation osteotomy may either force the leg into external rotation or dislocate the head posteriorly. For a femoral osteotomy, there should be a concentric, congruent reduction, near-normal hip range of motion, and near-normal cartilage space.

After 3 or 4 years of age, a femoral osteotomy can be performed to correct the proven proximal femoral deformity, but the acetabular response is much less reliable. A Salter osteotomy is able to provide the correction needed, not only with respect to the acetabular dysplasia but also by supplying anterior coverage to a moderately anteverted femoral head. In older children, an acetabular procedure is needed to correct acetabular deformity.

Assuming no remodeling potential, when does residual dysplasia warrant surgical correction? Many of the criteria have been extrapolated from the CE angle and acetabular index data in adults, with the goal being a normal hip with a CE angle greater than 25°. In the very young child (younger than 5 years of age), the acetabular index is the most valuable radiographic indicator. The upper limit of normal is 30° at less than 1 year of age, 25° from 1 to 3 years of age, and less than 20° from 3 years of age to adulthood. The standard deviation, however, is large for normal patients.

The CE angle is not useful below 5 years of age. The center of the femoral head is not the center of the ossific nucleus, so that the measurement can be inaccurate in the young child. The center is best determined using a template of concentric circles, such as that used by others to determine sphericity in Perthes disease. According to Tonnis' study,[108] the lowest normal CE angle for children 5 to 8 years of age is 19°; that for children 9 to 12 years of age is 25°; that for children 13 to 16 years of age is 26° to 30°; and that for adults is 26° to 30°. The normal mean values are 25° from 5 to 8 years of age, 30° from 9 to 12 years of age, and 35° for 13 years of age or older. Wiberg[119] was more generous in his

limits of normality. An abnormal CE angle for an adult was less than 20°, and that for children 3 to 17 years old was less than 15°.

There are, however, no clear-cut guidelines on how to use these data in decision making. The decision to be made is who should be operated on and when. On review of the literature dealing not with what has been suggested but with what has been done, the CE angle is less than 20°, and the acetabular index is greater than 20° (most often greater than 25°) (Table 4–2).

In the young child, persisting dysplasia often results because of an inadequately reduced hip. If the hip is stable and concentric on arthrography, one can delay acetabuloplasty until the age of 8 years without compromising the results of surgery, because many hips will improve spontaneously. If the acetabular index is abnormal but improving after reduction, surgery can also be delayed. The improvement, most rapid for the first 6 months, often plateaus after 1 to 2 years. Abduction bracing may be used as long as the index is improving. Initially, this is full-time bracing, weaned to night wear only after approximately 2 years and continued if needed until 4 to 5 years of age. If the index has failed to progress over 9 to 12 months despite treatment, if the arthrogram shows persisting instability with subluxation or dislocation, if the femoral head is deformed, or if hip range of motion is being lost, delay in surgery cannot be justified. Usually, this treatment program will take the child with a persisting problem to the age of 3 to 4 years, when femoral osteotomies are still, to some, a reasonable option.

An equally logical treatment plan, based on early pelvic osteotomies, has been advocated by Hall.[36] This assumes that the acetabulum has a poor remodeling potential, and thus, nothing is to be gained by delaying a pelvic osteotomy past 18 months of age. At times, early pelvic osteotomies

TABLE 4–2. *Preoperative Criteria, Acetabular Index (AI), and Center-Edge (CE) Angle for Patients Receiving Innominate Osteotomies for Acetabular Dysplasia*

Study	Average Patient Age (years)	Average AI (range)	Average CE Angle (range)	Operation
Kumar, et al.[59]	13.9	32° (28–35°)	5° (−5–15°)	Triple osteotomy
Barrett, et al.[7]	4.0	33° (—)	— (—)	Salter osteotomy
Sutherland and Greenfield[103]	14.3	36.5° (30–60°)	6° (10–18°)	Double osteotomy
Kalamchi[50]	5.7	31.8° (25–38°)	5° (−8–15°)	Salter osteotomy
Tonnis, et al.[109]	21.9	30.6° (—)	−3° (—)	Triple osteotomy

are performed with open reduction to stabilize the reduction. This is rarely required for reductions performed at less than 18 months of age but may be needed in 20% of open reductions between the ages of 18 and 36 months. In this case, the osteotomy must be used only to maintain the reduction and must never be used to obtain one. Although not without risk of avascular necrosis, proper technique can minimize this complication while avoiding the need to resort to the technique of pinning across the joint to stabilize the head in the socket.

For acetabular reconstruction, the goal is to rotate the roof of the acetabulum to establish a normal femoral-acetabular relationship with hyaline cartilage in the weight-bearing superior position. The three most common procedures are the pericapsular (Pemberton) osteotomy, the innominate osteotomy (Salter osteotomy and its modifications), and the triple innominate osteotomy. The Pemberton technique is an acetabuloplasty, designed to

change the shape of the acetabulum. The innominate osteotomies act by purely redirecting the acetabulum. For successful reconstruction, whether innominate osteotomy or acetabuloplasty, three prerequisites must be met: the hip must be concentrically reduced and congruous, the range of motion of the hip must be essentially normal, and the cartilage space must be near normal.

The Pemberton acetabuloplasty (Fig. 4–16) was designed as an incomplete pericapsular innominate osteotomy to lower the anterolateral acetabular roof, to provide anterolateral coverage, and to reduce acetabular volume. This could be used in treating dysplasia or to stabilize the reduction at the time of an open reduction. The acetabuloplasty assumes a plasticity of the acetabular roof and an open triradiate cartilage. Because the triradiate cartilage is completely fused by approximately 10 to 12 years of age and starts to lose some pliability at approximately 6 to 8 years of age, the upper age

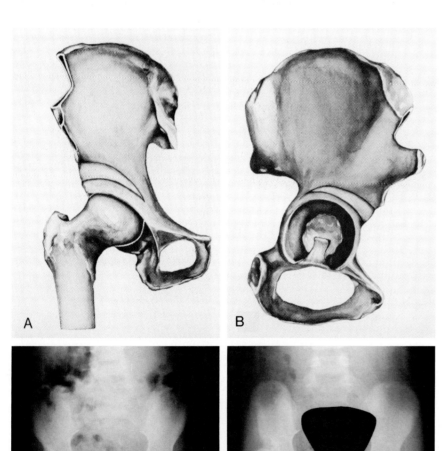

FIG. **4–16.** The Pemberton acetabuloplasty. **A.** Anterior view. **B.** Lateral view. This is an incomplete periacetabular osteotomy, improving anterior and superior coverage but not affecting posterior coverage. **C.** Preoperative radiograph of dysplastic right hip. **D.** Postoperative radiographs of dysplastic right hip. The Pemberton acetabuloplasty improved both the acetabular index and the center-edge angle. (A and B, from Tachdjian MO (ed): Congenital Dislocation of the Hip. New York, Churchill Livingstone, 1982. C and D, courtesy of D. Kehl, M.D., Scottish Rite Children's Hospital, Atlanta, Georgia.)

limit for this procedure is approximately 6 years old. The reader is referred to Pemberton's description of the procedure for technical details.[82] The procedure is technically demanding, requiring precise placement of pericapsular cuts extending back to the posterior branch of the triradiate cartilage.

This procedure has several advantages. Because it is incomplete, the osteotomy has inherent stability, with no pin fixation required. The posterior wall is left unrotated. A criticism of the Salter osteotomy is that the anterolateral coverage is achieved by rotation of the entire acetabulum, decreasing the posterior coverage. There are, however, disadvantages to the Pemberton procedure. The cut must be precise, otherwise the osteotomy may fracture the thin fragment distally or extend posteriorly into the triradiate cartilage, producing a growth arrest. Occasionally, the bone graft may be unstable in the osteotomy site and may require pin fixation. Avascular necrosis also has been reported.

Most importantly, by definition, the acetabulo-

plasty produces an acetabulofemoral incongruity. This change in acetabular configuration, even if toward a state of increased sphericity, is poorly tolerated by older children and produces cartilage damage. It is assumed that the younger child will be able to tolerate the change through plasticity of the hip and remodeling.

The single innominate osteotomy (Fig. 4–17) (Salter osteotomy or any of its modifications) can be performed from 18 months of age through adulthood. Because resistance to rotation through the symphysis pubis increases with age, the correction may be limited, and a double or triple osteotomy and possibly a shelf augmentation may be required. The indications for a Salter osteotomy are the same as those for a Pemberton procedure. For the patient younger than 6 years of age, the techniques are interchangeable to most surgeons, with the innominate osteotomy preferred by many because it is technically easier. The innominate osteotomy does not change the acetabular configuration, as the

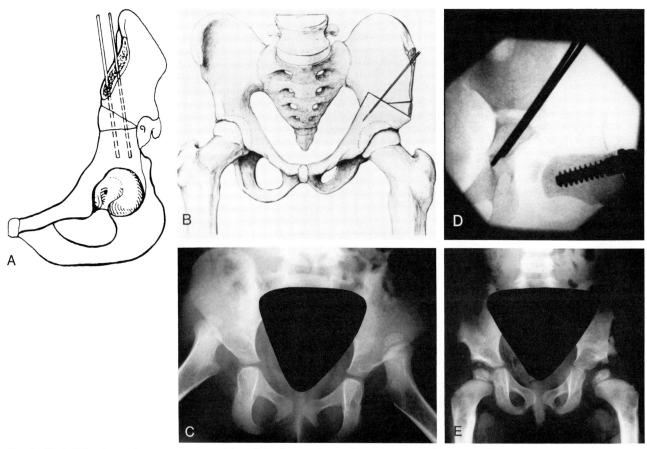

Fig. 4–17. **A.** Salter innominate osteotomy, with graft in the opening wedge and two Kirschner wires for fixation. There is no displacement of the osteotomy posteriorly in the sciatic notch. **B.** Kalamchi modification with posterior triangular notch and a single Kirschner wire for fixation. **C.** Preoperative radiograph of bilateral dislocated hips with acetabular dysplasia. **D.** Intraoperative radiograph showing varus femoral osteotomy. **E.** Postoperative radiograph after removal of instrumentation. (A, from Tachdjian MO (ed): Congenital Dislocation of the Hip. New York, Churchill Livingstone, 1982. B, from Kalamchi A: Modified Salter osteotomy. J Bone Joint Surg 64A:183–187, 1982.)

Pemberton procedure does, and it can be performed up to 15 years of age.

The osteotomy and rotation of the distal fragment produce an extension and adduction of the acetabulum, providing increased anterior and lateral coverage. Rab[86] predicts an upper limit of 25° of extension and 10° of adduction. This suggests that if a subluxated hip is still unstable in 25° of flexion and 10° of abduction, a Salter osteotomy would fail to rotate the acetabulum enough to provide stability in the neutral position.

In practice, how much rotation can be achieved? In the children in Barrett and colleagues' study,[7] who were 1.5 to 11.5 years old at surgery, the acetabular indices improved by 14 to 17°, with an average CE angle at followup examination of 27 to 30°. Kalamchi's modified Salter osteotomies improved the acetabular index by 13 to 28° (average, 17°), with the CE angle improving by 18 to 32°.[50] In Utterback and MacEwen's series,[111] however, the index improved only an average of 10°. Millis[72] reported an average improvement in the index of 20° until the age of 10 years, thereafter seeing only an 8° change; others also have seen improvement of only approximately 12°.

With these results, the Rab criteria appear conservative. Kumar and coworkers[59] suggest obtaining a concentric reduction of the hip by abduction in extension. If the abduction required is less than 25°, a single innominate osteotomy will probably be successful. In general, the indications for a Salter osteotomy are limited to an acetabular index of 40° or less (some suggest 30°), a CE angle of 10° or more, less than 20% uncoverage of the femoral head (if coxa magna), and concentric reduction with less than 25° of abduction.

The techniques are well described by Salter and Dubos[90] and Kalamchi.[50] The Salter osteotomy may lengthen the leg by 1 cm, a discrepancy that can be minimized by using the Kalamchi technique. The Salter innominate osteotomy is an opening wedge osteotomy. In the Kalamchi modification, a triangular notch is cut in the superior iliac fragment. The acetabular fragment is rotated and displaced into the notch. The Salter osteotomy is inherently unstable, often displacing posteriorly or medially. Pin fixation is required, with the attendant need for a second procedure to remove the pins and the risk of joint penetration by the pins. The Kalamchi notch provides some increased stability to displacement, although pin fixation is still needed. If it is unclear whether a Salter osteotomy will be sufficient in an older child, one can perform an ischial osteotomy, which is the first step of a Steel triple osteotomy. If the rotation is insufficient

when the superior innominate osteotomy is done, the pubic osteotomy can be performed. The Salter osteotomy carries a risk of avascular necrosis because of increased pressure of the rotated acetabulum on the femoral head. Occasionally, an intertrochanteric or subtrochanteric osteotomy may be indicated, either to normalize the pressures or to correct secondary femoral deformity and reestablish normal hip congruence.

If 25 to 45° of abduction is required to center the hip, a Salter osteotomy alone will not suffice. A shelf procedure added to an innominate osteotomy usually will add 10° to the final CE angle,[58,59] but for a shelf procedure to be effective, the CE angle formed by the acetabular rim alone must be greater than 0°. The usual solution is to use a more complex pelvic osteotomy. Many osteotomies have been described, such as the Sutherland double osteotomy,[103] the Steel triple osteotomy,[107] and various dial and spherical osteotomies. All of these osteotomies are technically demanding, with potentially severe complications.

For us, the triple innominate osteotomy has been the standard (Fig. 4–18). The degree of rotation is good, allowing mobilization in almost any direction to cover the head and to allow medialization of the acetabulum. There is no age limit. The greater freedom of movement of the inferior fragment, however, has its drawback in that the osteotomy is unstable and requires secure internal fixation. In Kumar and coworkers' patients with preoperative CE angles of 10° or less and an age range of 9 to 21 years, CE angles improved an average of 32° (range, 20° to 40°).[59] If more than 45° of abduction is needed preoperatively to center the head in extension, a triple innominate osteotomy is often adequate. Occasionally, a shelf could be used laterally, providing further coverage and an average improvement in the CE angle by an extra 10°. If extremes of abduction (50 to 60°) are needed, the femur is usually deformed, and a varus proximal femoral osteotomy is indicated to supplement the pelvic osteotomy.

Various shelf procedures[58,97] have been advocated to provide lateral coverage and to prevent superior migration of the femoral head. The shelf procedure alone is unreliable in improving the stability of a subluxated hip. It is helpful when coxa magna is present, because it is the only procedure that increases the volume of the acetabulum. Graft placement is critical, as a poorly buttressed graft or one placed too high will resorb because of lack of weight-bearing.

Combined procedures are still controversial, predominantly because of the risk of avascular necro-

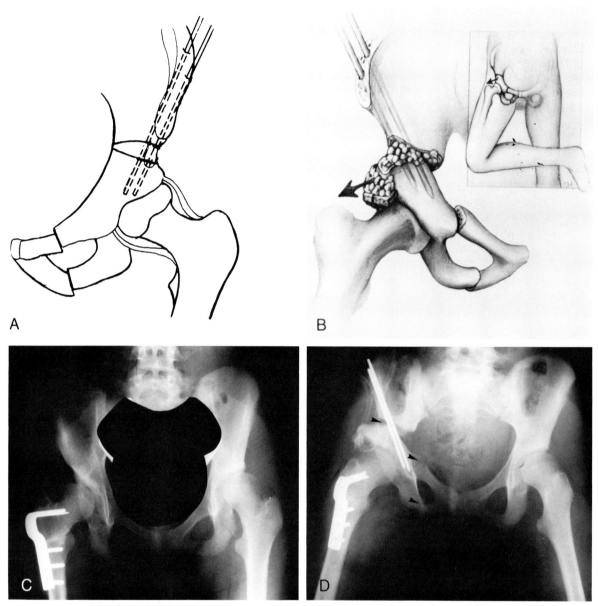

FIG. 4–18. **A.** Steel triple osteotomy **B.** Kumar's modification, with removal of a segment of the ischium to facilitate medial displacement. A shelf also has been added superiorly. **C.** Preoperative radiograph of an older child with sublaxation and severe dysplasia. **D.** A triple osteotomy with lateral shelf augmentation. The osteotomy sites are marked with arrowheads. (A, from Tachdjian MO (ed): Congenital Dislocation of the Hip. New York, Churchill Livingstone, 1982. B, from Kumar SJ, et al.: Triple osteotomy of the innominate bone for the treatment of congenital hip dysplasia. J Pediatr Orthop 6:393–398, 1986.)

sis. Obviously, it would be attractive to correct all deformities at the time of an open reduction in order to minimize the number of interventions. At times, a femoral shortening is indicated to obtain a reduction, just as some advocate a pelvic osteotomy to stabilize a reduction. However, Tonnis[107] reported an 8.4% incidence of avascular necrosis with open reduction alone, a 10.3% incidence with a concurrent pelvic osteotomy, and a 22.2% incidence with an intertrochanteric osteotomy, with or without a pelvic osteotomy. The reported incidence

of avascular necrosis is from 8 to 30% for concurrent open reductions and femoral shortening osteotomies.[15,18,57] In Mardam-Bey and MacEwen's series,[68] however, the incidence of necrosis was lower in those who had concurrent pelvic or femoral osteotomies than in those with open reduction alone. Presumably, the femoral shortening osteotomy decreased the pressure on the femoral head. According to some reports, intertrochanteric osteotomies pose a greater risk of avascular necrosis than do diaphyseal shortening osteotomies. We have noted osteopenia of the femoral head and neck after intertrochanteric osteotomies but no apparent increased incidence of avascular necrosis.

The only objective of an open reduction is a deep concentric reduction of the femoral head. In most cases, pelvic and femoral osteotomies can be done as separate procedures, delayed 6 months or more (probably up to 8 years of age for the pelvic osteotomy[67]). Concurrent pelvic and femoral osteotomies can be done at the time of open reduction but add significantly to the difficulty of the operation. Secondary procedures contribute to postoperative stiffness and, if poorly done, contribute to redislocation of the hip. Furthermore, they also increase the incidence of avascular necrosis. If a pelvic osteotomy is performed, the soft tissue tension must be released. When the femoral head is reduced under appropriate tension and is followed by a pelvic osteotomy, such as a Salter procedure, the distal displacement of the acetabulum may again make the tension on the reduced head unacceptably high. The adductor and psoas tenotomies that accompany innominate osteotomies are usually adequate, but a subtrochanteric femoral osteotomy may be needed. Although operating on both sides of the hip joint at the time of open reduction may be necessary on the rare occasion and may be done with relative safety by the experienced surgeon, in general it should be avoided if possible.

It already has been shown that all forms of treatment, closed or open reduction, are associated with avascular necrosis. The ischemic event has two basic patterns. It may involve the femoral ossific nucleus alone (Group 1) (Fig. 4–19), or it also may damage the physis (Figs. 4–20 to 4–22). These patterns have been described by Salter and coworkers,[91] Tonnis,[107] and Kalamchi and MacEwen.[51,52] The changes confined to the ossific nucleus alone may manifest themselves as a delay in the appearance of the center, failure of the ossific nucleus to grow over a year, or disappearance of the ossific nucleus after it has formed. The neck may widen, and the epiphysis may appear sclerotic, cystic, or fragmented. Usually, the ossific nucleus regains its spherical shape, with only a mild residual flattening of the head, or coxa magna.

The ischemic events that affect the growth plate result in more severe deformities. If the plate damage is limited to the lateral portion (Group 2) (Fig. 4–20), a short femoral neck with a progressive valgus deformity will occur. The femur is an average of 2.5 cm short. Although the head is normal, the valgus position may lead to subluxation and lateral uncovering. Theoretically, an isolated medial or posteromedial arrest can occur, leading to a short varus neck and trochanteric overgrowth. The more usual picture, which includes the medial plate, is a central arrest (Group 3) (Fig. 4–21). The growth of the neck is arrested, but the neck-shaft angle is unchanged. The femoral head is usually round, but because of incongruity or acetabular dysplasia, arthritis is likely. Trochanteric overgrowth and leg length inequality (average, 5 cm) can be a problem. The totally involved femur (Group 4) (Fig. 4–22)

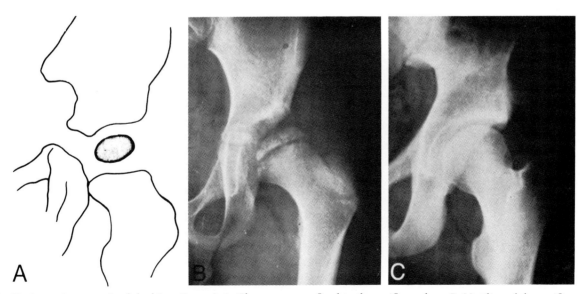

Fig. 4–19. Avascular necrosis of the hip—Group I. **A.** Changes are confined to the ossific nucleus. **B.** Mottling of the ossific nucleus, with fragmentation and flattening. **C.** At maturity, minimal deformity. (A, from Kalamchi A, MacEwen GD: Avascular necrosis following treatment of hip dislocation. J Bone Joint Surg 62A:876–888, 1980. B and C, from Tachdjian MO (ed): Congenital Dislocation of the Hip. New York, Churchill Livingstone, 1982.)

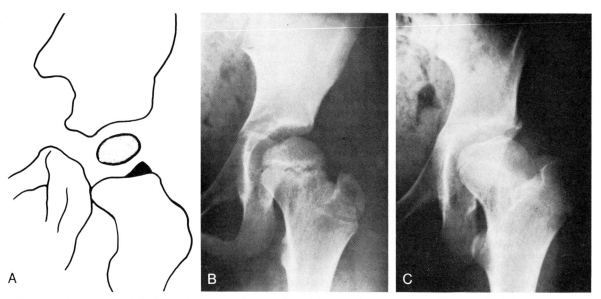

Fig. 4–20. Avascular necrosis of the hip—Group II. **A.** Lateral physeal damage. **B.** Irregularity of lateral half of physis. **C.** At maturity, short, valgus femoral neck. (A, from Kalamchi A, MacEwen GD: Avascular necrosis following treatment of hip dislocation. J Bone Joint Surg 62A:876–888, 1980. B and C, from Tachdjian MO (ed): Congenital Dislocation of the Hip. New York, Churchill Livingstone, 1982.)

has severe damage to both the head and physis. Residual femoral head deformity can be severe. The neck is in varus position, with significant overgrowth of the greater trochanter. Acetabular dysplasia is usual, with progressive deterioration of the joint and subluxation.

When greater trochanteric overgrowth appears likely, as with a central arrest or total involvement,

an epiphysiodesis of the greater trochanter[60] can prevent progressive overgrowth and abductor weakness. Although the upper age limit is cited to be 8 to 10 years, the earlier the recognition of the problem and treatment, the greater the likelihood that a more physiologic trochanter-head relationship can be preserved. Early in the course of the disease, the asymmetry of the metaphyseal growth arrest lines

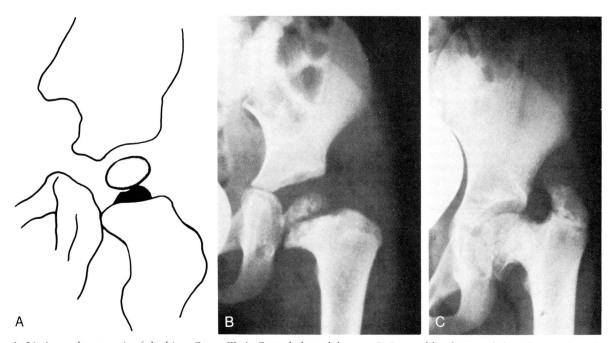

Fig. 4–21. Avascular necrosis of the hip—Group III. **A.** Central physeal damage. **B.** Femoral head is mottled, with metaphyseal irregularity adjacent to physis. **C.** At maturity, short neck with relative overgrowth of greater trochanter. (A, from Kalamchi A, MacEwen GD: Avascular necrosis following treatment of hip dislocation. J Bone Joint Surg 62A:876–888, 1980. B and C, from Tachdjian MO (ed): Congenital Dislocation of the Hip. New York, Churchill Livingstone, 1982.)

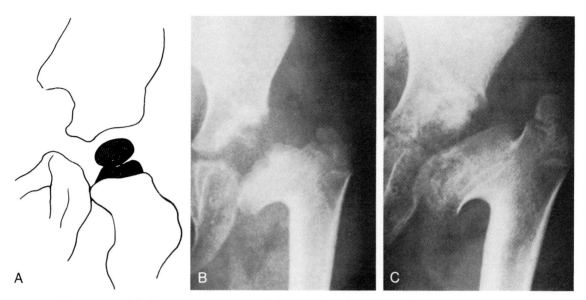

Fɪɢ. 4–22. Avascular necrosis of the hip—Group IV. **A.** Total damage to head and physis. **B.** Delayed ossification of the femoral head, with beaking and varus deformity of the neck. **C.** Later, physis is closed, with severe deformity of both head and neck. (A, from Kalamchi A, MacEwen GD: Avascular necrosis following treatment of hip dislocation. J Bone Joint Surg 62A:876–888, 1980. B and C, from Tachdjian MO (ed): Congenital Dislocation of the Hip. New York, Churchill Livingstone, 1982.)

seen radiographically has been suggested as an indicator of physeal damage.[78] At a later age, a greater trochanteric transfer is required to normalize this relationship and restore abductor strength.[29,56]

Salvage procedures are reserved for the patient who cannot be expected to achieve a normal hip.[42] In such a patient, the hip is irreversibly deformed or has cartilage damage. The joint surfaces are incongruous, and the head may be subluxated. Other procedures have failed, and the hip is often stiff from fibrous or osseous ankylosis. Symptoms of pain, limp, or fatigue may be present. Surgical intervention can be delayed until the onset of symptoms. The relief of pain by many of these procedures is dramatic but short-lived. Arthroplasty may be needed, but this eventuality should be delayed. Many will respond to the same nonoperative treatments used for coxarthrosis, such as antiinflammatory medications, weight reduction, abductor strengthening, cane ambulation, and restriction of activities.

When incongruity with coxarthrosis is a problem, varus or valgus intertrochanteric osteotomies to place the head in a position of greater congruity and the osteophytes in a weight-bearing position have been advocated.[12,69] Often, the procedure of choice is a valgus extension osteotomy. The varus osteotomy is rarely used, although it can be indicated for the valgus deformity associated with physeal arrest. Arthrodesis is also an option for the unilaterally involved hip.[96]

Salvage procedures on the pelvic side involve extending a bony shelf laterally over the superior portion of the capsule. This graft provides support to a weight-bearing portion of the head and redistributes the pressures of weight-bearing. The interposed capsule undergoes a metaplastic change to fibrocartilage.

The Chiari osteotomy[17,66] is a shelf procedure that both medializes the acetabulum and provides lateral osseous coverage of the femoral head (Fig. 4–23). This procedure can be used for any CE angle. The simple shelf procedure discussed previously is limited because the preoperative CE angle cannot be less than 0°. However, both work under the same principle. In the Chiari procedure, the cut in the pelvis must be close to the capsule, so that the displaced iliac fragment forms a roof in contact with the capsule. If the simple shelf or the Chiari roof is placed too high, the shelf will not be weight-bearing and will not act in a load-sharing configuration. If the CE angle is less than 0°, the simple shelf cannot bear the load and may fail. The indication for a Chiari osteotomy is pain with instability when the prerequisites for reconstructive procedures cannot be met. It is best if some hip motion is preserved, usually at least 60° of flexion and extension.

Although the Chiari procedure will not improve a Trendelenburg gait, the relief of pain is often dramatic. Pre-existing arthritis usually will downgrade the results, but approximately 90% of the patients can expect some improvement. How long the pain relief lasts is unknown, although it is probably limited to less than 15 to 20 years. This limitation in part is a reflection of the fact that the fibrocartilage

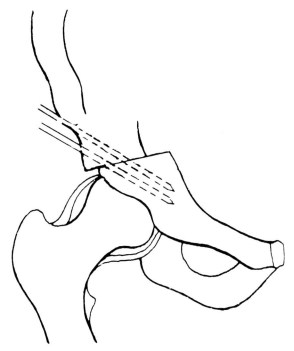

Fig. 4–23. Chiari pelvic osteotomy. The osteotomy is immediately superior to the capsule and slopes medially upward to allow for displacement of the fragments. (From Tachdjian MO (ed): Congenital Dislocation of the Hip. New York, Churchill Livingstone, 1982.)

in the weight-bearing portion of the hip has a shorter lifetime than hyaline cartilage.

References

1. Aarskog D, Stoa KF, Thorsen T: Urinary oestrogen secretion in newborn infants with congenital dysplasia of the hip joint. Acta Paediatr Scand, 55:394–397, 1966.
2. Andren L, Borglin NE: A disorder of oestrogen metabolism as a causal factor of congenital dislocation of the hip. Acta Orthop Scand, 30:169–171, 1960.
3. Artz TD, Levine DB, Lim WN, et al: Neonatal diagnosis, treatment and related factors of congenital dislocation of the hip. Clin Orthop, 110:112–136, 1975.
4. Arzimanoglu A: Treatment of congenital hip dislocation by muscle release, skeletal traction and closed reduction in older children. Clin Orthop, 119:70–75, 1976.
5. Barlow TG: Congenital dislocation of the hip in the newborn. Proc R Soc Med, 59:1103–1106, 1966.
6. Barlow TG: Early diagnosis and treatment of congenital dislocation of the hip. J Bone Joint Surg, 44B:292–301, 1962.
7. Barrett WP, Staheli LT, Chew DE: The effectiveness of the Salter innominate osteotomy in the treatment of congenital dislocation of the hip. J Bone Joint Surg, 68A:79–87, 1986.
8. Berkeley ME, Dickson JH, Cain TE, Donovan MM: Surgical therapy for congenital dislocation of the hip in patients who are 12 to 36 months old. J Bone Joint Surg, 66A:412–420, 1984.
9. Bialik V, Fishman J, Katzir J, Zeltzer M: Clinical assessment of hip instability in the newborn by an orthopedic surgeon and a pediatrician. J Pediatr Orthop, 6:703–705, 1986.
10. Bjerkreim I, Van Der Hagen CB: Congenital dislocation of the hip joint in Norway. Acta Orthop Scand (Suppl), 157:1–88, 1974.
11. Boal DKB, Schwentker EP: The infant hip: Assessment with real-time ultrasound. Radiology, 157:667–672, 1985.
12. Bombelli R: Osteoarthritis of the Hip. New York, Springer-Verlag, 1976.
13. Bos CFA, Slooff TJJH: Treatment of failed open reduction in congenital dislocation of the hip. Acta Orthop Scand, 55:531–535, 1984.
14. Bradley J, Wetherill M, Benson MKD: Splintage for congenital dislocation of the hip. J Bone Joint Surg, 69B:257–263, 1987.
15. Browne RS: The management of late diagnosed congenital dislocation and subluxation of the hip. J Bone Joint Surg, 61B:7–12, 1979.
16. Carter C, Wilkinson J: Persistent joint laxity and congenital dislocation of the hip. J Bone Joint Surg, 46B:40–45, 1964.
17. Chiari K: Iliac osteotomy in young adults. In The Hip. Proceedings of the 7th Meeting of the Hip Society. St. Louis, Mosby, pp. 260–277, 1979.
18. Coleman SS: Congenital Dysplasia and Dislocation of the Hip. St. Louis, Mosby, 1978.
19. Cooperman DR, Wallensten R, Stulberg SD: Acetabular dysplasia in the adult. Clin Orthop, 175:79–85, 1983.
20. Crawford A, Slovek R: Fate of the untreated congenitally dislocated hip. Orthop Trans, 2:73, 1978.
21. Czeizel A, Szentpetery J, Tusnady G, Vizkelety T: Two family studies on congenital dislocation of the hip after early orthopaedic screening in Hungary. J Med Genet, 12:125–130, 1975.
22. Czeizel A, Tusnady G, Vaczo G, Vizkelety T: The mechanism of genetic predisposition in congenital dislocation of the hip. J Med Genet, 12:121–124, 1975.
23. Dahlstrom H, Oberg L, Friberg S: Sonography in congenital dislocation of the hip. Acta Orthop Scand, 57:402–406, 1986.
24. Davies SJM, Walker G: Problems in the early recognition of hip dysplasia. J Bone Joint Surg, 66B:479–484, 1984.
25. Dunn PM: Perinatal observations on the etiology of congenital dislocation of the hip. Clin Orthop, 119:11–22, 1976.
26. Ferguson A: Primary open reduction of congenital dislocation of the hip using a median adductor approach. J Bone Joint Surg, 55A:671–689, 1973.
27. Finlay HVL, Maudsley RH, Busfield PI: Dislocatable hip and dislocated hip in the newborn infant. Br Med J, 4:377–381, 1967.
28. Finsterbush A, Pogrund H: The hypermobility syndrome. Musculoskeletal complaints in 100 consecutive cases of generalized joint hypermobility. Clin Orthop, 168:124–127, 1982.
29. Fletcher RR, Johnston CE: Greater trochanteric advancement for the treatment of coxa brevis associated with congenital dislocation of the hip. Orthopedics, 8:519–525, 1985.
30. Fredensborg N, Nilsson BE: Overdiagnosis of congenital dislocation of the hip. Clin Orthop, 119:89–92, 1976.
31. Gage JR, Winter RB: Avascular necrosis of the capital femoral epiphysis as a complication of closed reduction of congenital dislocation of the hip. J Bone Joint Surg, 54A:373–388, 1972.
32. Galasko CSB, Galley S, Menon TJ: Detection of congenital dislocation of the hip by an early screening program, with

particular reference to false negatives. Isr J Med Sci, 16:257–259, 1980.

33. Graf R: Classification of hip joint dysplasia by means of sonography. Arch Orthop Trauma Surg, 102:248–255, 1984.

34. Gross RH, Wisnefske M, Howard TC III, Hitch M: Infant hip screening. *In* The Hip. Proceedings of the 10th Meeting of the Hip Society. St. Louis, CV Mosby, pp. 50–67, 1982.

35. Haas SS, Epps CH, Adams JP: Normal ranges of hip motion in the newborn. Clin Orthop, 91:114–118, 1973.

36. Hall JE: Pelvic osteotomy in the early treatment of CDH. Adv Orthop Surg, 10:3–11, 1986.

37. Harcke HT, Grissom LE: Sonographic evaluation of the infant hip. Semin Ultrasound, CT, MR, 7:331–338, 1986.

38. Harris NH: Acetabular growth potential in congenital dislocation of the hip and some factors upon which it may depend. Clin Orthop, 119:99–106, 1976.

39. Harris NH, Lloyd-Roberts GC, Gallien R: Acetabular development in congenital dislocation of the hip. J Bone Joint Surg, 57B:46–52, 1975.

40. Harris WH: Etiology of osteoarthritis of the hip. Clin Orthop, 213:20–33, 1986.

41. Heikkila E: Congenital dislocation of the hip in Finland (an epidemiologic analysis of 1035 cases). Acta Orthop Scand, 55:125–129, 1984.

42. Herold HZ: Salvage operations for failure of previous surgery in congenital dislocation of the hip. Isr J Med Sci, 19:824–827, 1983.

43. Hiertonn T, James U: Congenital dislocation of the hip: experiences of early diagnosis and treatment. J Bone Joint Surg, 50B:542–545, 1968.

44. Ilfeld FW, Westin GW, Makin M: Missed or developmental dislocation of the hip. Clin Orthop, 203:276–281, 1986.

45. Ilfeld FW, Westin GW: "Missed" or late diagnosed congenital dislocation of the hip. Isr J Med Sci, 16:260–266, 1980.

46. Jensen BA, Reimann I, Fredensborg N: Collagen type III predominance in newborns with congenital dislocation of the hip. Acta Orthop Scand, 57:362–365, 1986.

47. Jessee EF, Owen DS, Sagar KB: The benign hypermobile joint syndrome. Arthritis Rheum, 23:1053–1056, 1980.

48. Jones D: An assessment of the value of examination of the hip in the newborn. J Bone Joint Surg, 59B:318–322, 1977.

49. Jones DA: Sub-capital coxa valga after varus osteotomy for congenital dislocation of the hip. J Bone Joint Surg, 59B:152–158, 1977.

50. Kalamchi A: Modified Salter osteotomy. J Bone Joint Surg, 64A:183–187, 1982.

51. Kalamchi A, MacEwen GD: Avascular necrosis following treatment of congenital dislocation of the hip. J Bone Joint Surg, 62A:876–887, 1980.

52. Kalamchi A, MacEwen GD: Classification of vascular changes following treatment of congenital dislocation of the hip. *In* Tachdjian MO (ed): Congenital Dislocation of the Hip. New York, Churchill Livingstone, pp. 705–711, 1982.

53. Kalamchi A, MacFarlane R III: The Pavlik harness: results in patients over three months of age. J Pediatr Orthop, 2:3–8, 1982.

54. Kalamchi A, Schmidt TL, MacEwen GD: Congenital dislocation of the hip. Open reduction by the medial approach. Clin Orthop, 169:127–132, 1982.

55. Kasser JR, Bowen JR, MacEwen GD: Varus derotation osteotomy in the treatment of persistent dysplasia in congenital dislocation of the hip. J Bone Joint Surg, 67A:195–202, 1985.

56. Kelikian AS, Tachdjian MO, Askew MJ, Jasty M: Greater tro-

chanteric advancement of the proximal femur: a clinical and biomechanical study. *In* The Hip. Proceedings of the 11th Meeting of the Hip Society. St. Louis, Mosby, pp. 77–105, 1983.

57. Klisic P, Jankovic L: Combined procedure of open reduction and shortening of the femur in treatment of congenital dislocation of the hips in older children. Clin Orthop, 119:60–69, 1976.

58. Kumar SJ, MacEwen GD: Shelf operation. *In* Tachdjian MO (ed): Congenital Dislocation of the Hip. New York, Churchill Livingstone, pp. 695–704, 1982.

59. Kumar SJ, MacEwen GD, Kumar ASJ: Triple osteotomy of the innominate bone for the treatment of congenital hip dysplasia. J Pediatr Orthop, 6:393–398, 1986.

60. Langenskiold A: Growth arrest of the greater trochanter for prevention of acquired coxa vara. *In* Tachdjian MO (ed): Congenital Dislocation of the Hip. New York, Churchill Livingstone, pp. 713–719, 1982.

61. Lehmann ECH, Street DG: Neonatal screening in Vancouver for congenital dislocation of the hip. Can Med Assoc J, 124:1003–1008, 1981.

62. Lindstrom JR, Ponseti IV, Wenger DR: Acetabular development after reduction in congenital dislocation of the hip. J Bone Joint Surg, 61A:112–118, 1979.

63. Lorenz A: Die sogenannte angeborene Huftverrenkung, ihre Pathologie und Therapie. *In* Deutsche Orthopaede. Herausgegeben von H. Gocht. Band 3. Stuttgart, F. Enke, 1920.

64. MacEwen GD, Bunnell WP, Ramsey PL: The hip. *In* Lovell W, Winter R (eds): Pediatric Orthopaedics, Vol 2. Philadelphia, JB Lippincott, pp. 703–735, 1986.

65. MacKenzie IG, Wilson JG: Problems encountered in the early diagnosis and management of CDH. J Bone Joint Surg, 63B:38–42, 1981.

66. Malefijt MCD, Hoogland T, Nielsen HKL: Chiari osteotomy in the treatment of congenital dislocation and subluxation of the hip. J Bone Joint Surg, 64A:996–1003, 1982.

67. Marafoti RL, Westin GW: Factors influencing the results of acetabuloplasty in children. J Bone Joint Surg, 62A:765–769, 1980.

68. Mardam-Bey TH, MacEwen GD: Congenital hip dislocation after walking age. J Pediatr Orthop, 2:478–486, 1982.

69. Maquet PGJ: Biomechanics of the Hip. New York, Springer-Verlag, pp. 76–133, 1985.

70. McKinnon B, Bosess MJ, Browning WH: Congenital dysplasia of the hip: the lax (subluxatable) newborn hip. J Pediatr Orthop, 4:422–426, 1984.

71. Milgram JW: Morphology of untreated bilateral congenital dislocation of the hips in a 74 year old man. Clin Orthop, 119:112–115, 1976.

72. Millis MB: Congenital hip dysplasia: Treatment from infancy to skeletal maturity. *In* Tronzo RG (ed): Surgery of the Hip Joint, 2nd Ed. New York, Springer-Verlag, p. 366, 1984.

73. Mitchell GP: Problems in the early diagnosis and management of congenital dislocation of the hip. J Bone Joint Surg, 54B:4–12, 1972.

74. Monk CJE, Dowd GSE: Monthly screening for the first 6 months of life for congenital hip dislocation. Isr J Med Sci, 16:253–256, 1980.

75. Morel G: The treatment of congenital dislocation and subluxation of the hip in the older child. Acta Orthop Scand, 46:364–399, 1975.

76. Mubarak S, Garfin S, Vance R, et al: Pitfalls in the use of the Pavlik harness for treatment of congenital dysplasia, sub-

luxation, and dislocation of the hip. J Bone Joint Surg, 63A:1239–1248, 1981.

77. Noble TC, Pullan CR, Craft AW, Leonard MA: Difficulties in diagnosing and managing congenital dislocation of the hip. Br Med J, 2:620–623, 1978.

78. O'Brien T, Millis MB, Griffin PP: The early identification and classification of growth disturbances of the proximal end of the femur. J Bone Joint Surg, 68A:970–980, 1986.

79. Ogden J: Dynamic pathobiology of congenital hip dysplasia. In Tachdjian MO (ed): Congenital Dislocation of the Hip. New York, Churchill Livingstone, pp. 93–144, 1982.

80. Palmen K: Preluxation of the hip joint. Acta Paediatr Scand 129(Suppl 50):1–71, 1961.

81. Paterson DC: The early diagnosis and treatment of congenital dislocation of the hip. Clin Orthop, 119:28–38, 1976.

82. Pemberton PA: Pericapsular osteotomy of the ilium for treatment of congenital subluxation and dislocation of the hip. J Bone Joint Surg, 47A:65–86, 1965.

83. Ponseti IV: Growth and development of the acetabulum in the normal child. J Bone Joint Surg, 60A:575–585, 1978.

84. Ponseti IV: Morphology of the acetabulum in congenital dislocation of the hip. J Bone Joint Surg, 60A:586–599, 1978.

85. Powell EN, Gerratana FJ, Gage JR: Open reduction for congenital hip dislocation: the risk of avascular necrosis with three different approaches. J Pediatr Orthop, 6:127–132, 1986.

86. Rab GT: Biomechanical aspects of Salter osteotomy. Clin Orthop, 132:82–87, 1978.

87. Race C, Herring JA: Congenital dislocation of the hip: an evaluation of closed reduction. J Pediatr Orthop, 3:166–172, 1983.

88. Ramsey P, Lasser S, MacEwen GD: Congenital dislocation of the hip: Use of the Pavlik harness in the child during the first six months of life. J Bone Joint Surg, 58A:1000–1004, 1976.

89. Renshaw TS: Inadequate reduction of congenital dislocation of the hip. J Bone Joint Surg, 63A:1114–1121, 1981.

90. Salter RB, Dubos J-P: The first fifteen years' personal experience with innominate osteotomy in the treatment of congenital dislocation and subluxation of the hip. Clin Orthop, 98:72–103, 1974.

91. Salter RB, Kostuik J, Dallas S: Avascular necrosis of the femoral head as a complication of treatment for congenital dislocation of the hip in young children. Can J Surg, 12:44–60, 1969.

92. Salter RB, Kostuik J, Schatzker J: Experimental dysplasia of the hip and its reversibility in newborn pigs. J Bone Joint Surg, 45A:1781, 1963.

93. Scaglietti O, Calandriello B: Open reduction of congenital dislocation of the hip. J Bone Joint Surg, 44B:257–283, 1962.

94. Schoenecker PL, Strecker WB: Congenital dislocation of the hip in children. Comparison of the effects of femoral shortening and of skeletal traction in treatment. J Bone Joint Surg, 66A:21–27, 1984.

95. Severin E: Contribution to the knowledge of congenital dislocation of the hip joint: late results of closed reduction and arthrographic studies of recent cases. Acta Chir Scand 84(Suppl 63):1–142, 1941.

96. Sponseller PD, McBeath AA, Perpich M: Hip arthrodesis in young patients: a long-term follow-up study. J Bone Joint Surg, 66A:853–859, 1984.

97. Staheli LT: Slotted acetabular augmentation. J Pediatr Orthop, 1:321–327, 1981.

98. Staheli LT, Dion M, Tuell JI: The effect of the inverted limbus on closed management of congenital hip dislocation. Clin Orthop, 137:163–166, 1978.

99. Stanisavljevic S: Etiology of congenital hip pathology. In Tachdjian MO (ed): Congenital Dislocation of the Hip. New York, Churchill Livingstone, pp. 27–33, 1982.

100. Stanisavljevic S, Mitchell CL: Congenital dysplasia, subluxation, and dislocation of the hip in stillborn and newborn infants. J Bone Joint Surg, 45A:1147–1158, 1963.

101. Steel HH: Triple osteotomy of the innominate bone. Clin Orthop, 122:116–127, 1977.

102. Stulberg SD, Harris WH: Acetabular dysplasia and development of osteoarthritis of the hip. In The Hip. Proceedings of the Hip Society. St. Louis, CV Mosby, p. 82, 1974.

103. Sutherland DH, Greenfield R: Double innominate osteotomy. J Bone Joint Surg, 59A:1082–1091, 1977.

104. Szoke N, Kuhl L, Heinrichs J: Ultrasound examination in the diagnosis of congenital hip dysplasia of newborns. J Pediatr Orthop, 8:12–16, 1988.

105. Thieme WT, Wynne-Davies R, Blair HAF, et al: Clinical examination and urinary oestrogen assays in newborn children with congenital dislocation of the hip. J Bone Joint Surg, 50B:546–550, 1968.

106. Tonnis D: Congenital Dysplasia and Dislocation of the Hip in Children and Adults. New York, Springer-Verlag, 1987.

107. Tonnis D: Congenital Hip Dislocation: Avascular Necrosis. New York, Thieme-Stratton, Inc, 1982.

108. Tonnis D: Normal values of the hip joint for the evaluation of x-rays in children and adults. Clin Orthop, 119:39–47, 1976.

109. Tonnis D, Behrens K, Tscharani F: A modified technique of the triple pelvic osteotomy: Early results. J Pediatr Orthop, 1:241–249, 1981.

110. Tredwell SJ, Bell HM: Efficacy of neonatal hip examination. J Pediatr Orthop, 1:61–65, 1981.

111. Utterback TD, MacEwen GD: Comparison of pelvic osteotomies for the surgical correction of the congenital hip. Clin Orthop, 98:104–110, 1974.

112. von Rosen S: Early diagnosis and treatment of congenital hip luxation. Acta Orthop Scand, 29:164, 1960.

113. von Rosen S: Further experience with congenital dislocation of the hip in the newborn. J Bone Joint Surg, 50B:538–541, 1968.

114. Voutsinas SA, MacEwen GD, Boos ML: Home traction in the management of congenital dislocation of the hip. Arch Orthop Trauma Surg 102:135–140, 1984.

115. Wedge JH, Wasylenko MJ: The natural history of congenital disease of the hip. J Bone Joint Surg, 61B:334–338, 1979.

116. Weiner DS, Hoyt WA, O'Dell HW: Congenital dislocation of the hip. The relationship of premanipulation traction and age to avascular necrosis of the femoral head. J Bone Joint Surg, 59A:306–311, 1977.

117. Weinstein SL, Ponseti IV: Congenital dislocation of the hip: open reduction through a medial approach. J Bone Joint Surg, 61A:119–124, 1979.

118. Westin GW: Acetabular development after closed or open reduction. Presented at the Fall Seminar, Alfred I. duPont Institute, Wilmington, DE, October 22, 1983.

119. Wiberg G: Shelf operation in congenital dysplasia of the acetabulum and in subluxation and dislocation of the hip. J Bone Joint Surg, 35A:65–80, 1953.

120. Wiberg G: Studies on dysplastic acetabula and congenital subluxation of the hip joint. Acta Chir Scand (Suppl), 83:58, 1939.

121. WILKINSON JA: A post-natal survey for congenital displacement of the hip. J Bone Joint Surg, 54B:40–49, 1972.

122. WILKINSON JA: Congenital Displacement of the Hip Joint. New York, Springer-Verlag, 1985.

123. WILKINSON JA: Prime factors in the etiology of congenital dislocation of the hip. J Bone Joint Surg, 45B:268–283, 1963.

124. WILLIAMSON J: Difficulties of early diagnosis and treatment of congenital dislocation of the hip in Northern Ireland. J Bone Joint Surg, 54B:13–17, 1972.

125. WYNNE-DAVIES R: A family study of neonatal and late-diagnosis congenital dislocation of the hip. J Med Genet, 7:315–333, 1970.

126. WYNNE-DAVIES R: Acetabular dysplasia and familial joint laxity: two etiologic factors in congenital dislocation of the hip. J Bone Joint Surg, 52B:704–716, 1970.

127. ZIONTS LE, MACEWEN GD: Treatment of congenital dislocation of the hip in children between the ages of one and three years. J Bone Joint Surg, 68A:829–846, 1986.

CHAPTER FIVE

Legg-Calve-Perthes Disease

J. RICHARD BOWEN
GARY MILLER

Legg-Calve-Perthes disease (Perthes' disease) is a pathologic condition of the immature hip caused by necrosis of the capital femoral bony epiphysis, and frequently, of the capital femoral physis. As the necrotic bone of the femoral epiphysis is replaced by living bone, the femoral head may deform. In three separate studies in 1910, Legg,[39] Calve,[10] and Perthes[49] distinguished this condition from tuberculosis, but it was Waldenstrom[62–65] who outlined the clinical stages of the disease process. Based on femoral head biopsies, Phemister[50] showed the histology of this disease to be bone necrosis. More recently, Catterall[13] reported the natural history and described prognostic factors.

The incidence of Perthes' disease varies from 1 in 12,500 in England[1] and 1 in 4750 in South Wales[27] to 1 in 1400 in British Columbia[22] and 1 in 1200 in Massachusetts.[44] The age at onset of symptoms ranges from 2 years to maturity; however, the most common age at onset is between 4 and 8 years.[4,13] The ratio of females to males is 1:4. Left and right hip involvement is almost equal, and bilateral involvement occurs in approximately 15% of affected children. Premature closure of the proximal femoral physis occurs in approximately 21% of affected hips.[6]

terosuperior femoral neck to enter the femoral epiphysis.[48] These vessels enter the femoral head to supply the bony epiphysis and the growth plate of the femoral neck.[61] However, vascular occlusion does not explain many of the observations reported in Perthes' disease. Some patients have delayed skeletal bone age,[38] short stature,[19,66] high incidence of breech presentation, increased incidence of genitourinary abnormality,[12] pyloric stenosis, congenital heart disease,[25] retarded growth in the distal segments of the extremities, and abnormal hormonal control of growth.[7,28,44] There is a reported predominance in patients born into low-income families and to parents whose ages are above the average childbearing age.[66] Recent studies have demonstrated elevated levels of somatomedin in the serum of young boys with Perthes' disease.[8] More recently, Mackenzie and colleagues have described femoral head necrosis in patients with multiple epiphyseal dysplasia.[40] It is possible that patients who develop Perthes' disease have a developmental or growth defect that predisposes the femoral head to infarction. Perthes' disease must be differentiated from a variety of clinical diseases that have similar clinical and radiographic appearances (Table 5-1).

Cause

The cause of the entire or partial necrosis of the bony epiphysis of the immature femoral head remains obscure. Proposed possible causes include endocrine disturbance, trauma, inflammation, inadequate nutrition, and genetic factors.[8,17,22,69] The most popular theory is occlusion of the arterial supply to the epiphysis with multiple episodes of infarction.[36,56] The normal blood supply to the femoral head arises from the profunda femoris artery, which branches to the medial femoral circumflex artery that arcs posteriorly to the hip joint and ascends the lateral retinacular arteries along the pos-

Clinical Features

Early in the course of Perthes' disease, the most common symptoms are pain and stiffness in the involved hip. The onset is generally insidious, and symptoms are enhanced by strenuous exercise. Frequently, the pain occurs in the groin area and radiates to the anteromedial area of the thigh; occasionally, the pain is referred to the knee area. Up to 12% of children with Perthes' disease have episodes of toxic synovitis of the hip (irritable hip syndrome).[16] Early signs of Perthes' disease include limp, abnormal hip motion, and muscle atrophy. The involved hip generally has decreased internal

TABLE 5–1. *Differential Diagnosis of Perthes' Disease*

1. Hypothyroidism*
2. Multiple epiphyseal dysplasia*
3. Slipped capital femoral epiphysis
4. Hemaglobinopathies (e.g., sickle-cell disease)
5. Tumors (e.g., osteoid osteoma, lymphoma, eosinophilic granuloma, pigmented villonodular synovitis, and chrondroblastoma)
6. Gaucher's disease
7. Infections (e.g., rheumatic fever, rheumatologic diseases, and tuberculosis)
8. Transient synovitis of the hip (toxic synovitis, irritable hip syndrome)

*Hypothyroidism and multiple epiphyseal dysplasia classically occur with bilateral hip involvement, whereas the remaining conditions occur as unilateral hip disease.

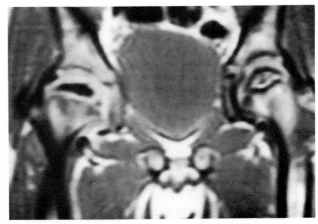

FIG. 5–1. Magnetic resonance image (T-weighted) of a right hip with early avascular necrosis.

rotation, as shown by the leg-roll test; a mild flexion contracture, as shown by the Thomas test; and limited abduction. The limp is usually antalgic; therefore, the pelvis dips on the involved side, and the stride is short. Some degree of muscle atrophy usually is observed in the thigh and buttock areas.

Although most patients present relatively early in the disease course, this is not always the case. In a series conducted at the Alfred I. duPont Institute, Wilmington, DE, 75% of patients presented during the early phases of necrosis or fragmentation, 18% presented during the reossification stage, and 7% presented at or near skeletal maturity.[4] The most common signs and symptoms of patients presenting later in the disease course include pain in the hip area, functional limitations of activities, and a limp that may be of the antalgic, stiff-hip, short-leg, or Trendelenburg type.

Differential Diagnosis

If a patient presents with the signs and symptoms of Perthes' disease but has normal radiographs, toxic synovitis must be considered. In toxic synovitis, radiographic signs of increased inferomedial joint space and lateral bulging of the capsule occur in 50% of the patients.[18] However, if the white blood cell count and sedimentation rate are significantly elevated, the possibility of infection should be considered. The hip should be aspirated to obtain cultures if infection is suspected, and an arthrogram should be performed in order to verify the adequacy of aspiration. When the diagnosis cannot be discerned clearly, a technetium polyphosphate bone scan or magnetic resonance image generally can show avascularity seen in Perthes' disease (Fig. 5–1).[15,60] Recently, it has been shown by magnetic resonance imaging (MRI) and technetium polyphosphate scanning that some patients

with multiple epiphyseal dysplasia[40] or trichorhinophalangeal syndrome[14] develop necrosis of the femoral capital epiphysis.

Radiographic and Pathologic Findings

Phemister[50] reported the primary pathologic process to be bone necrosis of the capital femoral epiphysis with an intact overlying articular cartilage. The infarction may also involve the proximal capital femoral physis, resulting in premature physeal closure. Waldenstrom divided the natural history of Perthes' disease into four radiographic stages: necrosis, fragmentation (resorption), reossification, and remodeling (Fig. 5–2).[62–65] The time duration for each stage varies among patients, but the average time is 5.7 months for the necrotic stage, 7.0 months for the fragmentation stage, and 20 to 38 months for the reossification stage. The remodeling stage continues until skeletal maturity.[4]

Necrotic Stage

Radiographically, the earliest sign of Perthes' disease may be the bulging of the hip capsule secondary to synovitis; however, this is rarely seen. Occasionally, a small, round osteopenic area develops medially in the metaphysis of the femoral neck. One of the more commonly seen early radiographic changes consists of a small capital epiphysis and the appearance of mild hip subluxation (Waldenstrom's sign) (Fig. 5–3).[64] The bony epiphysis, and possibly the capital femoral growth plate, are infarcted early in the disease process; however, the articular cartilage, which receives its nutrition from synovial fluid, continues to grow.[11] The articular cartilage growth is asymmetric with an increased thickness on the medial and lateral aspects

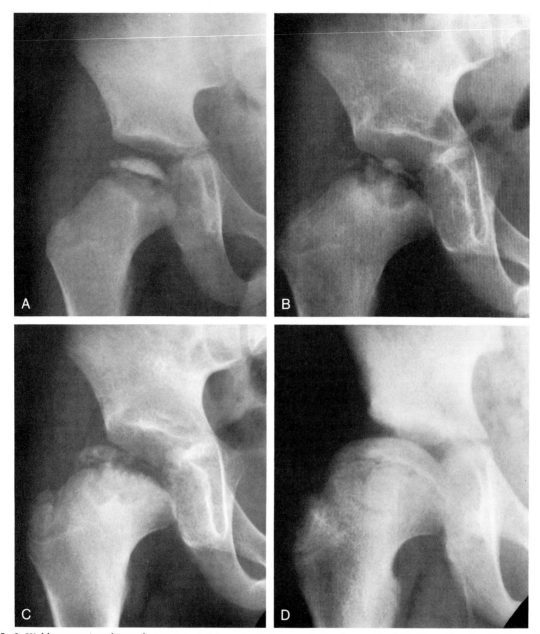

Fɪɢ. 5–2. Waldenstrom's radiographic stages. **A.** Necrosis. **B.** Fragmentation (resorption). **C.** Reossification. **D.** Remodeling.

of the femoral head.[21] This asymmetric growth results in the appearance of lateral subluxation (Waldenstrom's sign).[62–65] Subsequently, the necrotic bone of the femoral epiphysis becomes radiopaque because of relative osteopenia of the surrounding viable bone, increased calcification of the necrotic bone, and apposition of new bone on necrotic trabeculae (creeping substitution).[50] Theoretically, it is believed that the initial infarction heals by creeping substitution, in which the woven bone grows over the necrotic lamellar bone. Subsequently, repetitive infarctions result in the process repeating itself several times, creating an increase in the trabecular thickness.[36,43] Histologically, areas of fatty replace-

ment of marrow and, occasionally, areas of cellular infiltrates of lymphocytes and plasma cells develop under the growth plate and adjacent to areas of epiphyseal necrosis. These metaphyseal changes result in radiographically apparent osteopenia under the growth plate. Fibrocartilaginous areas with reactive bony borders extend into the metaphysis below the physis and radiographically give the appearance of a metaphyseal cyst (Fig. 5–4).[51]

The avascular epiphyseal bone becomes unable to support the mechanical stress, and vertical compression of the trabeculae occurs. The bony femoral epiphysis is reduced in height, and a subchondral fracture is seen radiographically as a lucent zone

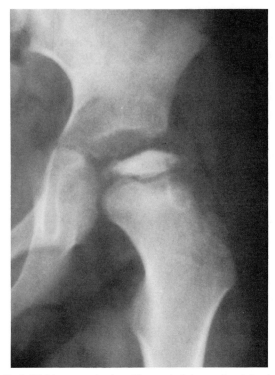

FIG. 5–3. Waldenstrom's sign. The capital femoral epiphysis appears smaller and the joint appears laterally subluxated because of asymmetric growth of the cartilage.

(crescent sign) (Fig. 5–5).[9,55] Further collapse may result in epiphyseal extrusion from the hip joint that generally occurs in an anterolateral direction.

Fragmentation Stage (Resorption Stage)

Osteoclasts subsequently resorb the necrotic, crushed trabeculae of bone, and fibrocartilage fills in the resorbed area (Fig. 5–2B).[43] The osteoclastic resorption generally begins at the periphery of the epiphysis and proceeds in an irregular fashion, but, occasionally, marked lysis of bone occurs at the su-

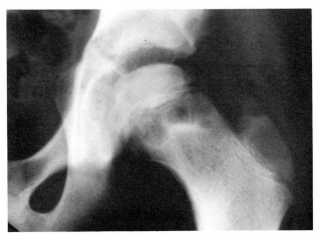

FIG. 5–4. Metaphyseal osteopenia and cysts.

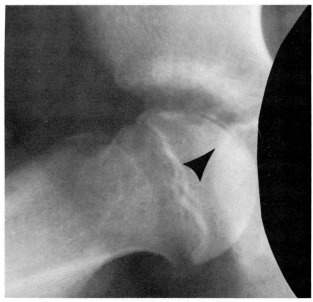

FIG. 5–5. Crescent sign. Lucent zone produced by a subchondral fracture.

perolateral portion of the femoral neck (Gage's sign) (Fig. 5–6). The extruded fibrocartilage and articular cartilage may calcify or ossify lateral to the acetabulum, given the radiographic appearance of femoral head extrusion. In the late necrotic stage and throughout the entire resorption stage, the femoral epiphysis may deform, with associated femoral neck widening (Fig. 5–7).

Reossification Stage

Following resorption of the necrotic trabeculae, an ingrowth of fibrovascular tissue occurs and sub-

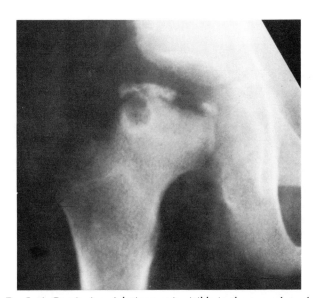

FIG. 5–6. Gage's sign. A lytic zone is visible in the superolateral femoral neck.

Remodeling Stage

Once the necrotic epiphysis has reossified, the femoral head continues to remodel until the patient reaches skeletal maturity (Fig. 5–2D). Infarction and subsequent ossification across the proximal femoral growth plate may impair later growth of the femoral neck, resulting in a shortened extremity and relative overgrowth of the greater trochanter (coxa brevis) (Fig. 5–8). In some hips with a deformed femoral head, acetabular growth over several years may result in a more congruent hip joint.

Deformities at Maturity

In skeletally mature patients who have had Perthes' disease, four patterns of deformity exist: coxa magna, coxa brevis, coxa irregularis, and osteochondritis dissecans (Fig. 5–9). In Perthes' disease, these four patterns of deformities occur in 58, 21, 18 and 3% of cases, respectively.[4]

Coxa Magna (congruent joint, enlarged femoral head)

Coxa magna is a hip deformity characterized by enlargement of the femoral head, widening of the femoral neck, and varying degrees of depression of epiphyseal height (Fig. 5–10). The femoral head may be spherical or oval, but the hip joint is congruent, with little tendency toward early degenerative joint disease.[45] Clinically, patients with spherical coxa magna are asymptomatic and have full

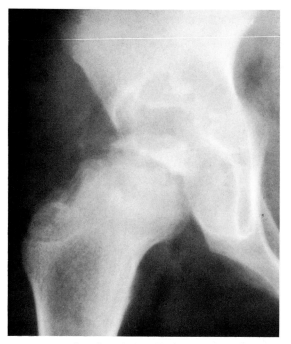

FIG. 5–7. Femoral neck widening during early Perthes' disease.

sequently ossifies (Fig. 5–2C). Occasionally, ossification occurs through the growth plate, which may create a bony bridge between the epiphysis and metaphysis, resulting in a growth arrest of the proximal capital femoral physis. The reossification generally progresses until the entire necrotic epiphysis is reconstituted, but, occasionally, small areas of the epiphysis fail to reossify by maturity, resulting in residual osteochondral defects (osteochondritis dissecans).

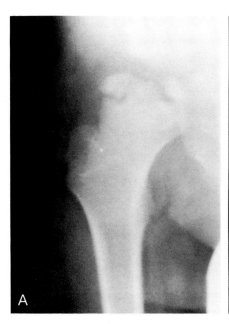

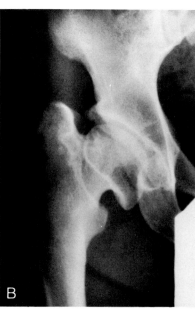

FIG. 5–8. Coxa brevis. Symmetric or central premature physeal closure begins as a bony bridge at the center of the physis, resulting in a shortened femoral neck with relative trochanteric overgrowth. **A.** Radiograph at adolescence. **B.** Radiograph at maturity.

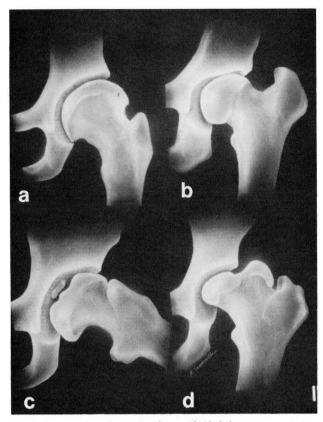

FIG. 5-9. Paintings depicting the residual deformities at maturity often noted in Perthes' disease. **a.** Coxa magna. **b.** Coxa brevis. **c.** Osteochondritis dissecans. **d.** Coxa irregularis. (From Abrams JS, Bowen JR: Legg-calve-perthes disease. Contemp Orthop 10:27–39, 1985.)

functional range of motion of the hip, whereas patients with oval coxa magna have excellent flexion and extension of the hip joint, but limited rotation and abduction.

Coxa Brevis

Coxa brevis is characterized by a shortened femoral neck length and a relative overgrowth of the greater trochanter in relation to the femoral head (Fig. 5–8). There is no true overgrowth of the greater trochanter, but the lack of femoral neck growth results in a shortened head-neck distance in relation to the height of the greater trochanter.[2,37] Coxa brevis occurs as a result of premature arrest of the proximal femoral physis.[6,37] The premature physeal closure may occur early in the remodeling stage, whereas in other cases, the growth plate remains radiographically visible for years prior to eventual premature closure. This premature physeal closure results in varying degrees of severity of deformity.[58]

Two patterns of premature physeal closure exist:

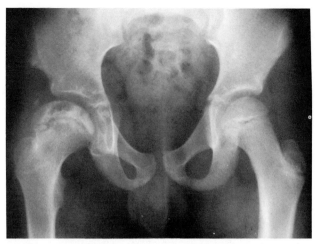

FIG. 5-10. Coxa magna. Most hips with Perthes' disease are somewhat enlarged at completion of healing.

symmetric and asymmetric. The most common pattern is symmetric closure, in which a bony bridge initially begins at the center of the physis and then progresses symmetrically to the periphery (Fig. 5–8). The symmetric physeal closure pattern occasionally can be recognized as early as the fragmentation phase, in which a central metaphyseal bony beak projects across the physis into the epiphysis.[6] Ossification of the central portion of the physis may take several years; at skeletal maturity, the femoral neck is short, and the neck-shaft angle remains normal, with relative overgrowth of the greater trochanter.

In the course of asymmetric premature physeal closure, a bony bridge forms asymmetrically near the peripheral margin of the physis. With subsequent growth, normal areas of the physis continue to grow and tilt the femoral head. The most common area of asymmetric premature physeal closure is at the lateral or anterolateral peripheral margin of the physis (Fig. 5–11).[6] Subsequent growth of the medial area of the physis tilts the femoral head laterally or anterolaterally, and the femoral head becomes oval. The lateral margin of the acetabulum becomes deficient, the medial joint space widens, and the greater trochanter continues to grow normally, resulting in a relative overgrowth of the shortened head and neck.

Coxa Irregularis (incongruent, enlarged femoral head)

Coxa irregularis (coxa magna) is caused by collapse and lateral extrusion of the femoral head, and lack of acetabular remodeling to the shape of the deformed femoral head, resulting in hip joint incon-

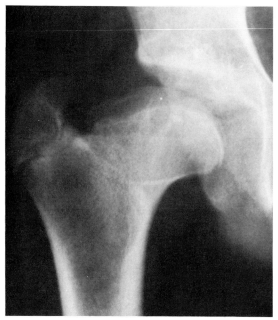

Fig. 5–11. Asymmetric physeal closure starts as a bony bridge at the anterolateral margin of the physis. Normal growth of the remaining physis tilts the femoral head.

gruency (Fig. 5–12).[70] During hip motion, the deformed femoral head impinges on the acetabulum, predisposing the hip to premature degenerative joint disease. The most obvious impingement occurs when the lower limb is abducted and the anterolateral corner of the acetabulum impinges against the superolateral side of the deformed femoral head forming a trench or groove (hinge abduction) (Fig. 5–13).

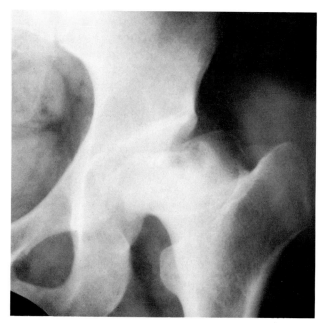

Fig. 5–12. Coxa irregularis. This hip has marked lateral extrusion and a flattened femoral head.

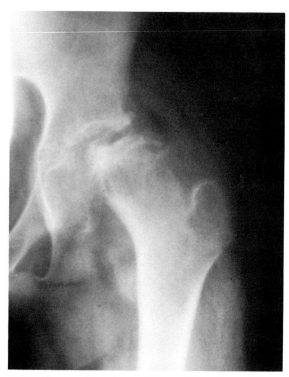

Fig. 5–13. Extreme lateral extrusion results in hinge abduction.

Osteochondritis Dissecans

Incomplete reossification of the infarcted epiphysis by maturity results in osteochondritis dissecans (Fig. 5–14). The area of osteochondritis dissecans may remain asymptomatic but, occasionally, may result in locking of the hip joint, "giving out" symptoms, or vague hip pain (internal derangement of the hip). Osteochondritis dissecans occurs most frequently in patients who develop Perthes' disease at an older age, and the area of osteochondritis dissecans is frequently in the weight-bearing portion of the femoral head.[48]

Prognosis

Several authors evaluating the long-term results of Perthes' disease have reported sphericity of the femoral head and joint congruity at maturity as important factors in determining prognosis.[24,32,42] Mose[45,46] developed a method of measuring sphericity of the weight-bearing surface of the femoral head by superimposing a transparent template with concentric circles 2 mm apart over radiographs (Fig. 5–15). If the weight-bearing surface of the femoral head varied from the concentric circles on the template by more than 2 mm, the results were considered poor. In general, patients who have a spherical femoral head at maturity tend to have an excellent long-term prognosis, whereas patients with signifi-

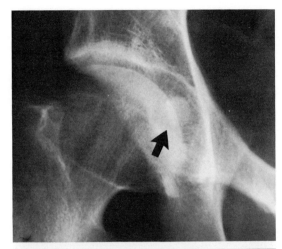

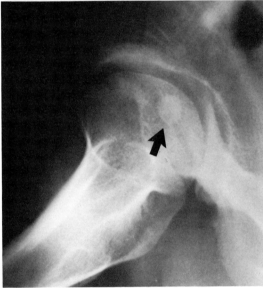

Fig. 5–14. Osteochondritis dissecans (loose body) is the result of incomplete reossification.

cant deformity and incongruity of the femoral head are predisposed to premature degenerative osteoarthritis of the hip.[42] Factors that have the greatest prognostic significance in developing a deformity of the femoral head in Perthes' disease are (1) age at onset of the disease; (2) the extent of necrosis of the capital epiphysis; (3) premature closure of the capital femoral physis and (4) persistent stiffness of the hip with deformity of the femoral head.[4,13]

Children less than 6 years of age at the onset of symptoms tend to have a good prognosis, whereas those with onset of symptoms at an age greater than 9 years tend to have a poor prognosis.[31] Younger patients appear to have less deformity of the femoral epiphysis and have a greater potential for remodeling any deformity before reaching maturity. Using the Mose method, it has been shown that only 15% of the patients younger than 6 years

of age at onset of symptoms will have poor results, whereas 70% of those greater than 9 years of age will tend to have poor results.[4,6]

The extent of epiphyseal necrosis also affects prognosis. In separate studies, Ralston[52] and O'Garra[47] reported a partial necrosis of the femoral epiphysis, and Catterall[13] divided the extent of epiphyseal necrosis into four categories (Table 5–2).

Catterall's classification frequently is used. However, it is difficult to apply, especially early in the disease process, and some investigators believe that not enough distinction is made between each group to justify the classification.[26] Salter and Thompson[55] classified the extent of epiphyseal necrosis into two groups: Group A, with less than 50% of the epiphysis involved, and Group B, with greater than 50% of the epiphysis involved. In the authors' evaluation of patients seen at the Alfred I. duPont Institute, there appear to be three distinct prognostic groups. Group A patients with less than 50% necrosis of the epiphysis generally have a good prognosis. Group B patients with between 50 and 100% epiphyseal necrosis tend to have a better prognosis than Group C patients, who have total epiphyseal necrosis (Fig. 5–16).[4] Premature closure of the capital femoral physis is associated with a high percentage of unsatisfactory results.[6] Fifty-seven percent of the patients with symmetric premature closure of the growth plate had a nonspherical femoral head at maturity, whereas 68% of the patients with asymmetric closure of the growth plate had a nonspherical femoral head at maturity. Patients with premature closure of the capital femoral physis frequently had leg-length discrepancies, a Trendelenburg gait, and occasional pain. Patients who have persistent stiffness of the hip and significant loss of sphericity of the femoral head after intensive therapy tend to have poor results. Extrusion

Table 5–2. *Catterall's Classification of Perthes' Disease**

Group I	Necrosis of the anterior part of the epiphysis
	No metaphyseal reaction
	No subchondral fracture line or sequestrum
Group II	Necrosis larger than Group I
	Sequestrum present
	Anterolateral metaphyseal reaction
	Subchondral fracture present
	Viable bone over growth plate
Group III	Large sequestrum
	Diffuse metaphyseal reaction
	Subchondral fracture extends to posterior half
	of the epiphysis
Group IV	Whole head necrosis

*Adapted from Catterall, A.: The natural history of Perthes' disease. J Bone Joint Surg, 53B:37–53, 1971.

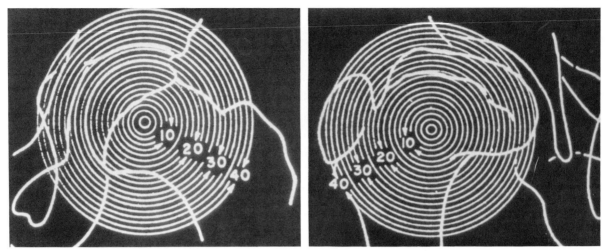

Fɪɢ. 5–15. The Mose template is superimposed over the femoral head. A spherical femoral head indicates a good result. A nonspherical femoral head indicates a poor result.

of the proximal femoral epiphysis, flattening of the femoral head, and incongruity of the joint surfaces may restrict motion as the femoral head abuts the acetabulum on abduction (hinge abduction) (Fig. 5–13). If the deformed femoral head cannot be repositioned into the acetabulum to allow remodeling, or if joint incongruity persists into adult life, poor prognosis may be anticipated.[23,42,59] Catterall[13] has listed several radiographic signs that indicate a risk of developing femoral head deformity including subluxation, lateral calcification, significant metaphyseal reaction, and Gage's sign.

Treatment

The goal of treatment in Perthes' disease is to minimize deformity of the femoral head and acetabulum. Prolonged bed rest, bed rest with immobilization, bed rest with traction, and non-weight-bearing without containment have all been proven unsatisfactory methods of treatment. Currently, popular methods of treatment include maintaining a full range of motion of the hip and containing the femoral head within the acetabulum. In containment treatment, the normally shaped acetabulum is used as a mold to prevent deformity of the femoral head (Fig. 5–17).[35] The weight-bearing surface femoral head can be directed into the depths of the acetabulum in one of the following ways: (1) positioning the leg in internal rotation and abduction; (2) positioning the leg in flexion and abduction; (3) redirecting the femoral head into the acetabulum by a varus osteotomy;[30] (4) redirecting the acetabulum over the femoral head with an innominate osteotomy; or (5) enlarging the acetabulum with a

shelf procedure. Containment appliances commonly used include the Toronto brace, the Scottish Rite orthosis, the trilateral socket hip abduction orthosis, the Birmingham brace, and the Petrie cast.

Patients with Perthes' disease typically present with pain in the hip that may radiate to the knee area, decreased motion of the hip, or a limp; however, these same symptoms may occur at various times during the disease process. For example, the symptoms may be caused by either synovitis early in the disease process, by crushing and extrusion of the femoral head during revascularization, by incongruity and hinge abduction during reossification, by a torn femoral labrum, or persistent osteochondritis dissecans as the patient approaches maturity. When the patient presents, the physician must determine the stage of the disease process as described by Waldenstrom and evaluate any deformity of the hip joint.

Most patients present early in the disease process, but a small percentage do so after the femoral head has begun reossification. Few patients present at or about the time of maturity. In order to aid in planning treatment protocols, the following classification system has been developed (Table 5–3).

Class I (Predeformity)

Class I patients present with pain and stiffness in the hip during Waldenstrom's stages of necrosis or fragmentation and a spherical epiphysis that generally can be seen on radiographs, arthrograms, or by MRI. The femoral head is considered spherical if it is within 2 mm of Mose concentric circles (Fig. 5–18).

The goals of treatment in patients with Class I

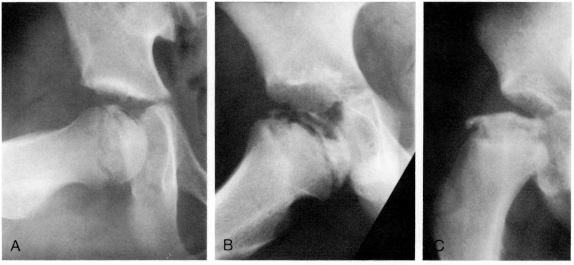

FIG. 5–16. **A.** Less than 50% of the femoral head involved. **B.** Greater than 50% involved. **C.** total epiphyseal necrosis.

hips are to relieve pain and prevent deformity of the epiphysis until the necrotic bone can be replaced by viable weight-supporting tissue. Initially, the pain is thought to be caused by synovitis, and evaluation of the hip with ultrasound often shows a small effusion. The first aspect of treatment in Class I patients is to obtain a painless, full range of motion of the hip. If the hip is mildly painful and stiff, treatment is aimed at obtaining full range of motion by physical therapy, and pain generally can be relieved by administering nonsteroidal anti-inflammatory drugs such as aspirin and placing the patient in a non-weight-bearing position. If the patient has severe pain and stiffness, hospitalization may be required. Hospitalized patients are placed in bed rest, the hips are held in wide abduction by skin traction, and physical therapy is used to increase range of motion with emphasis on abduction and internal rotation.[57] The majority of Class I patients have a moderate limp and pain and limited abduction and internal rotation, which can be treated on an outpatient basis by serial abduction casting (broomstick or Petrie cast) to obtain motion (Fig. 5–19). The cast is applied with the patient's lower limbs near maximal abduction and internal rotation as tolerated by pain. Excessive tension is relieved by reducing abduction approximately 10°, which relieves the pain. The patient should perform sit-ups and toe-touching exercises to increase flexion and extension of the hips. The casts are adjusted by gradually increasing abduction every 2 to 3 days on an outpatient basis until radiographs demonstrate that the lateral margin of the growth plate is within the lateral margin of the bony ace-

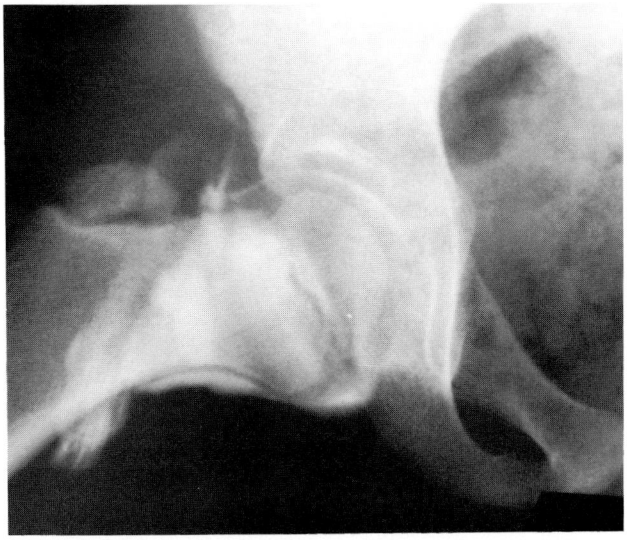

FIG. 5–17. This femoral head is contained, as shown by arthrography.

TABLE 5-3. *Treatment Classification**

Class I (Predeformity):	Presenting with a spherical epiphysis with the Waldenstrom signs of necrosis or fragmentation of the femoral head (Fig. 5–18)
Class II (Deforming):	Presenting with a deformed epiphysis with the Waldenstrom signs of necrosis or fragmentation of the femoral head (Fig. 5–21)
Class III (Remodeling):	Presenting after the femoral epiphysis has begun to reossify, and before skeletal maturity (Fig. 5–25)
Class IV (Maturity):	Presenting near or after skeletal maturity (Fig. 5–9)

*Adapted from Bowen JR, Foster BK, Hartzell CR: Legg-Calve-Perthes Disease. Clin Orthop, 185:97–108, 1984.

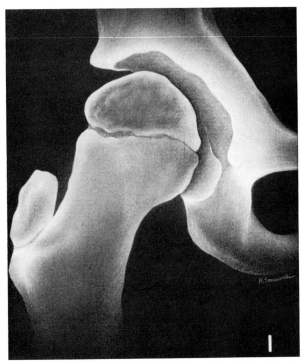

FIG. 5–18. Painting depicting Class I (predeformity). Spherical epiphysis in the stage of necrosis or fragmentation. (From Abrams JS, Bowen JR: Legg-calve-perthes disease. Contemp Orthop 10:27–39, 1985.)

tabulum (about 45° of abduction). During the progressive abduction casting, non-weight-bearing is maintained to reduce hip irritation and subsequent synovitis. After full range of motion has been obtained, a daily range of motion therapy program is emphasized throughout the entire healing period.

The second aspect of treatment in Class I pa-

tients is prevention of deformity of the femoral head that may occur from crushing or extrusion of the epiphysis. Patients in whom greater than 50% of the femoral head is necrotic or those who are greater than 6 years of age have a high probability of developing a deformity if left untreated. The extent of epiphyseal necrosis may be demonstrated radiographically as the area of increased density, the area of epiphysis under the crescent sign, and the area of the epiphysis undergoing fragmentation. Early in the disease process, the extent of necrosis is difficult to determine radiographically, and a bone scan or magnetic resonance imaging can delineate the area of avascularity.

If a patient has a high probability of developing a deformity (greater than 6 years of age or greater than 50% of the epiphysis necrotic), a containment weight-bearing orthosis such as the Scottish Rite orthosis (Atlanta brace) (Fig. 5–20) is recommended until the anterolateral margin of the epiphysis has reossified. The period from the onset of symptoms until early reossification of the anterolateral margin of the epiphysis typically takes approximately 13 months, after which time further epiphyseal deformity is unlikely.

Patients who have a decreased chance of developing a deformity may be treated by an intensive range of motion program, as previously described, and periodic radiographs obtained to evaluate

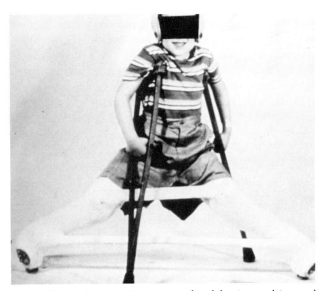

FIG. 5–19. Petrie cast. Containment by abduction and internal rotation.

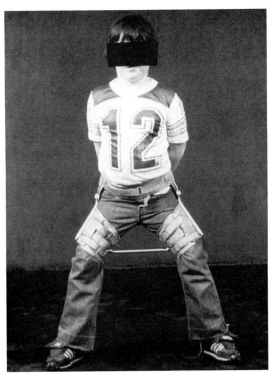

FIG. 5–20. Scottish Rite orthosis (Atlanta brace).

progress. When determining those patients who should be treated by containment, the "half and half" rule is helpful: contain hips when more than half the epiphysis is necrotic and in patients who are more than half-a-dozen years of age.

In summary, Class I patients present with a spherical femoral head in the necrotic or revascularization stage and must be treated as follows. (1) Reduce painful synovitis by keeping the patient nonambulatory until hip motion is restored and administering nonsteroidal anti-inflammatory drugs such as aspirin. (2) obtain and maintain full motion of the hip by either physical therapy, progressive abduction traction, or progressive abduction casting. And (3) hips with a high probability of deformity should be treated by containment therapy until the anterolateral aspect of the epiphysis reossifies ("half and half" rule).

Class II (Deforming Epiphysis)

Class II patients present with a deformity of the epiphysis of 2 mm or greater from sphericity using the Mose circle method during the Waldenstrom stage of necrosis or fragmentation (resorption) (Fig. 5–21). Two characteristic types of deformities of the epiphysis are seen in Class II hips: (1) lateral ex-

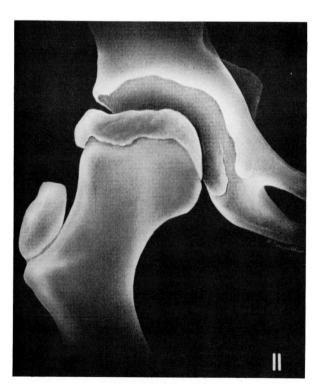

Fig. 5–21. Painting depicting Class II (deforming epiphysis). Nonspherical epiphysis during the stage of necrosis or fragmentation. (From Abrams JS, Bowen JR: Legg-calve-perthes disease. Contemp Orthop 10:27–39, 1985.)

trusion of the epiphysis with hinge abduction (Fig. 5–22), and (2) vertical compression of the epiphysis (crushing) (Fig. 5–16C). All patients in Class II require containment treatment.

If the patient presents with crushing of the epiphysis without hinge abduction, full range of motion should be obtained, as described for Class I patients, and the hip should be contained until the anterolateral margin of the epiphysis reossifies. Verification of compression of the epiphysis generally can be demonstrated radiographically by (1) flattening of the weight-bearing surface of the epiphysis, (2) decreased height of the epiphysis from the growth plate to the superior acetabular margin, and (3) lateral subluxation. Containment may be by cast, brace, orthosis, or surgery.

If the patient presents with lateral extrusion and hinge abduction, radiographs may show calcification of the epiphysis lateral to the acetabular margin, and arthrographic evaluation generally shows the extruded portion of the epiphysis. Lateral extrusion may cause hinging of the hip on abduction as the extruded cartilaginous material abuts the anterosuperior border of the acetabulum. If the hinge abduction is not corrected, a groove will form on the anterolateral corner of the epiphysis, resulting in significant irregularity of the femoral head. Persistent hinging may result in incongruent joint surfaces and coxa irregularis at maturity. Patients presenting with lateral extrusion and hinging should be treated by longitudinal skin traction to reduce the hinging, and subsequently, the hip should be gradually abducted until the extruded epiphysis can be reduced in the acetabulum.[53] The traction may take several weeks and, in some patients with persistent stiffness, an operative adductor tenotomy may be necessary to allow the extruded portion of the epiphysis to be redirected into the acetabulum. An arthrogram performed at this stage of treatment will show the extruded epiphysis and groove, which was caused by hinge abduction, to be reduced into the depths of the acetabulum. The hip should then be contained with the extruded epiphysis reduced into the acetabulum by cast, orthosis, or surgery until the epiphysis reossifies in the anterolateral weight-bearing part. When surgical containment is anticipated, an abduction plaster cast may be applied for several weeks before operation until the epiphysis "settles" into the acetabulum, which makes subsequent operative containment considerably easier.

Nonoperative containment is recommended for most patients, because it produces comparable results without the risk of operative procedures.[35] Younger patients (generally less than 6 to 7 years of

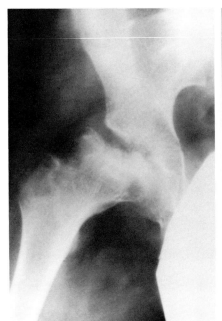
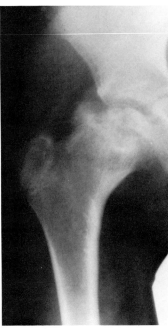

Fɪɢ. 5–22. Lateral extrusion with hinge abduction.

age) tolerate orthoses well, whereas older patients are less tolerant. Nonoperative containment is discontinued when reossification of the anterolateral portion of the epiphysis occurs; reossification takes place an average of 13 months after onset of symptoms.

In those patients who cannot tolerate nonoperative treatment, an operative procedure is indicated. The extruded epiphysis must be reduced into the acetabulum and hinging of the hip must be relieved prior to the operative procedure, as described previously. There is no definitive operative treatment of Perthes' disease; each method has disadvantages and some poor results.[54,67] The varus osteotomy (Fig. 5–23) offers adequate containment.[29] However, this procedure is less useful in those patients who show signs of proximal femoral growth plate closure (coxa brevis). The varus osteotomy accentuates a limb-length discrepancy and may accentuate relative overgrowth of the greater trochanter. The innominate osteotomy of Salter also offers good containment but theoretically increases the hip joint pressure by elongating the pelvis.[41] The Kalamchi modification of the Salter innominate osteotomy (Fig. 5–24) provides adequate containment and prevents pelvic elongation.[33] In general, the authors prefer the varus osteotomy unless the growth plate shows irregularity and impending premature physeal closure, in which case, the Kalamchi modification of the Salter innominate osteotomy is utilized.

In summary, the authors suggest containment treatment of all patients who present with a defor-

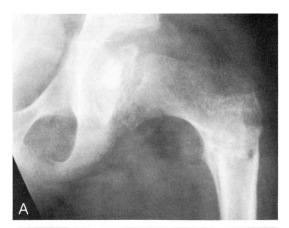
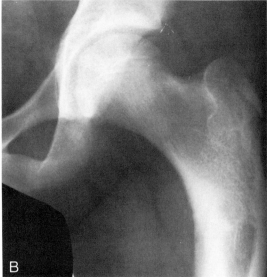

Fɪɢ. 5–23. **A.** Varus osteotomy. **B.** Remodeling of varus osteotomy.

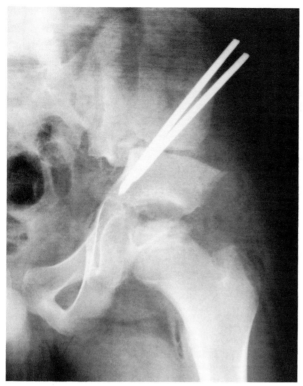

Fig. 5–24. Kalamchi modification of the Salter innominate osteotomy for containment.

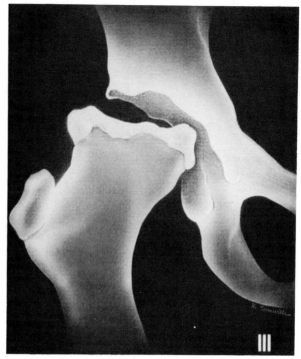

Fig. 5–25. Painting depicting Class III (remodeling). (From Abrams JS, Bowen JR: Legg-calve-perthes disease. Contemp Orthop 10:27–39, 1985.)

mity of the epiphysis, that is, in the necrotic or resorption stage (Class II) (Fig. 5–21). Noncontainment orthoses work well for the young patient; however, older patients often refuse braces, and operation is indicated. An active range of motion therapy program is necessary throughout the healing phase of Perthes' disease. For nonoperative containment, the Scottish Rite orthosis is preferred; for surgical containment, the varus osteotomy is preferred, unless there appears to be a probable premature closure of the capital femoral physis, at which time a Kalamchi modification of the Salter innominate osteotomy is recommended.[33]

Class III (Remodeling)

Class III patients present for treatment later in the disease course when the femoral head is undergoing reossification but prior to maturity (Fig. 5–25). Because further epiphyseal deformity generally does not occur during reossification, any treatment is therefore considered reconstructive. Patients whose femoral head and acetabulum are congruent and who are asymptomatic should be encouraged to perform a daily range of motion exercise with emphasis on flexion and extension. No further treatment is required unless the hip becomes painful.

The authors have become encouraged by a relatively small group of patients who present at a young age (typically, less than 7 years) with an incongruent femoral head that has already entered the reossification stage of Waldenstrom. Typically, the femoral head is irregular, is larger than the volume of the acetabulum, and shows hinge abduction. In these young patients who have open capital femoral growth plates, prolonged containment may result in increased sphericity of the femoral head during the remaining growth phases. The hip should be placed in longitudinal skin traction until the epiphysis can be reduced into the acetabulum by gradual abduction. A shelf procedure is then performed to cover the large femoral head and prevent subsequent hinge abduction (Fig. 5–26). The patient is maintained postoperatively with the leg in abduction casting for 6 weeks. After cast removal, non-weight-bearing crutch ambulation and range of motion therapy to the hip is performed until the ossification of the shelf procedure has matured. Although this procedure has shown some early encouraging results, few patients meet the criteria for this type of treatment: irregular femoral head, hinge abduction, open capital femoral physis, and less than 7 years of age.

A large percentage of Class III patients with hip pain have internal derangement of the hip such as a

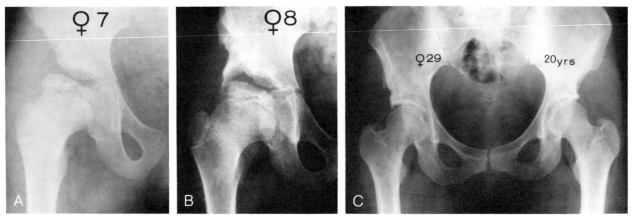

Fɪɢ. 5–26. Sequence showing excellent result from shelf procedure for containment. A Preoperative. B. Postoperative. C. 20-year followup. (From Bowen JR, Abrams JS, Hartzell CR: Legg-calve-perthes disease. Clin Orthop 185:97–108, 1984.)

torn acetabular labrum, an osteocartilaginous loose body, or joint incongruity with hinge abduction. Joint incongruity with hinge abduction is the most frequent cause of pain, and the goal of treatment is to restore joint congruity with a reconstructive procedure. An arthrogram frequently will show the hinge abduction, and often the most congruent position is obtained with the hip held in mild adduction and flexion. Typically, the articular surface of the medial and anterior portion of the femoral head will be preserved. In such patients, a valgus extension osteotomy may be beneficial in redirecting the femoral head by externally tilting the femoral head to reduce the hinge abduction, and repositioning

the biologically healthy articular surface into the weight-bearing area of the acetabulum (Fig. 5–27). The Garceau procedure, in which the lateral one third of the femoral head is removed, also eliminates hinge abduction;[20] however, in the authors' opinion, the long-term results of this procedure have not been encouraging.

Class IV (Mature)

Class IV patients are mature or approaching maturity and present with a residual deformity of Perthes' disease (Fig. 5–9), including a limp, limb-

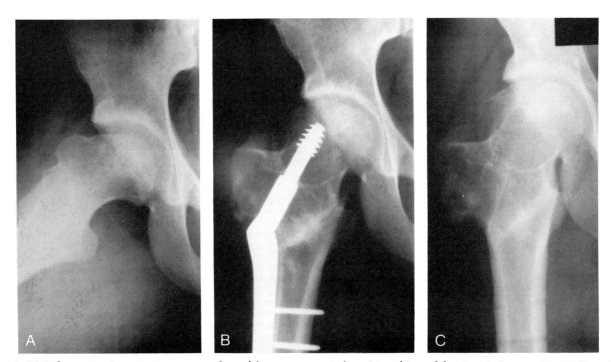

Fɪɢ. 5–27. Valgus-extension osteotomy was performed for management of persistent hinge abduction. A. Preoperative. B. Operative. C. Postoperative.

length discrepancy, or internal derangement of the hip. Treatment is directed toward correcting the existing deformity that causes symptoms. A limb-length discrepancy can be treated by an appropriately timed epiphysiodesis of the contralateral femur if the patient is immature, or by femoral shortening in the mature patient. A severe Trendelenburg gait or trunk shift caused by premature closure of the capital femoral physis may be treated by lateral and distal transfer of the greater trochanter. Symptomatic osteochondritis dissecans may be excised operatively.[34] Recently, osteocartilaginous fragments, as well as tears of the femoral labrum, have been treated by arthroscopy.[5] Early degenerative joint disease is seldom seen in Perthes' disease during early adulthood but may occur in middle and later life (Fig. 5–28).[42,59] Reconstructive osteotomies of the femur or acetabulum that redirect the more favorable biological structures into weight-bearing positions and realign the mechanical forces are helpful in treating early degenerative disease.[3]

Conclusion

Even though the cause and a totally effective treatment of Legg-Calve-Perthes disease are not available, advances have been made to reduce the harmful effects of this condition. Patients with little risk of developing a permanent deformity (less than 6 years old with an undeformed capital femoral epiphysis and less than 50% of epiphyseal necrosis) may be symptomatically treated. Patients with a higher risk of developing a permanent hip deformity may require range of motion therapy to reduce contractures and may need containment of the femoral head to prevent deformity. Even with the most diligent treatments, some patients develop deformities that require reconstructive procedures, such as equalization of limb-length inequality, osteotomies to reduce painful hinge abduction in adolescence, operative removal of symptomatic osteochondritis dissecans, and various techniques to address early degenerative joint disease.

The authors would like to thank James T. Guille and Cynthia Brodoway at the Alfred I. duPont Institute, Wilmington, DE, for their assistance in the preparation of this chapter.

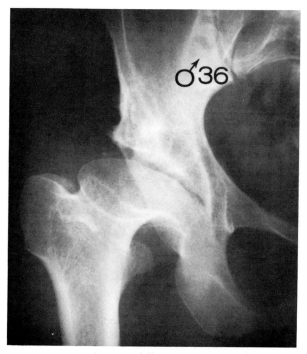

FIG. 5–28. Osteoarthrosis at followup in a patient (age 36 years) who had adolescent onset of total epiphyseal necrosis.

References

1. BARKER DJP, DIXON E, TAYLOR JF: Perthes' disease of the hip in three regions of England. J Bone Joint Surg, 60B:478–480, 1978.
2. BARNES JM: Premature epiphyseal closure in Perthes' disease. J Bone Joint Surg, 62B:432–437, 1980.
3. BOMBELLI R: Osteoarthritis of the Hip: Pathogenesis and Consequent Therapy. New York, Springer-Verlag, 1976.
4. BOWEN JR, FOSTER BK, HARTZELL CR: Legg-Calve-Perthes disease. Clin Orthop, 185:97–108, 1984.
5. BOWEN JR, KUMAR SJ, JOYCE JJ III, BOWEN JC: Osteochondritis dissecans following Perthes' disease: arthroscopic-operative treatment. Clin Orthop, 209:49–56, 1986.
6. BOWEN JR, SCHREIBER FC, FOSTER BK, WEIN BK: Premature femoral neck physeal closure in Perthes' disease. Clin Orthop, 171:24–29, 1982.
7. BURWELL RG, et al.: Perthes' disease: an anthropometric study revealing impaired and disproportionate growth. J Bone Joint Surg, 60B:461–477, 1978.
8. BURWELL RG, et al.: Raised somatomedin activity in the serum of young boys with Perthes' disease revealed by bioassay: a disease of growth transition? Clin Orthop, 209:129–138, 1986.
9. CAFFEY J: The early roentgenographic changes in essential coxa plana: their significance in pathogenesis. Amer J Roentgen, 103:620–634, 1968.
10. CALVE J: Sur une forme particuliere de pseudocoxalgie greffee sur les deformations caracteristiques de l'extremite superieure du femur. Rev Chirurgie, 42:54, 1910.
11. CATTERALL A: Legg-Calve-Perthes Disease. New York, Churchill Livingstone, 1982.
12. CATTERALL A, LLOYD-ROBERTS GC, WYNNE-DAVIES R: Association of Perthes' disease with congenital anomalies of genitourinary tract and inguinal region. Lancet, 1:996–997, 1971.
13. CATTERALL A: The natural history of Perthes' disease. J Bone Joint Surg, 53B:37–53, 1971.
14. COWELL HR, WEIN BK: Genetics in orthopaedics. Orthop Surg Update Series 1(28):1–8, 1981.
15. DANIGELIS JA, FISHER RL, OZONOFF MB, SZIKLAS JJ: 99MTc-

polyphosphate bone imaging in Legg-Perthes disease. Radiology, 115:407–413, 1975.

16. DEVALDERRAMA JAF: The "observation hip" syndrome and its late sequelae. J Bone Joint Surg, 45B:462–470, 1963.

17. EDGREN W: Coxa plana: a clinical and radiological investigation with particular reference to the importance of the metaphyseal changes for the final shape of the proximal part of the femur. Acta Orthop Scand (Suppl 84), 1965.

18. FERGUSON AB, Jr: Synovitis of the hip and Legg-Calve-Perthes disease. Clin Orthop, 4:180–188, 1954.

19. FISHER RL: An epidemiological study of Legg-Perthes disease. J Bone Joint Surg, 54A:769–778, 1972.

20. GARCEAU G, RAPP G, LIDGE RT: Coxa plana (a surgical approach). J Bone Joint Surg, 55A:1313, 1973.

21. GERSHUNI-GORDON DH, AXER A: Synovitis of the hip joint—an experimental model in rabbits. J Bone Joint Surg, 56B:69–77, 1974.

22. GRAY IM, LOWRY RB, RENWICK DHG: Incidence and genetics of Legg-Perthes disease (osteochondritis deformans) in British Columbia: evidence of polygenic determination. J Med Genet, 9:197–202, 1972.

23. GREEN NE, BEAUCHAMP RD, GRIFFIN PP: Epiphyseal extrusion as a prognostic index in Legg-Calve-Perthes disease. J Bone Joint Surg, 63A:900–905, 1981.

24. GOWER WE, JOHNSTON RC: Legg-Perthes disease, long-term follow-up of thirty-six patients. J Bone Joint Surg, 53A:759–768, 1971.

25. HALL DJ, HARRISON MHM, BURWELL RG: Congenital abnormalities and Perthes' disease: clinical evidence that children with Perthes' disease may have a major congenital defect. J Bone Joint Surg, 61B:18–25, 1979.

26. HARDCASTLE PH, ROSS R, HAMALAINEN M, MATA A: Catterall grouping of Perthes' disease: an assessment of observer error and prognosis using the Catterall classification. J Bone Joint Surg, 62B:428–431, 1980.

27. HARPER PS, BROTHERTON BJ, COCHLIN D: Genetic risks in Perthes' disease. Clin Genet, 10:178–182, 1976.

28. HARRISON MHM, TURNER MH, JACOBS P: Skeletal immaturity in Perthes' disease. J Bone Joint Surg, 58B:37–40, 1976.

29. HARRY JD, GROSS RH: A quantitative method for evaluating results of treating Legg-Perthes syndrome. J Pediatr Orthop, 7:671–676, 1987.

30. HOIKKA V, LINDHOLM TS, POUSSA M: Intertrochanteric varus osteotomy in Legg-Calve-Perthes disease: a report on 112 hips. J Pediatr Orthop, 6:600–604, 1986.

31. IPPOLITO E, TUDISCO C, FARSETTI P: Long-term prognosis of Legg-Calve-Perthes disease developing during adolescence. J Pediatr Orthop, 5:652–656, 1985.

32. IPPOLITO E, TUDISCO C, FARSETTI P: The long-term prognosis of unilateral Perthes' disease. J Bone Joint Surg, 69B:243–250, 1987.

33. KALAMCHI A: Modified Salter osteotomy. J Bone Joint Surg, 64A:183–187, 1982.

34. KAMHI E, MACEWEN GD: Osteochondritis dissecans in Legg-Calve-Perthes disease. J Bone Joint Surg, 57A:506–509, 1975.

35. KELLY FB, CANALE ST, JONES RR: Legg-Calve-Perthes disease: long-term evaluation of non-containment treatment. J Bone Joint Surg, 62A:400–407, 1980.

36. KEMP HBS: Perthes' disease: an experimental and clinical study. Ann R Coll Surg Engl, 52:18–35, 1973.

37. KERET D, HARRISON MHM, CLARKE, NMP, HALL DJ: Coxa plana—the fate of the physis. J Bone Joint Surg, 66A:870–877, 1984.

38. KRISTMUNDSDOTTIR F, BURWELL RG, HARRISON MHM: Delayed skeletal maturation in Perthes' disease. Acta Orthop Scand, 58:277–279, 1987.

39. LEGG AT: An obscure affection of the hip joint. Boston Med Surg J, 162:202, 1910.

40. MACKENZIE WG, BASSETT GS, MANDELL GA, SCOTT CI Jr.: Avascular necrosis of the hip in multiple epiphyseal dysplasia. J Pediatr Orthop 9:666–671, 1989.

41. MAXTED MJ, JACKSON RK: Innominate osteotomy in Perthes' disease: a radiological survey of results. J Bone Joint Surg, 67B:399–401, 1985.

42. MCANDREW MP, WEINSTEIN SL: A long-term follow-up of Legg-Calve-Perthes Disease. J Bone Joint Surg, 66A:860–869, 1984.

43. MCKIBBIN B, RALIS Z: Pathological changes in a case of Perthes' disease. J Bone Joint Surg, 56B:438–447, 1974.

44. MOLLOY MK, MACMAHON B: Birth weight and Legg-Perthes disease. J Bone Joint Surg, 49A:498–506, 1967.

45. MOSE K, et al.: Legg-Calve-Perthes disease, the late occurrence of coxarthrosis. Acta Orthop Scand (Suppl 169), 1977.

46. MOSE K: Legg-Calve-Perthes disease: a comparison between three methods of conservative treatment. Thesis, Copenhagen, Universitetsforlaget I Aarhus, 1964.

47. O'GARRA JA: The radiographic changes in Perthes' disease. J Bone Joint Surg, 41B:465–476, 1959.

48. OGDEN JA: Changing patterns of proximal femoral vascularity. J Bone Joint Surg, 56A:941–950, 1974.

49. PERTHES G: Uber arthritis deformans juvenilis. Dtsch Z Chir, 107:11, 1910.

50. PHEMISTER DB: Repair of bone in the presence of aseptic necrosis resulting from fractures, transplantations, and vascular obstruction. J Bone Joint Surg, 12:769–787, 1930.

51. PONSETI IV: Legg-Perthes disease. Observations on pathological changes in two cases. J Bone Joint Surg, 38A:739–750, 1956.

52. RALSTON EL: Legg-Perthes disease and physical development. J Bone Joint Surg, 37A:647, 1955.

53. RICHARDS BS, COLEMAN SS: Subluxation of the femoral head in coxa plana. J Bone Joint Surg, 69A:1312–1318, 1987.

54. SALTER RB: The present status of surgical treatment for Legg-Perthes disease. J Bone Joint Surg, 66A:961–966, 1984.

55. SALTER RB, THOMPSON GH: Legg-Calve-Perthes disease: the prognostic significance of the subchondral fracture and a two-group classification of the femoral head involvement. J Bone Joint Surg, 66A:479–489, 1984.

56. SANCHIS M, ZAHIR A, FREEMAN MAR: The experimental simulation of Perthes' disease by consecutive interruptions of the blood supply to the capital femoral epiphysis in the puppy. J Bone Joint Surg, 55A:335–342, 1973.

57. SERLO W, HEIKKINEN E, PURANEN J: Preoperative Russell traction in Legg-Calve-Perthes disease. J Pediatr Orthop, 7:288–290, 1987.

58. SHAPIRO F: Legg-Calve-Perthes disease: a study of lower extremity length discrepancies and skeletal maturation. Acta Orthop Scand, 53:437–444, 1982.

59. STULBERG SD, COOPERMAN DR, WALLENSTEIN R: The natural history of Legg-Calve-Perthes disease. J Bone Joint Surg, 63A:1095–1108, 1981.

60. SUTHERLAND AD, SAVAGE JP, PATERSON DC, FOSTER BK: The nuclide bone-scan in the diagnosis and management of Perthes' disease. J Bone Joint Surg, 62B:300–306, 1980.

61. TRUETA J: The normal vascular anatomy of the human femoral head during growth. J Bone Joint Surg, 39B:358–394, 1957.

62. WALDENSTROM H: Coxa plana, osteochondritis deformans

coxae: Calve-Perthessche Krankheit, Legg disease, Zentral-blatt Chirurgie, 47:539, 1920.

63. WALDENSTROM, H.: On coxa plana, osteochondritis deformans coxae juvenilis: Legg's disease, maladie de Calve, Perthes Krankheit. Acta Chirurg Scand, 55:557–590, 1923.

64. WALDENSTROM H: The first stage of coxa plana. Acta Orthop Scand, 5:1–32, 1934.

65. WALDENSTROM H: The first stages of coxa plana. J Bone Joint Surg, 20:559–566, 1938.

66. WEINER DS, O'DELL, HW: Legg-Calve-Perthes disease: observations on skeletal maturation. Clin Orthop, 68:44–49, 1970.

67. WENGER DR: Selective surgical containment for Legg-Perthes disease: recognition and management of complications. J Pediatr Orthop, 1:153–160, 1981.

68. WYNN-DAVIES R: Some etiologic factors in Perthes' disease. Clin Orthop, 150:12, 1980.

69. WYNN-DAVIES R, GORMLEY J: The aetiology of Perthes' disease. Genetic, epidemiological and growth factors in 310 Edinburgh and Glasgow patients. J. Bone Joint Surg, 60B:6–14, 1978.

70. YNGVE DA, ROBERTS JM: Acetabular hypertrophy in Legg-Calve-Perthes disease. J Pediatr Orthop, 4:416–421, 1985.

CHAPTER SIX

Slipped Capital Femoral Epiphysis

PETER PIZZUTILLO

Slipped capital femoral epiphysis was recognized by Pare in 1572 as a pathologic condition that differed from traumatic dislocation of the hip. Muller later described this condition as "bending of the neck of the femur" and presented a case report with pathologic and microscopic findings that he believed suggested rickets as the primary cause.[43] To the present time the cause of slipped capital femoral epiphysis remains elusive. Ischemia with resultant weakening of the proximal femoral growth plate,[52,72] repeated microtrauma, thinning of the periochondrial ring,[15] and loss of integrity of the cartilagenous bridge between trochanteric apophysis and the proximal femoral ossification center, and collagen deficiency[2,60] have been proposed as possible causes. Extrinsic factors such as pelvic irradiation have been associated with slipped capital femoral epiphysis.[5,22,58]

As the child enters adolescence there is increased obliquity of the plane of the physis of the proximal femur that creates greater shear stress at the proximal femoral growth plate. Concomitantly, thinning of the periosteum of the femoral neck occurs that weakens resistance to shear stress and may allow failure. Ponseti studied biopsy specimens from patients with slipped capital femoral epiphysis and noted significant widening of the zone of hypertrophy of the physis with irregularity and disruption of the morphology, irregular septal formation with young collagen fibrils, and loss of the normal columnar architecture of the growth plate.[45,67] Chondrocyte degeneration has been reported at proliferative and hypertrophic zones.[3] It has not yet been established whether these changes reflect primary process or secondary changes caused by mechanical disruption of the physis.[36]

The phenotypic profile for individuals with slipped capital femoral epiphysis has suggested an association with endocrine disorders with the cherubic, obese, and hypogonadal appearance similar to the Frohlich syndrome. In 1950, Harris demonstrated in rat studies that growth hormones weaken the growth plate, whereas sex hormones strengthen the growth plate.[37] Subsequent reports have documented the association of slipped capital femoral epiphyses with endocrinopathies such as hypopituitarism, cretinism, growth hormone deficiency, juvenile hypothyroidism, hyperparathyroidism, hypogonadism, and renal rickets that suggest causal relationship between endocrine dysfunction and slipped capital femoral epiphysis.[9,12,14,20,39,40,42,58,63,70,90]

Hypothyroidism should be suspected in the young child with slipped capital femoral epiphysis, especially when associated with significant delay in skeletal maturation and bilateral hip involvement. Children with known hormonal deficiencies who are in the early phases of replacement therapy of thyroid hormone or growth hormone[26,73] may demonstrate marked hypertrophy of the proximal femoral physis with intrinsic physeal weakness. These children are at risk for slipped epiphysis and should be carefully monitored and limited in their activities until radiographic evidence of a more normal physeal structure is demonstrated. It should be noted that no primary hormonal dysfunction has been demonstrated in the vast majority of children with slipped capital femoral epiphysis,[71] and no variance from expected growth rates has been documented.[25,33]

Heredity is also considered a significant factor. Rennie reported 14 families each with more than one member with slipped capital femoral epiphysis.[74] No mode of inheritance has yet been established, however, a genetic predisposition to this problem must be considered. Genetic factors may be more important than has been realized in the past because of the recent recognition of "silent slips" that have only come to clinical attention during middle age with the emergence of symptoms related to osteoarthritis of the hip. Interestingly, an association has been established between slipped epiphysis and Down's Syndrome[80] and tibia vara.[78]

Slipped capital femoral epiphysis is more commonly seen in blacks[7] and has a higher incidence in the eastern sector of the United States.[49] It appears

152

to be more common in males than females.[32,34] The common age of onset of symptoms is between 11 and 14 years of age in females, and between 10 and 16 years of age in males. The left hip is involved with a frequency of twice that of the right hip and bilateral involvement is seen in a minimum of 25% of patients.[32,34]

The presentation of patients with slipped capital femoral epiphysis is varied. Unfortunately, the duration of pain has been used as the primary parameter in establishing a classification system and has proved to be extremely unreliable. By definition, an acute slipped capital femoral epiphysis is one in which the duration of pain is less than 3 weeks.[1,4,17] This is rare in actual practice, because on close questioning many patients may admit to an exacerbation of pain in a period of time less than 2 weeks, but frequently have pain of a low grade nature that has existed for many months. This patient must be distinguished from the patient with an acute epiphyseal fracture of the proximal femur that is caused by severe trauma, such as a fall or vehicular injury, and is associated with a high incidence of avascular necrosis.

The majority of patients with chronic slipped epiphysis have a prodromal symptomatic phase of low-grade aching pain that is related to activity. The patient may perceive pain at the medial aspect of the distal thigh, at the knee, or may complain of intermittent painless limp or a sense of lower extremity fatigue. The low-grade symptoms may only be brought to conscious attention by an acute episode of severe pain following trivial trauma, such as slipping on a floor, with consequent inability to stand because of the pain. The latter situation has been described as the acute-on-chronic form of slipped capital femoral epiphysis. The design of a safe treatment program demands that the individual's history of pain be diligently sought in order to determine its true duration. The mechanical reduction of a chronic slipped capital femoral epiphysis, as well as the acute on chronic slipped femoral epiphysis has resulted in avascular necrosis with poor results.[13,51,56,61] In the immature individual, complaint of knee pain necessitates a detailed evaluation of range of motion of the hip in order to rule out referred pain from the hip. The low grade nature of pain, its relationship to increased activity, and its radiation to the distal, medial thigh and knee have frequently resulted in significant delay of diagnosis. Educational efforts in the last several decades have resulted in earlier diagnosis by both pediatricians and orthopaedic surgeons.

The physical examination of a child with slipped capital femoral epiphysis will reveal an antalgic gait with the involved limb in external rotation. In the more acute expressions of the problem, the patient will not be able to bear weight on the involved leg and may not be able to actively flex and extend the involved hip. If the suspicion of a chronic slipped capital femoral epiphysis exists, physical examination should be performed in a gentle manner. The range of motion of the involved hip will reveal limitation in range of motion of the hip in flexion, internal rotation, and abduction when compared to the more normal opposite hip. With more advanced degrees of deformity, attempts to flex the involved hip result in obligatory external rotation of the hip.

An interesting observation has been made in recent years that documents limited internal rotation of the uninvolved hip as well as the involved hip. In addition, contrary to observation in normal hips, rotation of the hip is greater when the hip is in extension than at 90° of flexion. CT evaluation of the hip joint in patients with slipped capital femoral epiphysis suggests the existence of premorbid femoral retroversion (Fig. 6–1).[18,30]

When presented with a patient with more acute pain, range of motion should be tested gently and only within the range of comfort. No attempt should be made to forcefully flex or internally rotate the involved hip for fear of inadvertent reduction of an unstable proximal femoral segment.

Radiographic evaluation should include an anteroposterior view of both hips and pelvis with a cross-table lateral view of the involved hip.[8] Traditionally, the frog lateral view of the hip has been used, but in a symptomatic hip, pain and limited range of motion will not permit a tangential view of the proximal femur by "frog" position and may result in mechanical reduction of the unstable displaced proximal femoral ossification center. The cross-table lateral view of the hip will more precisely document the extent of posterior displacement of the proximal femoral physis in relation to the metaphysis. The changes noted on anteroposterior radiographs of the hips and pelvis may include nothing more than widening and irregularity of the involved growth plate suggestive of the "preslip" condition. With progressive deformity, there is loss of overhang of the epiphysis on the femoral neck (Fig. 6–2), decreased height of the crescent-shaped epiphysis, and exclusion of the superior aspect of the metaphysis from acetabular coverage (Fig. 6–3). In the acute slipped capital femoral epiphysis, no widening or irregularity of the physis is seen and no rounding of the junction of the medial aspect of the femoral neck and the displaced epiphysis are noted to suggest a more chronic process.

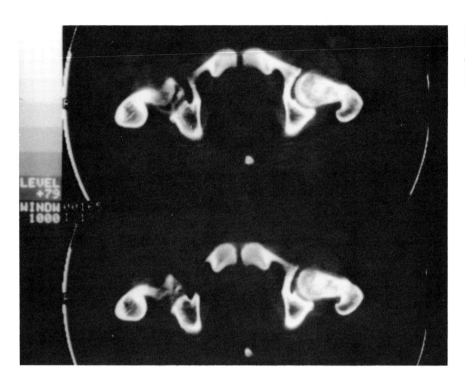

FIG. 6–1. CT scan demonstrates posterior displacement of the proximal femoral epiphysis of the right hip and also indicates relative retroversion of the uninvolved left hip.

It is extremely important to distinguish between the acute and the chronic slipped capital femoral epiphysis. In the absence of radiographic signs that suggest a chronic process, and with a detailed history to support a diagnosis of acute slip, reduction of the deformity may be accomplished and is supported by medical literature. The incidence of avascular necrosis in acute slipped epiphysis appears to relate primarily to the severity of the imposed trauma. The concern with reduction of the acute

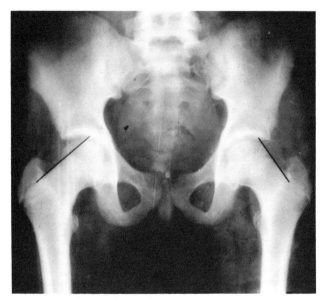

FIG. 6–2. Early slip detected with anteroposterior view of the hips and pelvis, which demonstrates loss of overhang of the epiphysis on the femoral neck as demonstrated by Kline's line.

on chronic slip is that the anatomic deformation that existed prior to the acute component of injury is not known. Gross instability at the physeal-metaphyseal junction would allow over-reduction that could compromise the vascular supply, resulting in avascular necrosis. On this basis, reduction of the acute on chronic, as well as the chronic slipped capital femoral epiphysis, is an uncontrolled and risky maneuver and is not indicated.

The natural history of slipped capital femoral epiphysis is difficult to define. However, small groups of untreated patients included as subsets of larger studies may be evaluated. Oram, in 1953,[65] and Jerre, in 1950,[47] reported two groups of untreated patients with slipped capital femoral epiphysis. Their long-term evaluations revealed that few hips were normal by radiographic analysis or function. Degenerative changes, as well as ankylosis, were frequently noted. Avascular necrosis of the femoral head was not documented in these untreated hips; however, chondrolysis did occur. The results were better than hips that had been treated.[66,76]

The treatment of slipped capital femoral epiphysis is varied. Bedrest with traction was recommended by Sabatier in 1768. Surgical treatment by subtrochanteric wedge osteotomy was described by Keetley in 1888; Sturrock was the first to describe pin fixation of slipped epiphyses in 1894. Reconstructive surgical procedures evolved and included femoral neck osteotomy by Bradford in 1895 and cheilectomy by Pullen in 1898. In 1931, Ferguson

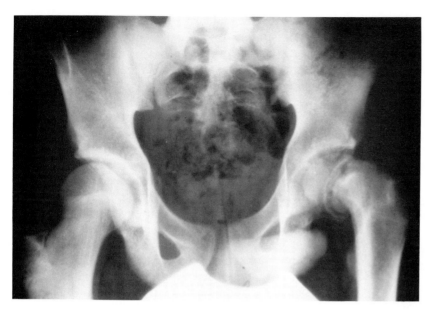

Fig. 6–3. More advanced degrees of slipped capital femoral epiphysis demonstrate chronic changes at the superior and inferior aspect of the femoral neck, decreased height of the crescent-shaped epiphysis, and exclusion of the superior aspect of the metaphysis from the acetabular cover.

and Howarth described the "bone pegging" procedure for epiphysiodesis of the proximal femur. Since that time, casting has been popularized by Steel, however, no other significant advance in the treatment of slipped capital femoral epiphysis has developed since the first half of this century.

The goal of treatment of chronic slipped capital femoral epiphysis is stabilization of the epiphysis in order to halt progression of the deformity, to promote early physeal closure, to relieve pain, and to improve range of motion. Casting has been successful without an increased incidence of avascular necrosis, but is associated with chondrolysis. Problems with the casting technique involve the nursing care problems of a large, obese teenager, and more importantly, the difficulty in determining the point at which immobilization can be safely discontinued. In the older teenager, the endpoint of casting would coincide with radiographic evidence of physeal closure that would confer a degree of confidence that is not realized in the younger child whose physes remain open. It must be remembered that these are abnormal growth plates and are at risk for increased displacement and progressive deformity.

The use of pins to stabilize the proximal femur has been the most common form of treatment of slipped capital femoral epiphysis. Pinning not only prevents further progression of slip, but also fosters early closure of the physis. A variety of fixation devices including Steinman pins, Hagie pins, hook-pins,[35] and cannulated screws[53] have been used to stabilize the physis. The use of a Smith-Peterson nail is contraindicated because of the significant incidence of complications following its usage. Pin fixation of a slipped epiphysis may be performed in mild, moderate, or severe degrees of displacement and requires good three-dimensional appreciation of deformity with technical skills to accomplish the operative goals. Depending on the direction and severity of displacement, a more anterior starting position on the thigh for pin placement usually is required to transfix the slipped epiphysis. Multiple penetrations of the anterior lateral femoral cortex must be avoided in order to decrease the stress-riser effect that may result in fracture of the femur with weight-bearing. Multiple pins frequently are not required and are contraindicated in the superior quadrant of the femoral head. Brodetti and others have described the interosseous blood supply of the femoral head and note that segmental necrosis of the femoral head in the superior quadrant may be created by clustered multiple pins (Fig. 6–4).[11,16] The pin or pins are directed across the physis and enter the proximal capital epiphysis at its inferior quadrant.[81] This position minimizes the risk of joint penetration and vascular embarassment in the superior weight-bearing area. Because severe displacement results in a small window for transfixion between the metaphysis and epiphysis, usually only one or two pins are required. Pin advancement should be followed by frequent fluoroscopic monitoring.[68] Once the physis is crossed, range of motion of the hip through its complete range under fluoroscopic examination should be accomplished in order to determine the true distance of the pin tip from the subchondral bone. This examination may be easily performed on an image table. In those patients with significant instability at the physeal metaphyseal junction, the use of a fracture table is discouraged in order to avoid inadvertent reduction of the physis.

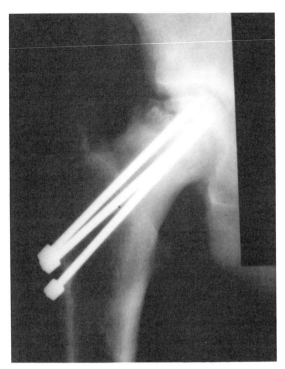

Fɪɢ. 6–4. Multiple pins involving the superior quadrants of the femoral head may result in segmental necrosis as described by Brodetti.

Complications have been reported with the technique of pinning of slipped capital femoral epiphysis and include avascular necrosis and chondrolysis. Avascular necrosis is related to reduction of the slipped epiphysis and to clustering of multiple pins in the superior quadrant of the femoral head, whereas chondrolysis is reported with higher incidence in patients who have persistent pin penetration of the joint.

The use of small caliber pins may result in fracture of the pins either at intraosseous locations or at the bone-pin interface. The removal of multiple pins may be difficult with resultant retained pin segments. Vigorous bone removal to retrieve pins may create a significant stress riser at the cortex that could result in fracture of the femur. Although threaded pins placed across the proximal femoral physis usually result in early closure of the physis, the proximal femoral epiphysis may actually grow off the tips of these pins in children with a significant amount of remaining growth. Prophylactic pinning of the opposite uninvolved hip cannot be recommended because of reported complications.[48]

Once the proximal femoral epiphysis has been mechanically stabilized, the pins bridging the physis should not be removed until the growth plate has been bridged with bone. If pin penetration of the joint is recognized intraoperatively or postoperatively, the offending pin should be withdrawn to a

safer area or replaced. Safeguards must be taken during surgery to avoid this pitfall by placing the hip through a complete range of motion under fluoroscopic evaluation.[6,54,75,83,86,89]

Surgical treatment of chronic slipped capital femoral epiphysis includes the biplane osteotomy,[69,79] as well as open or closed epiphysiodesis of the proximal femoral physis.[59,87] The biplane osteotomy has been associated with the complication of chondrolysis[28,77] and is technically challenging.[19] Open epiphysiodesis involves a large operative approach with increased blood loss. The reported results of treatment by this technique, however, indicate a significant improvement in the incidence of avascular necrosis and chondrolysis and may thus justify the more extensive procedure.

The risks of closed epiphysiodesis technically reproduce the problems of pin fixation of the slipped capital femoral epiphysis with additional concerns regarding the use of a bone graft in a graft channel. Violation of the joint with the bone graft and loss of mechanical stabilization after graft fracture compromise the results of this technique.

Once bony bridging of the physis has been accomplished by pinning, remodeling of the proximal femur has been documented with the development of a more functional range of motion of the hip.[10,62] Occasionally, remodeling does not occur to an acceptable degree and cheilectomy or subtrochanteric osteotomy may be required to improve the existing range of motion. The base of femoral neck osteotomy, as well as the femoral neck osteotomy, have only few reports of satisfactory results[27,50] and are more commonly associated with a high incidence of avascular necrosis and thus cannot be recommended.[29,51,88]

The major complications encountered in the treatment of slipped capital femoral epiphysis are avascular necrosis and chondrolysis. Avascular necrosis is associated with reduction of the femoral head on the femoral neck. Many surgeons agree that reduction is contraindicated in chronic slipped capital femoral epiphysis but recommend "gentle" reduction of the acute on chronic slipped capital femoral epiphysis. Difficulty arises in the latter circumstance because no good endpoint exists to signal completion of reduction. If an acute-on-chronic process is postulated by the treating surgeon, then reduction to an anatomic position would almost always be excessive. Vascular insult to the femoral head may occur resulting in an immediate, permanent, and serious physical disability in the young patient. No good treatment options exist for total head necrosis. Segmental necrosis of the femoral head may be improved by reconstructive procedures, such as rotational osteotomy of the proximal femur as described by Sugioka[57,82] or by valgus osteotomy of the proximal femur. When extensive necrosis of the femoral head develops with severe degenerative changes, marked limitation of motion and pain, arthrodesis of the hip is the preferred option in the young patient (Fig. 6–5). Arthrodesis of the hip should be performed without violation of the abductor and extensor muscle groups of the hip in order to preserve an effective motor system for subsequent prosthetic replacement at an older age. Because of the immediate disability associated with avascular necrosis of the hip, reduction of acute-on-chronic or chronic slipped capital femoral epiphysis is not recommended. It should be emphasized that these comments refer to the chronic slipped capital femoral epiphysis and not to acute injury, which

usually reflects an epiphyseal fracture of the proximal femur.

Chondrolysis was first described by Elmslie in 1913 and histologically related to impaired nourishment of joint cartilage by Waldenstrom in 1930.[85] Chondrolysis has been reported in the slipped capital femoral epiphysis that is untreated, following cast immobilization, with persistent pin penetration of the joint, following femoral neck or subtrochanteric osteotomy, and following both closed and open epiphysiodesis of the proximal femur. It occurs more frequently in black patients.[41,44,84] Typically, patients with chondrolysis present with a progressive loss of motion of the hip with the development of fixed deformity in flexion and adduction. Radiographic evaluation demonstrates a narrowing of the joint space of the hip with osteopenia

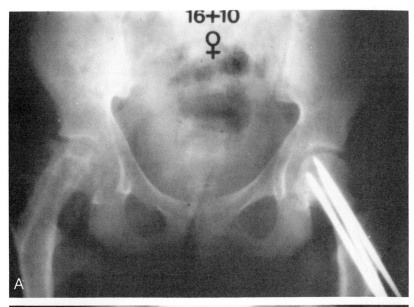

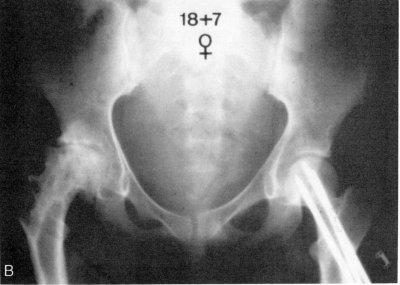

FIG. 6–5A,B. Pin fixation of slipped capital femoral epiphysis may result in excellent results with maintenance of normal range of motion. The development of avascular necrosis compromises the entire joint and usually leads to rapid degeneration.

on both the acetabular and femoral side of the joint (Fig. 6–6).[24,31] Bone scan reveals generalized increased uptake in the area of the hip joint. In 1963, Cruess' studies confirmed the existence of synovial fibrosis with impaired nutrition of hyaline cartilage.[21] Morrissey identified increase in serum immunoglobulins and C3 component of complement in patients who developed chondrolysis. An autoimmune etiology has been implicated on this basis and is under investigation.[23]

The treatment of chondrolysis demands a persistent program that obtains and maintains an improved range of motion of the hip joint. Internal and external rotation of the joint are frequently difficult to recover, however, flexion and extension of the hip may be obtained in a functional range. If necessary, controlled manipulation of the hip joint under anesthesia with adductor tenotomy, and occasionally capsulotomy, should be done in order to increase flexion, decrease flexion contracture, and foster abduction. These maneuvers place the lower extremity in a more functional position for gait. Prolonged nonweight-bearing with traction, the use of continuous passive motion, vigorous physical therapy, and pain relieving techniques have been successful in reconstituting a more normal joint surface and developing a functional range of motion of the hip.[38,46] Ogden has documented a variable response of the hyaline cartilage of the hip to injury that is varied by race and sex.[64] Black females tend to sustain the greatest degree of narrowing of the cartilage and, unfortunately, experience the least degree of rebound of the cartilage. Ogden's observations parallel the experience in chondrolysis of the hip joint in slipped capital femoral epiphysis and suggest that persistence in active treatment, rather than passive acceptance, is essential in restoring joint function. This involves commitment to a long-term program of one to two years duration in order to realize beneficial results. In the absence of substantial improvement in pain and functional activity, arthrodesis of the hip allows for improved limb position and the relief of pain.

References

1. AADALEN RJ, WEINER DS, HOYT W, HERNDON CH: Acute slipped capital femoral epiphysis. J Bone Joint Surg, 56A(7):1473–1487, 1974.
2. AGAMANOLIS DP, WEINER DS, LLOYD JK: Slipped capital femoral epiphysis: a pathological study I. A light microscopic and histochemical study of 21 cases. J Pediatr Orthop 5(1):40–46, 1985.
3. AGAMANOLIS DP, WEINER DS, LLOYD JK: Slipped capital femoral epiphysis: a pathological study II. An ultrastructural study of 23 cases. J Pediatr Orthop, 5(1):47–58, 1985.
4. BARASH HL, GALANTE JO, RAY RD: Acute slipped capital femoral epiphysis. Clin Orthop, 79:96–103, 1971.
5. BARRETT IR: Slipped capital femoral epiphysis following radiotherapy. J Pediatr Orthop, 5(3):268–273, 1985.
6. BENNET GC, KORESKA J, RANG M: Pin placement in slipped capital femoral epiphysis. J Pediatr Orthop, 4:574–578, 1984.
7. BISHOP JO, OLEY TJ, STEPHENSON CT, TULLOS HS: Slipped capital femoral epiphysis: a study of 50 cases in black children. Clin Orthop, 135:93–96, 1978.
8. BLOOMBERG TJ, NUTTALL J, STOKER DJ: Radiology in early slipped femoral capital epiphysis. Clin Radiol, 29:657–667, 1978.
9. BONE LB, ROACH JW, WARD WT, WORTHEN HG: Slipped capital femoral epiphysis associated with hyperparathyroidism, J Pediatr Orthop, 5:589–592, 1985.
10. BOYER DW, MICKELSON MR, PONSETI IV: Slipped capital femoral epiphysis. J Bone Joint Surg, 63A(1):85–95, 1981.
11. BRODETTI A: The blood supply of the femoral neck and head in relation to the damaging effects of nails and screws. J Bone Joint Surg, 42B(4):794–801, 1960.
12. CARLIOZ H, VOGT JC, BARBA L, DOURSOUNIAN L: Treatment of slipped upper femoral epiphysis. J Pediatr Orthop, 4:153–161, 1984.
13. CASEY BH, HAMILTON HW, BOBECHKO WP: Reduction of acutely slipped upper femoral epiphysis, J Bone Joint Surg, 54B(4):607–614, 1972.
14. CHIROFF RT, SEARS KA, SLAUGHTER WH: Slipped capital femoral epiphyses and parathyroid adenoma. J Bone Joint Surg, 56A(5):1063–1067, 1974.
15. CHUNG SMK, BATTERMAN SC, BRIGHTON CT: Shear strength of the human femoral capital epiphyseal plate. J Bone Joint Surg, 58A(1):94–103, 1976.
16. CLAFFEY TJ: Avascular necrosis of the femoral head. J Bone Joint Surg, 42B(4):802–809, 1960.

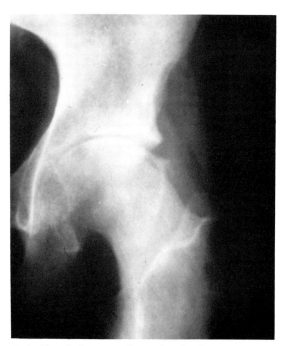

FIG. 6–6. Chondrolysis is radiographically demonstrated by osteopenia and narrowing of the hip joint space.

17. CLEVELAND M, ROSWORTH DM, DALY JN, HESS WE: Study of displaced capital femoral epiphyses. J Bone Joint Surg, 33A(4):955–967, 1951.
18. COHEN MS, et al: Slipped capital femoral epiphysis: assessment of epiphyseal displacement and angulation. J Pediatr Orthop, 6:259–264, 1986.
19. COLYER RA: Compression external fixation after biplane femoral trochanteric osteotomy for severe slipped capital femoral epiphysis. J Bone Joint Surg, 62:557–560, 1980.
20. CRAWFORD AH, MACEWEN GD, FONTE D: Slipped capital femoral epiphysis co-existent with hypothyroidism. Clin Orthop, 122:135–140, 1977.
21. CRUESS RL: The pathology of acute necrosis of cartilage in slipping of the capital femoral epiphysis. J Bone Joint Surg, 45A(5):1013–1024, 1963.
22. DICKERMAN JD, NEWBERG AH, MORELAND MD: Slipped capital femoral epiphysis (SCFE) following pelvic irradiation for rhabdomyosarcoma. Cancer, 44:480–482, 1979.
23. EISENSTEIN A, ROTHSCHILD S: Biochemical abnormalities in patients with slipped capital femoral epiphysis and chondrolysis. J Bone Joint Surg, 58A(4):459–467, 1976.
24. EL-KHOURY GY, MICKELSON MR: Chondrolysis following slipped capital femoral epiphysis. Diagn Radiol, 123:327–330, 1977.
25. EXNER GV: Growth and pubertal development in slipped capital femoral epiphysis: a longitudinal study. J Pediatr Orthop, 6:403–409, 1986.
26. FIDLER MW, BROOK CGD: Slipped upper femoral epiphysis following treatment with human growth hormone. J Bone Joint Surg, 56A(8):1719–1722, 1974.
27. FISH JB: Cuneiform osteotomy of the femoral neck in the treatment of slipped capital femoral epiphysis. J Bone Joint Surg, 66:1153–1168, 1984.
28. FRYMOYER JW: Chondrolysis of the hip following Southwick osteotomy for severe slipped capital femoral epiphysis. Clin Orthop, 99:120–124, 1974.
29. GAGE JR, et al: Complications after cuneiform osteotomy for moderately or severely slipped capital femoral epiphysis. J Bone Joint Surg, 60A(2):157–165, 1978.
30. GELBERMAN RH, et al: The association of femoral retroversion with slipped capital femoral epiphysis. J Bone Joint Surg, 68:1000–1007, 1986.
31. GOLDMAN AB, SCHNEIDER R, MARTEL W: Acute chondrolysis complicating slipped capital femoral epiphysis. Am J Roentgenol, 130:945–950, 1978.
32. HAGGLUND G, HANSSON LI, ORDEBERG G: Epidemiology of slipped capital femoral epiphysis in southern Sweden. Clin Orthop 191:82-94, 1984.
33. HAGGLUND G, et al: Longitudinal growth of the distal fibula in children with slipped capital femoral epiphysis. J Pediatr Orthop, 6:274–277, 1986.
34. HALL JE: The results of treatment of slipped femoral epiphysis. J Bone Joint Surg, 39B(4):659, 1957.
35. HANSSON LI: Osteosynthesis with the hook-pin in slipped capital femoral epiphysis. Acta Orthop Scand 53:87–96, 1982.
36. HARRIS WR: The endocrine basis for slipping of the upper femoral epiphysis. J Bone Joint Surg, 32B(1):5, 1950.
37. HARRIS WR, HOBSON KW: Histological changes in experimentally displaced upper femoral epiphyses in rabbits. J Bone Joint Surg, 38B(4):914–921, 1956.
38. HARTMAN JT, GATES DJ: Recovery from cartilage necrosis following slipped capital femoral epiphysis. Orthop Rev, 1(2):33–37, 1972.
39. HEATLEY FW, GREENWOOD RH, BOASE DL: Slipping of the upper femoral epiphyses in patients with intracranial tumours causing hypopituitarism and chiasmal compression. J Bone Joint Surg, 58B(2):169–175, 1976.
40. HENNESSY MJ, JONES KL: Slipped capital femoral epiphysis in a hypothyroid adult male. Clin Orthop, 165:204–208, 1982.
41. HEPPENSTALL RB, MARVEL JP Jr, CHUNG SMK, BRIGHTON CT: Chondrolysis of the hip. Clin Orthop, 103:136–142, 1974.
42. HEYERMAN W, WEINER D: Slipped epiphysis associated with hypothyroidism. J Pediatr Orthop, 4(5):569–573, 1984.
43. HOWORTH B: History of slipping of the capital femoral epiphysis. Clin Orthop, 48:11, 1966.
44. INGRAM AJ, CLARKE MS, CLARK CS, MARSHALL WR: Chondrolysis complicating slipped capital femoral epiphysis. Clin Orthop, 165:99–109, 1982.
45. IPPOLITO E, MICKELSON MR, PONSETI IV: A histochemical study of slipped capital femoral epiphysis. J Bone Joint Surg, 63A(7):1109–1113, 1981.
46. IPPOLITO E, RICCIARDI-POLLINI PT: Chondrolysis of the hip. Ital J Orthop Traumatol. 7:335–344, 1981.
47. JERRE T: A study in slipped upper femoral epiphysis with special reference to late functional and roentgenological results and to value of closed reduction. Acta Orthop Scand Suppl, 6:3, 1950.
48. JOHNSTON CE, HERNANDEZ AA: Prophylactic pinning in slipped upper femoral epiphysis. 7(9):1502–1507, 1984.
49. KELSEY JL, KEGGI KJ, SOUTHWICK WE: The incidence and distribution of slipped capital femoral epiphysis in Connecticut and the southwestern United States. J Bone Joint Surg, 52A:1203, 1970.
50. KRAMER WG, CRAIG WA, NOEL S: Compensating osteotomy at the base of the femoral neck for slipped capital femoral epiphysis. J Bone Joint Surg, 58:796–800, 1976.
51. KULICK RG, DENTON JR: A retrospective study of 124 cases of slipped capital femoral epiphysis. Clin Orthop, 162:87–90, 1982.
52. LACROIX P, VERBRUGGE J: Slipping of the upper femoral epiphysis. J Bone Joint Surg, 33A(2):371–381, 1951.
53. LEHMAN WB, et al: A method of evaluating possible pin penetration in slipped capital femoral epiphysis using a cannulated internal fixation device. Clin Orthop, 186:65–70, 1984.
54. LEHMAN WB, et al: The problem of evaluating in situ pinning of slipped capital femoral epiphysis: An experimental model and a review of 63 consecutive cases. J Pediatr Orthop 4:297–303, 1984.
55. LITCHMAN HM, DUFFY J: Slipped capital femoral epiphysis: factors affecting shear forces on the epiphyseal plate. J Pediatr Orthop, 4(6):745–748, 1984.
56. LOWE HG: Avascular necrosis after slipping of the upper femoral epiphysis. J Bone Joint Surg, 43B(4):688–699, 1961.
57. MASUDA T, et al: Transtrochanteric anterior rotational osteotomy for slipped capital femoral epiphysis: a report of 5 cases. J Pediatr Orthop, 6:18–23, 1986.
58. McAFEE PC, CADY RB: Endocrinologic and metabolic factors in atypical presentations of slipped capital femoral epiphysis. Clin Orthop, 180:188–197, 1983.
59. MELBY A, HOYT WA Jr, WEINER DS: Treatment of chronic slipped capital femoral epiphysis by bone-graft epiphyseodesis. J Bone Joint Surg, 62A(1):119–125, 1980.
60. MICKELSON MR, PONSETI IV, COOPER RR, MAYNARD JA: The ultrastructure of the growth plate in slipped capital femoral epiphysis. J Bone Joint Surg, 59:1076–1081, 1977.
61. MICKELSON MR, EL-KHOURY GY, CASS JR, CASE KJ: Aseptic necrosis following slipped capital femoral epiphysis. Skeletal Radiol, 4:129–133, 1979.

62. O'Brien ET, Fahey JJ: Remodeling of the femoral neck after in situ pinning for slipped capital femoral epiphysis. J Bone Joint Surg, 59:62–68, 1977.
63. Ogden JA, Southwick WO: Endocrine dysfunction and slipped capital femoral epiphysis. Yale J Biol Med, 50:1–16, 1977.
64. Ogden JA, Simon TR, Southwick WO: Cartilage space width in slipped capital femoral epiphysis: the relationship to cartilage necrosis. Yale J Biol Med, 50:17–30, 1977.
65. Oram V: Epiphysiolysis of the head of the femur. Acta Orthop Scand, 23:100, 1953.
66. Ordeberg G, Hansson LI, Sandstrom S: Slipped capital femoral epiphysis in southern Sweden. Clin Orthop, 191:95–104, 1984.
67. Ponseti IV, McClintock R: The pathology of slipping of the upper femoral epiphysis. J Bone Joint Surg, 38A(1):71–83, 1956.
68. Rab GT, Simon SR: An improved method for pinning of chronic slipped capital femoral epiphysis. J Pediatr Orthop, 5:212–213, 1985.
69. Rao JP, Francis AM, Siwek CW: The treatment of chronic slipped capital femoral epiphysis by biplane osteotomy. J Bone Joint Surg, 66:1169–1175, 1984.
70. Rappaport EB, Fife D: Slipped capital femoral epiphysis in growth hormone-deficient patients. AJDC, 139:396–402, 1985.
71. Razzano CD, Nelson C, Evershan J: Growth hormone levels in slipped capital femoral epiphysis. J Bone Joint Surg, 54:1224–1226, 1972.
72. Rennie AM: The pathology of slipped upper femoral epiphysis. J Bone Joint Surg, 42B(2):273–279, 1960.
73. Rennie W, Mitchell N: Slipped femoral capital epiphysis occurring during growth hormone therapy. J Bone Joint Surg, 56B(4):703–705, 1974.
74. Rennie AM: The inheritance of slipped upper femoral epiphysis. J Bone Joint Surg, 64B:180–184, 1982.
75. Rooks MD, Schmitt EW, Drvaric DM: Unrecognized pin penetration in slipped capital femoral epiphysis. Clin Orthop, 234:82–89, 1988.
76. Ross PM, Lyne ED, Morawa LG: Slipped capital femoral epiphysis long-term results after 10–38 years. Clin Orthop, 141:176–180, 1979.
77. Salvati EA, Robinson HJ Jr, O'Dowd TJ: Southwick osteotomy for severe chronic slipped capital femoral epiphysis: results and complications. J Bone Joint Surg, 62:561–570, 1980.
78. Schmidt TL, Mallo GJ: Slipped capital femoral epiphysis in a patient with infantile tibia vara. Orthopedics, 1(6):471–473, 1978.
79. Southwick WO: Osteotomy through the lesser trochanter for slipped capital femoral epiphysis. J Bone Joint Surg, 49A(5):807–835, 1967.
80. Stack RE, Peterson LFA: Slipped capital femoral epiphysis and Down's disease. Clin Orthop, 48:111–117, 1966.
81. Stambough JL, Davidson RS, Ellis RD, Gregg JR: Slipped capital femoral epiphysis: an analysis of 80 patients as to pin placement and number. J Pediatr Orthop, 6:265–273, 1986.
82. Sugioka Y: Transtrochanteric rotational osteotomy in the treatment of idiopathic and steroid induced femoral head necrosis. Clin Orthop, 184:12–23, 1984.
83. Swiontkowski MF: Slipped capital femoral epiphysis. Orthopedics, 6(6):705–712, 1983.
84. Tillema DA, Golding JSR: Chondrolysis following slipped capital femoral epiphysis in Jamaica. J Bone Joint Surg, 53(A):1528–1540, 1971.
85. Waldenstrom H: On necrosis of the joint cartilage by epiphysiolysis capitis femoris. Acta Chir Scand, 67:935–946, 1930.
86. Walters R, Simon SR: Joint destruction: a sequel of unrecognized pin penetration in patients with slipped capital femoral epiphyses. Hip society award papers, 8:145–164.
87. Weiner DS, Weiner S, Melby A, Hoyt WA Jr: A 30-year experience with bone graft epiphysiodesis in the treatment of slipped capital femoral epiphysis. J Pediatr Orthop, 4:145–152, 1984.
88. Wilson PD, Jacobs B, Schecter L: Slipped capital femoral epiphysis. J Bone Joint Surg, 47A(6):1128–1145, 1965.
89. Zahrawi FB, Stephens TL, Spencer GE, Clough JM: Comparative study of pinning in situ and open epiphysiodesis in 105 patients with slipped capital femoral epiphyses. Clin Orthop, 177:160–167, 1983.
90. Zubrow AB, Lane JM, Parks JS: Slipped capital femoral epiphysis occurring during treatment for hypothyroidism. J Bone Joint Surg, 60A(2):256–258, 1978.

CHAPTER SEVEN

Septic Arthritis of the Hip in Childhood

PETER PIZZUTILLO

Acute infection of the hip in infancy and childhood is truly a medical and surgical emergency. Prior to the advent of antibiotic therapy, septic arthritis of the hip resulted in significant mortality with 13 of 21 patients succumbing to this infection in the report by Thomas Smith in 1874.[20] With the introduction of antibiotic therapy, lives were spared, and the goal of treatment shifted from preservation of life to preservation of limb[12,17] and, more currently, to improved quality of limb function.

The most common method of infection of the immature hip is hematogenous spread.[32,34] Although the primary site of infection can be identified in most patients, there remains a significant number of children with septic arthritis of the hip with no identifiable source of infection. In the medically compromised neonate, infection may initally develop at parenteral routes, such as the umbilical catheter, and spread to the hip joint. In the infant and toddler, ears and throat are the most common sources of infection. The hip is the most common joint involved with septic arthritis in the infant and toddler[36] followed in frequency by the knee, which is the most commonly infected joint in the adolescent and adult.

Hematogenous seeding of bacteria directly to the hip joint or via transphyseal vessels[31] to the chondroepiphysis are common methods of involvement in those less than one year of age. Between 18 months and 16 years of age, the proximal femoral metaphysis is more commonly involved[18,33] allowing infection at this site to secondarily spread to the hip joint. Less commonly, osteomyelitis of the ossification center of the proximal femur or of the acetabulum may result in secondary joint involvement.

Septic arthritis of the infant hip may have lifelong tragic effects. The fluid boundary that normally exists between the femoral head and the acetabulum is destroyed, promoting subluxation and eventual dislocation of the femoral head. Increasing intracapsular pressure, combined with the mechanical stretching of vessels in a dislocated hip, may result in avascular necrosis of the proximal femur and complete destruction of the femoral head and neck. Lysosomal enzymes from white blood cells, in combination with bacterial toxins, cause chondrocyte damage and injury to the matrix of hyaline cartilage that is not apparent at the time of surgery.[4] Gross morphologic changes in hyaline cartilage develop later as a consequence of mechanical stress imposed on impaired cartilage matrix. Lavage of an infected joint dilutes enzymes and other breakdown products to diminish their effects within the joint.[5] When avascular necrosis develops in combination with toxic articular changes, the result is a destructive process of such magnitude that normal hip function is rarely regained.

The clinical presentation of septic arthritis of the hip in infants is usually acute and commonly associated with infection of the ears or throat. In the neonate, anorexia and lethargy may be the only signs of sepsis with no acute constitutional signs.[2,9,10,15,29,30,34,37] The infant may become irritable, anorexic, and febrile, and the child's parents may notice that passive movement of the affected lower extremity is painful and resisted. The older child, who is able to walk, will voluntarily discontinue weight-bearing. As the severity of pain increases, the child will not be able to rest and will become more irritable. Irritability is exacerbated by fever and dehydration. Once infection of the hip has become well established, the child will lie supine with the involved hip held in a position of flexion, abduction, and external rotation (Fig. 7–1). Swelling and heat are noted at the anterior aspect of the groin and severe spasm and guarding prohibit passive range of motion of the hip.

Attention and concern for the involved hip should not distract the clinician from consideration of other diagnoses such as trauma, discitis, infec-

161

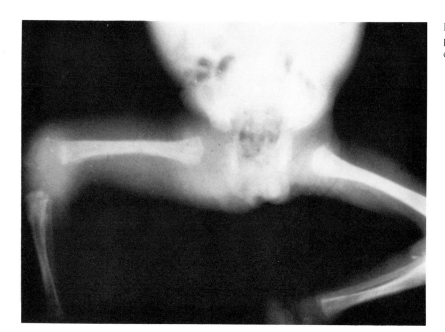

FIG. 7–1. The infant's hip is laterally displaced and held in a position of flexion abduction and external rotation.

tion of the sacroiliac joint, and retroperitoneal mass or infection.[22,33] After complete examination of the entire child, examination of the lower extremity should be accomplished by specifically isolating the foot, ankle, lower leg, knee joint, femur, and hip joint (Fig. 7–2). In the presence of pain and sig-

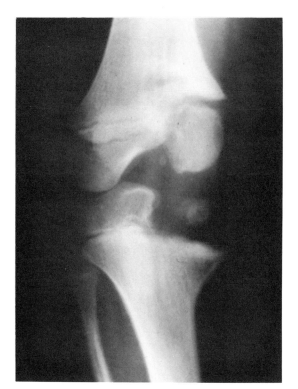

FIG. 7–2. Concomitant septic arthritis of the knee resulted in marked alteration in growth of the proximal tibial epiphysis and physis.

nificant restriction of passive motion of the hip joint, radiographic evaluation of the hips and pelvis, as well as of the entire involved femur, is helpful in eliminating trauma as the cause. Radiographic demonstration of capsular distension of the hip joint had been considered an important diagnostic sign, but is easily reproduced by flexion, abduction, and external rotation of a normal hip. Early radiographic evaluation of the hip may be normal.[37] Widening of the medial aspect of the hip joint and osteopenia of the proximal femoral metaphysis are radiographic signs that indicate an established pathologic process of septic arthritis.[39] In the absence of adequate treatment, radiographs progressively reveal decrease in size of the proximal femoral ossification center, subluxation of the hip joint, and lucency of the proximal femoral metaphysis.

While the child is in the imaging department, aspiration of the hip should be performed with sterile technique under fluoroscopic control. In the presence of significant capsular distention of the hip joint, aspiration of the joint is easily accomplished; however, with little intracapsular fluid, aspiration becomes more difficult. If the needle is successfully positioned within the capsule, the injection of 2 ml of air will result in an air arthrogram of the hip joint. If injection of air yields only a dark shadow around the tip of the needle, the capsule has not yet been entered. If no fluid or purulent material is aspirated from the joint once penetration of the capsule has been established, lavage with sterile saline may be sent for Gram stain, culture, and sensitivity tests. If clear synovial fluid is aspirated, it should also be sent for Gram stain, culture, and sensitivity tests and should not be taken as a sign that infection does not exist. In the presence of osteomyelitis of the proximal femur, a sympathetic effusion of the hip joint will frequently occur. If purulent material is aspirated from the hip joint, it should be analyzed immediately by Gram stain, culture, sensitivity, and cell count with differential. The aspirate from an infected hip joint will reveal a leukocyte count in excess of 50,000 cells with a differential of 95% polymorphonuclear cells. Glucose analysis of the aspirated fluid will reveal levels 30% lower than serum glucose; protein levels will be elevated. Finally, a poor mucin test is noted in the face of infection. Distant sites of possible infection, e.g., throat, as well as blood cultures, should also be sent to the laboratory. Peripheral blood studies will reveal a leukocytosis with a shift to the left and an elevated erythrocyte sedimentation rate. It should be cautioned that the latter studies may be normal in the neonate and may then delay diagnosis.[24]

Early infection of the hip joint may be difficult to prove by routine laboratory studies or by evaluation of the synovial fluid. This is especially true with concomitant osteomyelitis of the proximal femoral metaphysis, proximal femoral ossification center, or acetabulum. The constitutional signs and symptoms and the restriction of motion that occurs with early osteomyelitis are more subtle than with joint disease. A reactive synovial fluid may be produced with a low white cell count, normal glucose and protein levels, and a normal mucin test. No organisms are usually noted on Gram stain. In this circumstance, technetium bone scan may be helpful in determining whether primary bone involvement exists. Early osteomyelitis is characterized by increased intramedullary pressure and thrombosis of vessels with a transient decrease in circulation and a resultant "cold spot" on the later phases of bone scan (Fig. 7–3). Later in the disease, hyperemia results in increased uptake in the area of infection. Gallium scan has been used in confusing clinical presentations, but has a significant disadvantage because it takes 72 hours for completion of the test.

Early osteomyelitis of the proximal femur, in the absence of joint involvement, may be appropriately treated with parenteral antibiotics without surgical drainage. The patient must be closely observed, and if significant clinical improvement is not noted in the first 24 hours of antibiotic therapy, further evaluation and surgical decompression may become necessary.

A variety of micro-organisms may be involved in the production of osteomyelitis or septic arthritis. In the neonate, although staphylococcus aureus is

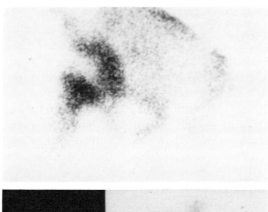

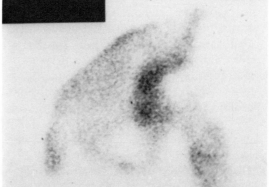

FIG. 7–3. Technetium bone scan demonstrates normal uptake in the upper uninvolved hip, whereas significant decrease in circulation is documented in the lower involved hip.

common, Group B Streptococcus and Gram negative organisms are also frequently involved. In the infant from six months to four years of age, Staphylococcus aureus again is common, but Haemophilus influenzae must be suspected[26] and treated until the results of culture are available. In the older child, Staphylococcus aureus is the most common offending organism.

Acute septic arthritis of the hip is a problem which may lead to permanent disability of the involved limb and death if not recognized early and treated appropriately. Once the diagnosis is established, supportive measures must be instituted to reverse dehydration and stabilize the child for surgical decompression of the hip joint. After the hip joint has been aspirated and fluid has been sent for Gram stain, culture, and sensitivity tests, an appropriate antibiotic should be started parenterally. In more advanced cases, aspiration of purulent material from the hip joint not only retrieves material for more specific diagnosis, but also decompresses the intracapsular pressure and decreases the risk of vascular compromise of the femoral head.

Arthrotomy of the hip may be accomplished either by anterior or posterior approach. Concerns exist regarding the increased risk of vascular injury when the posterior approach is used, however, increased morbidity after posterior approach to the hip joint has not been substantiated and remains a hypothetical concern. Surgical treatment includes the creation of a large window in the hip capsule that will permit complete irrigation of the joint and continued drainage. Lavage of the hip joint dilutes destructive enzymes and removes thickened debris that could further compromise articular cartilage. A drain is sutured to the capsule to allow continued drainage. If posterior surgical drainage of the hip joint has been performed, the patient is placed in a posterior splint in order to immobilize the joint and to rest the inflamed soft tissues about the hip. If the hip had progressed to subluxation or frank dislocation, gentle abduction positioning in a posterior frame is helpful for a short period of time. This may be followed by abduction bracing. In the absence of subluxation, posterior splinting is used for five days or until the early acute symptomatic phase of the process has subsided. If anterior surgical drainage of the hip is performed, the child is placed in a hip spica and nursed in the prone position to foster drainage. Early surgical intervention can result in continued growth and development of a normal hip joint. The following have been identified in multiple studies of septic arthritis of the hip as significant factors in patients with poor results: age less than one year, especially the neonate; delay in treatment of more than four days from the onset of symptoms; concurrent osteomyelitis of the acetabulum or of the proximal femur; and hip dislocation (Fig. 7–4).[1,2,6–10,12,13,16–18,21,25,28–30,34,35]

Repeat aspiration of the hip joint has been suggested as effective treatment for septic arthritis of the hip in nonorthopaedic literature. It has been our experience that even after careful aspiration of the hip joint under fluoroscopy, a significant residual amount of purulent material remains within the capsule at the time of surgical drainage. The morbidity of surgical arthrotomy of the hip joint has been reduced to minimal levels, whereas the risk of incomplete lavage of the hip joint is of such magnitude that permanent disability may be expected.

Controversy also surrounds the duration of antibiotic treatment. It is well known that the hyperemia associated with septic arthritis of the hip allows for excellent levels of antibiotic in the joint fluids. Clinical and laboratory parameters serve as useful guidelines in the determination of duration of treatment. When septic arthritis of the hip exists in the absence of osteomyelitis, parenteral antibiotics may be continued for one week or until the patient's clinical status has improved and the erythrocyte sedimentation rate has been reduced by 20%.

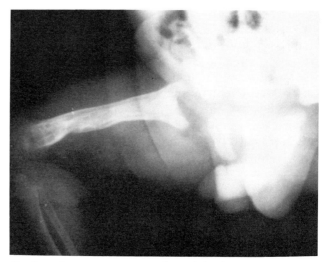

FIG. 7–4. Concurrent osteomyelitis of the femur in association with septic arthritis has a high incidence of poor results as demonstrated in this radiograph.[27]

The patient may then be treated with a 6-week course of oral antibiotics. When osteomyelitis coexists with septic arthritis, parenteral antibiotics are given for 2 weeks followed by oral antibiotics for a 6- to 12-week period as long as adequate serum bacteriocidal levels of antibiotics can be achieved and can be checked on a regular basis.[27]

Past clinical studies of septic arthritis of the hip have identified factors associated with poor results and have emphasized the need for early diagnosis, expedient surgical drainage, and appropriate antibiotic treatment. The sequelae of septic arthritis of the hip are varied and complicated, and many have no good treatment options. The delay in diagnosis that is associated with infants under the age of one year significantly increases the risk of a poor result. Ogden and Trueta have shown a diffuse network of blood vessels that cross the physis in the first 15 months of life.[31] During this time, infection may spread directly from the metaphysis into the epiphysis with the possibility of direct physeal destruction.[32] Infection of the hip joint has resulted in closure of both the proximal femoral physis as well as the triradiate cartilage of the pelvis.[6] The degree of destruction of the hip joint is variable and depends on the virulence of the organism,[14] the delay in treatment, the performance of adequate surgical drainage, and the use of appropriate antibiotics. Hunka, et al., have published a radiographic classification of septic arthritis of the hip that describes sequelae and suggests prognosis.[16] Under the best conditions, early treatment and surgical intervention result in continued normal growth of a congruent femoral head with an open, growing physis (Class I). Hunka's Class II hip has mild deformity of

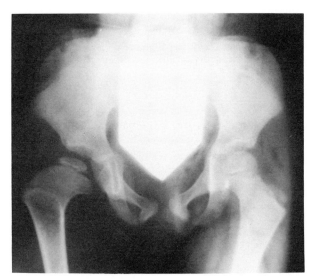

Fɪɢ. **7−5.** Class II hips demonstrate mild deformity of the femoral head and neck with a possibility of early physeal closure.

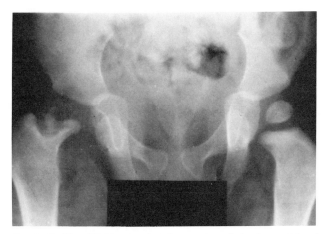

Fɪɢ. **7−7.** Class IV hips involve destruction of the femoral head and neck with a remnant of the femoral neck in apposition with the acetabulum.

the femoral head with either an open physis or a physis undergoing premature closure (Fig. 7−5). The Class III hip involves pseudarthrosis of the femoral neck that may be stable or unstable as demonstrated by push-pull radiographic views (Fig. 7−6). Valgus osteotomy of the proximal femur with bone grafting of the defect is indicated in the face of instability at the pseudarthrosis. Class IV hips demonstrate complete destruction of the femoral head with a remnant of the femoral neck that remains either stable within the acetabulum or is dislocated from the acetabulum (Fig. 7−7). Class V hips exhibit total destruction of the femoral head and neck with no remaining articulation (Fig. 7−8).

Results in addition to the development of an incongruous hip joint include progressive leg length discrepancy, relative overgrowth of the greater trochanter, unstable pseudarthrosis of the femoral neck, unstable articulation of the remnant of the femoral neck within the acetabulum, and complete loss of joint articulation.

Evidence of incongruency or avascular necrosis of the ossification center of the proximal femur may be treated by abduction bracing in the same mode as Perthes disease. If early closure of the proximal femoral physis occurs, epiphysiodesis of the greater trochanter should be accomplished early in order to maintain a mechanically efficient abductor mechanism. At later ages, relative overgrowth of the greater trochanter may be treated by distal transfer of the trochanter. Pseudarthrosis of the femoral neck, when unstable, may be addressed through direct bone grafting of the defect and valgus osteotomy of the proximal femur. A more complex set of problems is created when the articulation is compromised by loss of the femoral head. In Class IV the femoral neck remnant may be either stable within the acetabulum or unstable outside of the

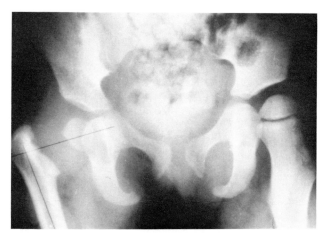

Fɪɢ. **7−6.** Class III hips demonstrate pseudarthrosis of the femoral neck.

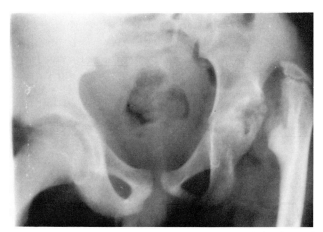

Fɪɢ. **7−8.** Class V hips exhibit total destruction of the femoral head and neck.

acetabulum. In the stable circumstance, arthrography may reveal a rounded cartilagenous anlage covering the remnant of the femoral neck. The anlage may be congruent or incongruent in neutral weight-bearing position. If it is incongruent, it may become more congruent by varus or valgus positioning. Improved congruence could then be created by appropriate varus or valgus osteotomy of the proximal femur.[3,11,19,28] When the femoral neck remnant resides outside of the confines of the acetabulum, push-pull radiographs are helpful in determining whether instability exists. In the face of instability, varus osteotomy of the proximal femur may be indicated to create a more stable articulation.[20,23]

The most severely afflicted hips have sustained complete loss of the femoral head and neck (Class V). Trochanteric arthroplasty has been proposed by Salvati and others as a successful method of treatment in the child under three years of age.[10,35,37,38] The greater trochanter is placed within the acetabulum by varus osteotomy and stabilized by advancement of the abductor musculature. Frequently, pelvic osteotomy is required to create a more competent acetabulum. In the face of marked instability and dysplasia of the acetabulum, arthrodesis of the hip becomes an option.[3]

In both Class IV and Class V hips, the growth potential of the proximal femur has been destroyed at an early age. Progressive leg length discrepancy may be managed by shoe lifts or by lengthening procedures of the ipsilateral lower leg, epiphysiodesis of the opposite distal femur or proximal tibia, or by a combination of procedures.

The sequelae of septic arthritis of the hip in infants may be of such severity that disability will permanently alter the character of the child's life with psychologic, recreational, and vocational ramifications. Early suspicion and diagnosis of this problem must be followed by expedient surgical drainage and parenteral antibiotics. Although the reconstructive procedures noted for more advanced problems may provide initial satisfactory results, there is significant concern that these individuals will eventually suffer disabling degenerative hip disease at a relatively young age with no good lifelong solutions.

References

1. BADGLEY CE, YGLESIAS L, PERHAM WS, SNYDER CH: Study of the end results in 113 cases of septic hips. J Bone Joint Surg, 18(4):1047–1061, 1936.

2. BORELLA L, GOOBAR JE, SUMMITT RL, CLARK GM: Septic arthritis in childhood. J Pediatr, 62(5):742–747, 1963.

3. BRYSON AF: Treatment of pathological dislocation of the hip joint after suppurative arthritis in infants. J Bone Joint Surg, 30B(3):449–453, 1948.

4. CURTISS PH Jr: Cartilage damage in septic arthritis. Clin Orthop Rel Res, 64:87–90, 1969.

5. DANIEL D, et al.: Lavage of septic joints in rabbits: effects of chondrolysis. J Bone Joint Surg, 58A:393–395, 1976.

6. DIAS L, TACHDJIAN MO, SCHROEDER KE: Premature closure of the triradiate cartilage. J Bone Joint Surg, 62B(1):46–48, 1980.

7. EYRE-BROOK AL: Septic arthritis of the hip and osteomyelitis of the upper end of the femur in infants. J Bone Joint Surg, 42B(1):11–20, 1960.

8. GILLESPIE R: Septic arthritis in childhood. Clin Orthop, 96:152–159, 1973.

9. GRIFFIN PP, GREEN WT Sr: Hip joint infections in infants and children. Orthop Clin North Am, 9(1):123–134, 1978.

10. HALLEL T, SALVATI EA: Septic arthritis of the hip in infancy. Clin Orthop, 132:115–128, 1978.

11. HARMON PH: Surgical treatment of the residual deformity from suppurative arthritis of the hip occurring in young children. J Bone Joint Surg, 24(3):576–585, 1942.

12. HARMON PH, ADAMS CO: Pyogenic coxitis: end-results and considerations of diagnosis and treatment. Surg Gynecol Obstet, 371–390, 1944.

13. HEBERLING JA: A review of two hundred and one cases of suppurative arthritis. J Bone Joint Surg, 23(4):917–921, 1941.

14. HOWARD JB, HIGHGENBOTEN CL, NELSON JD: Residual effects of septic arthritis in infancy and childhood. JAMA, 236(8):932–933, 1976.

15. HOWARD PJ: Sepsis in normal and premature infants with localization in the hip joint. Pediatrics, 279–289, 1957.

16. HUNKA L, et al.: Classification and surgical management of the severe sequelae of septic hips in children. Clin Orthop, 171:30–36, 1982.

17. INGE GAL, LIEBOLT FL: The treatment of acute suppurative arthritis (report of thirty-six cases treated by operation). Surg Gynecol Obstet, 86–101, 1935.

18. KAHN DS, PRITZKER KPH: The pathophysiology of bone infection. Clin Orthop, 96:12–19, 1973.

19. L'EPISCOPO JB: Stabilization of pathological dislocation of the hip in children. J Bone Joint Surg, 18(3):737–742, 1936.

20. LLOYD-ROBERTS GC: Suppurative arthritis of infancy (some observations upon prognosis and management). J Bone Joint Surg, 42B(4):706–720, 1960.

21. LUNSETH PA, HEIPLE KG: Prognosis in septic arthritis of the hip in children. Clin Orthop, 139:81–85, 1979.

22. MARCH AW, RILEY LH, ROBINSON RA: Retroperitoneal abscess and septic arthritis of the hip in children (a problem in differential diagnosis). J Bone Joint Surg, 54A(1):67–74, 1972.

23. MITCHELL GP: Management of acquired dislocation of the hip in septic arthritis. Orthop Clin of North Am 11(1):51–64, 1980.

24. MORREY BF, BIANCO AJ, RHODES KH: Septic arthritis in children. Orthop Clin North Am 6(4):923–934, 1975.

25. MORREY BF, BIANCO AJ, RHODES KH: Suppurative arthritis of the hip in children. J Bone Joint Surg, 58A(3):388–392, 1976.

26. NELSON JD, KOONTZ WC: Septic arthritis in infants and children: a review of 117 cases. Pediatrics, 38(6):966–971, 1966.

27. NELSON JD, HOWARD JB, SHELTON S: Oral antibiotic therapy for skeletal infections of children. J Pediatr, 92(1):131–134, 1978.

28. NICHOLSON JT: Pyogenic arthritis with pathologic dislocation of the hip in infants. JAMA, 141(12):826–831, 1949.

29. OBLETZ BE: Acute suppurative arthritis of the hip in the neonatal period. J Bone Joint Surg, 42A(1):23–30, 1960.

30. OBLETZ BE: Suppurative arthritis of the hip joint in infants. Clin Orthop, 22:27–33, 1962.

31. OGDEN JA: Changing patterns of proximal femoral vascularity. J Bone Joint Surg, 56A(5):941–950, 1974.

32. OGDEN JA, LISTER GL: The pathology of neonatal osteomyelitis. Pediatrics, 55(4):474–478, 1975.

33. PATERSON D: Septic arthritis of the hip joint. Orthop Clin North Am 9(1):135–142, 1978.

34. ROSS DW: Acute suppurative arthritis of the hip in premature infants. JAMA, 156(4):303–307, 1954.

35. SALVATI EA: Septic arthritis of the hip in infancy: treatment of the sequelae and long-term results. *The Hip*, 105–124, 1979.

36. SIFFERT RS: The effect of juxta-epiphyseal pyogenic infection on epiphyseal growth. Clin Orthop, 10:131–139, 1957.

37. STETSON JW, DEPONTE RJ, SOUTHWICK WO: Acute septic arthritis of the hip in children. Clin Orthop, 56:105–116, 1968.

38. WEISSMAN SL: Transplantation of the trochanteric epiphysis into the acetabulum after septic arthritis of the hip. J Bone Joint Surg, 49A(8):1647–1651, 1967.

39. WHITE H: Roentgen findings of acute infectious disease of the hip in infants and children. Clin Orthop, 34–42, 1962.

CHAPTER EIGHT

Hip Abnormalities in Dwarfism

GEORGE S. BASSETT
CHARLES I. SCOTT, Jr.

Introduction

Hip deformities are frequent disabling sequelae of dwarfing conditions. These hip abnormalities are a result of a generalized disturbance in the growth of cartilage and bone variously affecting the axial and appendicular skeleton. By definition, dwarfs are disproportionately short statured. The disproportions are determined by the relative predominance of trunk versus limb involvement. Hence, certain dwarfing conditions have greater shortening of the limbs with respect to the trunk and vice versa. For example, the limb involvement relative to trunk involvement is more severe in achondroplasia, pseudoachondroplasia, and the metaphyseal dysplasias leading to the appearance of short-limbed dwarfism. In contrast, the significant spinal involvement present in metatropic dwarfism, Kniest syndrome, and spondyloepiphyseal dysplasia congenita results in short-trunk dwarfism. Involvement of the limb segment is likewise variable. Rhizomelic (upper), mesomelic (middle), or acromelic (distal) shortening of the limbs may be present. The spinal involvement is also variable, including platyspondyly, atlantoaxial instability, kyphosis, scoliosis, or stenosis. These various distinctions are useful for identification purposes but not for classification.

The heterogeneity of the short-statured syndromes demands an accurate diagnosis, which frequently requires a thorough evaluation by a geneticist. For instance, differentiation of the various subtypes of spondyloepiphyseal dysplasia tarda or pseudoachondroplasia generally is not possible for the orthopaedic surgeon. In addition, the natural history and prognosis for each of the skeletal dysplasias are highly variable, which may influence decision making for treatment of the hip disorder. Thus, the evaluation of the hip deformity must be made in conjunction with a proper identification of the specific skeletal dysplasia. For example, the apparent diminished walking tolerance or pain presumed to be originating in the hip of an achondroplastic patient is more likely to be secondary to a myelopathy originating from lumbar spinal stenosis or a severe thoracolumbar kyphosis. Therefore, the initial evaluation of the short-statured individual must consist of a complete history, including family history, physical examination, appropriate radiographs, including the spine and the upper and lower extremities, and consultation with a geneticist.

Rubin made an early attempt to characterize skeletal dysplasias based upon the radiographic region of predominant growth disturbance, that is, epiphysis, physis, metaphysis, or diaphysis.[8,21] Although these anatomic divisions may be useful in order to classify the dysplasia radiographically according to traditional nomenclature, that is, multiple epiphyseal dysplasia, metaphyseal chondrodysplasia, and so on, this terminology does not completely reflect the extent of histopathologic involvement. For example, biopsies from patients with multiple epiphyseal dysplasia reveal not only epiphyseal involvement but also significant alterations of the chondrocytes in all four zones of the physis and abnormal cartilage bars in the metaphysis.[14] Similarly, in a patient with metaphyseal chondrodysplasia, abnormalities have been observed originating in the physis consisting of nests of cartilage cells proliferating into the hypertropic zone, disorganized cell columns, and irregular provisional calcification.[11] The widely used classification and nomenclature of intrinsic skeletal dysplasia was developed in Paris in 1969, was revised in 1983,[1] and is now considered the standard.

This classification separates the intrinsic diseases of bone into broad categories based upon knowledge of pathogenesis. Further subdivision is based upon morphologic distinction. For instance, "osteochondrodysplasias," meaning abnormalities

TABLE 8–1. *Osteochondrodysplasias (abnormalities of cartilage or bone growth and development)—Defects of Growth of Tubular Bones or Spine**

Identifiable at Birth
  Usually lethal before or shortly after birth
    Achondrogenesis
    Hypochondrogenesis
    Fibrochondrogenesis
    Thanatophoric dysplasia
    Atelosteogenesis
    Short rib syndromes
  Usually nonlethal dysplasia
    Chondrodysplasia punctata
    Campomelic dysplasia
    Kyphomelic dysplasia
    Achondroplasia
    Diastrophic dysplasia
    Metatropic dysplasia
    Chondroectodermal dysplasia (Ellis-van Creveld)
    Asphyxiating thoracic dysplasia (Jeune)
    Spondyloepiphyseal dysplasia congenita
    Kniest dysplasia
    Dyssegmental dysplasia
    Mesomelic dysplasias
    Acromesomelic dysplasia
    Cleidocranial dysplasia
    Oto-palato-digital syndromes
    Larsen syndrome

Identifiable in Later Life
  Hypochondroplasia
  Dyschondrosteosis
  Metaphyseal chondrodysplasias
  Spondylometaphyseal dysplasias
  Multiple epiphyseal dysplasia
  Arthro-ophthalmopathy (Stickler)
  Pseudoachondroplasia
  Spondyloepiphyseal dysplasia tarda (X-linked recessive)
  Progressive pseudorheumatoid chondrodysplasia
  Brachyolmia
  Dyggve-Melchior-Clausen dysplasia
  Spondyloepimetaphyseal dysplasias
  Oto-spondylo-megaepiphyseal dysplasia (OSMED)
  Myotonic chondrodysplasia (Catel-Schwartz-Jampel)
  Para-stenotic dysplasia
  Tricho-rhino-phalangeal dysplasia
  Acrodysplasia with retinitis pigmentosa and nephropathy (Saldino-Mainzer)

*Adapted from Lenzi L, Capilupi B: International nomenclature of constitutional diseases of bone. Revision 1983. Ital J Orthop Traumatol, 11(2)249–256, 1985.

of cartilage or bone growth and development, are differentiated from "dysostoses," malformations of individual bones, singly or in combination. There are more than one hundred specific intrinsic dysplasias that are fairly well defined. This chapter will deal with those hip abnormalities observed in the dwarfing disorders. These consist of conditions categorized as osteochondrodysplasias Group I: defects of growth of tubular bones or spine (Table 8–1).

Achondroplasia

Achondroplasia is the most common form of short-limbed dwarfism. It is transmitted as an autosomal dominant trait. The majority of affected individuals are the result of spontaneous new mutations. Clinical features are recognizable at birth, including an enlarged neurocranium with frontal bossing, midface hypoplasia with depression of the nasal bridge and malar area, rhizomelic shortening of the extremities, "trident" hand, relatively normal trunk length, ligamentous laxity, exaggerated lumbar lordosis, and a protuberant abdomen. Radiographic features are characteristic and include neurocranial enlargement with a shortened base of the skull, a small, narrow foramen magnum, interpedicular narrowing in the lumbar spine, thoracolumbar kyphosis with posterior scalloping of the vertebral bodies, and a broad, short pelvis with wide iliac wings, horizontal superior acetabular margins, and small, acutely angulated sacrosciatic notches. The long bones are short, thick, and mildly bowed at birth. The distal femoral physis has an inverted "V" configuration.[15,18]

Ponseti has demonstrated that the alterations of skeletal growth are predominantly at the physeal region of long bones.[6] The growth plate of the iliac crest apophysis is virtually normal, whereas the triradiate cartilage, an enchondral growth plate, is affected. This results in a deep, horizontal acetabulum. Epiphyseal and articular cartilage is not affected. The hips are congruous, although the femoral necks are shortened, with mild overgrowth of the greater trochanters. This is consistent with an abnormality of growth in the physis sparing the appositional growth plate of the greater trochanter. Coxa vara is not a usual feature of the achondroplastic hip (Fig. 8–1).

Osteoarthritis is uncommonly observed in the adult achondroplastic dwarf. Hip pain in these patients is more likely to be secondary to spinal canal stenosis, which affects a majority of patients in varying degrees. This usually leads to diminished walking and standing tolerance. Surgery is rarely necessary for hip abnormalities in achondroplasia. Extension osteotomy of the proximal femur has been used occasionally in an attempt to improve excessive lumbar lordosis and relieve symptoms of spinal stenosis. The short-term benefits of this procedure are variable, and the long-term effectiveness is not known. Generally, most lower extremity surgery in achondroplasia is performed distally in order to restore proper alignment of the hip-knee-ankle mechanical axis.

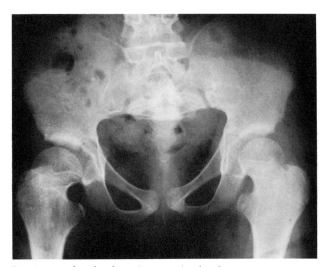

Fɪɢ. 8–1. Achondroplasia (10 years). The iliac wings are small and square with horizontal acetabular roofs. The sacrosciatic notches are small. The hips are congruous, with short, broad femoral necks and mild trochanteric overgrowth.

Chondrodysplasia Punctata

Chondrodysplasia punctata appears to be a heterogeneous group of disorders characterized by extraepiphyseal calcification and stippling of the epiphyses. A rhizomelic type (autosomal recessive), which is usually lethal, a sex-linked dominant form, and the more common Conradi-Hunermann type (autosomal dominant) have been identified.[17,19] The typical Conradi-Hunermann type is characterized by flat facial features with depression of the nasal bridge, congenital cataracts, alopecia, icthyosiform skin changes, and congenital heart disease. At birth, multiple punctate asymmetric extraepiphyseal calcifications and stippling of the epiphyses may occur involving the long bones, spine, and tarsal and carpal bones. These calcifications ordinarily disappear by one year of age. Spinal deformities, including kyphosis, scoliosis, and kyphoscoliosis, may develop rapidly in the first year of life from congenital anomalies or abnormal vertebral growth. Frequently, early spinal surgery is required. Odontoid hypoplasia may lead to significant atlantoaxial instability, requiring posterior cervical fusion.

Asymmetric involvement of the extremities is common, with varying degrees of limb shortening and joint contracture. Typically, there may be bowing of the femur and flaring of the distal femoral metaphysis combined with shortening. Limb length discrepancy may be considerable, ranging in magnitude to 6 cm. Hip involvement is likewise asymmetric and variable. There may be mild irregularity or significant deformity, including progressive subluxation, depending on the severity of epiphyseal involvement. The development of the ossific nucleus of the femoral head is delayed. Coxa vara is commonly found in conjunction with the asymmetric shortening of the femur (Fig. 8–2). Indications for valgus osteotomy are similar to those reported for congenital coxa vara. These include a neck-shaft angle less than 100°, progressive varus deformity, and a large persistent defect in ossification of the femoral neck. However, valgus osteotomy carries the inherent risk of premature closure of the physis from excessive pressure.[9] This risk may be minimized if some femoral shortening is done with the osteotomy, thereby decreasing the forces across the hip joint. The presence of significant hip contracture, deformity, or leg length inequality must be assessed carefully when considering any surgical intervention for the involved femur. For example, in patients with chondrodysplasia punctata, femoral lengthening may be an attractive solution for a 4- to 6-cm limb length discrepancy. However, if significant hip deformity exists, as is often the case, this approach must not be used, because progressive subluxation or stiffness may occur (Fig. 8–3).

Metatropic Dwarfism

Metatropic dwarfs have significantly shortened limbs at birth with relatively long and narrow trunks. There is significant platyspondyly radiographically, with anterior tongue-like flattening of the vertebral bodies and relatively tall disc spaces. Severe kyphoscoliosis usually develops during the first several years of life, leading to progressive trunk shortening.[7] This change in body proportions from a short-limbed disproportion at birth to a

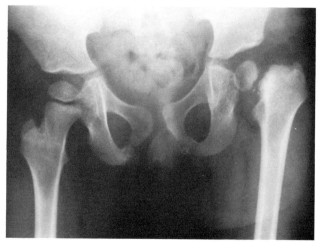

Fɪɢ. 8–2. Chondrodysplasia punctata (2 years). Coxa vara is present with a defect of ossification in the femoral neck. Stippled calcifications are still present in the ischial rami.

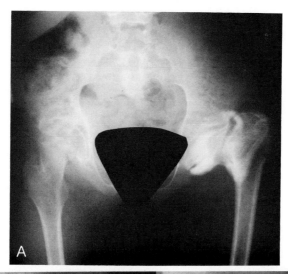

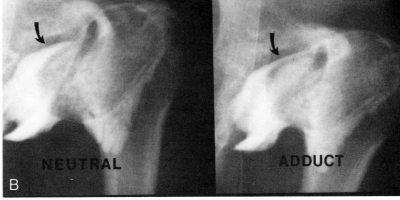

Fɪɢ. **8–3.** Chondrodysplasia punctata (14 years). **A.** A 4.5-cm femoral shortening occurred in association with coxa vara. Arthrography confirmed hip subluxation and incongruity. Femoral lengthening in this setting may result in further subluxation, leading to dislocation or stiffness from loss of articular cartilage. **B.** In this patient, adduction of the femur improves hip congruity. Note the diminished superior dye pool in adduction in comparison with neutral positioning. For reconstruction, valgus intertrochanteric osteotomy would be the procedure of choice.

short-trunk variety with growth and development led Maroteaux to suggest the term "metatropic," meaning "changing pattern," for this type of dwarfism.[3] Atlantoaxial instability is not uncommon secondary to odontoid hypoplasia and frequently requires posterior stabilization. Some patients have a small tail-like skin fold lying over the sacrum. Metatropic dwarfism is extremely rare, with an autosomal recessive mode of inheritance.

Significant metaphyseal flaring and epiphyseal involvement of the long bones lead to a "dumbbell" radiographic appearance. With a narrow diaphyses and pronounced metaphyseal widening, the joints appear enlarged radiographically and clinically. Ossification is delayed, and hence the epiphyses deform, leading to limited motion and premature osteoarthritis. The hips have small, deformed femoral heads, shortened femoral necks, and enlarged trochanteric regions. The acetabula are horizontal and deep, covering the small femoral heads

adequately in most instances. Protrusio acetabuli may be present. A distinctive iliac notch is usually present just superior to the attachment of the acetabular labrum (Fig. 8–4). Although the osteoarthritis may be significant, cardiopulmonary problems secondary to the progressive spinal deformities often predominate, precluding surgical intervention. Many patients fail to live beyond the second decade because of severe neurologic or cardiopulmonary symptoms secondary to the spinal deformity.

Diastrophic Dysplasia

Diastrophic dysplasia is an autosomal recessive disorder with short-limbed disproportion. It is characterized by severe kyphoscoliosis, resistant clubfeet, and contractures, subluxations, or dislocations of joints. Patients with this condition are further recognized by a shortened first metacarpal

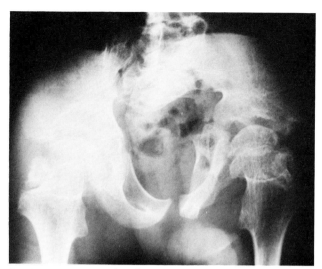

FIG. 8–4. Metatropic dwarfism (9 years). The femoral heads are enlarged with satisfactory congruity in this patient. The femoral necks are short, with broadened intertrochanteric regions and irregular ossification. Protrusion of the acetabula has distorted the pelvis.

with laxity of the metacarpophalangeal joint ("hitchhiker thumb"), synostosis of the proximal interphalangeal joints of the hand, and cystic swellings of the auricles, giving rise to cauliflower ear deformities. The head and skull are normal clinically, but calcifications of the pinnae and intracranial calcification may be found radiographically. The face has a peculiar appearance, with a narrowed nasal bridge, broad, flared nostrils, and circumoral fullness. Cleft palate is observed in 25% of cases. Cervical spine deformities are often severe, including a rapidly progressive cervical kyphosis secondary to hypoplasia of the C3 or C4 vertebral bodies in association with posterior element dysraphism. Atlantoaxial instability has not been observed, although the odontoid process may assume a horizontal orientation in patients with significant cervical kyphosis. Early recognition and surgical stabilization may be required to prevent progressive deformity and myelopathy if instability is present. If stable, resolution of the kyphosis may be anticipated. Basilar invagination also has been observed in diastrophism. Thoracic kyphoscoliosis frequently develops in the first five years of life. If bracing fails to control curve progression, early posterior spinal fusion is frequently necessary.

The hips are essentially universally involved in patients with diastrophic dysplasia. Anatomic abnormalities include coxa vara, subluxation, dislocation, and coxa valga with significant flexion contractures. Secondary osteoarthritis of the hips is virtually inevitable and is further complicated by severe valgus deformity of the knees with significant flexion contractures.

The epiphyses are often significantly involved in diastrophic dysplasia, leading to delayed ossification and early deformation of the femoral head. It has been reported that 25% of diastrophic dwarfs have bilateral hip dislocations.[22] These appear to be developmental dislocations rather than typical congenital hip dislocations. For these patients, femoral head ossification is delayed, with broadening of the femoral necks and metaphyses (Fig. 8–5). Initially, the acetabula may appear to contain the cartilaginous femoral heads properly. As the femoral head ossifies, a central area remains unossified, producing a saucer-shaped defect. This leads to a broad, flattened femoral head with a shortened metaphyseal region (Fig. 8–6). The growth disturbance and failure of ossification produce progressive coxa vara with a sequence of lateral extrusion of the femoral head, hinge abduction, subluxation, or, in many instances, dislocation (Fig. 8–7). These dislocations appear to result from a combination of femoral head deformity, severe flexion contractures, and a failure of the acetabula to contain the misshaped femoral heads. These hips tend to be the stiffest and progress to premature osteoarthritis most rapidly. Some hips, although contracted, do not deform rapidly but rather stay relatively well contained in the acetabulum. These hips appear to be more flexible, with less incongruity of the hip joint. Osteoarthritis results nevertheless, although not as rapidly.

Treatment of the hip in diastrophic dysplasia

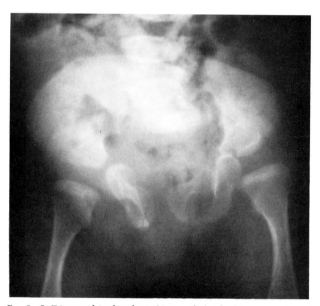

FIG. 8–5. Diastrophic dysplasia (6 months). The hips are reduced, although poorly contained by the small acetabula. The ossification of the femoral heads is delayed. Severe bowing and shortening of the femur are present in association with broadened femoral necks and metaphyses.

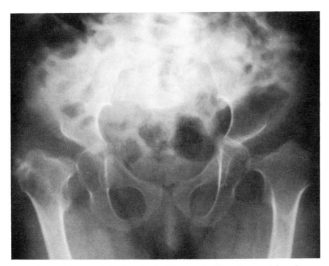

FIG. 8–6. Diastrophic dysplasia (4 years). The femoral heads are subluxated and poorly covered by the smaller acetabula. A central saucer-shaped defect of ossification persists. Hinge abduction is present frequently and is demonstrated best by arthrography.

must be planned in relation to the deformities involving the whole lower extremity if a functional result is to be achieved. Various considerations include evaluation of hip joint incongruity, the magnitude of the contractures present in the weight-bearing joints and degree of stiffness, as well as the overall alignment of the mechanical axis of the lower extremity.

Unfortunately, the severity of the spinal abnormalities and clubfoot deformities frequently requires early surgical intervention, necessitating a delay in treatment of the hips. Often, significant deformity and stiffness already are present, preclud-

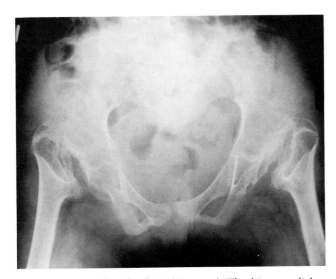

FIG. 8–7. Diastrophic dysplasia (11 years). The hips are dislocated bilaterally. Note the poor development of the acetabula and the dissolution of the femoral heads and necks distally to the intertrochanteric region.

ing any attempt at surgical reconstruction. Attention first should be directed at improving and maintaining motion of the hip and knee. If satisfactory motion is achieved, surgery may be considered to improve congruity of the hip joint. Arthrography may be helpful in the early assessment of these patients with poorly ossified femoral heads to determine the optimal position for congruity. For those hips with significant coxa vara, superolateral femoral head deformation, or hinge abduction, valgus intertrochanteric osteotomy may improve congruity, but should be performed only if the hip and knee have a functional range of motion.

Severe osteoarthritis is common in young adult life, and total hip replacement may be considered for the diastrophic dwarf if his or her general medical condition is acceptable. However, careful evaluation of the spine, neurologic function, and lower extremity alignment, contracture, and motion must be completed prior to surgical consideration. Hence, surgical reconstruction of the hip, whether it be osteotomy or arthroplasty, frequently will not be feasible in diastrophic dwarfs in light of their overall medical condition and functional limitations.

Chondroectodermal Dysplasia

Chondroectodermal dysplasia, otherwise known as Ellis-van Creveld syndrome, is characterized by acromesomelic limb shortening, postaxial polydactyly of the hands, and dysplastic nails, hair, and teeth.[13] Neonatal mortality occurs frequently because of severe cardiopulmonary complication of congenital heart disease. This rare short-limbed disproportionate dwarfing condition, frequently found among the Amish, is inherited in an autosomal recessive fashion.[4] Distinctive radiographic signs include a caudally directed spike observed rising below the sciatic notch in infants and fusion of the capitate and hamate bones of the hand. Chondroectodermal dysplasia generally is considered a disorder of the ectoderm and physeal growth. The lateral aspect of the proximal tibial epiphysis characteristically is severely involved, giving rise to a progressive genu valgum deformity. This usually requires early proximal tibial osteotomy for correction. Older patients require combined femoral and tibial osteotomies for reconstruction (Fig. 8–8). The femoral ossific nucleus ossifies early and is ordinarily present at birth. Thus, deformation of the epiphyseal cartilage of the femoral head does not occur. The hip is affected only mildly apart from slight broadening and

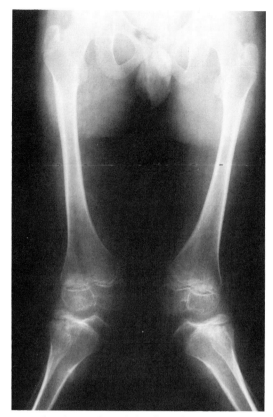

Fɪɢ. 8–8. Chondroectodermal dysplasia (12 years). Severe genu valgum deformities exist secondary to a lateral growth disturbance of the tibial epiphyses and overgrowth of the medial femoral condyle. Apart from the valgus deformity of the femoral necks, the hips are well contained and congruous.

valgus orientation of the femoral neck. Premature osteoarthritis of the hip is not typical.

Spondyloepiphyseal Dysplasia Congenita

Spondyloepiphyseal dysplasia congenita is an autosomal dominant condition characterized by extreme short stature with disproportionate shortening of the trunk and severe hip involvement.[20] The spine is severely diminished in height from platyspondyly, which is compounded in many instances by progressive early kyphoscoliosis. A fixed exaggerated lumbar lordosis is usually present along with pectus carinatum. Odontoid hypoplasia with resultant atlantoaxial instability is a common occurrence, necessitating posterior fusion, which should be considered as soon as the diagnosis is entertained. Cervical myelopathy was reported in one series to occur in 30% of patients with spondyloepiphyseal dysplasia. Clinical manifestations included respiratory symptoms in infancy, failure to achieve normal motor milestones of standing or walking, and various degrees of quadriplegia following minor trauma.[15] Associated extraskeletal ab-

normalities include retinal detachment in two thirds of the patients, severe myopia with cataracts, deafness, and cleft palate.

Involvement of the appendicular skeleton is less abnormal distally, although clubfoot deformity is not infrequent. The epiphyses are involved predominantly, with irregular ossification and diminished size. The metaphyses also are involved to a degree, with irregular margins and flaring. The most severely involved epiphyses are in the proximal femur. Significant delay in the ossification of the capital femoral epiphyses occurs, and these frequently do not appear until 4 or 5 years of age. Early deformation of the femoral head may be suspected if the "sagging rope" sign is observed radiographically.[10] If this sign is present, the femoral head usually is enlarged, with flattening and extrusion. Arthrography should be considered to assess congruity, subluxation, and hinge abduction (Fig. 8–9). Severe coxa vara often develops. The coxa vara is usually progressive, leading to flattening and deformation of the femoral head, shortening of the femoral neck, and eventual dislocation in those patients with severe growth disturbance of the capital femoral physis. There is overgrowth of the greater trochanter. The hips develop a significant flexion contracture in conjunction with the fixed lumbar lordosis. Premature osteoarthritis is a likely early sequela.

Assuming proper evaluation and treatment of any spinal deformities, hip reconstruction may be

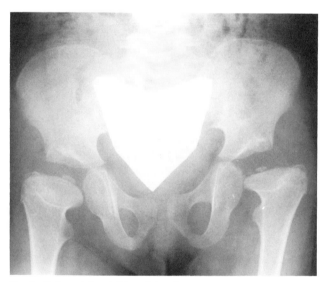

Fɪɢ. 8–9. Spondyloepiphyseal dysplasia congenita (4 years). Ossification of the capital femoral epiphysis is significantly delayed. The femoral neck is broad, with trochanteric overgrowth. The "sagging rope" sign is present, which is indicative of early deformation of the femoral head. The increased distance from the teardrop to the femoral neck is suggestive of subluxation. Arthrography confirmed subluxation with hinge abduction.

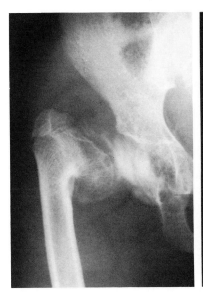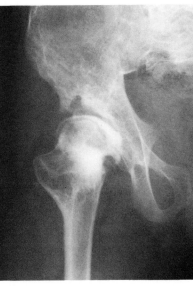

Fig. 8–10. Spondyloepiphyseal dysplasia congenita. **Left.** The preoperative arthrogram of a 10-year-old girl reveals severe coxa vara and dislocation. Symptoms included pain, waddling gait, and decreased walking endurance. **Right.** Two years after combined open reduction, valgus intertrochanteric osteotomy, and Chiari osteotomy, arthrography reveals satisfactory congruity and stability.

considered with a valgus intertrochanteric osteotomy and acetabuloplasty prior to dislocation. Hip arthrography is an invaluable aid in the preoperative assessment. If dislocation has occurred, walking tolerance may deteriorate, although coexisting myelopathy must be ruled out. In selected cases, the results of combined open reduction, valgus osteotomy, and capsulorrhaphy will be successful in obtaining reduction (Fig. 8–10). The valgus osteotomy improves the congruity of the hip joint and the function of the abductors through simultaneous advancement of the greater trochanter. Frequently, a Chiari osteotomy is required for coverage of the femoral head and stability because of severe acetabular insufficiency. These seemingly aggressive measures appear to be warranted in light of the significant risk of premature osteoarthritis and the difficulties of arthroplasty in this population of patients.

Spondyloepiphyseal Dysplasia Tarda

Spondyloepiphyseal dysplasia exists in a tarda form with X-linked recessive, autosomal recessive, and dominant modes of transmission in various families. A careful family history and evaluation of appropriate family members are thus important in distinguishing one disorder from another. The trunk is disproportionately shortened but is not as severely involved as in spondyloepiphyseal dysplasia congenita. Craniofacial abnormalities are not present in the tarda form. Atlantoaxial instability may be present secondary to odontoid hypoplasia or os odontoideum. Scoliosis is unusual in spondyloepiphyseal dysplasia tarda. The epiphyseal involvement is similar to that observed in multiple epiphyseal dysplasia, but in the latter, not to the extent of spinal involvement that is present in spondyloepiphyseal dysplasia tarda. There may be mild brachydactyly but not the degree observed in pseudoachondroplasia.

Generally, hip involvement is anatomically less severe compared to spondyloepiphyseal dysplasia congenita. Mild coxa vara may exist, but it is not progressive and does not result in dislocation. However, the epiphyseal involvement of the hip frequently leads to osteoarthritis in early adult life because of coxa vara or flattening, incongruity, or extrusion of the femoral head. Frequently, the clinical appearance of a patient with spondyloepiphyseal dysplasia tarda may be altered so mildly that the diagnosis is not made until late adolescence. Patients often are referred to an orthopaedic surgeon for mild hip symptoms or after a radiograph of the pelvis has been obtained for unrelated complaints. These changes may simulate bilateral Perthes disease, but the involvement is symmetric (Fig. 8–11). Furthermore, a skeletal survey will reveal obvious radiographic changes involving multiple epiphyses and the spine.[12]

Surgical reconstruction of these hips must be considered when the patient presents in adolescence or young adult life. Premature osteoarthritis is such a common sequela that treatment is warranted unless the femoral head is properly contained by the acetabulum. Arthrography is useful in the evaluation process. Generally, mild to moderate coxa vara is present with coxa magna. If coverage of the femoral head is poor, with no extrusion or flattening, pelvic osteotomy will facilitate containment. Shelf augmentation may be required in

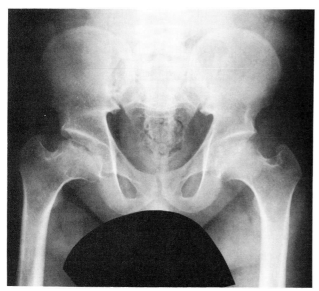

Fɪɢ. **8–11.** Spondyloepiphyseal dysplasia tarda (19 years). Mild coxa vara and coxa magna with ossification irregularities of the capital femoral epiphyses. The acetabula are virtually normal, adequately containing the femoral heads.

addition to the pelvic osteotomy because of femoral head enlargement. If extrusion, significant flattening, or hinge abduction is evidenced by arthrogram, valgus intertrochanteric osteotomy is usually the primary surgical procedure. Occasionally, a Chiari osteotomy or shelf procedure will be performed in conjunction with the valgus osteotomy to improve coverage of the femoral head. This is particularly warranted if the femoral head is not completely ossified, because the acetabular procedure adds lateral support and may prevent further flattening.

In juvenile patients, before satisfactory ossification of the capital femoral epiphysis has occurred, a "sagging rope" sign frequently is observed on the radiograph.[10] If this sign is present, the possibility of coxa magna with early deformity and lateral extrusion or subluxation must be considered. This is evaluated readily by arthrography. If arthrographic confirmation of extrusion or subluxation is obtained, abduction bracing or pelvic osteotomy should be considered provided that the femoral head is reducible in abduction and only minimal flattening is present. At this stage, the cartilaginous femoral head still may be remodeled by containment. However, if hinge abduction is present, pelvic osteotomy should not be performed unless preceded by valgus osteotomy, as in the older patient.

Cleidocranial Dysplasia

This is an autosomal dominant condition predominantly affecting membrane bones such as the

clavicle and skull with widening of the symphysis pubis. Short stature may be present but usually is not marked in degree. The capital femoral epiphysis ossifies early and is often present at birth, giving the appearance of a widened physis and short neck (Fig. 8–12). In spite of the widened physis, discontinuity of the femoral head and neck has not been reported. Coxa vara may be observed, and if progressive, valgus osteotomy is warranted if joint incongruity is not a problem (Fig. 8–13). A valgus deformity in association with a short neck is observed more commonly in cleidocranial dysplasia. However, premature osteoarthritis is not common.

Metaphyseal Chondrodysplasia

This group of disorders is characterized by defective enchondral bone formation leading to mild short stature, relatively normal epiphyses, broadened metaphyses, and lateral bowing of the femur and tibia (Fig. 8–14). There are several distinct types, including the more common Schmid and McKusick (cartilage hair hypoplasia) types and the rare Jansen type.[16] In the Schmid type, inherited by autosomal dominant transmission, there is mild shortness of stature, increased lumbar lordosis, waddling gait, and varus deformities of the hips,

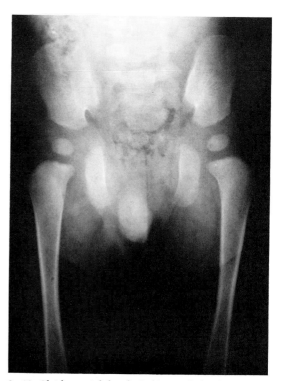

Fɪɢ. **8–12.** Cleidocranial dysplasia (4 months). Advanced maturation of the capital femoral epiphyses with a wide symphysis pubis and hypoplastic pubic rami.

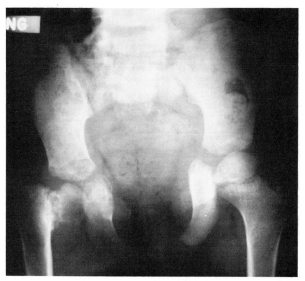

Fɪɢ. 8–13. Cleidocranial dysplasia (5 years). Severe coxa vara is present on the right with an ossification defect of the femoral neck. The symphysis pubis is wide, and the pubic rami are hypoplastic.

knees, and ankles. The McKusick type, otherwise known as cartilage hair hypoplasia, is characterized by autosomal recessive inheritance, shortness of stature, and ligamentous laxity and may be associ-

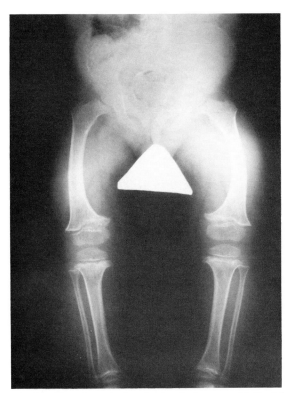

Fɪɢ. 8–14. Metaphyseal chondrodysplasia, type McKusick (4 years). Bilateral coxa vara, with bowing and shortening of the femurs and tibias. The metaphyses are flared and mildly irregular. The epiphyses are normal.

ated with disorders of malabsorption, Hirschsprung's disease, and abnormal cellular immunity. Hip involvement is less severe than in the Schmid type. However, the hands are significantly involved in the McKusick type, with shortening of metacarpals and phalanges with cone-shaped epiphyses.[5] The Jansen type is extremely rare and is characterized by marked expansion of the metaphyses with irregular ossification and widening of the physes. It is characterized by significant shortness of stature, angular deformities of extremities, decreased joint mobility, significant hand involvement with cupped metaphyses, and autosomal dominant mode of inheritance.

Hip involvement in the metaphyseal chondrodysplasias is usually a mild coxa vara. A progressive varus deformity is not common unless a triangular metaphyseal fragment exists in the inferior femoral neck. Valgus osteotomy is indicated if there is progressive varus deformity of the presence of a triangular metaphyseal fragment. Hip joint congruity is usually normal, because epiphyseal involvement is minimal. Osteoarthritis may develop early as a consequence of malalignment of the joints but not to the extent or frequency observed in the epiphyseal or spondyloepiphyseal dysplasias.

Multiple Epiphyseal Dysplasia

Multiple epiphyseal dysplasia is one of the more common forms of skeletal dysplasia leading to mild shortness of stature in varying degrees. It is usually transmitted as an autosomal dominant trait, and many patients are first referred to the orthopaedic surgeon with complaints referable to premature degenerative arthritis or "bilateral Perthes disease." The hallmark of this disorder is bilateral symmetric involvement of multiple joints, including the hands and feet, with only minor spinal involvement. Secondary centers of ossification appear fragmented and are late in developing. Crossan and associates have emphasized the importance of differentiating bilateral failure of the capital femoral epiphysis from Perthes disease.[12] In those instances of bilateral symmetric Perthes disease, the probability of another disorder is high, including multiple epiphyseal dysplasia, spondyloepiphyseal dysplasia, or pseudoachondroplasia. However, unilateral avascular necrosis of the capital femoral epiphysis has been observed in patients with multiple epiphyseal dysplasia (Fig. 8–15).[23] This avascularity has been documented by nuclear radiographic and magnetic resonance imaging (MRI) techniques (Fig. 8–16). These hips appear to go through the

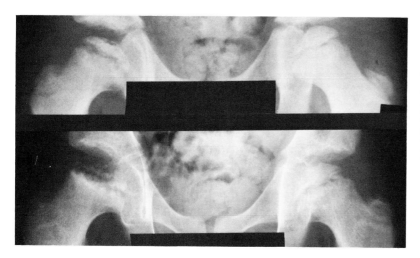

Fig. 8–15. Multiple epiphyseal dysplasia. **Top.** An 8-year-old boy with known multiple epiphyseal dysplasia (positive family history and skeletal survey) develops pain in the right hip. There is increased density in the right capital femoral epiphysis and a crescent sign. The left capital femoral epiphysis is small and irregular, but avascular changes are absent. **Bottom.** Six months later there is progressive resorption on the right, with normal growth on the left.

usual stages of injury and repair that are seen in Perthes disease. However, the time course for these changes may be prolonged compared with that in Perthes disease. If avascular necrosis is superimposed on multiple epiphyseal dysplasia, treatment consists of restoring motion followed by containment of the femoral head in the acetabulum. Motion is regained through traction and physical therapy, and containment is achieved by abduction bracing or surgery, depending on the age of the patient.

The delay in femoral head ossification results in poor support for the enlarging epiphyseal cartilage, resulting in a mushroom-shaped femoral head. Radiographically, a "sagging rope" sign is often present at this stage (Fig. 8–17). If the femoral head is poorly contained by the acetabulum, further deformation with flattening, extrusion, or subluxation may occur. Before significant deformation occurs, there appears to be a role for brace containment. We have been using an abduction-internal rotation orthosis at nighttime. With the delay in ossification, the cartilaginous femoral head

appears to remodel, with improved congruity and stability. Alternatively, acetabuloplasty may be considered for more severe deformities. If significant discrepancy in size exists between the femoral head and the acetabulum or if incongruity exists, innominate osteotomy should not be performed. Shelf augmentation or Chiari osteotomy may be considered to improve femoral head coverage and stability. Hip arthrography with neutral, abduction, and adduction views greatly facilitates the decision making process (Fig. 8–18). Varus osteotomy to improve containment is usually contraindicated because a mild varus deformity is usually present. If there is significant flattening or lateral extrusion, reconstruction is usually limited to valgus extension osteotomy for the young adult. Premature osteoarthritis is a common sequela of multiple epiphyseal dysplasia. At maturity, the femoral heads are enlarged, irregular, and often incompletely covered by the acetabula (Fig. 8–19). In addition to the coxa magna, varus deformity with femoral neck shortening and trochanteric overgrowth is usually present.

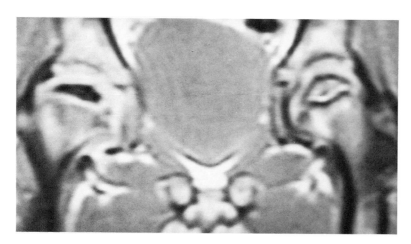

Fig. 8–16. Multiple epiphyseal dysplasia (8 years). An MRI scan of the patient in Figure 8–15 reveals an avascular capital femoral epiphysis on the right and normal vascularity on the left. (From Mackenzie WG, Bassett GS, Mandell GA, Scott CI: Avascular necrosis of the hip in multiple epiphyseal dysplasia. J Ped Orthop, 9:666–667, 1989)

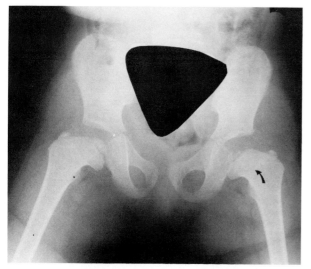

FIG. 8–17. Multiple epiphyseal dysplasia (5 years). The ossification of the capital femoral epiphyses is delayed, and mild coxa vara and trochanteric overgrowth are present. A "sagging rope" sign is present bilaterally, which is indicative of early deformation of the femoral head and frequently subluxation. Arthrography was performed (see Fig. 8–18). (From Mackenzie WG, Bassett GS, Mandell GA, Scott CI: Avascular necrosis of the hip in multiple epiphyseal dysplasia. J Ped Orthop, in press.)

Hereditary Arthro-ophthalmopathy

Hereditary arthro-ophthalmopathy (Stickler syndrome), inherited in an autosomal dominant mode, is characterized by severe myopia, retinal detach-

ment, mild platyspondyly, enlargement of joints, and epiphyseal changes. Clinical manifestations vary considerably within a given family. These patients usually do not have major shortness of stature, but because of the epiphyseal irregularities, they are prone to premature osteoarthritis. Frequently, the hips assume a valgus orientation, which may be quite significant (Fig. 8–20). In some instances, a varus osteotomy is warranted.

Pseudoachondroplasia

The entity termed "pseudoachondroplastic spondyloepiphyseal dysplasia" by Maroteaux and Lamy in 1959 historically has been confused with achondroplasia.[2] This is a heterogeneous group of disorders characterized by rhizomelic short-limbed dwarfism with a relatively normal-sized trunk, head, and facies and short hypermobile fingers. The skeletal dysplasia usually is not apparent at birth, but the growth retardation of the limbs becomes apparent by two to three years of age. Inheritance is autosomal dominant in the majority of families. In a few pedigrees, autosomal recessive transmission has been considered likely. Limb involvement is significant, with both angular deformities and premature osteoarthritis. This occurs because of severe ligamentous laxity and epiphyseal involve-

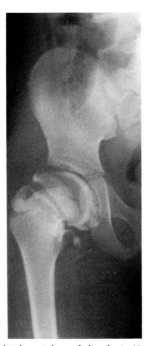 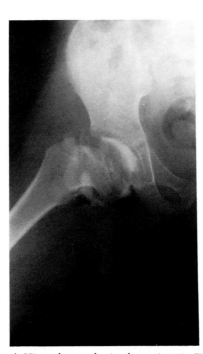 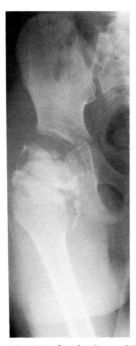

FIG. 8–18. Multiple epiphyseal dysplasia (5 years). Hip arthrography in the patient in Figure 8–17. **Left.** The femoral head is mushroom-shaped with mild subluxation. This should be treated. **Center.** The hip centers well with abduction-internal rotation positioning. There is a persistent superomedial dye pool. This mild incongruity is not a contraindication to nighttime brace management, as the cartilaginous femoral head will remodel. **Right.** The dye pool is obliterated with flexion-adduction of the hip. In the late adolescent or young adult patient who lacks remodeling potential, valgus intertrochanteric osteotomy will improve congruity.

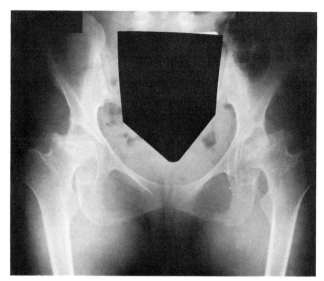

FIG. 8–19. Multiple epiphyseal dysplasia (23 years). Severe incongruity of the hips. The femoral heads are flattened, with substantial lateral extrusion and poor acetabular coverage. Cystic changes are developing in the femoral heads.

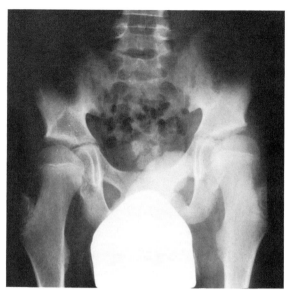

FIG. 8–20. Hereditary arthro-ophthalmopathy (14 years). Enlargement of the femoral heads and broadened femoral necks with significant valgus orientation with some loss of acetabular coverage.

ment. Varus deformities of the femur and tibia occur both proximally and distally, leading to major varus malalignment. Alternatively, genu valgum may be quite severe. Alignment of the lower extremities frequently requires multiple osteotomies for correction, and recurrent deformity is likely in the growing child. Scoliosis may occur as well as atlantoaxial instability related to odontoid hypoplasia. This condition should be distinguished from spondyloepiphyseal dysplasia congenita,

which is recognized at birth and usually has less involvement of the hands.

The hip joints are universally involved, although usually not to the extent present in spondyloepiphyseal dysplasia congenita. The capital femoral epiphysis ossifies late, and early deformation and subluxation may occur. The femoral necks are broad and shortened. The femoral heads enlarge and flatten and are poorly covered by the acetabula (Figs. 8–21 and 8–22). Severe coxa vara may result.

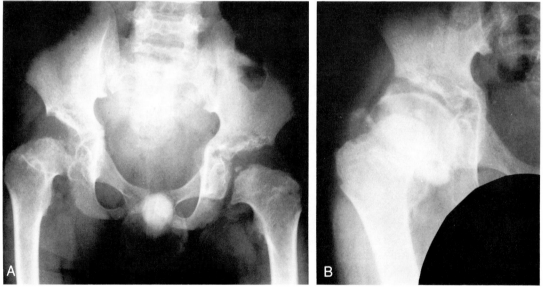

FIG. 8–21 Pseudoachondroplasia (11 years). A. The ossification of the capital femoral epiphyses is significantly delayed. The femoral necks are short, and the metaphyses are broad. The acetabula are shallow and irregular. B. Arthrography reveals a mushroom-shaped femoral head with satisfactory hip joint congruity. The acetabular labrum extends incompletely over the femoral head.

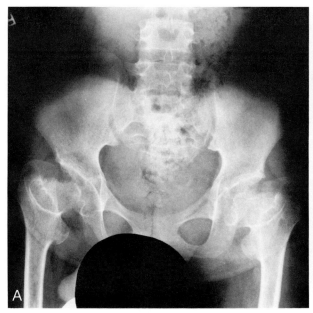
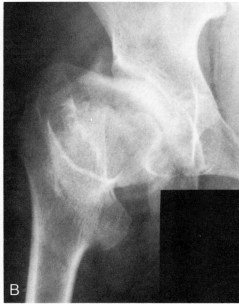

FIG. 8–22 Pseudoachondroplasia (14 years). Same patient as in Figure 8–21. **A.** Three years later, there is significant coxa vara, trochanteric overgrowth, and a "sagging rope" sign. Mild subluxation and shallow acetabula exist. **B.** Hip arthrography reveals increased femoral head deformity with flattening, extrusion, and subluxation.

These changes may simulate Perthes disease; however, Perthes disease rarely is symmetric. Late deformity occurring in adolescent and young adult years usually is treated by valgus osteotomy to improve congruity and lengthen the abductor moment arm. Varus osteotomy usually is contraindicated in late cases because of the lack of concentricity and relative trochanteric overgrowth. Hip arthrography

FIG. 8–23. Pseudoachondroplasia (47 years). The femoral heads are deformed and flattened, with shallow acetabula. Degenerative changes are present. The iliac crests are broad and square. There is moderate platyspondyly, but no narrowing of the interpedicular distance as in achondroplasia.

in children frequently reveals subluxation and early femoral head deformation. Consideration must be given to containment therapy by either bracing or surgery. We have utilized an abduction-internal rotation orthosis mimicking a Petrie cast at nighttime in the younger child. Surgically, a pelvic osteotomy may be performed and is preferable to a varus osteotomy for containment, because coxa vara usually develops in these children. If pseudoachondroplastic hip involvement is left untreated, premature severe osteoarthritis may develop in early adult years, necessitating total hip arthroplasty (Fig. 8–23). Thus, early intervention is required.

Summary

Hip involvement is common in various nonachondroplastic dwarfing conditions. The importance of accurate recognition of the specific type of skeletal dysplasia cannot be overstressed. For most orthopaedists, consultation with an experienced geneticist knowledgeable in intrinsic bone dysplasias is essential. Orthopaedic abnormalities requiring treatment must be prioritized. Atlantoaxial instability as well as other significant spinal deformities must be recognized and treated. Any treatment of the hips must be considered in light of the total alignment of the lower extremities, because lower extremity alignment must be corrected in order to restore a proper weight-bearing axis. Because premature osteoarthritis of the hips is a common sequela, early surgical intervention is frequently warranted in order to avoid total hip arthroplasty in the early adult years.

References

1. MAROTEAUX P: Bone Diseases of Children. Philadelphia, Lippincott, 1979.
2. MAROTEAUX P, LAMY M: Les formes pseudo-achondroplastiques de dysplasies spondyloepiphysaires. Presse Med, 67:383, 1959.
3. MAROTEAUX P, SPRANGER JW, WEIDEMANN H-R: Der Metatrophische Zwergwuchs. Arch Kinderheilk, 173:211, 1966.
4. McKUSICK VA, et al: Dwarfism in the Amish I: The Ellis-van Creveld syndrome. Bull Johns Hopkins Hosp, 115:306–336, 1964.
5. McKUSICK VA, et al: Dwarfism in the Amish II: Cartilage-hair hypoplasia. Bull Johns Hopkins Hosp, 116:285–326, 1965.
6. PONSETI IV: Skeletal growth in achondroplasia. J Bone Joint Surg, 52A:701–716, 1970.
7. RIMOIN DL, SIGGERS DC, LACHMAN RS, SILBERBERG R: Metatropic dwarfism, the Kniest syndrome, and pseudoachondroplastic dysplasia. Clin Orthop, 114:70–82, 1976.
8. RUBIN P: Dynamic Classification of Bone Dysplasias. Chicago, Year Book Medical Publishers, 1964.
9. SCHMIDT TL, KALAMCHI A: The fate of the capital femoral physis and acetabular development in developmental coxa vara. J Pediatr Orthop, 2:534–538, 1982.
10. APLEY AG, WIENTROUB S: The sagging rope sign in Perthes' disease and allied disorders. J Bone Joint Surg, 63B:43–47, 1981.
11. COOPER RR, PONSETI IV: Metaphyseal dysostosis: description of an ultrastructural defect in the epiphyseal plate chondrocytes. J Bone Joint Surg, 55A:485–495, 1973.
12. CROSSAN JF, WYNNE-DAVIES R, FULFORD GE: Bilateral failures of the capital femoral epiphysis: bilateral Perthes disease, multiple epiphyseal dysplasia, pseudoachondrodysplasia, and spondyloepiphyseal dysplasia congenita tarda. J Pediatr Orthop, 3:297–301, 1983.
13. ELLIS RWB, ANDREW JD: Chondroectodermal dysplasia. J Bone Joint Surg, 44B:626–636, 1962.
14. HUNT DD, PONSETI IV, PEDRINI-MILLE A, PEDRINI V: Multiple epiphyseal dysplasia in two siblings. J Bone Joint Surg, 49A:1611–1627, 1967.
15. KOPITS SE: Orthopaedic complications of dwarfism. Clin Orthop, 114:153–179, 1976.
16. KOZLOWSKI K: Metaphyseal and spondylometaphyseal chondrodysplasia. Clin Orthop, 114:83–93, 1976.
17. MANZKE H, CHRISTOPHERS E, WIEDEMANN H-R: Dominant sex-linked inherited chondrodysplasia punctata: a distinct type of chondrodysplasia punctata. Clin Genet, 17:97–107, 1980.
18. SCOTT CI: Achondroplastic and hypochondroplastic dwarfism. Clin Orthop, 114:18–30, 1976.
19. SPRANGER JW, OPITZ JD, BIDDER U: Heterogeneity of chondrodysplasia punctata. Humangenetik, 11:190–212, 1971.
20. SPRANGER JW, WEIDEMANN H-R: Dysplasia spondyloepiphysaria. Acta Paediatr Helv, 21:598, 1966.
21. STELLING FH: The hip in heritable conditions of connective tissue. Clin Orthop, 90:33–49, 1973.
22. WALKER BA, et al: Diastrophic dwarfism. Medicine, 51:41, 1972.
23. MACKENZIE WG, BASSETT GS, MANDELL GA, and SCOTT CI JR: Avascular necrosis of the hip in multiple epiphyseal dysplasia. J Pedi Orthop, 9:666–671, 1989.

PART III

Trauma

CHAPTER NINE

Fractures of the Acetabulum

JAMES KELLAM

Introduction

The acetabulum represents the pelvic portion of the hip joint, which is a major weight-bearing joint in the lower extremity. Displaced intra-articular fractures require anatomical reduction in order that post-traumatic osteoarthritis is minimized and function and mobility is maximized.[6,8,9] This is achieved in any joint by attaining congruity and stability through the appropriately chosen treatment modality. In the acetabulum both are extremely important goals to obtain. Congruity means that the femoral head is under the acetabular weight-bearing dome. Associated with this is stability of the hip, particularly in the posterior aspect.

The importance of congruity and stability has been confirmed by Rowe and Lowell. The results of their study on acetabular fractures directly correlate congruity of the dome and femoral head to good long-term results. Also associated is a relationship of femoral head damage and hip joint stability to long-term results. This is also confirmed by Larson,[5] Carnesali,[1] and Pennal.[7]

Judet and Letournel,[4] in their large series, have shown that an anatomical reduction gives 90% satisfactory long-term results. If the fracture is imperfectly reduced approximately 55% of patients have a satisfactory result; if protrusion occurs 11% have a good result. As a brief review, the major factors that determine the outcome of any acetabular fracture are:

1. Degree of displacement.
2. Damage of the articular surface, particularly the weight-bearing dome, femoral head, and retained intra-articular fragments.
3. The adequacy of reduction, particularly, joint congruity and stability.
4. Complications, e.g., avascular necrosis, heterotopic ossification, sepsis, and nerve palsies.

Therefore, to treat acetabular fractures it is imperative to know and understand the anatomy of the acetabulum and hence the pathoanatomy. In order for the surgeon to logically treat acetabular fractures a classification that correlates clinical results to fracture patterns is required. A knowledge of many operative approaches is needed. The method of reduction and fixation techniques in this area must be understood as well as a meticulous postoperative regime. These components of acetabular fracture management are discussed.

Anatomy

The acetabulum consists of two bony columns that approach each other like an inverted "Y," meeting at a notch known as the dome. The acetabulum faces laterally at approximately 60 to 70° to the axis of the iliac wing. The posterior column consists of a strong triangular piece of bone that runs from the ischium and ischial tuberosity up to the sciatic notch. The inner aspect of this is the posterior superior portion of the quadralateral plate and the anterior portion represents the posterior articular surface of the wall of the acetabulum. This component is functionally important for the stability of the hip joint. The anterior column consists of the iliac crest down to the pubic ramus and the symphysis. It meets at the dome of the posterior column.

The acetabulum can be broken down into five parts. The first and most important part is the superior portion of the acetabulum where the columns meet. This is a thick triangular piece of cancellous bone that is the weight-bearing dome of the acetabulum. This portion is extremely important in fracture work because this is where long-term problems occur in relation to osteoarthritis if malreduction occurs. The anterior portion, or anterior column, consists of the pubic rami, the anterior wall across the front of the hip joint as well as the iliac wing component portion of the anterior column. The posterior portion consists of the posterior wall, which is part of the posterior column. Therefore,

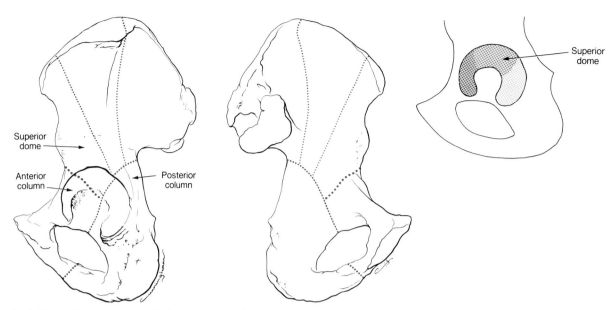

FIG. 9–1. Three views of the acetabulum, an inverted "Y" consisting of the posterior column and the anterior column meeting at the superior dome. Note that the anterior column extends well posteriorly onto the iliac wing. (From Schatzker J., Tile M.: The Rationale of Operative Fracture Care. Heidelberg, Springer-Verlag, 1989.)

fractures can be considered as one or a combination of any one of these five parts. A simple classification can be devised by consideration of which of the five parts is fractured (Fig. 9–1).

Mechanics of Acetabular Fractures

Acetabular fractures are a direct result of the vector of forces applied to the hip, modified through the femoral head position with regard to flexion, extension, rotation and abduction.

The fracture's force can be in the lateral compression vector or may be axially applied along the shaft of the femur. The lateral compressive forces are unaffected by flexion and extension of the hip but are affected by the rotation, abduction, and adduction of the femoral head. Neutral abduction and adduction create an anterior column fracture with perhaps a posterior undisplaced transverse component because of the nature of the antiversion of the femoral neck. As external rotation increases, more anterior column and anterior wall fractures occur. As internal rotation increases to 20°, T- and transverse fractures are more common; greater than 20° internal rotation results in a posterior column or wall fracture. (Fig. 9–2). Abduction and adduction simply change the position of the transverse fracture component. The greater the abduction the lower the transverse fracture occurs.

With an axially directed force along the femur, flexion and extension become more important than

rotation, abduction, or adduction. At 90° of flexion with neutral abduction and adduction, posterior wall fractures are common. As abduction is increased, the fracture becomes posterior column to transverse. With increasing adduction, posterior wall fractures are converted to pure dislocations. As flexion decreases under 90°, the chances of a dome fracture occurring increase.

As well as the acetabular fracture, one should

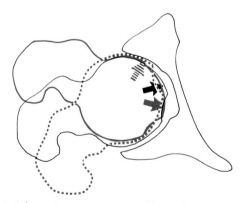

FIG. 9–2. Schematic representation of how a lateral compression injury, with the force directed through the femoral head, can change the fracture pattern by the varying degrees of rotation. Internal rotation, as shown by the solid red line and solid red arrow, has a force directed in the posterior aspect, thus creating a posterior-type fracture pattern. External rotation, represented by the dotted femoral head and hatched red arrow, shows that anterior fractures will occur. A purely directed lateral force, as shown by the black line and black arrow, basically produces transverse fracture patterns. (From Schatzker J., Tile M.: The Rationale of Operative Fracture Care. Heidelberg, Springer-Verlag, 1989.)

TABLE 9–1. *Classification of Acetabular Fractures*

Elementary Fractures
  Posterior wall
  Posterior column
  Anterior wall
  Anterior column
  Transverse

Combination Fractures
  T-fracture
  Posterior column and posterior wall
  Transverse and posterior wall
  Anterior column (or wall) with posterior hemitransverse
  Double-column

also think about the associated injuries that occur in the extremity and the patient secondary to the direction force vector.

The mechanism of injury is important to understand because it helps in interpreting x-rays. If an appropriate history can be obtained regarding what transpired with the patient and the injured limb, then as the x-rays are reviewed, a clearer understanding of the injury can be achieved.

Classification (Tables 9–1 to 9–3)

As can be seen from the mechanics of acetabular fractures, an infinite number of fractures can occur, depending on the position of the head with respect to flexion, extension, rotation, and sagittal position when the force is applied. In order to be helpful, a clinical decision making classification must aid treatment decisions, as well as highlight the poten-

TABLE 9–2. *Classification of Acetabular Fractures*

Undisplaced fractures
Displaced fractures

Type I
Posterior types±posterior dislocation
A. Posterior column
B. Posterior wall
  - associated with posterior column
  - associated with transverse fracture

Type II
Anterior types±anterior dislocation
A. Anterior column
B. Anterior wall
C. Associated anterior and transverse fracture

Type III
Transverse Types±central dislocation
A. Pure transverse
B. T-fractures
C. Associated transverse and acetabular wall fractures
D. Double column fractures

(From Tile M: Fractures of the Pelvis and Acetabulum. Baltimore, Williams & Wilkins, 1984.)

TABLE 9–3. *Classification of Acetabular Fractures. (According to AO Documentation Center)*

  I. Fractures involving one column or wall
 II. Fractures involving both columns with a portion of the dome attached to the axial skeleton
III. Fractures involving both columns with no portion of the dome attached to the axial skeleton

tial problems with each of the different injuries. Tile's classification,[10] which is a modification of Judet-Letournel's, defines the important prognostic factors in acetabular fractures, namely degree of displacement, degree of comminution, position of the fracture with particular emphasis on dome involvement, and most important, the presence of a dislocation, posteriorly, centrally or anteriorly.

Posterior Fractures with or without Posterior Dislocation (Type 1)

These fractures involve the posterior column, posterior wall or a combination of both, as well as a transverse fracture, associated with a posterior wall or column injury. The common feature of these injuries are mechanism, which usually is a blow to the flexed knee and, therefore, an axial load along the femur that can lead particularly to posterior cruciate disruptions. Also, posterior hip dislocations are common in this group of fractures. Therefore, the incidence of avascular necrosis and sciatic nerve injury increase, as well as superior gluteal artery bleeding.

Posterior Column Fractures (Fig. 9–3). A pure posterior column fracture is a rare injury. It begins at the greater sciatic notch, goes through the acetabular fossa and out the obturator foramen. It continues down through the ischium or ischial tuberosity. This is best seen on the iliac oblique view. It is commonly associated with a posteriorly displaced femoral head, either alone or in association with the column. These fractures are difficult to reduce anatomically and because they usually involve a major component of the weight-bearing dome anatomical reduction is mandatory and, therefore, open reduction and internal fixation is usually required.

Posterior Wall Fractures (Fig. 9–4). Posterior wall fractures are common, either involving the true posterior wall or the wall and part of the superior dome. These fractures also have been classified by Epstein,[3] in his classification of fracture dislocations of the hip. Marginal impaction of the acetabular articular surface is common. As the femoral head is driven out of the acetabulum, the head

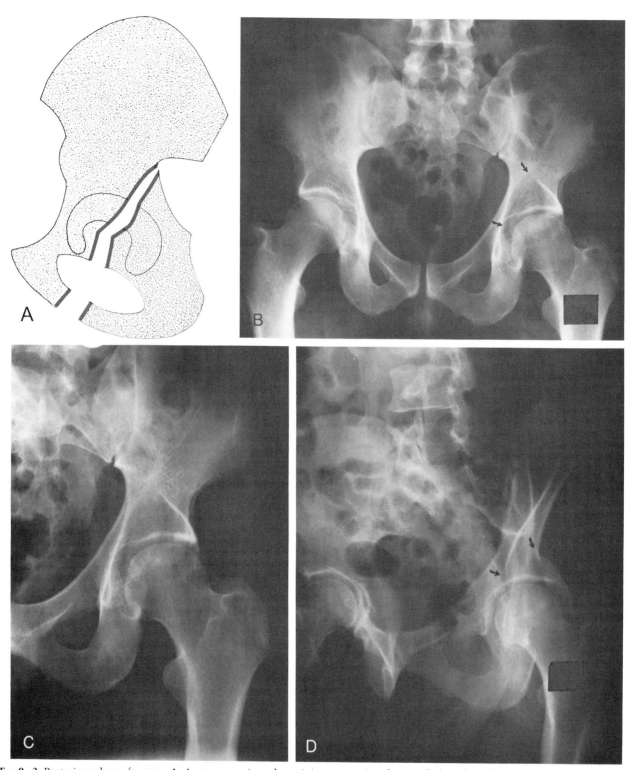

Fig. 9–3. Posterior column fracture. **A.** A pure posterior column injury traversing the acetabulum through the junction of the posterior and anterior columns crossing the weight-bearing dome. This fracture can exit through the notch thus injuring the superior gluteal artery. **B.** Anteroposterior radiograph of the pelvis demonstrating a posterior column fracture with a sharp spike shown by a black arrow. This spike can impale the superior gluteal artery or the sciatic nerve. Note also the associated posterior dislocation of the femoral head. **C.** Iliac oblique view showing the displaced posterior column and posterior dislocation. Note that the anterior wall is intact on this view. **D.** Obturator oblique view showing the fracture exiting through the ischial tuberosity, but most importantly showing that the anterior column is intact. Note the small fragments superior to the femoral head representing the posterior wall of the acetabulum. This view is ideal for showing the posterior wall displaced and the fracture fragment. (From Schatzker J., Tile M.: The Rationale of Operative Fracture Care. Heidelberg, Springer-Verlag, 1989.)

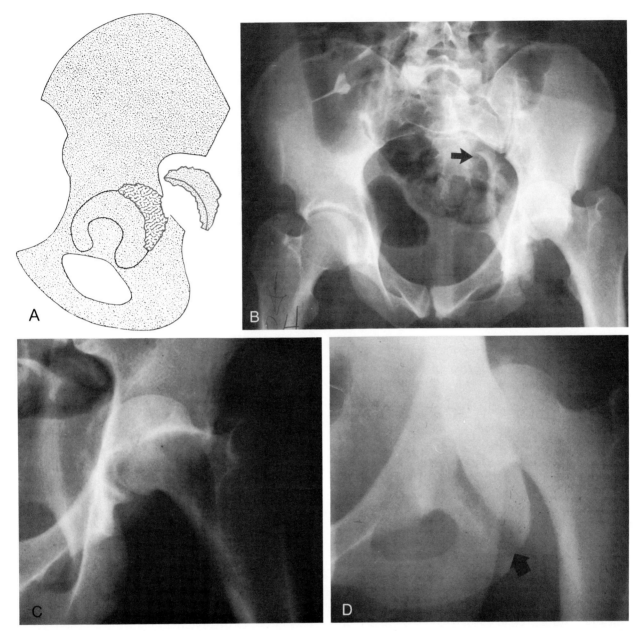

Fig. 9–4. Posterior wall fracture. **A.** Schematic representation of the location of the posterior wall fracture. Note that it directly involves a portion of the weight-bearing dome and the portion of the hip joint giving stability in the extended position. **B.** Posterior wall fracture fragment on an anteroposterior radiograph of the pelvis. In this position the hip is reduced and appears to be concentric as compared to the normal other side. The small black arrow shows the extent of the posterior wall fracture fragment. **C.** The Iliac oblique view again shows that the posterior column is intact, and one can note the posterior wall fracture. **D.** On the obturator oblique view one can see the large posterior wall fracture fragment as noted by the arrows. (From Schatzker J., Tile M.: The Rationale of Operative Fracture Care. Heidelberg, Springer-Verlag, 1989.)

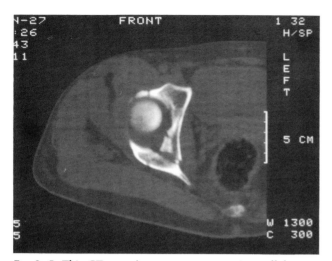

Fig. 9–5. This CT scan demonstrates a posterior wall fracture with marginal impaction. The arrow demonstrates the impacted fracture as it is bent back and impacted into the acetabulum. This is the equivalent of a depressed tibial plateau fracture.

bends the posterior fracture margin backwards depressing the edge of the intact acetabulum. This is important to recognize intraoperatively in order that it can be elevated to restore joint congruity. Stability of the hip joint is important with respect to these fractures. Studies by Vailas[11] and Calkins[2] have evaluated posterior fractures and posterior wall size with respect to hip stability. Less than 25% loss of the posterior wall would maintain stability in the hip. If greater than 33% of the posterior wall was lost and the posterior capsule was not intact, the hip tended to be unstable. With greater than 50% loss of the posterior wall of the acetabulum the hip joints were unstable. This is adequately evaluated by a CT scan (Fig. 9–5). Clinical evaluation and an examination under anesthesia also should be carried out to assess stability after reduction.

It should be recognized that in a great number of these cases a posterior wall fracture really involves the major component of a superior weight-bearing dome. This provides true instability of the hip joint as well as incongruity. These fractures must be anatomically reduced. Also associated with this is a transverse fracture or posterior column injury. These are usually undisplaced but must be recognized in order to make appropriate preoperative plans and decide upon a surgical approach. One must caution that these small fragments may become avascular if care is not taken to maintain soft tissue attachments of the capsule and consequently may resorb, leading to further long-term instability. As well, there is a tremendous force through this area and screw fixation alone is not suitable. These

types of fractures must all be buttressed with a plate.

Posterior Wall With Associated Transverse Fractures (Fig. 9–6). This injury is important to recognize when the major problem is related to the posterior wall fracture and not the transverse component. Usually, the transverse fracture is minimally displaced and does not require reduction. It is important to recognize this because if one makes an inappropriate choice of surgical approach, it may be difficult to treat this fracture. This is a common fracture pattern, seen in up to 20% of cases.

Anterior Fractures With or Without Anterior Dislocation (Type II)

Anterior fractures are relatively common if one considers the pubic ramus fractures seen in the lateral compression injury to the pelvis that usually occurs at the root of the superior ramus, and involves a small portion of the anterior wall of the acetabulum. Consequently, these injuries do need careful evaluation to make sure they do not extend into the dome (Fig. 9–7). Anterior dislocation of the hip is usually uncommon. One must also be aware of femoral nerve or femoral artery vein injury because the pubic ramus component of this fracture can tilt upward through the neurovascular structures and create significant limb threatening injuries.

Anterior Column Fractures (Fig. 9–8). Fractures through the anterior column can involve three common areas. It must be remembered that the anterior column usually consists of the majority of the iliac wing above the acetabulum. Consequently, an anterior column fracture may exit through the weight-bearing dome and up the iliac crest. It may also exit at the level of the anterior inferior spine or between it and the anterior superior iliac spine. Occasionally the fracture exits just below the anterior inferior spine of the pelvis. These are all anterior column fractures with variable degrees of dome involvement. The closer the fracture is to the anterior inferior spine, the less dome involvement occurs.

Anterior Wall Fractures (Fig. 9–9). These are not common fractures, as mentioned above, and usually are associated with a dislocation anteriorly as the wall is moved out of the way and the hip can slide forward. Because of instability, they usually require internal fixation. One problem associated with this type of fracture is that it tends to occur in osteoporotic bone, particularly seen in alcoholics

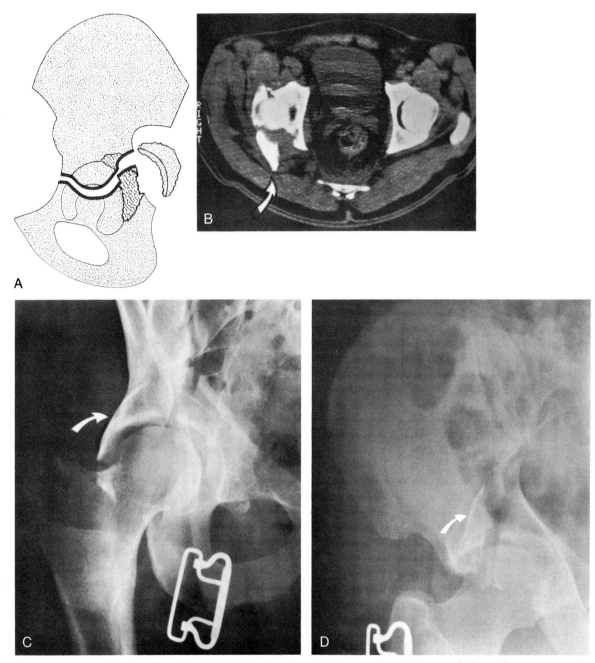

FIG. 9–6. **A** and **B.** A posterior wall fracture associated with a transverse fracture through the acetabulum. This common variant of a posterior wall injury is best seen on the CT scan on Figure 9–6B. The arrow points out the posterior wall fracture fragment and one can appreciate the transverse component going through the anterior column. **C.** The obturator oblique view demonstrating the anterior column fracture and the white arrow pointing to the posterior wall component. Note that the obturator ring is intact and thus there is no T component to this fracture. **D.** The iliac oblique view. The white arrow shows the posterior wall fracture and the posterior column component of the transverse fracture, which is displaced. (From Schatzker J., Tile M.: The Rationale of Operative Fracture Care. Heidelberg, Springer-Verlag, 1989.)

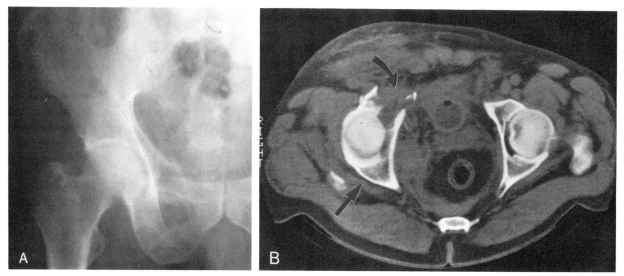

FIG. 9–7. **A.** Low anterior column fracture associated with a superior pubic ramus fracture. This is seen on the anteroposterior aspect of the pelvis. **B.** The CT scan of this injury demonstrates significant involvement of the anterior column although the dome is intact as well as the majority of the anterior column. This fracture is low and does not require operative intervention. It does demonstrate, however, that some superior pubic rami fractures associated with pelvic fractures do enter the acetabulum. (From Schatzker J., Tile M.: The Rationale of Operative Fracture Care. Heidelberg, Springer-Verlag, 1989.)

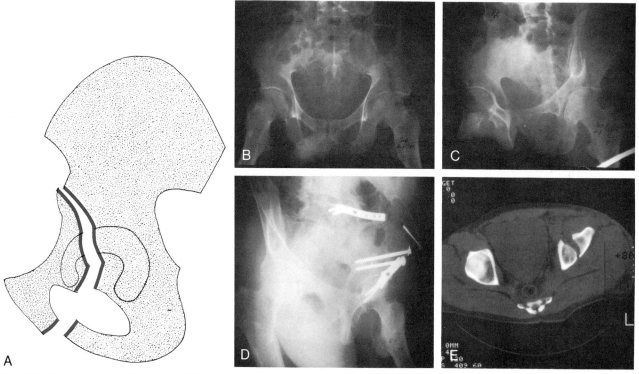

FIG. 9–8. Anterior column fracture. **A.** Schematic representation of the anterior column shows a common anterior column fracture in the mid portion between the low and the high fractures. The high fracture runs up into the iliac crest and the low fracture exists below the anterior inferior spine. **B.** Anteroposterior radiograph of the pelvis showing a high anterior column fracture. **C.** Obturator oblique view showing the displacement of the anterior column fracture. **D.** Iliac oblique view showing the posterior column intact. **E.** A representative CT section showing the involvement of the dome in this fracture. Note the rotation of the anterior column. (From Schatzker J., Tile M: The Rationale of Operative Fracture Care. Heidelberg, Springer-Verlag, 1989.)

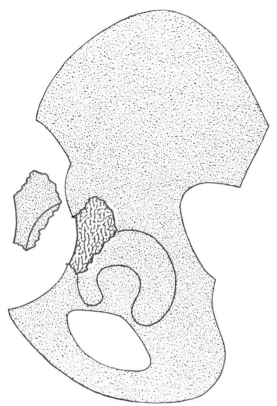

FIG. 9–9. Schematic representation of an anterior wall fracture. This uncommon fracture usually is associated with another injury to the acetabulum. (From Schatzker J., Tile M.: The Rationale of Operative Fracture Care. Heidelberg, Springer-Verlag, 1989.)

and the elderly, and may be associated with medial wall comminution. In this type of fracture it is difficult to obtain a solid fixation.

Anterior Column or Anterior Wall Fractures with an Associated Transverse Posterior Fracture (Fig. 9–10). Again, this is the reverse of the similar situation in the posterior wall. Close observation and attention to the details and diagnosis are important in order to make the appropriate surgical approach.

Transverse Fractures With or Without Central Dislocation of the Femoral Head (Type III) (Fig. 9–11)

Transverse fractures represent a split of the hemipelvis into two sections that occurs through the acetabulum. Both columns are fractured, but the dome of the acetabulum, however small, is not separated from the axial skeleton. This transverse fracture can occur at any level throughout the acetabulum and, depending on where it occurs, affects the prognosis of this injury. The lower the fracture,

the less dome involvement, and therefore, congruity and stability are much better. The head tends to migrate centrally with the lower portion of the transverse fracture. These fractures can be seen best on the iliac and obturator oblique views. The roof arc measurements help to determine stability.

Because both columns are attached to each fragment, reduction can usually be accomplished by surgically approaching this injury from either the anterior or posterior aspects and reducing the most displaced component of this injury. The other component will follow.

T-Fractures (Fig. 9–12). A T-fracture of the acetabulum represents a transverse fracture in which a split occurs in the medial wall of the acetabulum down to the obturator foramen and through the ischial ramus. This component now separates the anterior column from the posterior column. However, the dome or the remainder of the acetabulum superiorly is still connected to the axial skeleton through the pelvis. This is a complicated fracture because reduction of one column does not mean the other column will reduce. This fracture usually requires an extensile approach in order that both columns can be reduced at the same time. The T component of this fracture may occur anywhere along the medial aspect of the acetabulum, thus, involving any component of this joint. CT scanning is particularly helpful to define this vertical split.

Associated Transverse and Acetabular Wall Fractures. These injuries have been discussed under the particular areas of significant displacement.

Double Column Fractures or Associated Double Column Fractures (Type IV) (Fig. 9–13)

This fracture pattern is the most complex fracture pattern in the acetabulum. It usually represents a T-fracture with its transverse component occurring just above the acetabular dome. This means that the acetabulum is completely separated from the axial skeleton and what is important concerning this is the amount of involvement of the T component of the fracture through the dome. This fracture usually is displaced inward, leaving the posterior iliac wing intact, which leaves a large spike or spur that is seen on the obturator oblique view as a pathognomonic "spur" sign of this fracture. If dome involvement is minimal, these fractures usually can be treated nonoperatively in traction with early motion and thus, achieve secondary congruence. However if the dome is involved, operative management is required. The fractures usu-

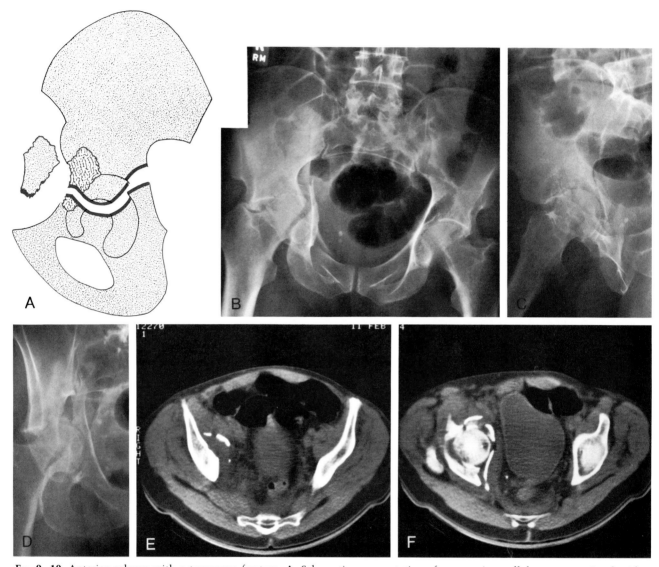

Fɪɢ. **9–10.** Anterior column with a transverse fracture. **A.** Schematic representation of an anterior wall fracture associated with a transverse fracture pattern. **B.** Anteroposterior radiograph showing an anterior wall fracture associated with a transverse fracture of the pelvis. **C.** Iliac oblique view with a minimally displaced posterior column injury. Note that the head appears dislocated centrally. **D.** Obturator oblique view showing the anterior central displacement of the head and the associated anterior wall fracture. The significant displacement of the anterior component of the transverse fracture is also noted. Note that the obturator ring is intact and that this represents a transverse fracture because there is no break in the ring representative of a "T" fracture. **E** and **F.** CT sections. Note in Figure 9–10F the transverse fracture through the dome portion of the acetabulum with a significant wall comminution. (From Schatzker J., Tile M.: The Rationale of Operative Fracture Care. Heidelberg, Springer-Verlag, 1989.)

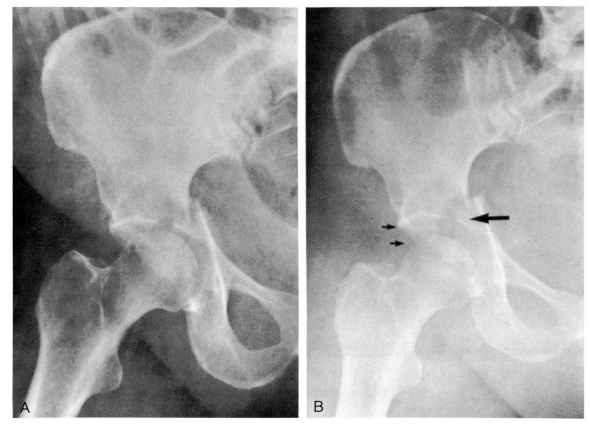

Fig. 9–11. Transverse fracture with or without central dislocation of the femoral head. **A** and **B.** Iliac oblique view. One can note a transverse fracture through the acetabulum. This is a high fracture. Note the subluxation of the hip and displacement of the fracture in Figure 9–11B, as shown by the arrows. (From Schatzker J., Tile M.: The Rationale of Operative Fracture Care. Heidelberg, Springer-Verlag, 1989.)

ally are associated with an iliac wing fracture that must be reduced first. The remainder of the acetabulum is then reconstructed.

Miscellaneous Fractures (Type V)

1. Acetabular fractures with associated pelvic ring and with associated iliac joint disruption.
2. Associated acetabular fractures with femoral neck; intertrochanteric and femoral shaft fractures.

This classification has dealt with displaced fractures. Other components or arms of the classification are undisplaced acetabular fractures. Undisplaced acetabular fractures can be classified in a similar fashion but do not require consideration for operative intervention.

Diagnosis

When one considers the diagnosis of acetabular fractures one must consider what has fractured,

how much displacement has occurred, if the fracture is congruous or if a congruous reduction can be obtained, if stability can be obtained, if there are intra-articular fragments, and what other injuries have occurred. The diagnosis is then made through clinical assessment and radiographic assessment.

Clinical Assessment

It is important to point out at this time that acetabular fractures are, in a sense, a major pelvic disruption, secondary to high energy trauma. Consequently, they have the same problems of blood loss and potential mortality from hypovolemic shock as pelvic ring injuries. An appropriate resuscitation routine based on the care of the airway, breathing, and circulation first must be obtained to stabilize the patient prior to intervention.

Physical examination is imperative to assess the vascular and neurologic status of the leg, with particular emphasis on the sciatic and femoral nerves. Their function must be documented exactly because one of the complications of operative treatment is sciatic and femoral nerve injuries. It is important to know the status of these nerves

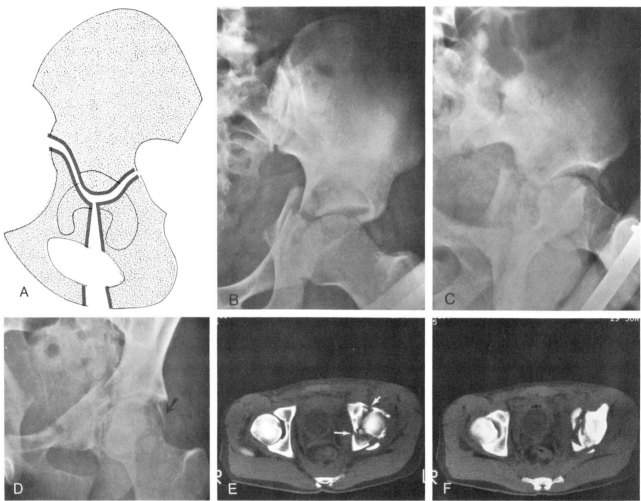

FIG. 9–12. **A.** Schematic representation of a "T" fracture of the acetabulum. Note that this is a transverse fracture with a vertical limb that extends through the medial aspect of the acetabulum and down through the obturator ring. Any fracture in the obturator ring is a clue that a transverse fracture may represent a "T" fracture. This is best evaluated with a CT scan. **B.** Anteroposterior radiograph of the pelvis demonstrating what appears to be a transverse fracture. **C.** The iliac oblique view confirms the displaced posterior component of this fracture. Note the subluxation of the head. **D.** The obturator oblique view showing the anterior component of a transverse fracture. There is also a posterior wall fracture as shown by the black arrow. Note that the obturator ring looks intact. **E** and **F.** Selected CT cuts of this fracture. Note the white arrow on the medial aspect of the acetabulum showing the "T" or vertical extension of this fracture. This is a "T" fracture, not a transverse fracture. This is significant because both the anterior and posterior columns are separated and care must be taken during the reduction and fixation to ensure that both are reduced. (From Schatzker J., Tile M.: The Rationale of Operative Fracture Care. Heidelberg, Springer-Verlag, 1989.)

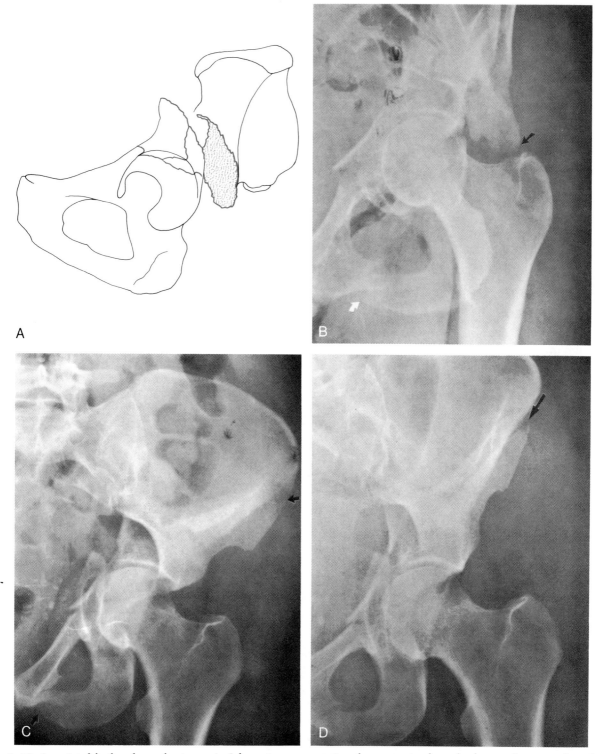

Fig. 9–13. Associated both column fractures. **A.** Schematic representation demonstrating how the fracture has gone through in a transverse pattern above the dome of the acetabulum. Extending down from this is a fracture line that may go all the way down into the obturator ring, representing a vertical extension or the dome involvement of the axial skeleton. **B.** The obturator oblique view. The black arrow points to the remaining portion of the iliac wing. This is the spur sign where the transverse component is noted. Note how the whole acetabulum and the femoral head have been pushed inward and appear relatively congruent on this x-ray. The white arrow shows a fracture through the obturator ring and is a clue to a "T" component to this fracture. **C.** The iliac oblique view. The posterior column is obviously displaced but the whole acetabulum appears relatively congruent. **D.** A post reduction x-ray in traction. The hip looks relatively congruent. A CT scan is required to define the exact involvement of the dome, and to decide whether this injury should be treated operatively or nonoperatively. (From Schatzker J., Tile M.: The Rationale of Operative Fracture Care. Heidelberg, Springer-Verlag, 1989.)

preoperatively. Associated injuries should be looked for as well. It is also important at this time to evaluate the soft tissue injury that has occurred with this fracture. Open fractures of the acetabulum should be handled according to the principles of handling for an open fracture of any joint. However, a soft tissue injury to the closed fracture, must be assessed carefully so that an inappropriate surgical approach is not carried out, compromising soft tissue healing, and thus internal fixation, through sepsis.

Radiographic Assessment

The radiographic assessment of an acetabular fracture requires an anteroposterior view of the complete pelvis. This view allows one to compare the fractured acetabulum with a normal acetabulum. This gives a general overview of the congruency of the hip, the amount of displacement, and a general understanding of the fracture. (Fig. 9–14) Inlet and outlet views of the pelvis are important in order that the sacrum and the sacroiliac joint as well as the posterior component of the pelvic ring injury, if there is one, can be assessed. Occasionally, the inlet view is helpful in documenting certain acetabular fractures, particularly associated both column fractures with an iliac wing injury.

Special Radiographic Investigations

In order to unravel the complexity of the anteroposterior x-ray, Judet and Letournel have described the two oblique x-rays taken at 45° to the horizontal plane.

The Obturator Oblique View (Fig. 9–15). This view is performed with the affected hip elevated so that a 45° angle between the pelvis and hip and the horizontal or radiographic film plane is developed. This effectively internally rotates the pelvis, thus, allowing the anterior column to be thrown into profile and best seen. This also places the posterior lip of the acetabulum in profile and it can be assessed. The spur sign is well seen on this as well as the obturator foramen, which helps to make the diagnosis of T-fractures.

The Iliac Oblique View (Fig. 9–16). This view is performed with the affected hip down and the unaffected hip turned up 45°. This, in effect, externally rotates the hemipelvis 45° with respect to the horizontal. The iliac wing is now seen directly onward and the posterior column is thrown into relief for full evaluation of the ischial component of the posterior column. The ischial spine is well seen, as is

the sciatic notch. In addition to the posterior column, the anterior wall or lip of the acetabulum is assessed.

Tomography

This may be useful in attempts to identify small intra-articular fragments or for further elucidating acetabular fractures if computer axial tomography is not present. It is important in the assessment of the dome fracture fragment if a CT scan is unavailable.

Computer Axial Tomography (Fig. 9–17)

The CT scan has revolutionized the assessment of acetabular fractures. It has allowed one to assess in a two-dimensional plane the acetabulum with respect to the dome, the weight-bearing portion, and most particularly the posterior column and posterior wall. Intra-articular fragments are easily seen and can be assessed regarding position and size.

Marginal impaction fractures can be looked for as well. T-fractures can be assessed, as can the acetabular wall or medial wall of the acetabulum with respect to comminution and displacement. Another important aspect of the CT scan is an appreciation of the rotational displacement of the fracture fragments. The posterior column fracture tends to rotate inward and thus when reduction is obtained must be rotated outward. These rotational malalignments are important to understand so that they can be transposed into action at the time of reduction in the operating suite.

The sacroiliac joint is important to assess as well because it may be involved in association with column fractures and transverse or T-fractures.

Three-Dimensional CT Scanning (Figs. 9–18 and 9–19)

A new CT scanning technique appears to produce good images allowing a three-dimensional understanding and perhaps will allow the surgeon to perform the operation on a computer screen and understand what is happening prior to performing the operation on the patient.

Following the radiographic assessment of acetabular fractures one can comment on the congruency and stability of the reduction. Joint congruity is assessed by comparing the parallelism of the acetabu-

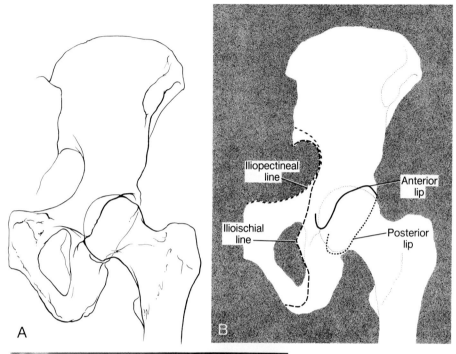

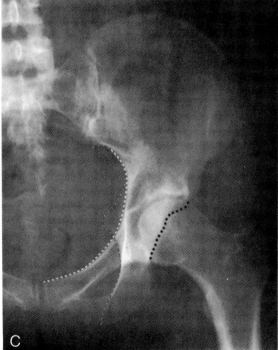

FIG. 9–14. A–C. The anterioposterior radiograph of the involved hip as well as the anteroposterior view of the pelvis is the first x-ray required. On the anteroposterior radiograph the iliopectineal line should be assessed to determine anterior column involvement. The ilioischial line should be assessed to determine posterior column involvement. Note that both lines coalesce at the notch. This area is difficult to evaluate on an anteroposterior x-ray. The anterior and posterior lips can also be assessed on an anteroposterior x-ray. Displacement of the femoral head, either posteriorly or centrally, also can be determined. Occasionally iliac wing fractures, as well as other fractures involving the sacrum and pubic rami may also be noted. (From Schatzker J., Tile M.: The Rationale of Operative Fracture Care. Heidelberg, Springer-Verlag, 1989.)

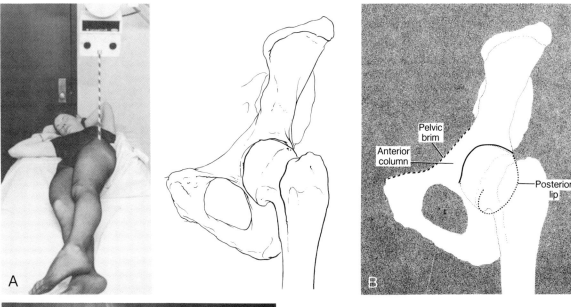

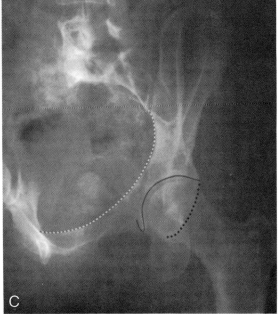

Fɪɢ. 9–15. Obturator oblique view. **A.** The position of the patient in order to obtain the obturator view. The involved hip is turned up approximately 45°. The radiographic beam is at right angles to the plate. This produces a view placing the iliac wing in profile and the anterior column is visualized extremely well. The obturator ring is also shown. **B.** On this view the iliopectineal line or pelvic rim is adequately assessed for fracture and displacement. This allows for assessment of the anterior column. This view also demonstrates the posterior lip. **C.** A radiographic of the obturator view. The iliopectineal line or pelvic brim is demonstrated in the alternating black and white dotted line. The black dotted line shows the posterior lip and the solid line shows the dome of the acetabulum and the medial wall and tear drop. (From Schatzker J., Tile M.: The Rationale of Operative Fracture Care. Heidelberg, Springer-Verlag, 1989.)

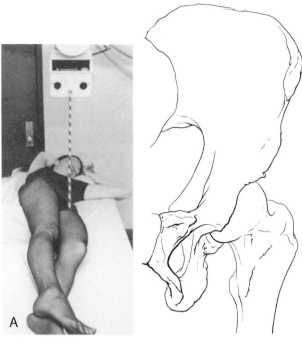

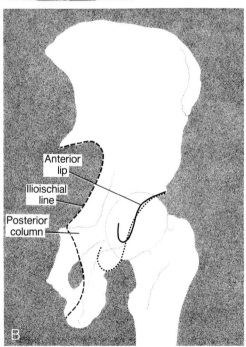

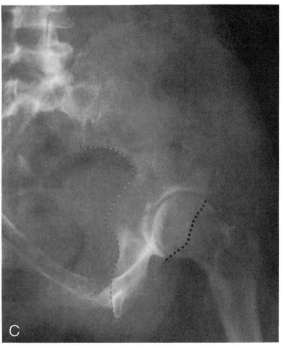

Fig. 9–16. Iliac oblique view. **A.** The patient positioned with the involved hip turned outward by 45° by rotating the patient up with the uninvolved hip on a cushion. This allows the radiographic beam to be at right angles to the complete iliac wing and posterior column. This is adequately shown in the schematic diagram. Note how well the iliac wing and posterior column are visualized. Note also the anterior wall is seen in excellent relief. **B.** On the iliac oblique view one can assess the ilioischial line from the sacroiliac joint down to the ischial tuberosity. It is easiest to try to pinpoint the notch and the ischial spine when developing this line. This will show any fracture through the posterior column. The anterior lip or wall is well visualized as is the medial wall, although this is more difficult to see on this view. **C.** Iliac oblique radiograph. Note the well demarcated black and white dotted line. The anterior wall is shown by the black dotted line. (From Schatzker J., Tile M.: The Rationale of Operative Fracture Care. Heidelberg, Springer-Verlag, 1989.)

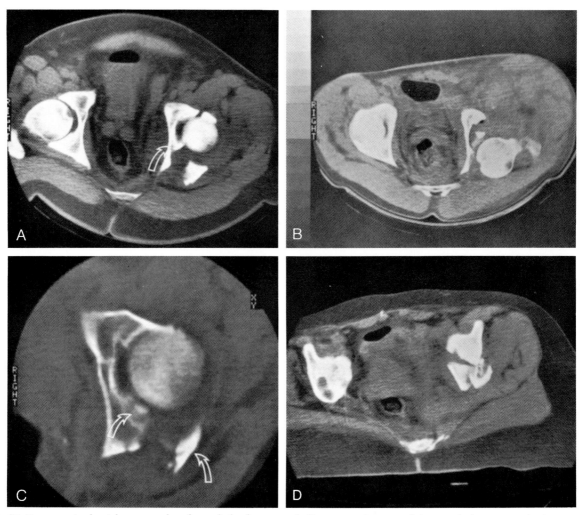

FIG. 9–17. Computerized axial tomography of acetabular fractures. **A.** Transverse fracture of the acetabulum. Note the large posterior wall fracture. The open arrow points to the rotated bony fragment. **B.** Posteriorly dislocated femoral head with a large fragment within the joint blocking reduction. **C.** Posterior wall fracture. Within the acetabulum there is an impacted fracture of the articular surface represented by the open arrow on the left. This represents marginal impaction. **D.** Comminuted acetabular fracture. This is an associated both-column fracture. Note to the right the intact iliac wing component representing the spur sign. The dome itself has a transverse fracture in it. (From Schatzker J., Tile M.: The Rationale of Operative Fracture Care. Heidelberg, Springer-Verlag, 1989.)

lar dome with that of the femoral head. The convex surfaces of both the dome and the superior portion of the head should be parallel and concentric. Lack of parallelism or concentricity in this area leads to a bad result. Care should be taken in the assessment of these fractures to ensure that there has not been a tilt through the dome fragment, thus leading to a lack of parallelism. Greater than a 2 mm step in any component of the dome or weight-bearing surface of the joint is significant and needs to be corrected in most circumstances.

The assessment of joint stability is determined on the three initial x-rays as well as the postreduction x-rays if a closed reduction is obtained. To find the roof arc angle, i.e., the angle described by Matta (Fig. 9–20), ascertain the center of the acetabulum and draw a perpendicular line through it and the acetabular dome. From this point draw a line through the fracture. The angle subtended between these two lines is the roof arc. This is a measurement of the amount of acetabulum remaining that will provide joint stability and thus stop subluxation of the hip posteriorly, medially, or anteriorly, depending on the view or fracture. If the roof arc angle is greater than 45° it indicates joint stability. This is a helpful technique in order to assess operability of acetabular fractures. It should not be used as a rigid criteria and is of no value in associated both column fractures.

After clinical and radiographic assessment one is able to commence to make a logical treatment decision based on present information.

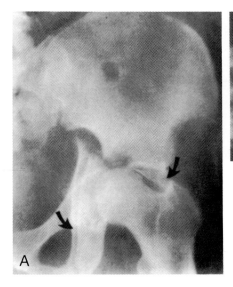

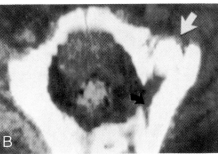

Fɪɢ. **9–18.** Reconstruction and three-dimensional CT views. **A.** Radiograph of a comminuted transverse fracture of the acetabulum with a subluxed sacroiliac joint. A large fragment is in the joint shown by the upper black arrow. One can appreciate a split in the medial wall by the lower black arrow. With CT reconstruction one can now appreciate the transverse component of the fracture through the pelvic ring of the SI joint shown by the black arrow. Note how the femoral head is wedged into the fracture pushing the iliac wing back, as shown by the white arrow. (From Schatzker J., Tile M.: The Rationale of Operative Fracture Care. Heidelberg, Springer-Verlag, 1989.)

Treatment Algorithm

First, determine the amount of displacement. All undisplaced acetabular fractures are treated nonoperatively.

Displaced Fractures

One must remember that in all displaced fractures incongruity and instability exist. This may exist for one type of fracture more than another, thus, leading to operative treatment more commonly in a particular group of fractures. The classi-

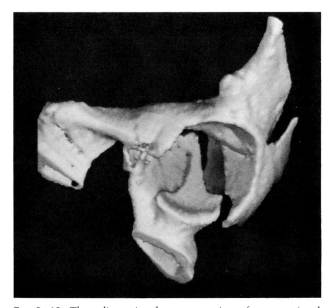

Fɪɢ. **9–19.** Three-dimensional reconstruction of an associated both column fracture showing how this kind of reconstruction is useful in assessment of joint involvement and congruency.

fication that has developed would tend to lead the surgeon to appropriate decision making (Fig. 9–21).

Therefore, the indications for surgery with respect to incongruity can be summarized by stating that posterior column or wall injuries, displaced fractures of the superior dome, and fractures in which a retained bony fragment is noted between the articular surfaces of the joint and not the fovea are almost mandatory indications for open reduction and internal fixation. Fractures following closed reduction when the head is congruous with the dome but the remainder of the fracture does not follow will remain unstable (roof arc angle <45°) no matter how long the fracture is kept in traction. Sciatic nerve injury, fractures of the ipsilateral femur, polytrauma, and the ipsilateral knee also are indications for operative treatment of acetabular fractures. Sciatic nerve injury that occurs during reduction or in traction requires a mandatory exploration and probably internal fixation.

Fractures of the acetabulum with ipsilateral femoral fractures are difficult to manage. The more proximal the fracture the more difficult the problem. Acetabular fractures associated with subcapital fractures are rare, but when they do occur require an anatomical reduction of both fractures, probably done at the same sitting. The approach determined probably will be an extensile approach using either a triradiate or extended iliofemoral, but mostly it depends on the acetabular fracture and what is required to achieve reduction. If an anterior column fracture is present two incisions probably will be required: an anterior ilioinguinal incision, with an associated second lateral approach to the hip.

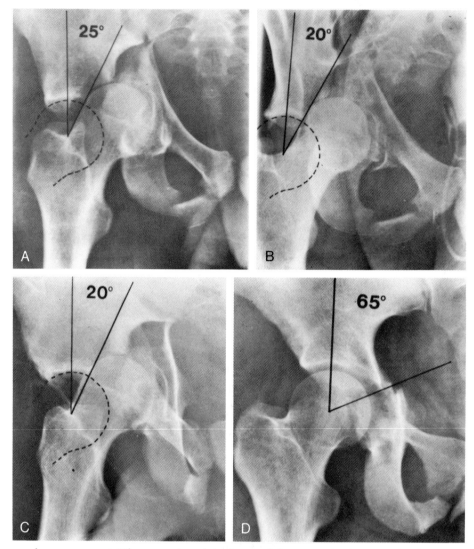

F_{IG}. 9–20. Roof arc angle measurement. When a portion of the fractured dome remains intact to the iliac wing, the use of roof arc angle measurements, as described by Matta, may be helpful in determining operability. These are performed on the three views. The femoral head is drawn into the acetabulum centering it under the remaining portion of the intact dome. The center of the femoral head is then determined and a vertical line drawn from this point. A line is then drawn to meet the fracture line medially. The angle between these two lines is the roof arc measurement. **A.** Obturator oblique view. **B.** Iliac oblique view. **C.** Anteroposterior view. These roof arc measurements are all below 45°, thus indicating relative incongruency in the joint and stability. **D.** Greater than 45° usually means that the fracture is stable and congruency will be maintained. (From Matta, J: Operative indications and choice of surgical approach for fractures of the acetabulum. Tech Orthop 1:17, 1986.)

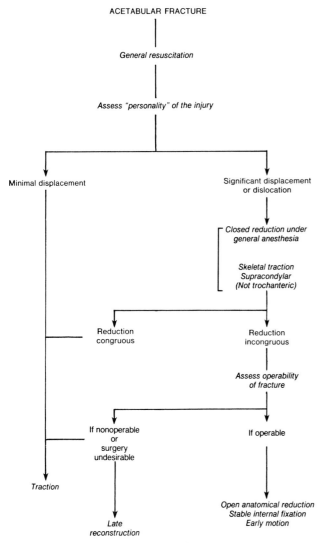

ACETABULAR FRACTURE

General resuscitation

Assess "personality" of the injury

Minimal displacement

Significant displacement or dislocation

Closed reduction under general anesthesia

Skeletal traction Supracondylar (Not trochanteric)

Reduction congruous

Reduction incongruous

Assess operability of fracture

If nonoperable or surgery undesirable

If operable

Traction

Late reconstruction

Open anatomical reduction Stable internal fixation Early motion

Fɪɢ. 9–21. Treatment algorithm for displaced fractures.

Intertrochanteric fractures again can be fixed either as a primary procedure with an acetabular fracture or the acetabular fracture can be delayed until the intertrochanteric fracture is fixed.

Femoral shaft fractures are probably best treated by the use of an intramedullary device, and with the advent of the locked intramedullary nail, one is able to nail the fracture closed and then proceed to do the appropriate exposure for the acetabular reconstruction. The starting position for the intramedullary nail is usually posterior to the greater trochanter tip and thus an osteotomy of the greater trochanter is still possible, fixed either with cancellous screws or a tension band method. The lateral decubitus position for nailing is preferred. This allows a smaller incision that can be directed more posteriorly without further surgical exposure.

Knee Disruptions

A patient with a knee disruption should be treated as required. Isolated injuries to the posterior cruciate and anterior cruciate could be left and functional stability determined at a later date. A major disruption probably should be treated operatively and immobilized either in a cast postoperatively or an external fixator, depending on the severity of the injury. However, the more important injury to be adequately treated is the acetabulum and this should take precedence.

Other Considerations

The age of the patient, the osteoporosis of the bone, and other social factors must be accounted for in these fractures.

Decision Making

When all has been taken into account, an appropriate algorithm can then be made in order that each acetabular fracture can be provided with individual appropriate management.

Undisplaced Acetabular Fractures

An acetabular fracture with 2 mm or less joint incongruity or step, or with medial roof arc angles greater than 45°, can adequately be managed nonoperatively. These require either skeletal or skin traction (depending on their stability) for a minimum of 6 weeks. Following this period if union is occurring, as confirmed by x-rays, mobilization of the patient using crutches and 30 pounds of weight-bearing is carried out for 6 further weeks. At this point, full weight-bearing is allowed. Throughout, emphasis on motion and muscle rehabilitation is maintained. It must be remembered that in the initial 2 to 4 weeks, a minimum of weekly x-rays are required to make sure that displacement does not occur through the fracture.

Displaced Acetabular Fractures

All fractures that do not fall into the above classification and are suitable and technically able to be treated operatively, would be fixed with open reduction and internal fixation. All dislocations or fracture and dislocations must be reduced as an emergency procedure before further assessment is carried out. This means that the head must be placed under the dome. This requires general anaesthesia, using an image intensifier to obtain the reduction. Assessment of the fracture and its stability is important.

Timing

These are complex operative procedures requiring appropriate decision making and investigation. Usually a delay of between 2 to 5 days is necessary to determine whether operative intervention is needed. This delay also is necessary in patients with high velocity injuries who are usually otherwise injured because it allows assessment and stabilization of the patient. However, the delay confines the patient to bed, usually in traction, and may not be suitable for the multiply injured patient. If all the appropriate information can be obtained so that an adequate decision can be made, immediate internal fixation of acetabular fractures may be carried out. This requires surgeons with excellent experience and adequate assistance. Appropriate blood and anaesthesia is important for this.

Until the definitive treatment decision is made, a greater trochanteric traction pin should *not* be inserted. If surgery is required, operative intervention through a greater trochanteric pin site may predispose the patient to a higher infection rate. Once the decision has been made to treat the patient nonoperatively in traction, a greater trochanteric pin may be inserted, if necessary.

The decision to carry out an open reduction also must be assessed thoroughly. Those fractures that are usually suitable for closed reduction and traction are low anterior column fractures, low transverse fractures, double column fractures without associated dome involvement, and medial wall comminuted fractures as long as the head remains congruent under the dome. Fractures that are not amenable to closed methods of treatment are posterior wall or posterior column fractures. The high transverse or T-fracture, which involves the dome, as well as both column fractures with significant dome involvement, and any fracture with a significant intra-articular fracture that destroys the congruity of the joint must be treated operatively.

Open Reduction and Internal Fixation of Acetabular Fractures

Approaches

As in all surgery, particularly intra-articular surgery, adequate exposure is mandatory for adequate visibility and to ensure that the joint can be adequately reconstructed. If one is to operate to reconstitute the hip joint or any joint it is mandatory that one can visually inspect this joint to determine the result of the surgical plan. Consequently, the approach to an acetabular fracture is a very important decision that must be made. It is based upon, first, the fracture pattern. Following determination of the fracture and its major displacement, assessment of the soft tissue injury must be carried out. The amount of damage to the underlying muscle and skin from the direct blow that has caused the acetabular fracture must be assessed. The approach through a contused area of muscle and skin may lead to significant postoperative complications, particularly if extensile exposures are used. Finally, the delay in performing the surgery also will determine the approach that will be used. If the delay is long and early healing is evident, an extensile approach to allow access to both the inner and outer aspects of the pelvis is required in order to mobilize these fracture fragments appropriately.

With respect to the fracture, the decision regarding the approach to use can be based on the previous classification. Posterior wall and column fractures can usually be approached through a standard posterior approach as described by Kocher and Langenbach. The Kocher-Langenbach incision gives adequate exposure to the posterior column and posterior wall. If, however, it is known that the dome is involved and that this must be repaired, serious consideration should be given to the use of a trochanteric osteotomy, associated with the Kocher-Langenbach incision. This allows reflection of the abductor muscles anteriorly and adequate exposure of the dome for reduction and fixation. (Fig. 9–22)

Anterior column fractures and anterior wall fractures require a significant amount of decision making, based on the fracture configuration. The anterior column fracture, which is a high iliac wing fracture, exiting along the wing itself, can usually, if noncomminuted, be fixed through an iliofemoral approach. However, low anterior column fractures and any fracture that involves the anterior wall usually require an anterior ilioinguinal approach. The ilioinguinal as described by Letournel does not allow visual inspection of the joint. The joint is reduced through an indirect reduction of the fracture fragments on the inner wall of the pelvis. If it is necessary for the joint to be inspected then an iliofemoral extension can be added to allow anterior exposure to the hip joint and capsule (Fig. 9–23).

The transverse and T-fractures usually require an extensile approach. Some transverse fractures can be reduced using either a simple Kocher-Langenbach approach or an iliofemoral approach,

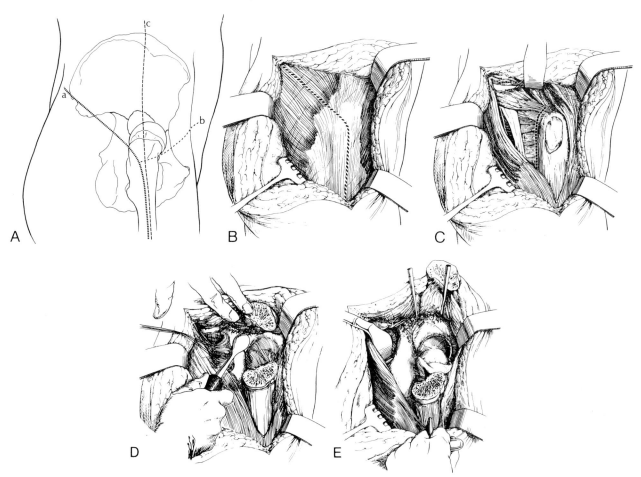

Fig. 9–22. The posterior approach with or without trochanteric osteotomy. **A.** The standard posterior approach to the hip is the Kocher-Langenbach approach, performed through incision (a). Incision (c) is performed for a more extensile approach as described by Ruedi. The anterior limb (b) may be used to convert a posterior approach to an extensile triradiate approach. **B–D.** Following the standard posterior incision from the posterior superior spine to the greater trochanter and down the shaft, the gluteus maximus muscle is identified with the fascia lata. This is then cut in the direction of the fibers to expose the posterior musculature of the hip and the sciatic nerve overlying the external rotators and quadratus femoris. The piriformis and external rotators are taken down. The obturator internus muscle is identified as the key to the posterior column because it exits from inside the pelvis around the lesser sciatic notch. If further exposure is required, trochanteric osteotomy as shown in fig. d, is performed. This allows access to the superior dome. **E.** Complete extensile exposure through the triradiate incision and radial capsulotomy of the hip. By sectioning the anterior limb through the fascia lata and turning back the attachments of the muscles from the anterior crest, one can now see the posterior column, the dome, and the anterior column. (From Schatzker J., Tile M.: The Rationale of Operative Fracture Care. Heidelberg, Springer-Verlag, 1989.)

depending on the nature of the displacement. Because the columns are attached reduction from one approach reduces the other column. However, one should also consider in planning these approaches what extensile approach can be used in order that the other column can be always reduced anatomically if necessary. The T-fractures demand an extensile approach. The extensile approaches that are available usually are the transtrochanteric or triradiate approach (Fig. 9–24) and the extended iliofemoral approach (Fig. 9–25).

Associated both column fractures again can be managed through an extensile approach, using the triradiate, extended iliofemoral, or anterior ilioinguinal approach.

As well as the approach, positioning of the patient should also be thought out. The posterior approaches can be done either in the prone or lateral decubitus position. It is difficult to move to a triradiate approach from a prone position. Therefore, the prone position is usually used for those fractures that do not require access to the anterior column. A lateral position should be used in all fractures in which an extensile triradiate extended iliofemoral approach will be required. The supine position can be used for the iliofemoral and anterior ilioinguinal approach. These approaches can be done on a standard operating table or on a traction table.

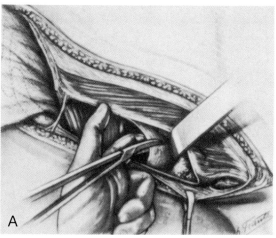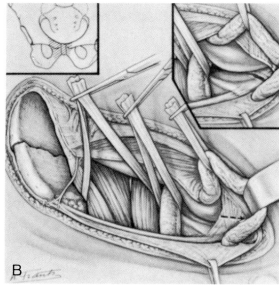

Fɪɢ. 9–23. **A.** Ilioinguinal approach with application to the "T" extension. For anterior fractures the ilioinguinal approach, with or without a "T" extension, is required. This approach requires identification of three major windows. These windows are the iliac wing under the iliopsoas, the interval between the iliopsoas and the vessels for the posterior column, and the medial window for pubic rami fractures. The key to this approach is the identification of the iliopsoas fascia and its complete division down under the pubic rami. Once this has been completed, all three windows can be identified, as shown in Figure 9–23B. If a joint must be visualized, the incision is extended down the limb using a modified Smith-Peterson nail. This will allow an anterior capsulotomy and inspection of the reduction in the joint. (From Schatzker J., Tile M.: The Rationale of Operative Fracture Care. Heidelberg, Springer-Verlag, 1989.)

Osteosynthesis

Prior to embarking on the internal fixation of any acetabular fracture, the fracture should be reviewed on a plastic pelvis. The fracture line should be drawn and the fixation visualized on the model. The placement of interfragmental screws, which is the cornerstone of all reconstructive surgery, must be planned well and the position of these screws visualized on the plastic pelvis. Review of the thick areas that will hold screws is important. The solid areas involve the iliac crest, the sciatic buttress, the brim of the true pelvis and the anterior border of the iliac wing. One must also be aware of the limits of the hip joint so that screws are not placed into this. The roof of the acetabulum is limited above by a line extending approximately one finger breadth above the posterior limit of the pelvic brim or above the superior margin of the greater sciatic notch, to the upper pole of the anterior inferior spine.

Instruments

Numerous bone holding forceps are required to reduce and hold the fractures in a reduced position. The use of large pointed reduction forceps and specialized pelvic reduction forceps are mandatory in these cases. The use of screws placed in the fracture fragments and then a Farabeouf-type clamp be-

tween these screws is sometimes helpful as well. Ball spikes are used to push the fragments into the reduced position. Deep retractors are also mandatory for this type of fixation. Screws are the standard screws of any internal fixation set and the plates that are used are usually 4.5 reconstruction and 3.5 reconstruction plates. These can be obtained either straight or in precurved formats. These plates must be contoured to lie directly on the bone surfaces. It is most common to use the 3.5 mm fragment sets because they give adequate purchase in the majority of situations (Fig. 9–26).

Specific Types of Fractures

Posterior Fractures: Reduction (Fig. 9–27)

Assessment of the acetabulum must be carried out for marginal impaction and these fractures can be reduced by elevation on to the femoral head and bone grafting performed behind them. Care must be taken to maintain the soft tissue attachments, particularly from the capsule to the posterior wall fragments. This means that one must operate through the fracture, rather than making appropriate capsular incisions. Fixation of posterior wall fractures is usually carried out by the means of interfragmental compression. Following completion of this the wall fragments must then be buttressed with a plate

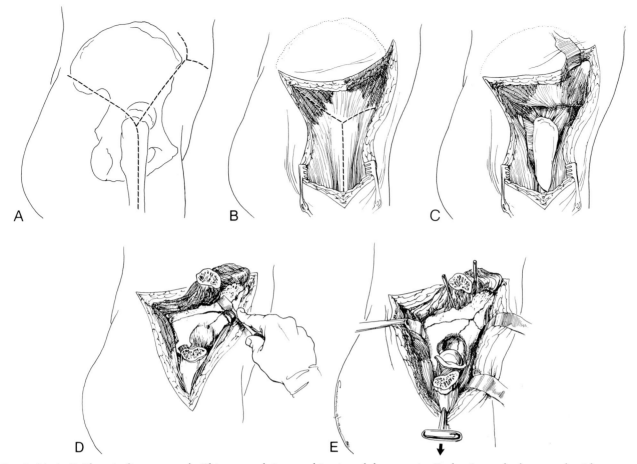

FIG. 9–24. A–E. The triradiate approach. This approach is a combination of the posterior Kocher-Langenbach approach with an anterior extension up to the iliac spine and along the anterior rim of the pelvis. Care must be taken not to create skin flaps. A subcutaneous dissection is limited only to the identification of the deep structures of the gluteus maximus, the fascia lata, and the tensor fascia. In Figure 9–24C these have been sectioned and the greater trochanter taken off, producing a large superior flap of gluteus muscles supplied by the skin vessels over the top of the pelvic brim. Continued dissection both anteriorly and posteriorly will allow adequate visualization of the iliac wing, posterior and anterior columns, and the internal aspect of the joint. (From Schatzker J., Tile M.: The Rationale of Operative Fracture Care. Heidelberg, Springer-Verlag, 1989.)

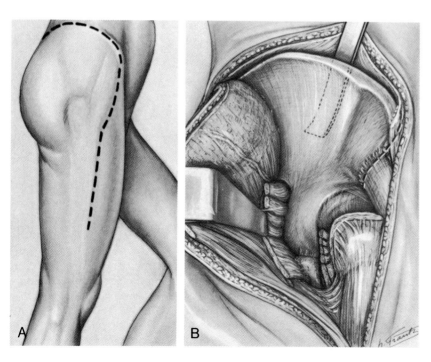

FIG. 9–25. The extended iliofemoral approach. The extended iliofemoral approach is described by Letournel. The superior gluteal artery supplies a large posterior-based flap. A and B. Incision extending from the posterior superior spine to the anterior spine and down the leg on the lateral aspect. The gluteal muscles as well as the rotators are taken off the greater trochanter. This exposes the iliac wing and the posterior column with access to the inner aspect of the pelvis and to the anterior column, as shown in Figure 9–25B. (From Schatzker J., Tile M.: The Rationale of Operative Fracture Care. Heidelberg, Springer-Verlag, 1989.)

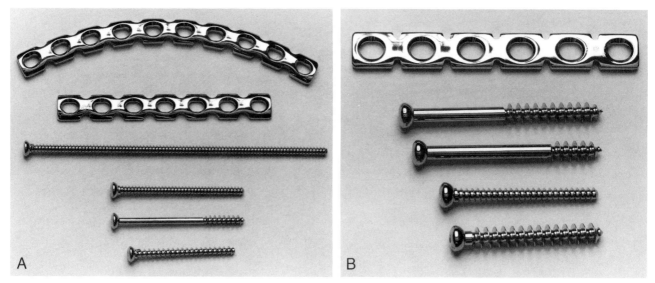

FIG. 9–26. Implants. **A.** The 3.5-mm reconstruction plate, both straight and curved, with the associated 3.5-mm screws. It is necessary to have nine fully threaded 3.5-mm cortical screws as well as the 4-mm cancellous screws as shown here. **B.** The 4.5-mm implants. This is the standard large fragment set. The plate, however, is a reconstruction plate. This system is rarely used, but may be necessary in large pelvii.

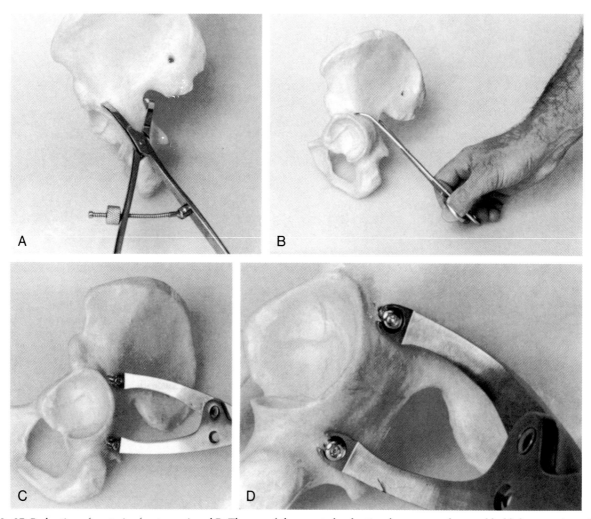

FIG. 9–27. Reduction of posterior fractures. **A** and **B.** The use of the serrated reduction forceps to reduce and hold the posterior column fracture. This also may be done with the large pointed reduction clamps as shown in Figure 9–27B. **C** and **D.** The use of the pelvic reduction clamps. These are fixed to bone through the use of cortical 4.5-mm screws. This achieves indirect reduction as well as stabilization of the fracture through compression. All instruments shown are needed for appropriate reduction. (From Schatzker J., Tile M.: The Rationale of Operative Fracture Care. Heidelberg, Springer-Verlag, 1989.)

molded to the posterior column. Care must be taken to direct the screws at the appropriate angle so that they do not enter the posterior aspect of the acetabulum. Screws should not be placed in the plate across the posterior fragments in the region of the acetabulum.

Posterior column fractures are the rotational malaligned. These are usually rotated about the vertical axis in an internal fashion and consequently must be externally rotated as well as pulled forward to maintain the reduction. One must visualize the reduction at the joint surface and at the greater sciatic notch as well as placing a finger through the greater sciatic notch along the quadrilateral plate to make sure that complete reduction is obtained. These must be stabilized with an interfragmental screw across the fracture line, as well as buttressed with a plate. (Fig. 9–28)

Anterior Fractures

Anterior wall fractures are reduced again by visualization of the joint and working through the fracture itself. Interfragmental screws and buttressing are necessary. Anterior column fractures again are treated in a similar fashion as the wall fracture. Interfragmental compression should be maintained across the iliac wing component of these fractures and buttressed using a plate. Fractures of the superior pubic ramus must be reduced anatomically and fixed, usually with a plate.

Transverse Fractures (Fig. 9–29)

Fixation of transverse fractures must again take into account the rotational component of the distal fracture fragment. This can only be assessed by palpation on the inner wall of the pelvis. Again, interfragmental compression must be achieved across the fracture line. Transverse T-fractures usually can be fixed in a transtrochanteric approach or posterior approach. The posterior column fracture fragment can be pushed out of the way to allow assessment of the anterior column fracture fragment. The hip is reduced under the remaining portion of the dome. The anterior column is held in position usually by a finger along the inner wall or by means of a hook across the anterior aspect. A long fixation screw can then be placed into the anterior fragment from the posterior iliac wing. This is a difficult screw to insert but usually can be placed with adequate visualization of the joint and anterior column. Following this the posterior column is re-

duced and fixed as a normal posterior column fracture.

Associated Both Column Fractures

The clue to these fractures is the reconstruction of the pelvis followed by the acetabulum reconstruction. Anatomical reductions must be performed of all fractures because a minor change or minor deformity in the iliac wing can lead to major displacements in the acetabulum itself. Normally, reduction commences at the posterior fracture and works forward.

Postoperative Care

When the operative procedure is complete the surgeon must assess: (1) the congruency of the reduction, and (2) its stability. Hopefully the congruence is normal and if not it must be as close as possible. What is most important, however, is the stability of the fixation. If adequate fixation is obtained with interfragmental compression and appropriate neutralization and buttress plates, postoperatively the patient can be placed on continuous passive motion for 5 to 7 days and then mobilized. There is no indication for postoperative traction. Weight-bearing should be the weight of leg for the first 6 weeks and then gradually increased to full weight-bearing by 3 months. During this phase active exercises to maintain the muscles and range of motion must be performed. Patients with greater trochanteric osteotomies should avoid abduction exercises for approximately 6 weeks, after which they should be commenced. The fixation of the greater trochanteric osteotomy, using interfragmental compression screw fixation is good and the problems of nonunion are rare.

If, however, the reduction is not stable or noncongruous but can be maintained by traction, the use of postoperative traction is mandatory. This can be combined through a femoral traction pin or tibial pin and the use of continuous passive motion. This traction should be maintained for 6 weeks until early union has begun. This is commonly seen in those fractures when comminution of the medial wall of the acetabulum exists. This is a difficult fracture to treat and although buttress plates can be placed over the inner brim of the acetabulum it is usually necessary to maintain traction on the hip joint to prevent medial subluxation and to maintain these fragments in their reduced

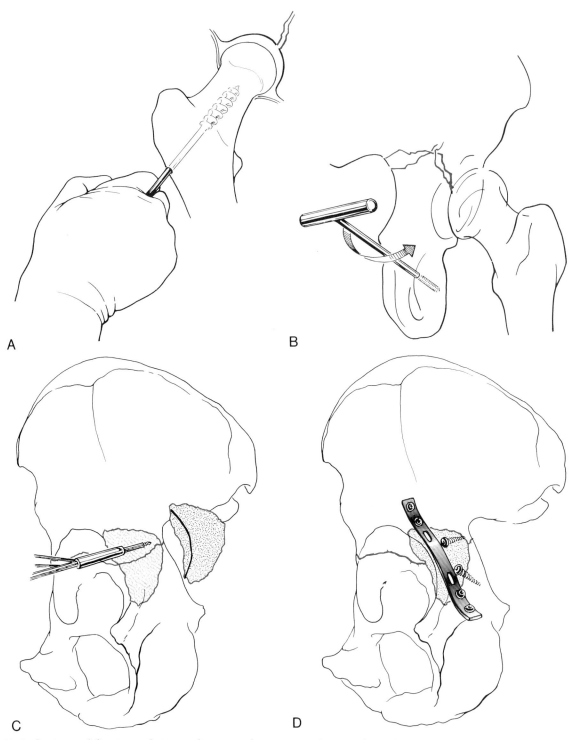

FIG. 9–28. Reduction and fixation techniques of posterior fractures. **A.** The use of a corkscrew in the femoral neck as a method of applying traction intraoperatively. This technique is helpful in enabling one to pull the head out of the acetabulum and thus maintain reduction and visually inspect the joint. **B.** The use of a Schanz screw or T handle placed into the ischial tuberosity. This allows one to control the posterior column particularly with regard to rotation. With this in place the rotational correction of the malrotated posterior column can then be controlled. **C.** The operative technique of internal fixation of a posterior wall fracture with lag screw fixation. **D.** The fracture fragment fixed with intrafragmental screw fixation taking care to avoid entry into the joint and then buttressing with a posterior plate. This is a similar technique that would be used for the fixation of a pure posterior column fracture. (From Schatzker J., Tile M.: The Rationale of Operative Fracture Care. Heidelberg, Springer-Verlag, 1989.)

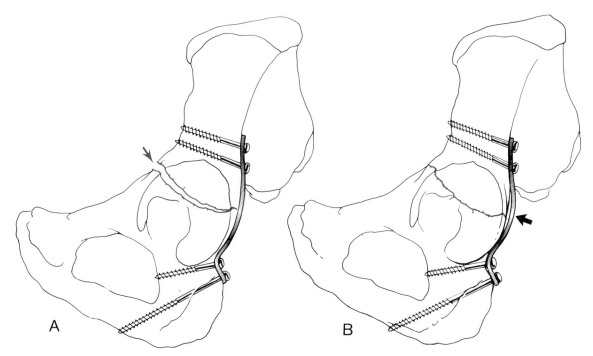

Fig. 9–29. Transverse fracture fixation. **A** and **B.** In a transverse fracture a plate that is improperly contoured will open the fracture anteriorly. It is important that the plate is slightly overcontoured so that when it is tightened down the anterior aspect is closed, as shown in Figure 9–29B. Note at the arrow that the plate is slightly contoured off the posterior aspect of the acetabulum to assure anterior compression. (From Schatzker J., Tile M.: The Rationale of Operative Fracture Care. Heidelberg, Springer-Verlag, 1989.)

position. As union occurs the hip becomes stable. Similarly, postoperative weight-bearing status is started at 6 weeks in this situation.

Complications

Acetabular fracture surgery is not without its complications. Postoperative infections can be minimized by the appropriate decision making with regard to incisions and soft tissue injuries in the region of the acetabulum. The use of prophylactic antibiotics is recommended. The management of postoperative infection is the same as in any intra-articular fracture. Early debridement and drainage with either closure over a suction irrigation system or the wound being left open and treated in this fashion with packing, and subsequent delayed closure is necessary. The average occurrence of infection in acetabular surgery is approximately 1 to 5%.

Sciatic nerve injury is a potential complication. Care must be taken throughout the operative procedure, in all of these situations, particularly from a posterior approach, that the knee is maintained in 90° of flexion. This relaxes the sciatic nerve and, with the hip in extension, should minimize its chances for damage. Appropriate retraction about the nerve must be carried out. If nerve injury oc-

curs, expectant treatment is performed. Seventy percent of these cases resolve and the patient becomes functional.

Hemorrhage

Involvement of the superior gluteal artery from posterior approaches and the femoral artery from anterior approaches can occur. In the anterior ilioinguinal approach proper dissection around the neurovascular bundle is mandatory. If this is carried out it is uncommon to see surgical problems of bleeding. The superior gluteal artery, however, may be damaged at the notch. This usually will be controlled by packing and if necessary one must open the retroacetabular area by sectioning the ischial spine or removing the sacrospinous ligament. This allows more access and the usual visualization of the artery as it comes through the notch. The common method of treating this is to pack the area until hemostasis is obtained.

Late Complications

The most common late complication is that of heterotropic ossification. This is significant in 20 to 35% of cases. It has been most commonly associated with the posterior approaches and particularly the extensile approach when either osteotomy or incision of the abductor muscles has been carried out. This can vary from mild to complete ankylosis of the hip. The prophylaxis for this is not well known. The use of Indocid at the present time seems to be beneficial. If significant limitation of hip joint motion occurs the heterotopic ossification can be excised. The use of a CT scan to evaluate its extent and position is important. The excision timing is usually approximately 1 year. The appropriate investigations of alkaline phosphatase and bone scanning are usually carried out. When the alkaline phosphatase has returned to normal and the bone scan shows decreasing activity, excision of the heterotopic ossification can be carried out. This should be done as early as possible in order that the hip can get back to its normal environment of motion.

Avascular Necrosis

Avascular necrosis is a complication that is inherent in the fracture pattern itself. Most posterior fractures and dislocations have approximately a 15 to 20% incidence. This may not be a complete head type and may not involve collapse. However, the treatment of this depends on the patient and his functional status.

Osteoarthritis

This complication depends on the ability to achieve a reduction. It is important to maintain a congruous hip in order that this does not occur.

Summary

The surgical management of acetabular fractures requires a complete understanding of the pelvis and the acetabulum with respect to anatomy and the pathomechanics of the injury. With this and a complete assessment involving the history, physical examination, appropriate plain x-rays, and CT scan an appropriate decision can be made regarding how to best manage it. An appropriate surgical approach to this is mandatory.

If the fracture can be adequately and safely approached it usually can be fixed. This provides the patient with the best ultimate result.

References

1. CARNESALE PG, STEWART MJ, BARNES SN: Acetabular disruption and central fracture dislocations of the hip. J Bone Joint Surg, 57A:1054–1059, 1975.
2. CALKINS MS, et al.: Computerized tomography evaluation of stability in posterior fracture dislocation of the hip. Presented at the American Academy of Orthopaedic Surgeons Annual Meeting, San Francisco, 1987.
3. EPSTEIN HC, Posterior fracture dislocations of the hip: comparison of open and closed methods of treatment in certain types. J Bone Joint Surg, 56A:1103–1127, 1974.
4. JUDET R, JUDET J, LETOURNAL E: Fractures of the acetabulum: classification and surgical approaches for open reduction. J Bone Joint Surg, 46A:1615–1647, 1964.
5. LARSON CB, Fractures dislocations of the hip. Clin Orthop, 92:147–150, 1973.
6. MATTA JM, ANDERSON LH, EPSTEIN HC, HENDRICKS P: Fractures of the acetabulum: a retrospective analysis. Clin Orthop, 205:230–240, 1986.
7. PENNAL GF, DAVIDSON J, GARSIDE H: Results of treatment of acetabular fractures. Clin Orthop, 151:115–123, 1980.
8. ROWE CR, LOWELL JD: Prognosis of fractures of the acetabulum. J Bone Joint Surg: 43A:30–59, 1961.
9. TILE M: Fractures of the Acetabulum: The Rationale of Operative Fracture Care. New York, Springer Verlag, 1986.
10. TILE M: Fractures of the pelvis and acetabulum. Baltimore, Williams and Wilkins, 177, 1984.
11. VAILAS JC, HURWITZ SR, WIESEL SW: Posterior acetabular fracture size: an experimental study with clinical applications. Presented at the American Academy of Orthopaedic Surgeons Annual Meeting, San Francisco, 1987.

CHAPTER TEN

Intracapsular Femoral Neck Fractures

JOHN J. CALLAGHAN

Approximately 250,000 hip fractures occur annually in the United States and result in health care costs of more than 1.25 billion dollars. With the advancing age of our population and better medical care, this number is likely to increase. One study showed that between the years 1965 and 1981 the number of hip fractures in the United States tripled. Other studies have predicted another threefold increase in the next two decades.[22]

The mortality rates associated with hip fractures vary from 13 to 30% within the first year after injury. After the first year, the life expectancy of patients returns to normal. Patients living in nursing homes prior to fracture have the highest morbidity and mortality rates and are the least likely to resume ambulation. Rehabilitation of these patients to their prefracture social status is difficult, with perhaps only one-half returning to their former degree of independence. The need to understand the nature and current treatment of hip fractures is essential after understanding the epidemiologic extent of the problem.[22]

Historical Review

The historical milestones in hip fracture treatment parallel those of orthopaedic principles themselves. Table 10–1 illustrates the development of hip fracture management from dynamic traction, to anatomic reduction and cast immobilization, to rigid internal fixation, and more recently implant arthroplasty.

Ambrose Pare,[61] in the 1500s was probably the first to recognize the hip fracture as a clinical entity. Internal fixation of femoral neck fractures was first discussed by von Langenbeck in 1850. However internal fixation was not practiced on a universal basis until Smith-Petersen developed the triflange nail in 1931.[74] The Judet brothers designed an acrylic femoral prosthesis in 1948 and this served as a prototype for the Moore,[56] Eicher, and Thompson femoral implants. Despite all of the ad-

vances noted in Table 10–1, the femoral neck fracture still remains the "unsolved fracture."

Anatomic Considerations
Vascular Supply

Critical to the success of surgical operations on the hip joint is the knowledge of the origins and distribution of the arteries supplying the head and the neck of the femur. The arterial blood supply of the proximal portion of the femur has been studied by Howe, et al., Trueta and Harrison,[82] Crock,[16] and Chung.[12] I endorse Crock's description because it is based on three-plane analysis and provides a standardization of anatomical nomenclature. Crock[16] describes three groups of arteries at the proximal end of the femur: (1) an extracapsular arterial ring located at the base of the femoral neck, (2) ascending cervical branches of the extracapsular arterial ring on the surface of the femoral neck and (3) the arteries of the round ligament (Fig. 10–1).

The extracapsular arterial ring is formed anteriorly by branches of the lateral femoral circumflex artery and posteriorly by a large branch of the medial femoral circumflex artery. The ascending cervical branches arise from the extracapsular arterial ring. They penetrate the capsule of the hip joint at the intertrochanteric line anteriorly and pass beneath the orbicular fibers of the capsule posteriorly. The ascending cervical branches pass upward under synovial reflections and fibrous prolongations of the capsule toward the articular cartilage that demarcates the femoral head from the neck. Weitbrecht[85] initially described these retinacular arteries. This close proximity of the retinacular arteries to bone puts them at risk of injury in any fracture of the femoral neck and especially in the superolateral area. These arteries penetrate the head and become the epiphyseal arteries. The metaphysis of the femoral neck is well vascularized with contributions from the extracapsular arterial ring, ascend-

TABLE 10–1. *Important Historical Dates in the Understanding and Treatment of Hip Fractures*

Date	Author	Advancement
1500s	Pare	Recognized hip fracture as a clinical entity
1823	Cooper	Classified hip fractures and recognized nonunion
1850	Von Langenbeck	First femoral neck nailing
1867	Phillips	Lateral-longitudinal traction
1883	Senn	Internal fixation animal studies
1902	Whitman	Closed reduction and casting
1916	Hey-Graves	Quadriflanged nail
1931	Smith-Petersen	Triflanged nail
1932	Johansson	Cannulated nail
1934	Moore	Multiple pin fixation
1936	Gaenslen	Multiple pin fixation
	Telson	
	Knowles	
1940	Moore	Stainless steel prosthesis
1944	Harmon	Sideplate and pins
1958	Deyerle	
1960	Charnley	Cemented femoral component
1972	Food and Drug Administration	Methyl methacrylate approved for general use in US

ing cervical branches, and the proximal femur nutrient artery. The artery of the ligamentum teres has variable contributions to the femoral head and it originates from the obturator artery or less frequently the medial femoral circumflex artery. When fractures of the femoral neck occur revascularization must take place from three sources: (1) the area of femoral head that has remained viable, (2) vascular ingrowth across the fracture site and (3) revascularization from vascular tissue growing in from that part of the femoral head not covered by articular cartilage.

Skeletal Anatomy

The femoral neck projects superiorly, anteriorly, and medially from the upper femoral shaft. The femoral head forms two-thirds of a sphere arising from the femoral neck and having an axis parallel to the neck. In the adult the axis between the neck and the shaft averages 135°; the femoral neck is anteverted from the transcondylar plane approximately 10°. Normally the axis of the femoral head is parallel to the axis of the femoral neck, but occasionally retroversion occurs. Recently, measurements have shown that the femoral head is not exactly round but that the meridians have longer radii than the radii of the equator. The internal trabecular system, described by Ward,[83] is pictured in Figure 10–2. These lines are the basis for determining the quality of bone when using the Singh index[71] (Table 10–2).

Mechanical Factors

Rydell,[65,66] using a femoral prosthesis with a strain gauge, has made considerable contributions regarding the forces acting on the femoral head. He showed that standing on one leg generated a force 2.5 times body weight in that hip. In one-leg support, with a cane in the contralateral hand, the force across the hip is reduced to body weight (40% reduction).[11] At rest with two-leg support, a force

TABLE 10–2. *Singh's Index*

Grade VI	All the normal trabecular groups are visible.
Grade V	Structure of the principal tensile and principal compressive trabeculae are accentuated.
Grade IV	Principle tensile trabeculae are significantly reduced but still present.
Grade III	There is a break in the continuity of the principal tensile trabeculae opposite the greater trochanter.
Grade II	Only the principal compressive trabeculae stand out prominently.
Grade I	The principal compressive trabeculae are significantly reduced in number and are no longer prominent.

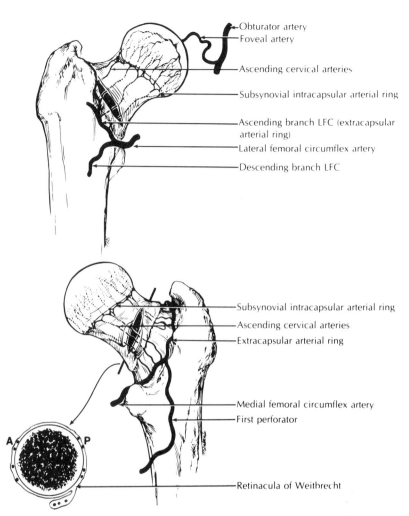

Fig. 10–1. Blood supply to the femoral head and neck from front (top) and back (bottom).

- Obturator artery
- Foveal artery
- Ascending cervical arteries
- Subsynovial intracapsular arterial ring
- Ascending branch LFC (extracapsular arterial ring)
- Lateral femoral circumflex artery
- Descending branch LFC

- Subsynovial intracapsular arterial ring
- Ascending cervical arteries
- Extracapsular arterial ring

- Medial femoral circumflex artery
- First perforator

- Retinacula of Weithbrecht

of approximately one-half body weight was exerted across each hip joint, whereas standing with the hip and knee flexed 90° increased the force to near body weight across the flexed hip. Running increased the hip forces to five times body weight. Lifting the leg from a supine position with a straight knee produces a force 1.5 times body weight across the hip joint. One should have an appreciation from these loads when considering the management of intracapsular hip fractures.

Classification of Intracapsular Hip Fractures

Two popular classifications have been used to describe femoral neck fractures. Pauwel's[62] classification is based on the angle the fracture forms with the horizontal plane, with Type I being 30° from the horizontal, Type II 50°, and Type III 70°, almost vertical (Fig. 10–3). Boyd[9,10] was unable to demonstrate an increasingly worse prognosis with a more

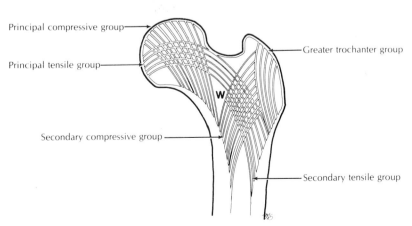

Fig. 10–2. Internal trabecular system of the head and neck with Ward's triangle (W).

- Principal compressive group
- Principal tensile group
- Greater trochanter group
- Secondary compressive group
- Secondary tensile group

Fig. **10–3.** Pauwel's classification of femoral neck fractures.

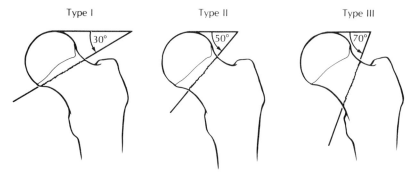

vertical fracture pattern, however. In his series, Type II fractures had 33% aseptic necrosis and 12% nonunion and Type III fractures 30% aseptic necrosis and 8% nonunion. Garden[26] described a classification based on the displacement (Fig. 10–4) rather than the angle of the fracture. He felt that the femoral neck fracture was a progression through four stages. The Garden I fracture is an impacted or incomplete fracture. The trabeculae of the inferior neck are still intact. The Garden II fracture is a complete fracture without displacement. There is a fracture line across the entire femoral neck. A Garden III fracture is a complete fracture with partial displacement. In the Garden III fracture the trabec-

ular pattern of the femoral head does not line up with that of the acetabulum, demonstrating incomplete displacement between the femoral fracture fragments. The retinaculum of Weibrecht may remain intact. The Stage IV fracture is complete fracture with total displacement of the fracture fragments. The trabecular pattern of the femoral head lines up with the trabecular pattern of the acetabulum. It must be remembered that the Garden classification and the Pauwel classification do not consider displacement in the lateral plane.

In addition to the angle of fracture and the amount of displacement the quality of bone and mechanism of energy are important.[2,3,78] In the el-

Fig. **10–4.** Garden's stages of femoral neck fractures. From upper left (stage I) clockwise to lower left (stage IV).

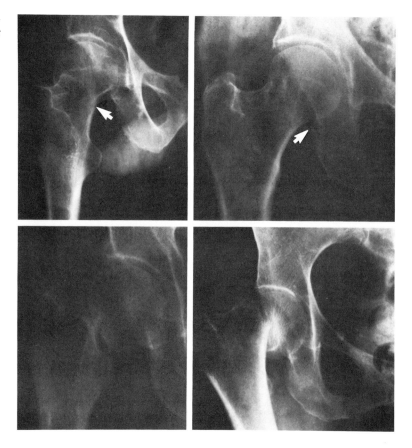

derly population studies have shown a high incidence of osteomalacia and osteoporosis[3] in patients with hip fractures whereas this is not usually a consideration in younger patients. Conversely, the energy necessary to produce a femoral neck fracture in patients under age 40 is much higher and creates greater soft tissue trauma than those in the elderly. Finally intracapsular fractures need to be separated by their anatomic location with subcapital fractures being those that occur immediately beneath the articular surface of the femoral head along the old epiphyseal plate and transcervical fractures being those passing across the femoral neck between the femoral head and the greater trochanter.

DeLee has classified femoral neck fractures based on patient characteristics and the treatment of intracapsular fractures in this chapter is structured on this classification (Table 10–3). Treatment is based on the philosophy of Boyd and Salvatore:[10] "The sacrifice of the head and neck and replacement by a metallic foreign object is not the answer for the majority of patients. In over half, the best available material is in the acetabulum and its indiscriminant removal should be avoided."

Impacted and Nondisplaced Fractures

Both operative and nonoperative treatment have been suggested for impacted femoral neck fractures (Garden Stage I).[1,2,3,5,10,15,20,24,26–30,34,37–39,44,45,47,49,63,69,73,80,87] Crawford's criteria for treating impacted fractures nonoperatively include: no shortening or external rotation of the limb, little discomfort on active or passive motion of the hip, the ability to perform active internal rotation of the limb, impaction on both anteroposterior and lateral radiographs, and a cooperative patient who can walk touch weight-bearing for at least 4 months.

There is some controversy concerning the opera-

TABLE 10–3. *DeLee Classification Based on Characteristics*

1. Femoral neck fracture in the elderly patient
   A. Impacted fractures
   B. Displaced fractures
2. Fractures of the femoral neck diagnosed late
3. Femoral neck fractures in the adult below 40 years of age
4. Stress fractures of the femoral neck
5. Ipsilateral fractures of the femoral neck and femoral shaft
6. Femoral neck fractures in patients with Paget's disease
7. Femoral neck fractures in patients with Parkinson's disease
8. Fractures of the femoral neck in patients with spastic hemiplegia
9. Post radiation fracture of the femoral neck
10. Pathologic femoral neck fractures secondary to metastatic disease of bone

tive reduction of impacted fractures. The cause of aseptic necrosis in impacted valgus fractures is thought to be kinking of the lateral epiphyseal vessels and tethering of the medial epiphyseal vessels in the ligamentum teres as the head assumes an extreme valgus position. Moore believed that fractures impacted in valgus should be reduced and nailed. However, Garden and others disagree with disimpaction because not all patients with aseptic necrosis develop symptoms. I recommend internal fixation with Hagie or Knowles pins of impacted fractures, even those that are recognized late, in all patients who can undergo anesthesia. I have even used percutaneous pins inserted under local anesthesia in medially disabled patients. We have used the newer cannulated pins (Richards and Asnis), but they have been difficult to remove and it usually is not possible to place more than three pins. Nondisplaced fractures (Garden II) are treated in a similar manner although occasionally we use a compression screw and side plate taking care not to spin the femoral head by putting a Steinmann pin through the head and across the acetabulum during drilling and screw insertion.

Displaced Fractures

In most patients nonoperative treatment for displaced fractures is not indicated. However, non-ambulatory patients with medical conditions or mental deterioration are candidates for the nonoperative approach. In these cases the patients are mobilized as soon as pain subsides with degree of mobilization dependent on the patient's pain.

Operative treatment of displaced Garden III and Garden IV fractures is based on the physiologic age of the patient. Other than the particular situations listed and discussed in the following sections the goal of primary treatment is to save the femoral head.[1–3,5,10,15,20,24,26–30,34,37–39,44,45,47,49,63,69,73,80,87] This philosophy is based on the fact that aseptic necrosis develops in only 15 to 30% of patients with displaced fractures and that not all aseptic necrosis that develops becomes symptomatic. Even though hemiarthroplasty provides immediate mobilization and eliminates the complications of aseptic necrosis, nonunion, and fixation failure, function following hemiarthroplasty is never equal to that of the patient's own femoral head and followup at 4 years demonstrates only 52% good or excellent results. Indications for bipolar replacement, which in the past have been shown to have no better clinical results than hemiarthroplasty, may be broader now that modular systems with trunion heads are being used. These modular systems should allow easier conversion of bipolar prostheses to total hip replacements by removing the femoral head to expose the acetabulum. In addition the newer modular unipolar replacements should be considered in older age groups.

Extension and flexion maneuvers both have been described for the closed reduction of displaced femoral neck fractures. Massie, Green,[30] Garden,[28,29] and McElvenny[44-47] have all described reduction in extension with distal traction and internal rotation of the leg. Leadbetter[41,42] popularized hip flexion for closed reduction of femoral neck fractures. I have found this maneuver of flexion to 90° with external rotation followed by extension and internal rotation helpful in hips that were irreducible by extension maneuvers.

In my practice, all traumatic displaced fractures in patients less than 50 years old are reduced and pinned even if it requires open reduction. With closed reduction an anterior capsulotomy is performed to evacuate the capsular hematoma. In patients 50 to 70 years of age, closed reduction is attempted and if unsuccessful a porous coated uncemented femoral component or a cemented femoral component with a bipolar head or uncemented acetabular component is used depending on the condition of the acetabular cartilage. If the patient is over 70 years of age cemented bipolar or total hip replacement is used unless the patient has less than 1 or 2 years life expectancy and has low demand, in which case an uncemented unipolar replacement is used.

Stress Fractures of the Femoral Neck

Since being described by Blecher[8] in 1905, stress fractures of the femoral neck have been recognized in two distinct populations: (1) young persons with normal bone experiencing strenuous activity and (2) older persons with osteopenic bone who experience minimal stress. Devas[19] classified femoral neck fractures as "distraction" or tension fractures with a transverse pattern that is perpendicular to the axis of the femoral neck (Fig. 10–5) and compression fractures that began as a haze of internal callus in the inferior part of the femoral neck (Fig. 10–6). Although most authors agree with internal fixation of femoral neck tension stress fractures some believe that the compression fractures can sometimes be treated nonoperatively. In my personal practice most are treated with pinning.

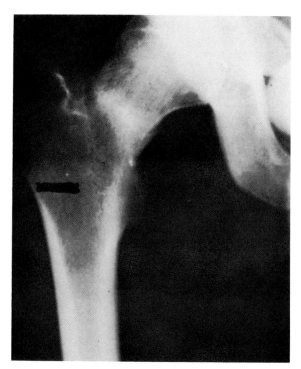

Fig. 10–5. Distraction type femoral neck stress fracture.

Fractures of the Femoral Neck with Ipsilateral Femoral Shaft Fractures

Fortunately, most femoral neck fractures associated with fractures of the femoral shaft are minimally displaced. However, this nondisplacement can lead to a delayed diagnosis. Fixation of the neck

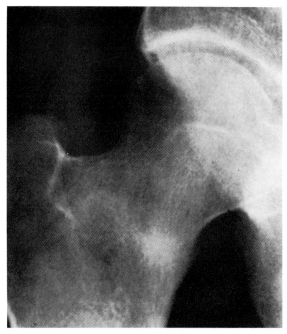

Fig. 10–6. Compression type femoral neck stress fracture.

fracture with nonoperative femoral shaft fracture treatment, intramedullary rodding (from above, through the knee, from the femoral condyle) with pinning of the neck fracture, plating the femur with pinning or compression screw fixation of the femoral neck, and Enders rodding have all been described as fixation methods for this fracture combination.[7,17,18,43,59,67,79] I find the use of the Russell Taylor (Richards) reconstruction nail the procedure of choice because of the ability to place femoral neck screws into the head going through the intramedullary nail. Occasionally, an anterior or posterior cannulated screw is needed for augmentation.

Femoral Neck Fractures in Patients with Paget's, Parkinson's Disease, and Spastic Hemiplegia

Failure of internal fixation devices has been reported in the treatment of femoral neck fractures associated with these three Ps: Paget's,[6,31,50,60,77] Parkinson's,[14,64,76] and spastic paralysis.[75] Use of endoprosthetic and total hip devices also has been associated with an increase complication rate, especially dislocation and loosening (particularly in Paget's disease), when used in these situations. When patients have mild forms of Parkinson's Disease or spastic hemiplegia, I continue to perform closed reduction and pinning of nondisplaced or minimally displaced fractures. For displaced fractures in patients without spasticity and rigidity and in all patients with spasticity and rigidity, I perform total hip arthroplasty or endoprosthetic replacement procedures through an anterolateral approach (to decrease the need for postoperative dislocation precautions in rehabilitation). In Paget's disease, unless the patient is under 50, I perform total hip replacement. Closed reduction and pinning has been associated with a high incidence of nonunion in these cases.

Pathologic Femoral Neck Fractures

Although internal fixation has been recommended in the past for fixation of impending as well as actual pathologic femoral neck fractures, the stresses across the hip joint in the area of the femoral neck are probably too great for any form of fixation used today to predictably prevent failure of the device. The main consideration in these fractures is to provide the patient pain relief first and

mobilization second.[33,36,40,59,68,70] Lane, et al.,[40] have shown that hemiarthroplasty or total hip procedures predictably accomplish these goals. Preoperative evaluation with radiographs and bone scanning is important to make certain that the acetabulum and distal femoral shaft are not involved with tumor. If there is no apparent acetabular involvement, I perform a cemented unipolar or bipolar replacement. If the patient has a predicted life expectancy of greater than 1 year (i.e., breast or prostate cancer) I use a long stem prosthesis (usually 200 mm 250 mm or 300 mm) to help prevent the possibility of later femoral shaft fracture (an entity that has occurred in my practice). If the acetabulum is involved, total hip replacement is performed using Steinmann pins into the pelvis[33] for support when necessary.

Summary

I feel strongly that a united femoral neck with a viable femoral head provides the most functional, painless hip no matter the age of the patient. In general, I recommend hemiarthroplasty or total joint arthroplasty only in patients with one of the five Ps: porosis (in the elderly), pathologic, paralysis (spastic), Parkinson's, and Paget's disease.

References

1. Ackroyd CE: Treatment of subcapital femoral fractures fixed with moore's pins: a study of 34 cases followed-up for up to 3 years. Injury, 5:100–108m, 1973–1974.
2. Arnold WD, Lyden JP, Minkoff J: Treatment of intracapsular fractures of the femoral neck. J Bone Joint Surg, 56A:254–262, 1974.
3. Arnold WD: The effect of early weight bearing on the stability of femoral neck fractures treated with Knowles pins. J Bone Joint Surg, 66A:847, 1984.
4. Asby ME, Anderson JC: Treatment of fractures of the hip and ipsilateral femur with the Zickel device. Clin Orthop, 127:156–160, 1977.
5. Bagby GW, Wallace GT: Femoral neck fractures in the elderly treated by multiple pins (Knowles). Northwest Med, 70:696–698, 1971.
6. Barry HC: Fractures of the femur in Paget's disease of bone in Australia. J Bone and Joint Surg, 46A:1359–1370, 1967.
7. Bernstein SM: Fractures of the femoral shaft and associated ipsilateral fractures of the hip. Orthop Clin North Am, 5:799–818, 1974.
8. Blecher A: Uber den Einfluss des Parade-Marsches auf die Entstehung der Fuss Geschwulst. Med Klin, 1:305–306, 1905.
9. Boyd HB, George LL: Complications of fractures of the neck of the femur. J Bone and Joint Surg, 29:13–18, 1947.

10. Boyd HB, Salvatore JE: Acute fracture of the femoral neck: internal fixation or prosthesis? J Bone and Joint Surg, 46A:1066–1068, 1964.

11. Brand RA, Crowninshield: The effect of cane use on hip contact force. Clin Orthop, 147:181, 1980.

12. Chung SMK: The arterial supply of the developing proximal end of the human femur. J Bone Joint Surg, 58A:961–970, 1976.

13. Cooper AP: A Treatise on Dislocations and on Fractures of the Joints, 2nd ed. London, Longman, Hurst, 1823.

14. Coughlin L, Templeton J: Hip fractures in patients with Parkinson's disease. Clin Orthop, 148:192–195, 1980.

15. Crawford HB: Experience with the non-operative treatment of impacted fractures of the neck of the femur. J Bone Joint Surg, 47A:830–831, 1965.

16. Crock HV: A revision of the anatomy of the arteries supplying the upper end of the human femur. J Anat (London), 99:77–88, 1965.

17. Delaney WM, Street DM: Fracture of the femoral shaft with fracture of neck of same femur. J Int Coll Surg, 19:303–312, 1953.

18. Dencker H: Femoral shaft fracture and fracture of the neck of the same femur. Acta Chir Scand, 129:597–605, 1965.

19. Devas M: Stress fractures of the femoral neck. J Bone Joint Surg, 47B:728–738, 1965.

20. Deyerle WM: Plate and periheal pins in hip fractures: two-plane reduction, total impaction and absolute fixation. Curr Pract Orthop Surg, 3:173–207, 1966.

21. Dorr L, et al.: Treatment of femoral neck fractures with total hip replacement versus cemented and noncemented hemiarthroplasty. J Arthroplasty, 1:21, 1986.

22. Fitzgerald: Orthopaedic Knowledge Update 2. American Academy of Orthopaedic Surgeons, pp. 360, 1987.

23. Francis KC, et al.: The treatment of pathological fractures of the femoral neck by resection. J Trauma, 2:465–473, 1962.

24. Gaenslen FJ: Subcutaneous spike fixation of fresh fractures of the neck of the femur. J Bone Joint Surg, 17:739–748, 1935.

25. Garden RS: The structure and function of the proximal end of femur. J Bone Joint Surg, 43B:576–589, 1961.

26. Garden RS: Stability and union in subcapital fractures of the femur. J Bone Joint Surg, 46B:630–647, 1964.

27. Garden RS: Scientific thinking and clinical research. Pro Mine Med Off Assoc (Johannesburg), 47:47–52, 1967.

28. Garden RS: Malreduction and avascular necrosis in subcapital fractures of the femur. J Bone Joint Surg, 53B:183–197, 1971.

29. Garden RS: Reduction and fixation of subcapital fractures of the femur. Orthop Clin North Am, 5:683–712, 1974.

30. Green JT, Gay FH: High femoral neck fractures treated by multiple-nail fixation: a survey of 100 cases. Clin Orthop, 11:177–183, 1958.

31. Grundy M: Fractures of the femur in Paget's disease of bone. J Bone Joint Surg, 52B:252–263, 1970.

32. Harmon PH: Treatment of trochanteric, subtrochanteric and transcervical fractures of the upper femur by fixation with plastic plate and stainless steel screws. Guthrie Clin Bull, 14:10–18, 1944.

33. Harrington KD, Johnston JO, Turner RH, Green DL: The use of methylmethacrylate as an adjunct in the internal fixation of malignant neoplastic fractures. J Bone Joint Surg, 54A:1665–1676, 1972.

34. Hey-Groves EW: Treatment of fractured neck of the femur with special regard to the results. J Bone Joint Surg, 12:1–14, 1930.

35. Hinchey JJ, Day PL: Primary prosthetic replacement in fresh femoral neck fractures. J Bone Joint Surg, 46A:223–240, 1964.

36. Jensen TM, Dillon WL, Reckling FW: Changing concepts in the management of pathological and impending pathological fractures. J Trauma, 16:496–502, 1976.

37. Johnansson S: On the operative treatment of medial fractures of the femoral neck. Acta Orthop Scand 3:362–385, 1932.

38. Knowles FL: Fractures of the neck of the femur. Wis Med J, 35:106–109, 1936.

39. Kofoed H, Alberts A.: Femoral neck fractures. Acta Orthop Scand, 51:127–136, 1980.

40. Lane JM, Sculco TP, Zolan S: Treatment of pathological fractures of the hip by endoprosthetic replacement. J Bone Joint Surg, 62A:954–959, 1980.

41. Leadbetter GW: A treatment for fracture of the neck of the femur. J Bone Joint Surg, 15:931–940, 1933.

42. Leadbetter GW: Closed reduction of fractures of the neck of the femur. J Bone Joint Surg, 20:108–113, 1938.

43. MacKenzie DB: Simultaneous ipsilateral fracture of the femoral neck and shaft: report of 8 cases. S Afr Med J, 45:458–467, 1971.

44. McElvenny RT: The roentgenographic interpretation of what constitutes adequate reduction of the femur neck fractures. Surg Gynecol Obstet, 80:97–106, 1945.

45. McElvenny RT: Management of intracapsular hip fractures. Surg Clin North Am, 29:31–58, 1949.

46. McElvenny RT: The immediate treatment of intracapsular hip fracture. Clin Orthop, 10:289–323, 1957.

47. McElvenny RT: Concepts and principles in the treatment of intracapsular fractures of the hip. Am J Orthop, 2:161–164, 1960.

48. McElvenny RT: The importance of the lateral x-ray film in treating intracapsular fractures of the neck of the femur. Am J Orthop, 4:212–215, 1962.

49. McQuillan WM, Abernethy PJ, Guy JG: Subcapital fractures of the neck of the femur treated by double-divergent fixation. Br J Surg, 60:859–866, 1973.

50. Milgram JW: Orthopaedic management of Paget's disease of Bone. Clin Orthop, 127:63–69, 1977.

51. Moore AT: Fracture of the hip joint (intracapsular): a new method of skeletal fixation. J S Carolina Med Assoc, 30:199–205, 1934.

52. Moore AT: Fracture of the hip joint: a new method of treatment. Int Surg Digest, 19:323–330, 1935.

53. Moore AT: Fracture of the hip joint: treatment by extra-articular fixation with adjustable nails. Surg Gynecol Obstet, 64:420–436, 1937.

54. Moore AT: Metal hip joint: a new self-locking Vitallium prosthesis. South Med J, 45:1015–1019, 1952.

55. Moore AT: Hip joint fracture (a mechanical problem) AAOS Instructional Course Lectures, 10:35–49; 1953.

56. Moore AT: The self-locking metal hip prosthesis. J Bone Joint Surg, 39A:811–827, 1957.

57. Moore AT, Bohlman HR: Metal hip joint: a case report. J Bone Joint Surg, 25:688–692, 1943.

58. Moore RH, Premer RF, Gustilo RB: Femoral neck fractures. Minn Med, 56:358–362, 1973.

59. Murray JA, Parrish FF: Surgical management of secondary neoplastic fractures about the hip. Orthop Clin North Am, 5:887–901, 1974.

60. Nicholas JA, Killoran P: Fracture of the femur in patients with Paget's disease. J Bone Joint Surg, 47A:450–461, 1965.

61. Pare A: The work of that Famous Chirurgeon, Ambroise Pare. Translated out of Latin and Compared with the French by Tho. Johnson, Book XV. London, Cotes Young, 1634.

62. Pauwels F: Der Schenkenholsbruck, em mechanicishes Prob-

lem. Grundlagen des Heilungsvorganges. Prognoses fur Orthopaedische Chirurgie, Ferdinand Enke, 1935.

63. PHILLIPS GW: Fracture of the neck of the femur: treatment by means of extension with weights, applied in the direction of the axis of limb, and also laterally in axis of neck: recovery without shortening of other deformity. Am J Med Sci, 58:398–400, 1869.

64. ROTHERMEL JE, GARCIA A: Treatment of hip fractures in patients with Parkinson's syndrome on levodopa therapy. J Bone Joint Surg, 54A:1251–1254, 1972.

65. RYDELL N: Forces acting on the femoral head-prosthesis. Acta Orthop Scand (Suppl), 88:7–132, 1966.

66. RYDELL N: Biomechanics of the hip joint. Clin Orthop, 92:6–15, 1973.

67. SCHATZKER J, BARRINGTON TW: Fractures of the femoral neck associated with fractures of the same femoral shaft. Can J Surg, 11:297–305, 1968.

68. SCHATZKER J, HAERI GB: Methylmethacrylate as an adjunct in internal fixation of pathologic fractures. Can J Surg, 22:179–182, 1979.

69. SENN N: Fractures of the neck of the femur with special reference to bony union after intracapsular fracture. Trans Am Surg Assoc, 1:333–441, 1883.

70. SIM FH, DAUGHERTY TW, IVINS JC: The adjunctive use of methylmethacrylate in the fixation of pathological fractures. J Bone Joint Surg, 56A:40–48, 1974.

71. SINGH M, NAGRATH AR, MAINI PSL: Changes in the trabecular pattern of the upper end of the femur as an index of osteoporosis. J Bone Joint surg, 52A:457–467, 1970.

72. SISK TD: Fractures. *In* Edmonson AS Crenshaw AH (eds): Campbell's Operative Orthopaedics. St. Louis, Mosby, 1980.

73. SMITH-PETERSEN MN: Treatment of fractures of the neck of the femur by internal fixation. Surg Gynecol Obstet, 64:286–295, 1937.

74. SMITH-PETERSEN MN, CAVE EF, VAN GORDER GW: Intracapsular fractures of the neck of the femur. Arch Surg, 23:715–759, 1931.

75. SOTO-HALL R: Treatment of transcervical fractures complicated by certain common neurological conditions. AAOS Instructional Course Lectures, 17:117–120, 1960.

76. STAEHELI JW, FRASSICA FJ, SIM FH: Prosthetic replacement of the femoral head for fracture of the femoral neck in patients who have Parkinson disease. J Bone Joint Surg, 70A:565, 1988.

77. STAUFFER RN, SIM FH: Total hip arthroplasty in Paget's disease of the hip. J Bone Joint Surg, 58A:476–478, 1976.

78. SWIONTKOWSKI MF, WINQUIST RA, HANSEN ST JR.: Fractures of the femoral neck in patients between the ages of twelve and forty-nine years. J Bone Joint Surg, 66A:837, 1984.

79. SWIONTKOWSKI MF, HANSEN ST JR., KELLAM J: Ipsilateral fractures of the femoral neck and shaft: a treatment protocol. J Bone Joint Surg, 66A:260, 1984.

80. TELSON DR, RANSOHOFF NS: Treatment of fractured neck of the femur by axial fixation with steel wires. J Bone Joint Surg, 17:727–738, 1935.

81. TRONZO RG: Surgery of the Hip Joint. Philadelphia, Lea & Febiger, 1973.

82. TRUETA J, HARRISON MHM: The normal vascular anatomy of the femoral head in adult man. J Bone Joint Surg, 35B:442–461, 1953.

83. WARD FO: Human Anatomy. London, Renshaw, 1838.

84. WATSON JONES R: Fractures and Joint Injuries, 4th ed. Baltimore, Williams & Wilkins, 1955.

85. WEITBRECHT J: Syndesmologiasive Historia Ligamentorum Corporis Humani guain Secundum. Observationes Anatomicas Concinnavit et Figuris ad Objecta Reentia Adumbratis Illustravit. Petropoli, Typographia Academiae Scientiari, pp. 139–141, 1742.

86. WHITMAN R: A new method of treatment for fractures of the neck of the femur, together with remarks on coxa vara. Ann Surg, 36:746–761, 1902.

87. WHITMAN R: The abduction method considered as the exponent of a treatment for all forms of fracture at the hip in accord with surgical principles. Am J Surg, 21:335–344, 1933.

CHAPTER ELEVEN

Extracapsular Hip Fractures

JEFFERY L. STAMBOUGH

Introduction

Extracapsular or intertrochanteric (trochanteric) hip fractures are one of the most common orthopaedic problems that have significant ramifications on society and on patients' lives. Introchanteric hip fractures are estimated to occur at a rate of over 200,000 per year, costing over $10 billion dollars.[1,177] Intertrochanteric fractures increase in frequency with increasing age, but occur most often in the seventh decade of life and affect females 80% of the time. Furthermore, the morbidity and mortality from these fractures are significant (mortality rates are variable but about one to two in ten patients are dead one year post fracture). Prevention, the most effective treatment for this problem, remains a hope for the future, despite advances in geriatrics, metabolic bone disease, and nutrition. The goals for the management of patients suffering from these fractures is to provide the most effective and quickest care at the lowest cost to society.

Except in rare circumstances, the management of intertrochanteric hip fractures is surgical. The days of prolonged bed rest, casting, and traction have passed, giving way to a variety of internal fixation devices to stabilize the fracture and allow early mobilization and rehabilitation.

Historical Perspective

Ambrose Pare (1510–1590) is credited with the first recognition of a fracture of the proximal femur distinguishing it from a hip dislocation.[137,138] Since then, the management of proximal femoral fractures has evolved in an attempt to improve results and decrease morbidity and mortality. Initial work in the late 1800s concentrated on improving fracture healing. By the turn of the century, traction methods were the accepted treatment resulting in adequate fracture healing in the majority of cases. Closer observation showed significant morbidity and mortality from the prolonged recumbency.[2,3,33,121,217,223,234] Although open reduction

and internal fixation techniques had been attempted earlier, it was the improvement in metallurgy, implant strength, and host implant reaction that most significantly affected the acceptance of internal fixation. The modern era of open reduction and internal fixation was begun with Smith-Peterson's introduction of a solid, four-flanged nail for fixation of proximal femoral fractures in 1931.[12,236]

Multiple reports comparing operative and nonoperative treatment began to clearly show superiority of open reduction and internal fixation, not in fracture healing or related complications, but in reducing patient morbidity. Multiple concurrent and nonconcurrent reports, some randomized, but none double-blind, have continued to support the efficacy of operative treatment in intertrochanteric hip fractures.[6,12,38,39,57,136,140,154,161,170,228] Mortality, a multifactorial problem in this elderly population, has not been totally eliminated though, and still remains a problem. Once open reduction and internal fixation demonstrated superiority, attention turned to improving fixation techniques because operative failures were common with solid screw or nail devices. Initially, side plates were added to these rigid devices and subsequently led to the development of a rigid nail and side plate.[19,40,64,72,93,110,111,119,193,194,244,246] Although these new devices were much stronger and a significant improvement, failures were still noted. This led to the introduction of the collapsable screw and side plate systems, one of the first of which was introduced in Germany.[212] The compression hip screw systems allow a "self-seeking equilibrium" and have become the standard in operative intertrochanteric fixation in the United States.[37,146,147,187] Concurrently in Europe, flexible, intermedullary nails modeled after the Kunscher intermedullary rod were introduced for fixation of these fractures. European experience has been relatively positive with the Ender's device, a finding that has not been widely corroborated in studies from the United States.[32,135,176,189,241] Kaufer, Singh, Laros, and others have further stressed the importance of the quality of bone and not only the biomechanical properties of the implant as being important variables in fracture fixation.[115,116,130–132,218,243]

Contemporary advances have centered around rehabilitation and biomechanical analyses.[105,106,145,157,159] End results have been attributed more to functional status of the patients rather than the fractures alone. Biomechanical analyses have lent support for early ambulation and weight-bearing without the need for prolonged or even limited bedrest.

Anatomy

It is not pertinent to this discussion to review the anatomy of the hip in great detail because this exists in multiple surgical texts. Rather, a review of the basic features key to the fracture treatment and surgical exposure is presented.[84] Two surgical approaches are used: lateral and anterolateral. The lateral is the most commonly used with the anterolateral (Watson-Jones) used in certain difficult and unstable fracture patterns (Fig. 11–1).

The greater trochanter is the key to the surface anatomy of the proximal femur. The greater trochanter is easily palpable in most patients and lies just below a line between the anterior superior iliac spine and the ischial tuberosity (Nealton's Line) in the normal extended hip. This anatomic relationship may be distorted in the intertrochanteric hip fracture and the most effective way to localize the greater trochanter relationships is to use a radiopaque guide with the image intensifier at the time of surgery.

The osteology of the entire proximal femur is geometrically complex. The head and neck join the proximal femoral shaft at the intertrochanteric crest (posterior) and line (anterior). These areas interconnect the posterolaterally situated greater trochanter and the posteromedially situated lesser trochanter. In the lateral extended femur, the anterior cortex of the femoral shaft is continuous with the femoral neck, which deviates from the shaft at an angle of about 135° from the shaft in the anteroposterior (AP) plane and 14° of anteversion in the coronal plane.[237] This basic relationship is important because the center of the greater trochanter is not the center of the shaft. The greater trochanter connects to the lateral femoral shaft through a raised bony ridge called the trochanteric ridge. A line through the center of the head and neck segment passes below the greater trochanteric ridge by about 2 to 3 cm.[211] The head of the femur has an average radius of 5 cm. The average neck radius is 2.5 cm in the AP plane and 3 cm in the vertical plane. The average length, from the lateral shaft to the articular surface of the femoral head is 10 cm (100 mm).[238]

The internal bony anatomy of the proximal femur consists of thin trabeculae that form distinct patterns in the AP and lateral projections. The anatomy is clinically applicable in determining screw placement and holding power during compression hip screw placement (Fig. 11–2). In 1970, Singh, et al., described the AP trabeculation as it relates to age-related bone loss.[218] These thickened cancellous bony plates form tension and compression trabeculae in accordance with the stresses on the proximal femur (Wolff's Law). It is not absolutely predictive of fracture, but it does relate directly to the ability of internal fixation devices to hold in the femoral head and neck. In general, screws placed in the femoral head and neck should be in the lower and posterior quadrants (Fig. 11–2).[235]

In the lateral plane, thickened trabeculation forms the calcar femorale, which is primarily posterior, spanning the lesser trochanter from the poste-

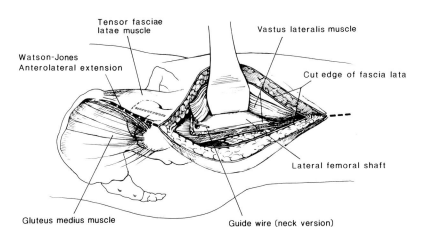

Tensor fasciae latae muscle

Vastus lateralis muscle

Watson-Jones Anterolateral extension

Cut edge of fascia lata

Lateral femoral shaft

Gluteus medius muscle

Guide wire (neck version)

Fɪɢ. 11–1. Surgical exposure. The lateral exposure to the femoral shaft usually allows adequate exposure to the fracture. The incision begins just below the greater trochanter and parallels the femoral shaft. The exposure may be enlarged by distal or proximal incisions. The vastus lateralis is elevated off the lateral femoral shaft and reflected anteriorly. A guide wire placed anteriorly along the femoral neck is a guide to the anteversion of the femoral head and neck.

Fig. **11–2.** Internal architecture of the proximal
femur. Left. The internal trabecular bone pattern is divided in compression and tension trabeculae; primary or secondary. They are progressively thinned and lost with osteoporosis
(disappear in order of numbers 1 to 6, sequentially). Right. The compression hip screw is best
placed inferiorly and slightly posteriorly in the
femoral head and neck to take advantage of the
stronger, more persistent primary compression
and tension trabecular.

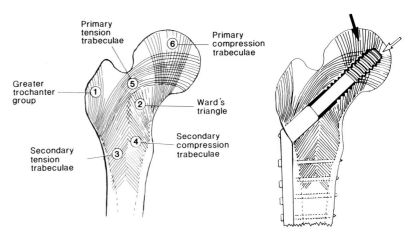

rior cortex of the neck to the posterior medial cortex of the femoral shaft. Other than the calcar
femorale, no specific trabeculation exists.[85] The
cancellous network is relatively uniform in the
femoral neck and head in this plane, making screw
and plate fixation straight down the middle or
slightly posterior, most acceptable.

The intertrochanteric line is defined as the line
interconnecting the two trochanteric prominences.
This line corresponds to the trochanteric crest posteriorly and the trochanteric line anteriorly. It is an
area of stress concentration because a rapid or sudden change in the shape produces a stress concentration and it is an area where the hip capsule and
muscles cross in their origin and insertions. Fractures which do not directly interconnect the two
trochanters but are near this are often referred to as
pertrochanteric fractures.

The blood supply to the femoral head and neck
comes from the medial femoral circumflex arteries
via the posterior and superior retinacular vessels
along the femoral neck (retinaculum of Weitbrecht).[35] At least 70% of patients derive their primary femoral head blood supply from these posterior vascular loops at the base of the neck. Care
should be taken to avoid this area during the surgical procedure. Posterior comminution of the fracture fragments may endanger these vessels, especially if overzealous reduction methods are used or
the superior and lateral retinacular vessels may be
injured by a poorly positioned screw.

The key to surgical approaches for extracapsular
hip fractures is the iliotibial band. This thickened
fibrous structure originates from the lateral iliac
crest and passes as a band, including the tensor fasciae latae muscle anteriorly, into the lateral proximal tibia at Gerty's tubercle. The iliotibial band encompasses the muscles of the proximal femur and
must be divided to gain access to the bony structures. The iliotibial band is thickest at the greater

trochanter where it covers the trochanteric bursa.
A straight lateral incision divides the iliotibial band
parallel to its fibers and makes repair easy.

The anterolateral approach divides the interval
between the tensor fasciae latae muscle and the
gluteus medius, dividing the iliotibial band slightly
posteriorly over the greater trochanter and then
along the middle of the femoral shaft laterally and
distally. The muscles protect the proximal femur
both as a covering, which has to be moved for adequate surgical exposure, and by dissipation of
forces, sparing the osseous structures. Once fracture has occurred, muscles provide tensile forces
that result in deformation of the lower extremity.
The anatomic axis of the hip to knee measures
about 7° valgus. Once fracture occurs in the proximal intertrochanteric region, the lower extremity
assumes a shortened and externally rotated position. The shortening is the direct result of muscle
shortening and the external rotation deformity is
caused by the pull of the adductor muscle group
(obturator nerve), which inserts posteriorly along
the linea aspera and loss of the abductor pull laterally. The pull of the iliopsoas, abductors, and vastus lateralis also contribute to the shortened and
externally rotated position.

The gluteus medius and minimus (superior gluteal nerve) originate from the lateral ilium and, in a
fan shaped manner, insert anterolaterally into the
greater trochanter. The gluteus medius is superficial to the minimus. The tensor fasciae latae muscle (superior gluteal nerve) is surrounded by the iliotibial band and originates from the ilium near the
anterior superior iliac spine. Innervation of these
muscles is posteriorly and near their origins.

The muscle inserts directly into the anterior portion of the iliotibial band. The iliopsoas muscle
(femoral nerve) inserts into the lesser trochanter
and is responsible for displacing this when the posterior medial cortex is fractured. The vastus later-

alis (femoral nerve) is a broad, thick muscle originating from the lateral proximal femur below the trochanteric ridge and inserting via the lateral retinaculum and quadriceps tendon into the patella. The muscle must be mobilized to gain access to the lateral femoral shaft. The vastus lateralis may be split parallel to the shaft or, more physiologically, reflected from the posterior shaft without denervating large portions of the muscle (1.5 cm from linea aspera).[171]

Biomechanics

Biomechanics of intertrochanteric hip fractures may be divided into three categories: (1) fracture production, (2) fracture fixation and stabilization, and (3) muscle and joint forces about the hip.

Intertrochanteric hip fractures are the result of direct and indirect forces involving the proximal femur. These extracapsular fractures are usually associated with a fall (direct force) but indirectly applied forces from surrounding muscles also play a definite role, although it is difficult to quantitate. A patient who falls from a standing height of 160 cm to 10 cm ground level generates a potential energy of 3700 kg/cm.[67,68] This is 40 times the energy needed to fracture the femoral neck. If this energy is not shared by the muscles and surrounding viscoelastic soft tissues, a fracture will inevitably occur. In many elderly people, the usual neuromuscular adaptations do not occur rapidly enough to protect the bone. This may be why fractures are increased in the elderly, especially patients with diabetes, cerebrovascular accidents, hemiplegia, or other diseases associated with neuromuscular disorders (Fig. 11–3).[44,149,167,197,215] For example, stroke patients preferentially suffer intertrochanteric hip fractures believed secondary to muscle weakness.[34]

Quality of bone is also an important factor.[60,129,153,243] It is generally accepted that over 65% of patients over the age of 60 and 90% of patients over the age of 70 will have some evidence of radiographic osteopenia. McLaughlin and Frankel have shown that osteopenic bone absorbs 25% less energy than younger bone.[151] This asymptomatic disease does not directly *cause* fracture, but it is a significant part of the equation, further predisposing the proximal femur to fracture because less energy can be absorbed by the bone prior to fracture (Fig. 11–3). Additionally, Niemann and Mankin have found about one-third of institutionalized patients with hip fractures also suffer from osteoma-

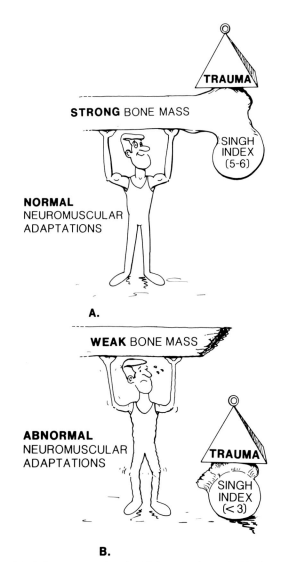

Fig. 11–3. Factors associated with intertrochanteric hip fracture. **A.** Decreased bone mass, altered neuromuscular adaptations, and trauma are factors relating to intertrochanteric hip fracture production. **B.** Alterations in any two of these significantly increases the patient's risk of fracture.

lacia, a metabolic bone disease that is correctible.[89,173] These considerations are all after the fact but become most important to the surgeon in regard to fracture stabilization.

The biomechanics of intertrochanteric hip fracture fixation has been extensively reviewed.[67,68,100,107,108,139] Early work has concentrated on the mechanical properties of the implant. With few exceptions, most implants are strong enough to withstand physiologic loads. Analyses do not take into account bone factors, which are equally critical in fracture fixation. Fracture fixation must resist varus and external rotation forces. Based on static moment analyses in the AP plane, intramedullary fixation is superior to the laterally placed rigid nail and side plates.

Compression hip screw devices have many advantages over intermedullary and rigid nail and side plate fixation systems. Gurtler, et al. showed in an in vitro unstable intertrochanteric hip cadaver model that compression hip screws were 2.5 times stiffer than Ender's nails and 3.5 times stiffer than the Harris condylocephallic nails.[75] When the compression hip screw failed, the device itself did not break, but the bone collapsed varusly. Furthermore, Jacobs has shown the compression hip screw acts as a tension band, converting tensile forces to compression forces related to the ability to slide laterally.[100] The lateral portion of the side plate is under a tensile force; the medial portion of the plate and medial cortex of the femur are under compression. The collapsibility or self-seeking equilibrium increases with increasing applied forces producing compression forces at the fracture site and shortening the AP moment arm. A further advantage is that it allows the screw to be inserted within .5 to 1 cm of subchondral bone, decreasing the chances of superior cutout.

Kyle, et al., have studied the sliding characteristics of the compression hip screw.[128] The coefficient of friction is similar, regardless of the material construction of the sliding hip screw, as long as the screw is adequately engaged within the barrel (more than 2 cm). Jamming of the construct was seen when inadequate engagement was present, especially at the 130 to 135° angles. Jenson, in a study of the yield point as a function of the angulation of the nail and metal composition, was unable to show significant advantages of stainless steel over cobalt-chromium-molybdium.[103] A 135° angled screw and side plate had a higher yield point than those at the 150° angle in their experiment. Static analyses of implant system failures show that most compression hip screw devices can withstand loads to failure in the range of 400 to 500 kg of force.[102,115,116] The telescoping screw and side plates are less stiff than the Holt rigid nail and side plate, but more stiff than the Jewett rigid nail and side plate, Ender's flexible intermedullary nails, and the Harris chondrocephallic intermedullary nail, respectively. Biomechanical and clinical studies have confirmed the superiority of this type of internal fixation in both stable and unstable intertrochanteric hip fractures.[98–100,102,105,159,227]

Fracture stability is defined as the ability of the proximal femur to withstand physiologic loads without fracture displacement, allowing for early weight-bearing and not resulting in late fracture failure. Fracture stability is judged clinically after closed reduction and depends on an intact column or cylinder of bone, especially in the medial and posteromedial cortices.[160] The proximal femur may be viewed as a two-column structure similar to the thoracolumbar spine. The lateral column consists of the greater trochanter and anterolateral proximal femur and is under tension. The medial column consists of the lesser trochanter and medial proximal femur and is under compression. The lateral column tensile loads have been estimated to be 900 pounds per square inch (psi) compared to compressive loads in the medial column of 1200 psi.[67,84] Unstable fractures of the intertrochanteric region usually comminute the medial cortices, giving way to a varus rotatory moment (this also relates to the anatomic versus mechanical axis). Whenever possible, anatomic reduction of the medial column is preferred.[49,127,188]

The application of static and dynamic analyses of the hip joint have applications to the postoperative care of these patients. Static, single leg analyses estimate joint reactive forces to be about 2.75 times body weight.[97] Dynamic analyses during gait estimate a much higher peak force (4 to 5 times body weight) especially during heel strike and toe off. Because our ultimate goal is to return the hip fracture patient to his premorbid activity and ambulation status, it might seem reasonable not to subject the recent hip fracture to these loads. In vivo studies using instrumented plates show that rising on and off of a bed pan, using the elbows, generates hip joint reactive forces approaching those of ambulation.[139] The use of a trapeze or other assistive devices reduces these forces slightly. On the other hand, in the horizontal position, the moments produced are half the moments compared to the upright position. Furthermore, forces can be reduced by the use of external assistive devices. It is well known that the proper use of a cane opposite to the symptomatic hip can decrease joint forces by 60%.[97] With this in mind, it seems preferable that the patient with an adequately fixed intertrochanteric hip fracture could be mobilized initially with assistance because the forces involved in mobilization are no greater than those associated with nursing activities. Clinical studies further support this approach.[103,191,195]

Patient Presentation and Evaluation

The typical intertrochanteric hip fracture patient presents to the emergency room after a fall. The patient, usually an elderly female, is transported by ambulance, because she usually has fallen at home or in an institutional facility. The details of this fall are often unclear, but the history of dizziness, syncope, or seizure may be obtained. A quick overview of the patient's lower extremity reveals the classic physical findings of a shortened and externally rotated leg, consistent with an extracapsular hip fracture.

The thigh is usually swollen and deformed and may even show signs of ecchymosis depending on the time from fracture to presentation in the emergency room. Movement of the leg to confirm the presence of a fracture is not only unkind, but may produce further comminution and should be avoided. The patient should be taken directly to x-ray for films of the involved hip as well as a routine chest x-ray, which inevitably is needed. The standard x-rays necessary to assess the intertrochanteric hip fracture are AP views of both hips and pelvis, and AP and true lateral views of the involved hip. The AP view of the pelvis is an important film to rule out any associated pelvic fractures and to allow assessment of true shortening, compared to the usually uninvolved side. The Singh index is best assessed from the uninjured side (15° internal rotation).[218] Once these elderly patients have fallen, associated fractures of the proximal humerus and distal radius should be looked for and radiographs obtained, if indicated.

Any patient who is suspected to have a serious medical illness should have a thorough evaluation by the internist or family physician. A thorough neurologic examination is essential because the patients often suffer from neuromuscular disorders. The neurovascular status of the injured leg should be carefully evaluated. It is rare to see a sciatic nerve palsy, but not uncommon to find the patient suffering from peripheral vascular occlusive disease. In one case when we placed the patient's foot in a foot holder on the fracture table, we observed that he had severe peripheral vascular occlusive disease with significant slough involving the entire dorsum of the foot. In these patients, it is preferable to place a distal femoral traction pin and to perform the surgery with skeletal traction. In addition, it is also important to look at the buttocks and sacral area for a decubitus ulcer.

The laboratory evaluation should include urinalysis, urine culture, and sensitivity (all patients should be suspected of a urinary tract infection until proven otherwise), renal profile, PT, PTT, CBC with differential and platelet counts, serum albumin, serum transfusion, and total protein. A 12-lead EKG should be standard. Special tests such as echocardiography are ordered as needed. An IV access line is started because most of these people are hypovolemic, either from not eating or secondary to blood loss. Consideration for nutritional support should also be given. Most of these patients have some clinical malnutrition that requires supplement, either by intravenous or alimental route.

If the patient is proceeding to the operating room within several hours, a single dose of cephalosporin should be given. If the patient will not have surgery for several days because of medical reasons, the patient's leg should be placed in traction, either Buck's extension traction or skeletal traction, depending on the surgeons preference.

Classification Schemes

Several classification schemes have been proposed for extracapsular hip fractures. The mere presence of multiple classifications indicates that clear method has been accepted to classify these common injuries. One such classification method simply divides trochanteric fractures by anatomic location into: (1) basal or basicervical, (2) intertrochanteric, (3) pertrochanteric, and (4) subtrochanteric.[101] Basicervical fractures are partially intracapsular but behave like intertrochanteric fractures. These are usually not comminuted and the oblique fracture line is just proximal to the intertrochanteric line. Intertrochanteric hip fractures are fractures that have a fracture line extending between the greater and lesser trochanters. These usually are simple fractures and have minimal to no comminution. The pertrochanteric fractures are usually designated as the fractures that have significant comminution of the intertrochanteric region, and at least part of the fracture line is an intertrochanteric type. There is usually significant posterior and posteromedial comminution. The subtrochanteric fractures begin at or below the lesser trochanter, involving the proximal 5 cm below the lesser trochanter of the proximal femur. These fractures may further be divided by the number of major fragments (e.g., four-part fracture). This fracture classification is descriptive and relates indirectly to treatment or prognosis.

Boyd and Griffin, reviewing 300 fractures at the Campbell Clinic, proposed a fracture classification of the intertrochanteric region into four types.[20] Type I is a linear fracture through the intertrochanteric region. Type II is a comminuted fracture through the same region. Type III is an intertrochanteric fracture with an associated subtrochanteric element. Type IV is an oblique fracture of the proximal portion of the femoral shaft involving the subtrochanteric region.

Tronzo proposed a five part classification based on fracture reduction.[219] The first type is an incomplete or nondisplaced intertrochanteric fracture. These are reduced with traction and anatomic reduction is easily achieved. A Type II fracture is a noncomminuted trochanteric fracture with or without significant displacement in which both trochanters are fractures. These two kinds of fractions are easily reduced by traction and anatomic reduction can be achieved. A Type III fracture is a comminuted fracture in which the lesser trochanteric piece is large. This kind of fracture is displaced by the iliopsoas pull, resulting in an unstable situation. The posterior wall is usually significantly comminuted with the beak of the inferior neck already displaced into the medullary fragment. A variant of the Type III involves complete fracture and separation of the greater trochanter. A Type IV fracture is a comminuted intertrochanteric fracture with disengagement of the two main fragments. Again, the posterior wall is significantly comminuted, but the spike of neck is displaced outside of or medial to the shaft, making reduction difficult. The Type V intertrochanteric fracture is the fracture associated with reverse obliquity of the fracture line. These are uncommon and significantly unstable. The fracture line starts in the posteromedial cortex and goes cephalad and laterally through the subtrochanteric region.

Ender divided these fractures into gaping and impacted types.[101] Rationale for this method is based on being able to achieve fracture stability by the use of flexible intermedullary nails.

Mueller divides intertrochanteric fractures into three groups (A, B, and C) based on fracture location and stability.[190] Type A are intertrochanteric with intact medial cortex, whereas Type B have comminution of the medial cortex. Type C are intertrochanteric with a subtrochanteric component (Gediz). This scheme is similar to the Boyd and Griffin classification.

The most widely used classification for intertrochanteric hip fractures is that proposed by Evans and confirmed by Jenson and Associates.[62,63,103–109] This system divides the intertrochanteric hip fractures into two types (Fig 11-4). Type I is a fracture with the primary fracture line extending into the intertrochanteric region. The Type II is a reverse obliquity or the Type V described by Tronzo.[219] The Type II or reverse obliquity fracture is uncommon and requires specific attention to restore stability. Evans' classification further divides the Type I fractures into two types, stable and unstable. It is this designation of stability that is most commonly used in discussions of surgical stabilization of intertrochanteric hip fractures. His classification of the Type I fracture into stable or unstable presumes that even if the fracture is comminuted, stability can be restored by the surgical procedure. Stable intertrochanteric hip fractures are easily treated by closed reduction through traction with internal fixation devices used to hold the fracture fragments in alignment until healing occurs.[140]

Unstable hip fractures are those involving significant medial and posteromedial cortex loss.[102] James and Hunter[101] have described five signs of instability. These are: (1) varus angulation with a vertical fracture line, (2) displaced lesser trochanter, (3) four-part fracture, (4) subtrochanteric extension, and, (5) absence of bone posteriorly (leg in internal rotation). If anatomic reduction cannot be achieved, these may require nonanatomic reduction, valgus osteotomy, medial displacement osteotomy, lateral displacement, varus reduction, or valgus reduction. Although fractures may be thought of in these groups, it is important to understand the "personality" of each individual's fracture pattern and adjust the treatment to achieve stability (intact medial column) accordingly.

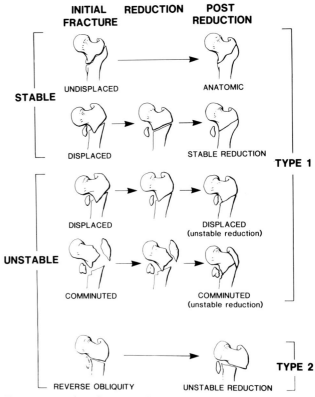

Fig. 11–4. Classification of intertrochanteric hip fractures. (Modified from Evans EM: The treatment of trochanteric fractures of the femur. J Bone Joint Surg 31B:190–203, 1949.)

Definitive Treatment

Decision making steps useful in intertrochanteric hip fracture management are several. The first issue is to determine whether the patient is a surgical candidate. These fractures require surgery to achieve and maintain fracture stability and reduce morbidity and mortality. On the other hand, not every patient with an intertrochanteric hip fracture is capable of undergoing surgery. Indications for nonoperative treatment are unclear. The majority of nonoperative treatments can be divided into two general categories. The first technique involves skillful neglect, allowing the fracture fragments to settle into a stable position in which healing can occur. This accepts a certain amount of varus deformity and shortening of the proximal femur. The second more popular applied nonoperative technique involves the use of traction.[178,214] This usually involves skeletal traction for 12 weeks, but a variety of other methods have been used. These require bedrest, although well leg traction, as described by Anderson, et al., and Childress, allow the patient to be mobilized.[2,3,33] If this method is to be applied, it is generally done so when the patient is not capable of undergoing operative stabilization. At the University of Cincinnati, this type of patient is most often a severely, multisystem injured patient with significant head injuries, who is not expected to survive. This patient usually is not capable of undergoing general or even spinal anesthesia. Occasionally, an elderly patient has such severe cardiovascular or pulmonary problems that anesthesia of any type cannot be undertaken safely. These situations are uncommon.

An intriguing but unproven alternative to bedrest and traction is external fixation. Anderson, et al., described a half pin frame using three Steinmann pins.[3] Clinical followup was lacking, but the technique allows bed to chair transfers. Gotfried, et al., reported 65 intertrochanteric fracture patients, 81% over the age of 80 years, who were treated with an AO external fixator.[74] This allowed immediate full weight bearing and was removed at 4.5 months. Mortality at 6 months was 36% and pin tract infections were the most common hardware related complication.

Because surgery is the treatment of choice, the issue of *when* to operate is important. It is a generally applied axiom that patients are in no better physical or nutritional health than when they first arrive in the emergency room. This principle has been applied to the polytraumatized younger patient. When dealing with the septagenerian and oc-

tagenarian population with intertrochanteric hip fractures, this is not always the case. Several authors have implied that these patients should be operated on immediately, whereas other authors have supported a careful medical workup and stabilization prior to surgery.[120,152,168] It has been the principle at the University of Cincinnati to operate on these patients as emergent or urgent cases when their medical status will allow. These patients are seen in the emergency room and prepared for surgery and are usually operated on within 6 to 12 hours after their presentation to the hospital. If there are extenuating medical circumstances, such as an unresolved heart condition, history of syncope with loss of consciousness necessitating a neurologic evaluation and CT scan, or other similar serious situations, surgery is postponed awaiting resolution. Once the patient's medical status has been cleared, the patient is operated on at the earliest convenient time.

The most appropriate type of anesthesia is controversial. McLaren, et al., reviewed a series of 75 patients treated in a prospective randomized but not double-blinded study.[150] Either general or spinal anesthesia was randomized. The average age of these patients was 75 years. The two groups were comparable in age, sex, hemoglobin, previous ambulatory status, and blood urea nitrogen (BUN). Surprisingly, they found a tenfold increase in mortality comparing general to spinal anesthesia. This work requires corroboration, but it suggests that preferentially, patients undergoing hip fracture treatment should be given spinal anesthesia. They hypothesized the cause of the increase in mortality to be pulmonary in origin (pulmonary embolus or bronchopneumonia). Other studies have found no correlation with results to type of anesthesia.[58] Although controversial at one time, the use of perioperative prophylactic antibiotics is well accepted. Burnett, et al., Boyd, et al., and Tengve and Kjellandr have published a series supporting the use of perioperative antibiotics.[22,24,233] Burnett, et al., reviewed 307 cases of fractures of the proximal femur who were given antibiotics in a double-blind, randomized fashion. The regimen consisted of preoperative antibiotics followed by 72 hours of postoperative IV first generation cephalosporin treatment. The cephalosporin treated group had a reduction in their wound infection rate, from 4.7% to 0.7%, which was statistically significant. There was, however, a strong trend toward colonization of cephalosporan resistant organisims. Tengve and Kjellandr studied 140 patients treated with a regimen of perioperative antibiotics followed by 48 hours postoperative treatment. Again, they used a first generation cephalosporin and found an 8-fold decrease in infection rate. Boyd, et al., also confirmed a decrease from 4.8% to 0.8% wound infection with prophylactic antibiotics. These studies support the use of first generation cephalosporins as a prophylaxis in the hip fracture patient. The duration of therapy may be somewhat controversial, but preoperative antibiotics followed by 24 to 48 hours of postoperative antibiotics is the standard. It may be that the colonization seen in the Burnett, et al., study was caused by the use of these antibiotics for 72 hours.

Hip fracture patients are commonly believed to be at risk for thromboembolism and pulmonary embolism. Prophylactic treatment is controversial.[17,47,69,83,158,162,185,202,230] Although several medications have been suggested, early mobilization is perhaps the best and most physiologic means of treatment. Risks and benefits of other prophylactic agents must be weighed in this predominantly elderly female population. Low doses of warfarin are effective in preventing pulmonary embolism, but wound problems are increased. On the other hand, aspirin has a low complication rate but reports on the efficacy of aspirin are conflicting. One randomized double-blind study found significant protective effect in patients with hip fractures of both sexes.[220] Controls experienced 60% deep vein thrombosis and 44% pulmonary embolism rates. The aspirin treated patients experienced only 26% deep vein thrombosis and 2% pulmonary embolism. We routinely use early mobilization and aspirin or coumarin combined with compression boots about the calves in our hip fracture patients.

The goal of operative treatment is to internally stabilize and reduce the fracture fragments. Kaufer, et al., emphasized that the strength of the fracture fixation system is determined by five variables: (1) bone quality, (2) fracture geometry, (3) reduction, (4) implant design, and (5) implant placement.[115] Laros refers to the first two factors as intrinsic because they are beyond the control of the surgeon.[132] The remaining three factors (extrinsic) can, at least in part, be controlled.

The contralateral proximal femur as seen in the preoperative AP view of both hips and pelvis should be quantitated by the Singh index.[218] When severe osteoporosis (Singh index of 3 or less) is noted, supplemental polymethyl methacrylate should be considered.[13,79,80,81,165] The technique for insertion of the polymethyl methacrylate has been described in detail by Laros.[13] Once the femoral head and neck segment have been reamed with the step cutting reamer, the cancellous portion in the

head and neck should be enlarged with a currette. The preassembled screw and side plate should then be inserted to confirm that it can be inserted with ease. Cement is then prepared in an injection gun and is slowly layered in the area in which the screw threads will be located. Care is taken not to inject the cement under pressure, nor to inject cement in such a way that once it hardens it will prevent sliding of the screw within the side plate barrel (Fig. 11–5).

The use of a fracture table has become commonplace. A wide variety of fracture table types are available. The table should include several features. It should have radiolucent peroneal post on which traction can be applied to the injured leg and variable positioning of the leg should be available. It is preferable if the extended leg can be held in a foot holder, but skeletal traction should also be available. The table should also allow biplanar image intensification so that the injured leg can be sterilely prepared and draped.

Fracture position has been somewhat controversial. The most common position is to treat the intertrochanteric hip fracture with the patient in the

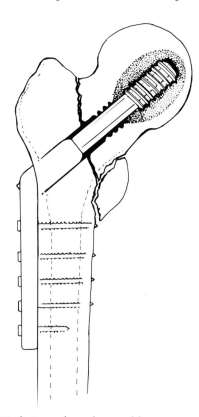

Fig. 11–5. Technique of supplemental bone cement fixation. In advanced osteopenia, the addition of polymethyl methacrylate (PMMA) around the screw threads helps increase purchase, decrease superior cut-out, and improve stability. Care should be taken not to allow the PMMA to cross the fracture site nor impede sliding of the screw in the barrel.

supine position. Several authors have discussed positioning the patient for intertrochanteric treatment in the lateral decubitus.[48] The injured leg is draped free and the surgical approach is similar. If this method is chosen, care should be taken to avoid varus positioning of the fracture.

The internal fixation of stable intertrochanteric hip fractures is well established.[50,174,175] A wide variety of fracture fixation alternatives are available. These divide into screw and side plate devices or intermedullary devices. The screw and side plate devices may be subdivided into telescoping and rigid types. Rigid devices largely have been abandoned because of their high complication rates. The compression hip screw systems are the most commonly used in the United States today. These can further be divided into those which are keyed and nonkeyed.[4] There is no strong evidence supporting the use of one of these types over another. At the University of Cincinnati, the dynamic hipsaw (DNS) hip system produced by the Swiss AO group is used in the majority of intertrochanteric hip fractures.[190]

Fracture treatment alternatives also includes intermedullary devices.[5,59,78,126,179,240] Intermedullary devices are divided into two groups, those that include flexible intermedullary nails and those with a condylocephalic nail.[82] The efficacy for intermedullary devices in stable hip fracture is numerous, but the results in unstable hip fractures have been less satisfactory. The European experience has not been duplicated in the United States, and most authors who have attempted prospective comparative series with compression hip screw devices with flexible intermedullary nails in unstable hip fractures have clearly shown a superiority of the compression hip screw. Therefore, the use of flexible intermedullary nails should be reserved for patients with stable intertrochanteric hip fractures for whom the benefits of the operative technique of short operative times, limited blood loss, and limited exposure are necessary. The operative technique has been reviewed in detail by several authors.

Other adjunctive internal fixation methods should be kept in mind for fixation and added stability of intertrochanteric hip fractures. In the basicervical type of intertrochanteric fractures, a superiorly placed cannulated screw or AO/ASIF cancellous screw adds rotational stability.[49] In unstable fractures that involve a large posteromedial lesser trochanteric fragment may benefit from additional screw placement to internally fix this fragment.[112,125] This may be done either through the plate, or independently of it. This requires a long

cortical screw. Finally, in unstable fractures requiring medial displacement osteotomy, it is often advantageous to have additional length to the side plate. An addition of two to four holes often increases the purchase and provides added stability. A long side plate is also indicated in intertrochanteric fractures with subtrochanteric extension.

Transiliac bone biopsy may be useful in all intertrochanteric hip fractures to: (1) differentiate osteoporosis, hyperostoidosis, and osteomalacia, (2) to qualitatively judge bone activity in order to guide postoperative treatment, and (3) to qualitatively judge the severity of the osteopenia. Ideally, double pulse tetracycline labeling would be preferred but cannot be used in these acute injuries. If surgery is delayed for several days, a single dose of tetracycline may be useful. This would consist of demeclocycline, 150 mg orally 3 times daily for a total of 3 days. The postoperative treatment should be directed at the underlying disease after 25 hydroxy vitamin D levels, thyroid function tests, and serum protein electrophoresis (SPEP). Techniques for bone biopsy have been reveiwed by Hodgson, et al.[88] Transiliac bone biopsy can be performed through the same position and same surgical preparation as the surgical procedure for internal fixation of the intertrochanteric hip fracture. A point 1 cm below and posterior to the anterior superior iliac spine is identified. The skin over this area is incised and soft tissue dissection is continued down to the outer cortex of the ilium. Using a biopsy trefine set, a tricortical bone graft is obtained (Fig. 11-6). Care must be taken in the severely osteopenic patient not to push the trefine but rather allow it to cut its way through the bone. This specimen should be sent for undecalcified analysis in 70% cthanol.

Operative Technique (Stable Fractures)

The patient is positioned supine on the fracture table.[190] Closed reduction is performed under image intensification. Reduction can usually be achieved by gentle longitudinal traction with the leg in 10 to 20° of abduction. The reduction maneuver is then completed by slight internal rotation and occasionally requires some flexion of the knee. May and Chacha have identified characteristics of the fracture pattern that influence reduction.[101] When significant posterior cortical loss exists in the proximal femur with separation of the greater trochanter fragment, reduction and fixation of the distal fragment in slight external rotation may be necessary.

The involved extremity is then draped freely to

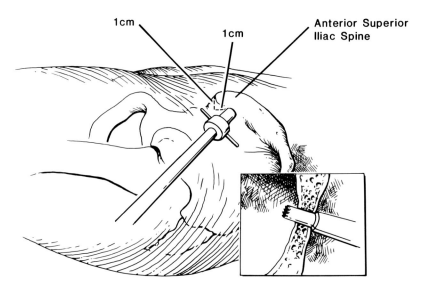

Fɪɢ. 11–6. Technique of transiliac bone biopsy. (Modified from Hodgson SF, et. al: Out-patient percutaneous biopsy of the iliac crest. Mayo Clin Proc, 61:28–33, 1986.)

allow easy biplanar image intensification. Exposure is accomplished through the anterior or anterolateral approach as discussed in the section on anatomy. A solid Kirschner wire is slid over the front of the femoral neck to identify the appropriate anteversion. The appropriate angled guide with T-handle is positioned along the lateral cortex (135° is most common). The point of introduction of the guide wire is determined by the position of the lesser trochanter or other landmarks. The level varies with the angle of the plate to be used, in the majority of cases the 135° plate is used, allowing the guide wire to be introduced about 2 to 3 cm below the trochanteric ridge. The angle guide is placed along the middle of the femoral shaft with the guide pointing to the center of the femoral head. The lateral cortex is opened with a 3.5 mm drill and the guide wire is inserted into the center of the femoral head at the level of the subchondral bone. The exact placement of the guide pin into the center of the head is the most important step in the surgical procedure. The pin must remain in place throughout the procedure. The guide pin must be in the center of the femoral head and neck or in the posterior and inferior quadrants. The guide wire position should be checked radiographically in both AP and lateral views. The tip of the guide wire must lie just short of the joint space to allow the correct position.

The length of the inserted guide pin is now measured. The DHS direct measuring device is slipped onto the guide pin and the length of the pin inserted into the proximal femur is read directly. The drill hole should end 10 mm short of the joint surface. To obtain this, subtract 10 mm from the reading and set the reamer to the correct depth. The depth of the DHS reamer may be adjusted in 5 mm

increments. When the different portions of the reamer enter the lateral cortex, the pressure exerted on the reamer should be diminished in order to avoid damage to the bone. This is particularly important when the entry point is close to the fracture.

For extremely hard cancellous bone, as encountered in young patients, the threads of the lag screw should be tapped using the shorter of the two centering sleeves. In osteoporotic bone, the screw is inserted as far as the 5 mm mark (the lag screw cutting itself at the last 5 mm of the thread). In hard bone, the screw is inserted as far as the zero mark on the wrench.

The DHS coupling screw is inserted into the hollow DHS shaft. The screw male thread is inserted into the female thread of the lag screw. The ridge and slot between the guide shaft and the lag screw must interdigitate. Slide the longer of the two centering screws over the DHS wrench. Glide the DHS wrench over the guide shaft-lag screw assembly and slip the centering sleeve over the guide wire into the bore hole. Insert the lag screw by turning the hand clockwise and exerting gentle pressure. If too much force is needed to introduce the screw, it is safer to check the position of the device with the image intensifier or back it out and use a tap first. The lag screw is inserted to the zero mark on the DHS wrench, reaches the lateral cortex, and remains 10 mm short of the joint line. The handle of the wrench must be placed parallel to the shaft of the femur before it is moved together with the centering piece. After removal of the wrench, the appropriate DHS plate is slid onto the assembly, the coupling screw is loosened and the guide shaft and guide pin are removed. The plate should be gently seated with the impactor. The 5-hole DHS plate is

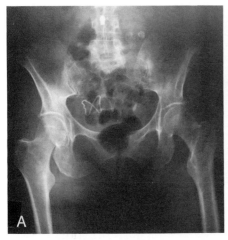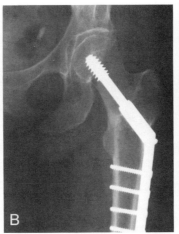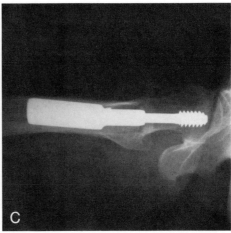

Fɪɢ. **11–7.** Nondisplaced, stable intertrochanteric hip fracture. **A.** A nondisplaced left intertrochanteric fracture in a healthy, 63-year-old professor with a Singh index of 5–6. **B.** Anteroposterior. **C.** Lateral. The stable fracture was easily reduced and stabilized with a DHS hip screw. Note the position of the hip compression screw in the inferior and posterior quadrants of the femoral head and neck.

fixed to the femur with 4.5 mm AO/ASIF cortical screws. The dynamic compression plate (DCP) neutral drill guide, 3.2 mm bit, and standard AO/ASIF technique should be used for insertion of the screws. A final impact on the fracture can be achieved with the DHS compression screw (Fig. 11–7).

In osteoporotic bone, the compression screw must be tightened carefully to avoid stripping of the thread of the DHS lag screw. Manual impaction of the fracture after the side plate has been attached to the shaft and impaction by early weight-bearing are probably much more effective than impaction with a compression screw. The compression screw should not be removed (Fig. 11–8).

Wound closure is then accomplished in layers. It is important to debride any nonviable muscle be-

cause it serves as a pabulum for infection. Suture closure of the vastus lateralis is recommended to obliterate dead space. Closed system drainage is used both deep and superficial to the iliotibial band. Subcutaneous layers should be carefully approximated with resorbable suture and skin approximation is usually accomplished with skin staples. A sterile dressing is applied with the drainage tubes directed distally to avoid the patient pulling these out inadvertently. The extremity is wrapped in a compressive dressing (Fig. 11–9).

Operative Technique (Unstable Fracture)

Unstable intertrochanteric hip fractures are defined as hip fractures in which the medial column

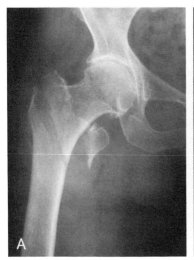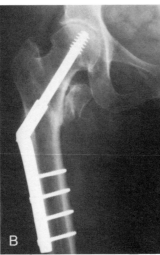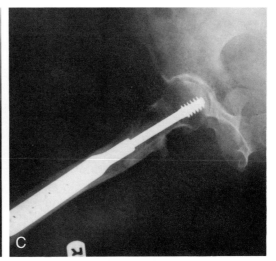

Fɪɢ. **11–8.** Displaced, stable intertrochanteric hip fracture. **A.** A displaced minimal comminuted three-part right intertrochanteric hip fracture in a 72-year-old nursing home patient. **B.** Anteroposterior. **C.** Lateral. The fracture was reduced and stabilized without reducing the avulsed lesser trochanter. The medial column was restored despite a nonanatomic position of the lesser trochanter.

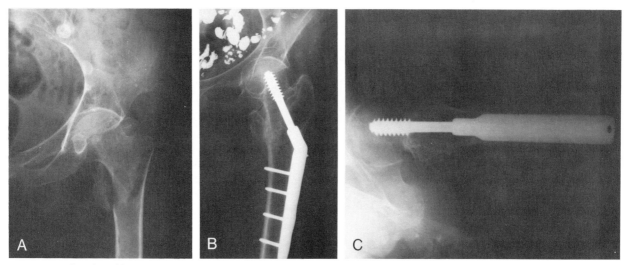

Fig. 11–9. Displaced, stable intertrochanteric hip fracture. **A.** A displaced, three-part intertrochanteric hip fracture in a 78-year-old retired school teacher. **B.** Anteroposterior. **C.** Lateral. The fracture was reduced and stabilized with a valgus reduction (150° side plate) and the displaced posteromedial fragment also went on to heal in a near-anatomic position.

stability cannot be restored by reduction technique. These fractures often require specific treatment techniques for a nonanatomic reduction.[45] Three such techniques are applicable in the management of unstable hip fractures. The goal is to restore medial column stability, which is accomplished in different ways in each technique. Sarmiento has popularized a valgus osteotomy.[141,164,204–207] The Wayne County reduction lateralizes the femoral shaft in relation to the head and neck segment, allowing for medial contact between the femoral head and neck segment and the medial cortex of the proximal femur.[51,207] The last method is that popularized by Dimon and Hughston and was first described by Aufranc and Lowell.[51,52] The Sarmiento valgus osteotomy and Wayne County reduction will not be discussed in detail here because they have been infrequently utilized at our institution. The Sarmiento technique is demanding and should be carefully studied before it is attempted.

Medial displacement osteotomy is indicated when anatomic reduction cannot be achieved. Kyle, et al., in reviewing 623 intertrochanteric hip fractures from Hennepin County found 96% satisfactory results with anatomic reduction in both stable and unstable hip fractures.[127] Others have observed that these intertrochanteric hip fractures tend to perform medial displacement osteotomy if one simply attempts as near an anatomic reduction as possible and allows for the compression screw device to collapse.

Many studies address the issue of medial displacement osteotomy.[51,52,91,94,96,123,222] This technique displaces the femoral shaft medially, allowing the head and neck fragment to settle within the proximal femoral medullary cavity. This provides both a lateral buttress as well as medial support for the proximal fragment. Dimon has reviewed the technical aspects in detail and only the highlights are discussed here.[51,52,94] The operative setup and approach are not significantly different from that of the treatment previously discussed for stable intertrochanteric hip fractures. Once the exposure has been completed, the first step in this technique is to perform or complete a trochanteric osteotomy. This allows one to visualize the proximal head and neck segment directly. A threaded Steinmann pin is then inserted superiorly in the head and neck segment to allow for control. A short compression screw measuring 4 to 5 cm is then inserted inferiorly and posteriorly in the head and neck segment (Fig. 11-10). The proximal femur is identified and a curette is used to open the medullary canal and to confirm that no significant medial fragmentation exists. The proximal femoral head and neck segment is then settled into the medullary cavity of the proximal femur. The side plate is attached to the compression screw and clamped to the femoral cortex. Traction is then released. Eccentrically drilling the holes in the side plate allows compression between the proximal fragment and the femoral shaft. One should not compress the fracture by tightening the compression screws because this tends to laterally displace the fracture rather than compress the osteotomy site (Fig. 11-11). Great care must be taken prior to attaching the plate to the femur to correct rotation. Neutral version should be the goal with the knee in slight internal rotation

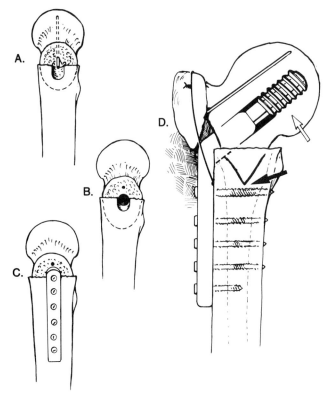

Fig. 11–10. Technique of medial displacement osteotomy. (Modified from Laskin, et.al: Intertrochanteric fractures of the hip in the elderly. Clin Orthop, 141:188–195, 1979.) **A.** The proximal fracture fragment in placed in the femoral canal. A superiorly placed Steinmann Pin helps in guiding the reduction. **B.** Traction is released to impact the two fragments. **C.** A short compression screw (open arrow) and long side plate are assembled. **D.** The side plate holes are drilled eccentrically to allow further compression. Care is taken not to allow the most proximal screw in the side plate from preventing impaction of the proximal fragment within the femoral canal (closed arrow). The greater trochanter may be reattached using a wire.

(10 to 15°). Alignment should be carefully confirmed by the image intensifier. The 135° side plate is usually adequate and results in a slight valgus reduction at the osteotomy site. A 5-hole DHS plate with a short barrel is a minimum. Occasionally, a long length side plate is required. The trochanter can be reapproximated and held with a separate 18-gauge stainless steel wire.

Post Operative Rehabilitation

Post operative rehabilitation of the intertrochanteric hip fracture must be individualized.[14,18,92,122,229] The goals of this program are not only to mobilize the patient, but also to return the patient to as near normal lifestyle as possible. Multiple variables must be considered in the postoperative rehabilitation of these patients. These factors include the patient's age, associated medical conditions, premorbid activity level, the presence of mental status changes, and the stability of the fracture and internal fixation. The ability to return the patient to his home with a good support system is an important prognostic factor in overall recovery.

Almost all hip fracture patients can be mobilized from bed to chair on the first postoperative day. From this, the patient should undergo a graduated weight-bearing program based on factors previously discussed. External supportive devices should start with parallel bars and a walker and advance as tolerated. All patients should be started with partial weight-bearing since nonweight-bearing is usually not possible in these fragile patients. Slight elevation of the contralateral leg with a half-inch, in-the-shoe lift often helps to achieve this goal. The speed of ambulation should be started at about 25% of normal and then advanced, as the patient tolerates, by increments of 25%. Most patients should also be instructed in transfer using the contralateral leg as a pivot point. A transfer platform may also help. Even in the debilitated patient or nonambulator, the patient may be able to perform only assisted transfer, but even in this case, bed to chair transfer should be encouraged to decrease the morbidity related with bedrest. These patients also benefit from a mobile lounge-type chair.

The initial exercise program should include isometric exercises of the involved extremity, pulmonary toilet, active range of motion and strengthening exercises of upper extremities, bed mobility exercises, and active assisted range of motion exercises. Upper extremity rehabilitation is important so that transfer ability can be maximized. The extent of involvement of each patient depends mostly on the patient's postoperative mental status and cognitive base line. More independent active range of motion should be advanced during the second and third weeks, depending on the fracture stability. With all other factors being equal, ambulation may be advanced as dictated by cardiovascular factors. Ambulation on stairs is the most difficult postoperative function to recapture and should be the last goal in the rehabilitation program.

The endpoint of rehabilitation is individually specific. The final results should maximize the post operative recovery and return the patient as near as possible to his preoperative functional and ambulatory levels. Finally, it must always be kept in mind that the ability to return the patient to his preoperative environment as soon as possible is a crucial factor and the continuation of a rehabilitation program in this environment is also preferred.[29,30]

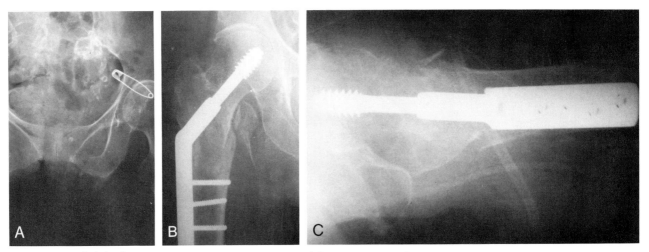

Fɪɢ. 11–11. Medial displacement osteotomy. **A.** A comminuted four-part intertrochanteric fracture in an osteopenic stroke patient (Singh index <3). **B.** Anteroposterior. **C.** Lateral. An anatomic reduction was not possible. A medial displacement osteotomy was performed.

Results

This chapter has primarily addressed the management of intertrochanteric hip fractures. Unfortunately, the end results are not solely related to the fracture, its fixation, or its ultimate healing. Rather, end results are most closely related to concomitant illness and the patient's functional status.[27,41,155] Patients with few concurrent illnesses, normal cardiovascular and pulmonary systems, normal mental status, stable fracture patterns, good bone quality, admission from home with the ability to return there, and no postoperative complications are the best prognostic indicators. The more of these factors that are absent, the less satisfactory the end result may be.

Although not a primary factor, failure of the fracture treatment will compromise the final result. Results of fracture treatment depend on the stability of the intertrochanteric hip fracture and are specific to the device used to stabilize the fracture.[28,129] In all comparative analyses, the compression hip screw has provided superior results[53,54,58,61,76,86,93,99,107,133,166,182,201,216,225,248,253] Stable fracture patterns are usually associated with better results when compared with unstable fractures. These stable fractures can be fixed with any of the available devices and good results as far as fracture healing and position can be expected. This is not the case with the unstable fracture, which has a higher complication rate and poorer end results.

The reasons for this are partly related to the fracture pattern which is also highly associated with increasing severity of osteopenia and more concurrent illnesses.

The ultimate goal of internal fixation of intertrochanteric hip fractures is a stable union and acceptable alignment. These fractures are clinically united in about 3 months in most cases, excluding associated problems known to alter fracture healing (e.g., Paget's Disease).[56] Fracture healing in this anatomic area proceeds by periosteal and endosteal callus formation.[84] Healing problems are usually related to distraction at the fracture site.

Percentages of satisfactory results have been variable in the reported series.[101] These results seem to be most influenced by the particulars of each patient cohort, which is difficult to compare from series to series. Considering only instrumentation problems by the type of internal fixation, the results also are variable. For example, instrumentation failure rates with the Jewett nail range from 4 to 9% in stable fractures and from 28 to 53% in unstable fractures. Complication rates of Ender's nailing have ranged from 1 to 64%. Results of compression hip screws have shown fixation failures in 2 to 9% of stable fractures and 5 to 21% of unstable fractures with anatomic reductions. Medial displacement osteotomy results have decreased complications in unstable fractures from 51 to 8% in one study.

Satisfactory healing of intertrochanteric hip fractures can be expected in approximately 95% of cases.[58,166] Internal fixation failures including nonunion and malunion are related in part to the fracture pattern as well as to the type of internal fixation device used. Fixation complications are higher in all series reported in unstable fractures and can be minimized in those situations in which anatomic reduction is not possible by performing a nonanatomic reduction. Morbidity and mortality rates continue to be high and have not been eliminated by internal fixation alone.[46]

Complications of Treatment

Complications of treatment of intertrochanteric hip fractures fall into two general categories: (1) patient-related complications, and (2) technical-related complications. Patient complications are patient-related problems such as wound infection, deep vein thrombosis, pulmonary embolus, decubitus, and urinary tract infection. Technical-related complications are problems related to the improper application of the surgical device.

Patient complications include morbidity and mortality. Most common morbidity includes infection, deep vein thrombosis, urinary tract infection, skin ulcers, and a multitude of possible medical complications from myocardial infarction to postoperative confusion.[70,198,210]

Mortality rates vary widely depending in part on the length of followup. Nonoperative mortality rates can approach 33%.[64,242] Intraoperative mortality is rare, but perioperative mortality occurs in from 10 to 20% of patients.[66,114,120] If the patient survives 6 months or more, the mortality rates generally equal age and sex match controls. Overall mortality is only about 6 to 7% higher when these factors are controlled.[73]

Infection rates ranging from 2 to 16% have been reported. Deep infection increases mortality.[11,173,133] Barr has divided infections into three catagories.[11] The first category of early superficial infections are primarily related to hematoma formation. The second category is early deep infections. The third category is late deep infections with or without joint involvement. Joint involvement is much less common in intertrochanteric hip fractures. The most common organism isolated in all series has been gram positive staphylococci, but bowel and bladder flora also have been found, especially in early superficial and deep infected cases. The causes of wound sepsis are multiple, but should be suspected in the patient with persistent hip pain, wound drainage, elevated sedimentation rate, and resistance to motion because of pain. Treatment consists of debridement, culture and sensitivity tests, organism-specific antibiotics, and delayed wound closure. Removal of the implant is indicated only in cases of late sepsis when the fracture healing is complete. For cases with extensive involvement of the hip joint, a Girdlestone may be considered as a salvage procedure.

Other patient-related complications have a variable incidence usually occurring in less than 5% of patients. These include skin sloughs over the dorsum of the foot, gangrene of the lower extremities caused by peripheral vascular occlusive disease, and pudendal nerve palsies caused by excessive traction over the perineal post.[90]

Technical complications have fortunately been rare. Several device-related complications have been reported, these include screw dislodgement from the barrel,[25,57,143] cutout of the implant superiorly (Fig. 11-12),[77] protrusion of the compression screw through the acetabulum,[113] vascular injuries secondary to excessive length and drilling of the screws for the side plate.[186] One case of peritonitis secondary to penetration of the guidewire has been reported.[49] Another case of vascular injury caused by a fracture fragment of the intertrochanteric hip fracture also has been reported.[221] Avascular necrosis is rare, but also has been reported after intertrochanteric hip fractures.[118,142] The cause for this remains unclear. Subcapital hip fractures have been identified more often in cases of rigid nail placement in which the nail stops in the neck region.[8,26,247] This produces a stress riser, predisposing the patient to subcapital hip fractures. Fracture malrotation also is a problem in comminuted frac-

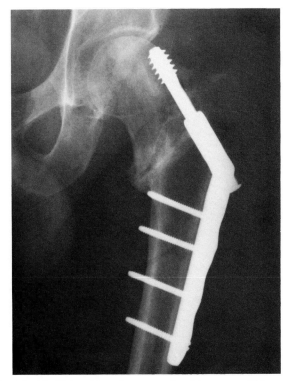

Fig. 11-12. Malpositioned compression hip screw. This compression hip screw was short and despite its superior and anterior cut-out fracture healing occurred.

tures. This generally results in an external rotation deformity that can be dramatic. Finally, fracture of the implant generally is associated with nonunion.[77] Bending of the implant suggests impending fracture failure and, because the majority of the load is being borne by the implant, resulting plastic deformation.

Special Considerations
Pathologic Fractures

Pathologic intertrochanteric hip fractures are most often caused by advanced osteopenia that has been addressed previously (Fig. 11–13). Metastatic carcinoma is the next most common causal factor with breast metastases being most frequent.[15] The indications for surgery in pathologic fractures are primarily for pain. The surgery is performed for quality of life, not quantity of life. Multiple studies have shown the efficacy of open reduction and internal fixation and radiation treatment in providing pain relief and improved function for these patients.[169,171] The use of supplemental polymethyl methacrylate has greatly enhanced the immediate stability. Because life expectancy is generally low, long-term failure has not been a clinical problem[13,43,55,79,80,81,144,156,181]

The indications for prophylactic fixation of impending pathologic fractures of the intertrochanteric region are similar to those in other long bones.[23,79,80,81,87,109,117] These indications include: (1) lesions that are painful after chemotherapy or radiotherapy, (2) lesions involving 50% or more of the cortex, (3) patients with life expectancy over 3 to 6 months, (4) lesions that are not responsive to chemotherapy or radiation therapy, producing significant pain, and (5) lack of a specific histologic diagnosis.

The application of the compression hip screw apparatus or other internal fixation is not different in these prophylactic circumstances, rather, the pathologic lesion is thoroughly curetted and the defect is then filled with polymethyl methacrylate.[13] It is important to delay the setting time of the polymethyl methacrylate and to insert it in a doughy state to prevent interposition of the polymethyl methacrylate in bony fragments risking delayed fracture healing.[134] This is most applicable to the completed fracture situation. If the medial cortex is destroyed or significant subtrochanteric extension has occurred, a cemented Zickel, reconstruction nail or endoprosthesis is a better alternative.[203,252] Radiographs of the entire femur are recommended before surgery to exclude synchronous bony metastases.

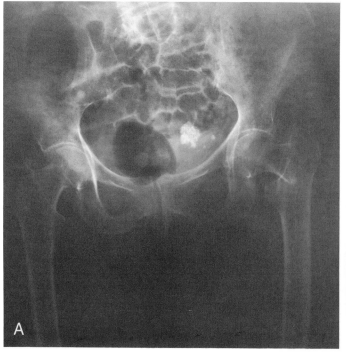 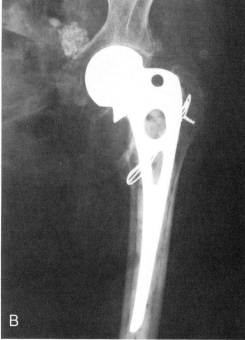

Fɪɢ. 11–13. Pathologic intertrochanteric hip fracture. **A.** A right pathologic fracture on an asthenic 95-year-old retired nurse with a history of rectal carcinoma. **B.** Because of her severe osteopenia, advanced age, and ambulation status, a cemented endoprosthesis with bone graft from fractured head and neck was performed.

Ipsilateral Femoral Shaft and Intertrochanteric Fracture

Ipsilateral femoral shaft fractures associated with an intertrochanteric or basicervical hip fracture are, fortunately, rare. In a large series of femoral shaft fractures, these associated proximal femoral shaft fractures were noted in about 3% of cases.[9] Unlike the standard intertrochanteric fracture, these tend to occur in younger patients as a result of motor vehicle accidents or other high velocity trauma. Priority in treatment rests first on restoring anatomic reduction to the proximal femur and then treating the femoral shaft fracture. The literature regarding this lesion is scanty and therefore no one good treatment method has emerged.[9,10,245]

There are various options to consider. The most commonly applied technique has been a compression hip screw with a long side plate. Other options include compression hip screw of the intertrochanteric fracture with supracondylar Ender's flexible

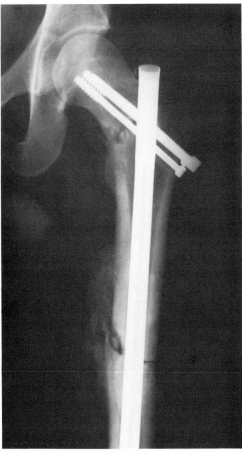

FIG. 11-14. Ipsilateral femoral shaft and basicervical fracture. These fractures were treated with a reamed reversed Grosse-Kempf nailing. Additional cannulated screws were used in the basicervical fracture and both fractures were primarily grafted with autogenous iliac bone.

nails or compression plate for the femoral shaft fracture, Ender's nails for both fractures, a Grosse-Kempf interlocking nail (opposite side) introducing the proximal interlocking nail into the femoral head and supplementing it with cortical compression screws (Fig. 11-14), and the modified "Y" Kuntscher nail. Several new intermedullary nails are available specifically for this fracture, such as the type designed by Russell and Taylor.[232] This is an intramedullary nail with proximal openings for the insertion of screws allowing fixation and compression of the intertrochanteric hip fracture as well as intramedullary fixation of the femoral shaft fracture.

Intertrochanteric and Subtrochanteric Fractures

This subtype of intertrochanteric hip fracture is often included in discussions of intertrochanteric hip fractures. The combination of subtrochanteric fracture associated with intertrochanteric fracture produces an unstable situation.[65,239] It is the subtrochanteric component of the fracture that is most difficult to handle. Wherever possible, anatomic reduction should be the goal with minimum reconstruction of the medial and posteromedial femoral cortices. A load sharing device, placed intermedullary, is the preferred method, but often the subtrochanteric component does not allow for placement of an intermedullary device such as a Zickel nail.[16,250,251] Options for this fracture pattern include a compression hip screw with long side plates, multiple flexible Ender's nails, or the AO blade plate.[124,192,200] Ruff and Lubbers reported satisfactory results in 43 of 45 patients with intertrochanteric subtrochanteric fractures using a sliding screw and long side plate device.[199] The AO blade plate is often difficult to apply to this situation, but offers several advantages.[209,213] (See Figure 11-19). The placement of the blade plate more perpendicular to the greater trochanter into the superior portion of the neck allows multiple areas for interfragmentary screw fixation through the plate. If the medial cortex cannot be adequately restored, weight-bearing should be delayed. Routine autogenous bone grafting is recommended.

Reverse Obliquity Fracture

This fracture was first described by Wright and is included as the Type II by Evans.[62,63,249] It is also called a reverse intertrochanteric fracture. The fracture line starts medially and superior to the lesser trochanter and extends slightly caudad and laterally

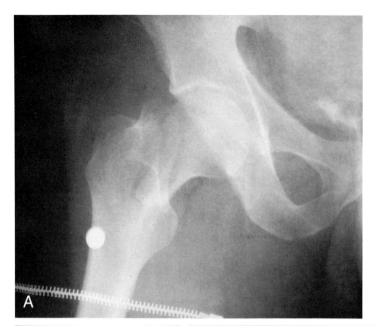

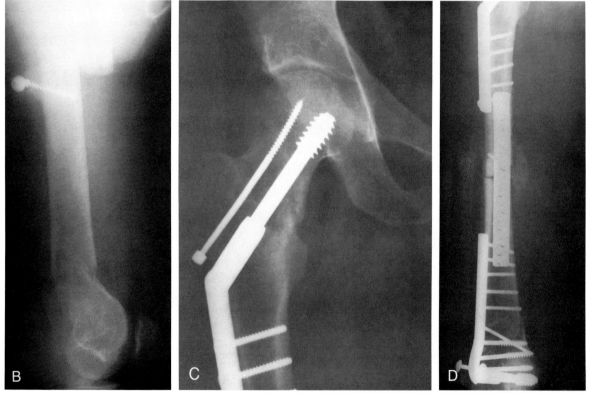

FIG. 11–15. Triple level ipsilateral femoral fracture. **A, B.** A left intertrochanteric fracture with associated ipsilateral transverse midshaft fracture and supracondylar fracture in a young polytraumatized man. **C.** The intertrochanteric hip fracture was reduced and stabilized with a compression hip screw and supplemental threaded screw to prevent rotation. **D.** The shaft and supracondylar fractures were plated and primarily bone grafted with autogenous iliac crest.

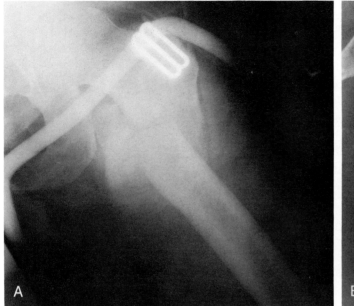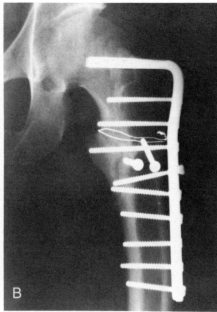

FIG. 11–16. Intertrochanteric/subtrochanteric fracture. **A.** A right unstable intertrochanteric hip fracture with subtrochanteric extension in a young male motor vehicle accident victim. **B.** The large posteromedial fragment must be repositioned for stability. A near anatomic reduction was obtained and internally fixed with AO blade plate with independent AO lag screws for the medial column. Note blade position in the head and neck and length of side plate.

to produce an unstable hip fracture. Furthermore, this fracture pattern is not stabilized by routine techniques. There is no lateral buttress once the compression hip screw is in place and the fracture fragments tend to displace by having the proximal portion slide laterally on the femoral shaft, resulting in pulling away of the femoral shaft from the plate. Several authors have advocated extension of an additional side plate above the side plate, which produces a lateral buttress. The method that Tronzo described is recommended (Fig. 11–18).[219]

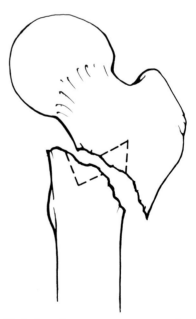

FIG. 11–17. Failed internal fixation in a reverse oblique fracture. This fracture pattern lacks a lateral buttress. If treated with routine techniques, medial displacement associated with fixation failure and nonunion are likely.

FIG. 11–18. Technique for step-cut osteotomy in the management of reverse obliquity fracture pattern. (Modified from Tronzo RG: Special considerations in management. Orthop Clin N Am, 5:571–583, 1974.)

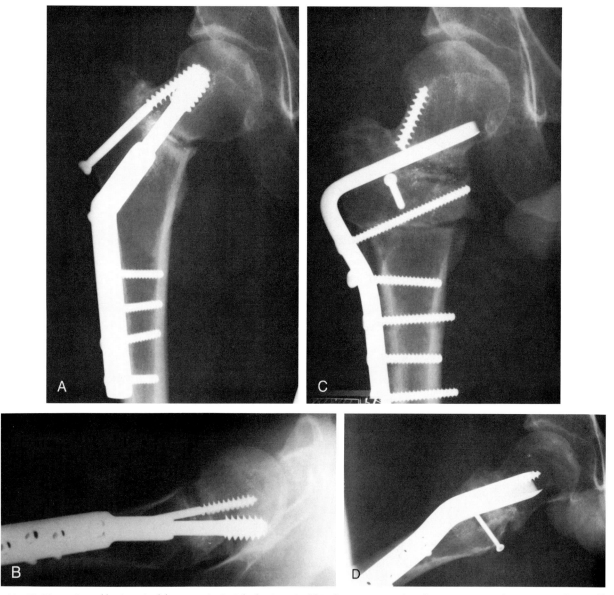

FIG. 11–19. Nonunion of basicervical fracture. **A.** A right basicervical hip fracture treated with a compresson hip screw and cancellous lag screw. **B.** On the lateral view, the compression screw was out the back of the femoral neck, preventing collapse of the screw within the barrel and resulting in nonunion. **C.** Anteroposterior. **D.** Lateral. This was managed by removal of old implant, valgus osteotomy, autogenous bone grafting, and AO blade plate fixation. The patient progressed to healing in six months.

This method establishes bony stability by resecting a wedge from the proximal femoral shaft, allowing interlocking of the fracture fragments. This produces bony stability, which is subsequently stabilized with a compression hip screw system. Medial displacement osteotomy is contraindicated (Fig. 11–17).

Salvage of the Failed Intertrochanteric Hip Fracture

Malunion

The most common deformity after intertrochanteric hip fracture is a varus malunion.[246] Minor degrees of varus shift at the fracture site usually have clinical sequelae. If the varus angulation is less than 110°, the potential for significant alterations in gait are noted. Fortunately, most of these situations are in the elderly patients who do not require revision surgery. Should the malunion occur in an active patient, a valgus intertrochanteric osteotomy may be needed.[183]

Nonunion

Nonunion rates range from 0 to 5% in large series.[231] The majority of intertrochanteric hip fractures will progress to bony union in 12 to 18 weeks,

regardless of the type of treatment. When nonunion occurs, it is usually a consequence of failure of the interal fixation device to allow the proximal head and neck segment to collapse onto the intertrochanteric region. This is usually produced by distractive force from a rigid nail and side plate or failure to slide in the compression hip screw situation. This ultimately leads to implant failure because the load is being transmitted primarily to the internal fixation device. The management of the nonunion depends on when it is recognized. If the internal fixation device is still relatively intact, although it may be slightly bent, it is best to remove this and replace it with a new compression hip screw with autogenous bone grafting. If the plate has already failed and there is significant deformity or destruction of the proximal femoral bone, a total hip arthroplasty or endoprosthesis is indicated (Fig. 11–20).[184,196,226]

Pain After Healed Intertrochanteric Fracture

Occasionally, despite a well performed compression hip screw procedure and healing of the patient's fracture, late pain develops. As more of the elderly population is surviving longer, the possibility for pain related to the procedure is increasing. Occasionally, pain will be caused by bursitis or other tissue irritation over the lateral plate. This

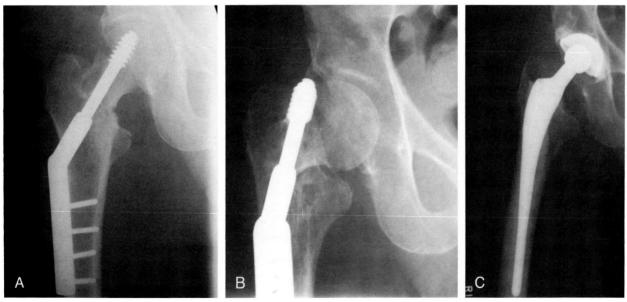

FIG. 11–20. Failure of hip compression screw secondary to osteopenia and poor screw fixation. **A.** A basicervical fracture in a retired elderly female school teacher treated with reduction and compression hip screw fixation. **B.** Stability was not adequately achieved and fixation failure occurred through her osteopenic bone. **C.** This was salvaged by cemented total hip replacement. This patient died 12 months postoperatively of cardiac arrest.

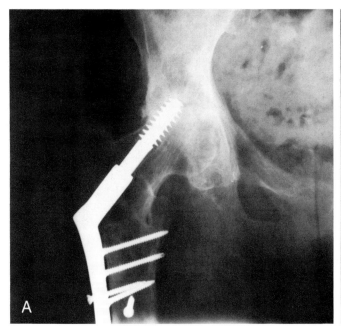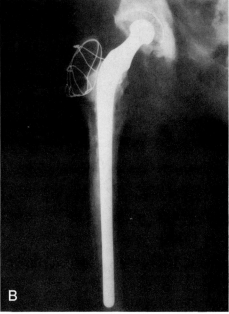

Fɪɢ. 11–21. Superior hip screw protrusion with late destructive arthritis. **A.** Collapse of the superior femoral head through to be avascular necrosis associated with screw protrusion and painful destructive arthritis is noted. **B.** This situation was easily remedied by cemented total hip replacement in this active, elderly female. This patient is 6 years postoperative and does well.

can be minimized by a careful closure of the vastus lateralis over the plate. If this is the case, it is preferable to try to correct the symptoms nonoperatively. It is not recommended to remove the internal fixation in these patients as a routine, but if necessary the implant may be removed 12 to 18 months postoperatively. Occasionally patients develop avascular necrosis with late segmental collapse or secondary degenerative arthritis. Depending on the quality of the acetabulum, an endoprosthesis or total hip replacement can be advocated. Stambough, et al., reported on a series of 140 conversion total hip replacements in a population with complications of fracture treatment.[224] Twenty-seven of these were caused by failures of the hip screw and side plate. Routine, cemented total hip replacement fared well functionally, but radiographically showed signs of early bone cement interface development in the femoral side caused by the multiple drill holes. A noncemented well fitting femoral component with a hybrid cemented acetabulum may be an alternative if the patient is under 65 years of age (Fig. 11–21).

Acknowledgment

The author would like to thank Drs. Edward V.A. Lim and Russell P. Clarke for allowing inclusion of several of their cases. The author also wishes to thank Mrs. Marci L. Nicholson for her excellent technical assistance and Mr. Stan M. Coffman for his outstanding medical illustrations.

References

1. Aʟꜰꜰʀᴀᴍ PA: An epidemiologic study of cervical and trochanteric fractures of the femur in the urban population. Acta Orthop Scand (Suppl), 65:1–109, 1964.
2. Aɴᴅᴇʀꜱᴏɴ R, McKɪʙʙɪɴ WB: Intertrochanteric fractures. J Bone Joint Surg, 25:153–168, 1943.
3. Aɴᴅᴇʀꜱᴏɴ RA: A new method for treating fractures, utilizing the well leg for countertraction. Surg Gynecol Obstet, 54:207–219, 1932.
4. Aɴᴛɪɴ ME: Key free compression hip screw in treatment of intertrochanteric hip fracture with early weight bearing: a clinical study. J Am Osteopath Assoc, 82:661–668, 1983.
5. Aᴘʀɪɴ H, Kɪʟꜰᴏʏʟᴇ RM: Treatment of trochanteric fractures with ender rods. J Trauma, 20:32–42, 1980.
6. Aᴜꜰʀᴀɴᴄ OE, Jᴏɴᴇꜱ WN, Tᴜʀɴᴇʀ RH: Severely comminuted intertrochanteric hip fracture. JAMA, 199:140–143, 1967.
7. Bᴀᴋᴇʀ DM: Fractures of the femoral neck after healed intertrochanteric fractures: a complication of too short a nail plate fixation. J Trauma, 15:73–81, 1975.
8. Bᴀᴋᴇʀ HR: Ununited intertrochanteric fractures of the femur. Clin Orthop, 18:209–219, 1960.
9. Bᴀʀqᴜᴇᴛ A, Fᴇʀɴᴀɴᴅᴇᴢ A, Lᴇᴏɴ H: Simultaneous ipsilateral trochanteric and femoral shaft fracture. Acta Orthop Scand, 56:36–39, 1985.
10. Bᴀʀqᴜᴇᴛ A, Mᴜꜱꜱɪᴏ A: Fracture dislocation of the femoral head and associated ipsilateral trochanteric and shaft fractures of the femur. Arch Orthop Trauma Surg, 102:61–63, 1983.
11. Bᴀʀʀ JS: Diagnosis and treatment of infections following internal fixation of hip fractures. Orthop Clin North Am, 5:847–864, 1974.
12. Bᴀʀᴛᴇʟꜱ WP: The treatment of intertrochanteric fractures. J Bone Joint Surg, 21:773–775, 1939.
13. Bᴀʀᴛᴜᴄᴄɪ EJ: The effect of adjunctive methyl methacrylate on failure of fixation and function in patient with intertro-

chanteric fracture and osteoporosis. J Bone Joint Surg, 67A:1094–1107, 1985.

14. BASMAJIAN JV (ed): Therapeutic exercise, 3rd ed. Baltimore, Williams & Wilkins, pp. 1–50, 1978.

15. BEALS RK, LAWTON ED, SNELL WE: Prophylactic internal fixation of the femur in metastatic breast carcinoma (338 cases). Cancer, 28:1350–1361, 1971.

16. BERGMAN GD, WINQUIST A, MAYO KA, HANSEN ST JR: Subtrochanteric fracture of the femur—fixation using the Zickel nail. J Bone Joint Surg, 69A:1032–1040, 1987.

17. BERGQVIST D, EFSING HO, HALLBOOK T, HEDLUND T: Thromboembolism after elective and post-traumatic hip surgery—a controlled prophylactic trial with dextran 70 and low-dose heparin. Acta Chir Scand, 145:213–218, 1979.

18. BOUMAN HD (ed): Exploratory and analytical survey of therapeutic exercises. Am J Phys Med, 46(1):25–43, 1967.

19. BOYD HB, ANDERSON LD: Management of unstable trochanteric fractures. Surg Gynecol Obstet, 112:633–638, 1961.

20. BOYD HB, GRIFFIN LL: Classification and treatment of trochanteric fractures. Arch Surg, 58:853–866, 1949.

21. BOYD HB, LIPINSKI SW: Nonunion of trochanteric and subtrochanteric fractures. Surg Gynecol Obstet, 104:463–470, 1957.

22. BOYD RJ, BURKE JF, COLTON T: A double blind clinical trial of prophylactic antibiotics in hip fractures. J Bone Joint Surg, 55A:1251–1258, 1973.

23. BREMNER RA, JELLIFFE AM: The management of pathological fracture of the major long bones from metastatic cancer. J Bone Joint Surg, 40B:652–659, 1958.

24. BURNETT JW, GUSTILO RB, WILLIAMS DN, KIND AC: Prophylactic antibiotics in hip fractures. J Bone Joint Surg, 62A: 457–461, 1980.

25. CAMERON HU, GRAHAM JD: Retention of the compression screw in sliding screw plate devices. Clin Orthop, 146:219–221, 1980.

26. CAMERON HU, PILLIAR RM, HASTINGS DE, FORNASIER VL: Iatrogenic subcapital fracture of the hip. Clin Orthop, 112:218–220, 1975.

27. CAMPION EW, JETTE AM, CLEARY PD, HARRIS BA. Hip fractures: a prospective study of hospital course complications and cost. J Gen Inter Med, 2:78–82, 1987.

28. CAUDLE RJ, HOPSON CN, CLARKE RP: Unstable intertrochanteric fracture of hip. Orthop Rev, 16:30–41, 1987.

29. CEDER L, THORNGREN KG, WALLDEN B: Prognostic indicators and early home rehabilitation in elderly patients with hip fractures. Clin Orthop, 152:173–184, 1980.

30. CEDER L, et al: Rehabilitation of hip fractures in the elderly. Acta Orthop Scand, 50:681–688, 1979.

31. CHANNON GM, WILEY AM: Aspirin prophylaxis of venous thromboembolic disease following fracture of the upper femur. Can J Surg, 22:468–472, 1979.

32. CHAPMAN MW, et al: The use of Ender's pins in extracapsular fractures of the hip. J Bone Joint Surg, 63A:14–28, 1981.

33. CHILDRESS HM: Well leg traction: an efficient but neglected procedure. Clin Orthop, 51:127–136, 1967.

34. CHRISTODOULON NA, PRETALEIS EK: Significance of muscular disturbance in the localization of fracutre of the proximal femur. Clin Orthop, 187:215–217, 1984.

35. CLAFFEY TJ: Avascular necrosis of the femoral head. J Bone Joint Surg, 42B:802–809, 1960.

36. CLAWSON DK: Intertrochanteric fracture of the hip. Am J Surg, 93:580–587, 1957.

37. CLAWSON DK: Trochanteric fractures treated by the sliding screw plate fixation method. J Trauma 4:737–756, 1964.

38. CLEVELAND M, BOSWORTH DM, THOMPSON FR: Intertrochanteric

fractures of the femur. J Bone Joint Surg, 29A:1049–1067, 1947.

39. CLEVELAND M, BOSWORTH DM, THOMPSON FR: Management of the trochanteric fracture of the femur. JAMA 137:1186–1190, 1948.

40. CLEVELAND M, et al: A ten year analysis of intertrochanteric fractures of the femur. J Bone Joint Surg, 41A:1399–1408, 1959.

41. COBEY JC, et al.: Indicators of recovery from fracture of the hip. Clin Orthop, 117:258–262, 1976.

42. CONRAD JJ: Medial displacement fixation of unstable intertrochanteric fractures of the hip. Bull Hosp Joint Dis, 32:54–62, 1971.

43. CORAN AG, BANKS HH, ALIAPOULIOS MA, WILSON RE: The management of pathologic fractures in patients with metastatic carcinoma of the breast. Surg Gynecol Obstet, 127:1225–1230, 1968.

44. COUGHLIN L, TEMPLETON J: Hip fractures in patients with Parkinson's disease. Clin Orthop, 148:192–195, 1980.

45. CRAM RH: The unstable intertrochanteric fracture. Surg Gynecol Obstet, 101:15–19, 1955.

46. DAHL E: Mortality and life expectancy after hip fractures. Acta Orthop Scand, 51:163–170, 1980.

47. DAVIS FM, QUINCE M, LAURENSON VG: Deep vein thrombosis and anaesthetic technique in emergency hip surgery. Br Med J, 281(6254):1528–1529, 1980.

48. DAVIS PH, FRYMOYER JW: The lateral position in the surgical management of intertrochanteric and subtrochanteric fractures of the femur. J Bone Joint Surg, 51A:1128–1134, 1969.

49. DELEE JC: Fracture and dislocation of the hip in R/G, Vol. 2. Edited by CA Rockwood and DP Green. Philadelphia, Lippincott, pp. 1257–1287, 1984.

50. DEYERLE WM: Surgical impaction over a plate and multiple pins for intertrochanteric fractures. Orthop Clin North Am, 5:615–628, 1974.

51. DIMON JH: The unstable intertrochanteric fracture. Clin Orthop, 92:100–107, 1973.

52. DIMON JH, HUGHSTON JC: Unstable intertrochanteric fractures of the hip. J Bone Joint Surg, 49A:440–450, 1967.

53. DOHERTY JH, LYDEN JP: Intertrochanteric fractures of the hip treated with the hip compression screw. Clin Orthop, 141:184–187, 1979.

54. DOPPELT SH: The sliding compression screw: today's best answer for stabilization of intertrochanteric hip fractures. Orthop Clin North Am, 11:507–523, 1980.

55. DOUGLASS HO, SHUKLA SK, MINDELL E: Treatment of pathologic fracture of long bones excluding those due to breast cancer. J Bone Joint Surg, 58A:1055–1061, 1976.

56. DOVE J: Complete fractures of the femur in Paget's disease of bone. J Bone Joint Surg, 62B:12–17, 1980.

57. DUNN EJ, SKINNER SR: Disengagement of a sliding screw plate. J Bone Joint Surg, 58A:1027–1028, 1976.

58. ECKER ML, JOYCE JJ, KOHL EJ: The treatment of trochanteric hip fractures using a compression screw. J Bone Joint Surg, 57A:23–27, 1975.

59. ELABDIEN BSA, OLERUD S, KARLSTRUM G: Enders nailing of pertrochanteric fracture. Clin Orthop, 191:53–63, 1984.

60. ELABDIEN BSA, OLERUD S, KARLSTRUM G: The influence of age on the morphology of trochanteric fracture. Arch Orthop Trauma Surg, 103:156–161, 1984.

61. ESSER MP, KASSAB JY, JONES DHA: Trochanteric fracture of the femur. J Bone Joint Surg, 68A:557–560, 1986.

62. EVANS EM: The treatment of trochanteric fractures of the femur. J Bone Joint Surg, 31B:190–203, 1949.

63. Evans EM: Trochanteric fractures. J Bone Joint Surg, 33B:192–204, 1951.

64. Fielding JW: Subtrochanteric fractures. Clin Orthop, 92:86–99, 1973.

65. Fielding JW, Cochran, GVB, Zickel RE: Biomechanical characteristics and surgical management of subtrochanteric fractures. Orthop Clin North Am, 5:629–649, 1974.

66. Fitts WT, Lehr HB, Schor S, Roberts B: Life expectancy after fracture of the hip. Surg Gynecol Obstet, 81:7–12, 1959.

67. Frankel VH: Mechanical fixation of unstable fractures about the proximal end of the femur. Bull Hosp Joint Dis, 24:75–84, 1963.

68. Frankel VH: Biomechanics of the hip joint. Instr Course Lect, 35:3–9, 1986.

69. Fredin HO, Nillius SA, Bergqvist D: Prophylaxis of deep vein thrombosis in patients with fracture of the femoral neck: a prospective comparison between dextran and a sulphated polysaccharide. Acta Orthop Scand, 53:413–417, 1982.

70. Freyberg RH, Levy MD: Medical management of the patient with a fracture of the hip. JAMA, 37:1190–1193, 1968.

71. Friedenberg ZB, Gentchos E, Rutt C: Fixation in intertrochanteric fractures of the hip. Surg Gynecol Obstet, 135:225–228, 1972.

72. Ganz R, Thomas RJ, Hammerle CP: Trochanteric fractures of the femur: treatment and results. Clin Orthop, 138:30–40, 1979.

73. Gordon AC: The probability of death following a fracture of the hip. Can Med Assoc J, 105:47–52, 1971.

74. Gotfried Y, Frisch E, Mendes DC, Roffman M: Intertrochanteric Fracture in High Risk Geriatric Patients Treated by External Fixation. Clin Orthop, 8:769–774, 1985.

75. Gurtler RA, Jacobs RR, Jacobs CR: Biomechanic evaluation of Ender's pins, the Harris nail, and the dynamic hip screw for unstable intertrochanteric hip fractures. Clin Orthop, 206:109–112, 1986.

76. Greider JL, Horowitz M: Clinical evaluation of the sliding compression screw in 121 hip fractures. South Med J, 73:1343–1348, 1980.

77. Harding AF: A clinical and metallurgical analysis of retrieved Jewett and Richards hip plate devices. Clin Orthop, 195:261–269, 1985.

78. Harper MC, Walsh T: Enders nailing for peritrochanteric fracture of femur. J Bone Joint Surg, 67A:79–88, 1985.

79. Harrington KD: The use of methyl methacrylate as an adjunct in the internal fixation of unstable comminuted intertrochanteric fractures in osteoporotic patients. J Bone Joint Surg, 57A:744–750, 1975.

80. Harrington KD, Johnston JO: The management of comminuted unstable intertrochanteric fractures. J Bone Joint Surg, 55A:1367–1376, 1973.

81. Harrington KD, Johnston JO, Turner RH, Green, DL: The use of methyl methacrylate as an adjunct in the internal fixation of malignant neoplastic fractures. J Bone Joint Surg, 54A:1665–1676, 1972.

82. Harris LJ: Closed retrograde intramedullary nailing of peritrochanteric fractures of the femur with a new nail. J Bone Joint Surg, 62A:1185–1193, 1980.

83. Hartman JT, et al.: Cyclic sequential compression of the lower limb in prevention of deep vein thrombosis. J Bone Joint Surg, 64A:1059–1062, 1982.

84. Harty M: The anatomy of the hip joint. *In* Surgery of the Hip Joint, Vol. 1. Edited by RG Tronzo. New York, Springer-Verlag, pp. 45–75, 1984.

85. Harty M: The calcar femorale and the femoral neck. J Bone Joint Surg, 39A:625–630, 1957.

86. Hayward J, Lowe LW, Tzevelekos S: Intertrochanteric fractures: a comparison between fixation of a two-piece nail plate and Ender's nails. Int Orthop, 7:153–158, 1983.

87. Heisterberg L, Johansen TS: Treatment of pathologic fractures. Acta Orthop Scand, 50:787–790, 1979.

88. Hodgson SF, et al.: Outpatient percutaneous biopsy of the iliac crest: methods, morbidity, and patient acceptance. Mayo Clinic Proc, 61:28–33, 1986.

89. Hodkinson HM: Fracture of the femur as a presentation of osteomalacia. Geront Clin, 13:189–191, 1971.

90. Hofmann A, Jones RE, Schoenvogel R: Pudendal nerve neuropraxia as a result of traction on the fracture table. J Bone Joint Surg, 64A:136–138, 1982.

91. Holland WR, Weiss AB, Daniel WW: Medial displacement osteotomy for unstable intertrochanteric femoral fractures. South Med J, 70:576–578, 1977.

92. Hollis M: Practical Exercise Therapy. Philadelphia, Lippincott, pp. 1–100, 1976.

93. Holt EP: Hip fractures in the trochanteric region: treatment with a strong nail and early weight-bearing. J Bone Joint Surg, 45A:687–705, 1963.

94. Hughston JC: Unstable intertrochanteric fractures of the hip. J Bone Joint Surg 46A:1145, 1964.

95. Hunter GA: The results of operative treatment of trochanteric fractures of the femur. Injury, 6:202–205, 1974.

96. Hunter GA, Krajbich IJ: The results of medical displacement osteotomy for unstable intertrochanteric fracture of the femur. Clin Orthop, 137:140–143, 1978.

97. Inman VT: Functional aspects of the abductor muscles of the hip. J Bone Joint Surg, 29A:607–619, 1947.

98. Jacobs RR, Armstrong HJ, Whitaker JH, Pazell, J: Treatment of intertrochanteric hip fractures with a compression hip screw and a nail plate. J Trauma, 16:599–603, 1976.

99. Jacobs RR, McClain O: In vitro strain patterns in "intertrochanteric fractures" internally fixed with nail plate or compression screw plate. Surg Forum, 27:511–514, 1976.

100. Jacobs RR, McClain O, Armstrong HJ: Internal fixation of intertrochanteric hip fractures: a clinical and biochemical study. Clin Orthop, 146:62–70, 1980.

101. James ETR, Hunter GA: The treatment of intertrochanteric fracture—a review article. Injury 14:421–431, 1982.

102. Jarrett PJ, Fleming LL, Whitesides TE: The stable internal fixation in peritrochanteric hip fractures. Instr Course Lect, 33:203–211, 1984.

103. Jenson JS: Mechanical strength of sliding screw plate hip implants. Acta Orthop Scand, 51:625–632, 1980.

104. Jenson JS: Classification of trochanteric fractures. Acta Orthop Scand, 51:803–810, 1980.

105. Jenson JS: Trochanteric fractures. Acta Orthop Scand (Suppl), 188:1–100, 1981.

106. Jenson JS, Sonne-Holm S: Critical analysis of Ender nailing in the treatment of trochanteric fractures. Acta Orthop Scand, 51:817–825, 1980.

107. Jenson JS, Sonne-Holm S, Tondevold E: Unstable trochanteric fractures: a comparative analysis of four methods of internal fixation. Acta Orthop Scand, 51:949–962, 1980.

108. Jenson JS, Tondevold E, Sonne-Holm S: Stable trochanteric fractures: a comparative analysis of four methods of internal fixation. Acta Orthop Scand, 51:811–816, 1980.

109. Jenson TM, Dillon WL, Reckling FW: Changing concepts in the management of pathologic and impending pathologic fractures. J Trauma, 16:496–502, 1976.

110. Jewett EL: One-piece angle nail for trochanteric fractures. J Bone Joint Surg, 23A:803–810, 1941.

111. Johnson LL, Lottes JO, Arnot JP: The utilization of the holt nail for proximal femoral fractures. J Bone Joint Surg, 50A:67–78, 1968.

112. Jones JB: Screw fixation of the lesser trochanteric fragment. Clin Orthop, 123:107, 1977.
113. Joseph KN: Acetabular protrusion of sliding screw. Acta Orthop Scand, 57:245–246, 1986.
114. Katz S, Ford AB, Heiple KG, Newill VA: Studies of illness in the aged: recovery after fracture of the hip. J Gerontology, 19:285–293, 1964.
115. Kaufer H: Mechanics of the treatment of hip injuries. Clin Orthop, 146:53–61, 1980.
116. Kaufer H, Matthews LS, Sonstegard D: Stable fixation of intertrochanteric fractures. J Bone Joint Surg, 56A:899–907, 1974.
117. Keene JS, Sellinger PS, McBeath AA, Engber, WD: Metastatic breast carcinoma in the femur. Clin Orthop, 203:282–288, 1986.
118. Kelbel JM, Connolly JF: Avascular necrosis following a routine intertrochanteric fracture of the femur. Nebr Med J, 12:156–159, 1984.
119. Kennedy J, McFarlene RM, McLaughlin AD: The moe plate in intertrochanteric fracture of the hip. J Bone Joint Surg, 38B:451–457, 1957.
120. Kenzora JE, McCarthy RE, Lowell JD, Sledge, CB: Hip fracture mortality. Clin Orthop, 186:45–56, 1984.
121. Key JA: Internal fixation of trochanteric fractures of the femur. Surgery, 6:13–23, 1939.
122. Kisner C, Colby LA: Therapeutic exercise: foundations and techniques. Philadelphia, Davis, pp. 8–63, 1985.
123. Kolind-Sorensen V: Comminuted intertrochanteric fracture of the femoral neck. Acta Orthop Scand, 46:651–653, 1975.
124. Kuderna H, Bohler N, Collon DJ: Treatment of intertrochanteric and subtrochanteric fractures of the hip by the Ender method. J Bone Joint Surg, 58A:604–611, 1976.
125. Kumar V: The syndrome of the fracture of the lesser trochanter in adults: a neglected aspect of the trochanteric fracture. Injury, 4:327–334, 1972–1973.
126. Kuokkanen H, Korzala O, Lauttamus L: Ender nailing of trochanteric fractures. Arch Orthop Trauma Surg, 105:46–48, 1986.
127. Kyle RF, Gustilo RB, Premer RF: Analysis of six hundred twenty-two intertrochanteric hip fractures. J Bone Joint Surg, 61A:216–221, 1979.
128. Kyle RF, Wright TM, Burstein AH: Biomechanical analysis of the sliding characteristics of compression hip screws. J Bone Joint Surg, 62A:1308–1314, 1980.
129. Lane JM, Vigorita VJ: Osteoporosis. J Bone Joint Surg, 65A:274–278, 1983.
130. Laros GS: The role of osteoporosis in intertrochanteric fractures. Orthop Clin North Am 11:525–537, 1980.
131. Laros GS: Intertrochanteric fracture. Arch Surg, 110:37–40, 1975.
132. Laros GS, Moore JF: Complications of fixation in intertrochanteric fractures. Clin Orthop, 101:110–119, 1974.
133. Laskin RS, Gruber MA, Zimmerman AJ: Intertrochanteric fractures of the hip in the elderly: a retrospective analysis of 236 cases. Clin Orthop, 141:188–195, 1979.
134. Lau HK, et al.: Treatment of comminuted trochanteric femoral fractures with Dimon-Hughston displaced fixation and acrylic cement—a preliminary report of 16 cases. Injury, 15:129–135, 1984.
135. Levy RN, Siegel M, Sedlin ED, Siffert RS: Complications of the Ender pin fixation in basicervical intertrochanteric and subtrochanteric fracture of the hip. J Bone Joint Surg, 65A:66–69, 1983.
136. Leydig SM, Brookes TP: Treatment of pertrochanteric fracture of the femur with a lag bolt. J Missouri Med Assoc, 37:354–357, 1940.
137. Lowell JD: Fractures of the hip. N Engl J Med, 274:1418–1425, 1966.
138. Lowell JD: Fractures of the hip (concluded). N Engl J Med, 274:1480–1490, 1966.
139. Lygre L: The loads produced on the hip joint by nursing procedures: a telemerization study. MS Thesis. (Nursing) CWRU, 1970.
140. MacEacherin AG, Heyse-Moore GH: Stable intertrochanteric femoral fractures. J Bone Joint Surg, 65B:582–583, 1983.
141. Malerich MM, Laros GS, Wade T, Yamada R: Four fragment intertrochanteric hip fractures: a biomechanical study. Trans Orthop Res Soc, 2:242, 1977.
142. Mann RJ: Avascular necrosis of the femoral head following intertrochanteric fractures. Clin Orthop, 92:108–115, 1973.
143. Manoli A: Malassembly of the sliding screw-plate device. J Trauma, 26:916–922, 1986.
144. Marcove RC, Yang DJ: Survival times after treatment of pathologic fractures. Cancer, 20:2154–2158, 1967.
145. Martinek H, Egkher E, Wielke B, Spangler H: Experimental tests concerning the biomechanical behaviour of petrochanteric osteosyntheses. Acta Orthop Scand, 50:675–679, 1979.
146. Massie WK: Extracapsular fractures of the hip treated by impaction using a sliding nail-plate fixation. Clin Orthop, 22:180–202, 1962.
147. Massie WK: Fractures of the hip. J Bone Joint Surg, 46A:658–690, 1964.
148. May JMB, Chacha PB: Displacements of trochanteric fractures and their influence on reduction. J Bone Joint Surg, 50B:318–323, 1968.
149. McClure J, Goldsborough S: Fracture neck of femur and contralateral intracerebral lesions. J Clin Pathol 39:920–922, 1986.
150. McLaren AD, Stockwell MC, Reid VT: Anesthesia techniques for surgical correction of fracture of femur. Anesthesiology, 33:10–14, 1978.
151. McLaughlin T, Frankel VH: A parametric study of the strength of the upper end of the femur. Unpublished Data, 1970.
152. McNeill DH: Hip fractures: influence of delay in surgery on mortality. Wis Med J, 74:129–130, 1975.
153. Melton LJ, et al.: Osteoporosis and the risk of hip fracture. Am J Epidemiol, 124:254–261, 1986.
154. Meyers MH: Trochanteric fracture. *In* Meyers MH (ed): Fracture of the hip. Chicago, Yearbook, pp. 66–73, 1985.
155. Meyn MA, Hopson C, Jayasankar S: Fractures of the hip in the institutionalized psychotic patient. Clin Orthop, 122:128–134, 1977.
156. Mickelson MR, Bonfiglio M: Pathologic fracture in the proximal portion of the femur: treatment by Zickel nail fixation. J Bone Joint Surg, 58A:1067–1070, 1976.
157. Mizrahi J, Kantarovski A, Najenson T, Susak Z: In vivo biomechanic evaluation of nail-plate fixation of femoral neck fracture of rehabilitation patient. Scand J Rehabil Med Suppl, 12:112–116, 1985.
158. Mok CK, et al.: The incidence of deep vein thrombosis in Hong Kong Chinese after hip surgery for fracture of the proximal femur. Br J Surg, 66(9):640–642, 1979.
159. Moller BN, Lucht U, Grymer F, Bartholdy NJ: Early rehabilitation following osteosynthesis with sliding hip screw for trochanteric fracture. Scand J Rehabil Med, 17:39–43, 1985.
160. Moller BN, Lucht U, Grymer F, Bartholdy NJ: Instability of trochanteric hip fracture following internal fixation. Acta Orthop Scand, 55:517–520, 1984.

161. Moore M: Treatment of trochanteric femoral fractures with special reference to complications. Am J Surg, 84:449–452, 1952.

162. Morris GK, Mitchell JR: Preventing venous thromboembolism in elderly patients with hip fractures: studies of low-dose heparin, dipyridamole, aspirin, and flurbiprofen. Br Med J, 1(6060):535–537, 1977.

163. Morris HD: Trochanteric Fractures. South Med J, 34:571–578, 1941.

164. Morrison D, Mrstik, LL, Weingarden TL: Management of unstable intertrochanteric fractures of the hip. J Am Osteopath Assoc, 77:793–802, 1978.

165. Muhr G, Tscherne H, Thomas R: Comminuted trochanteric femoral fractures in geriatric patients: the results of 231 cases with internal fixation and acrylic cement. Clin Orthop, 138:41–44, 1979.

166. Mulholland RC, Gunn DR: Sliding screw plate fixation of intertrochanteric femoral fractures. J Trauma, 12:581–591, 1972.

167. Mulley G, Espley AJ: Hip fracture after hemiplegia postgrad. Med J, 55:264–265, 1979.

168. Mullen JO: Death in hip fracture: a prospective approach to its prediction and minimization. 54th Annual AAOS Proceedings, San Francisco, p 167, 1987.

169. Murray JA, Parrish FF: Surgical management of secondary neoplastic fracture about the hip. Orthop Clin North Am, 5:857–901, 1974.

170. Murray RC, Frew JFM: Trochanteric fractures of the femur. J Bone Joint Surg, 31B:204–219, 1949.

171. Mussbichler H: Arterial supply of the head of the femur. Acta Radiol Scand, 46:533–546, 1956.

172. Naiman PT, Schein AJ, Siffert RS:Medial displacement fixation for severely comminuted intertrochanteric fractures. Clin Orthop, 62:151–155, 1969.

173. Neimann KMW, Mankin HJ: Fractures about the hip in an institutionalized patient population. II. Survival and ability to walk again. J Bone Joint Surg, 50A:1327–1340, 1968.

174. Nielsen P, Jelnes R, Rasmusser LB, Ebling A: Trochanteric fracture treated by the McLaughlin nail and plate. Injury, 16:333–336, 1985.

175. Norton PL: Intertrochanteric fractures. Clin Orthop, 66:77–81, 1969.

176. Olerud S, Stark A, Gilstrom P: Malrotation following Ender's nailing. Clin Orthop, 147:139–142, 1980.

177. Owen RA, Melton LJ, Gallagher JC, Riggs BL: The national cost of acute care of hip fracture associated with osteoporosis. Clin Orthop, 150:172–176, 1980.

178. Pandey S: A modified conservative treatment of trochanteric fractures. Int Surg, 53:201–205, 1970.

179. Pankovich AM, Tarabishy IE: Ender nailing of intertrochanteric and subtrochanteric fractures of the femur. J Bone Joint Surg, 62A:635–645, 1980.

180. Parrish FF, Murray JA: Surgical treatment of secondary neoplastic fracture. J Bone Joint Surg, 52A:665–686, 1970.

181. Perez CA, Bradfield JS, Morgan HC: Management of pathologic fracture. Cancer, 25:684–693, 1971.

182. Petersen CA, Pasternak HS, Kraus H: Use of 150 degree nail plate combination in intertrochanteric fractures of the hip. J Trauma, 14:236–241, 1974.

183. Phoenix OF: Internal fixation in intertrochanteric osteotomy. *In* The Fixation of Fractures Using Plates. The Institution of Mechanical Engineers, pp. 10–16, 1974.

184. Pinder RC, Durnin CW, Cook DA: The Leinbach prosthesis in the treatment of complex intertrochanteric fractures. Presented at AAOS Meeting, Las Vegas, March, 1981.

185. Pollack A, Harrison MH: Hip fractures and deep-vein thromboembolism (letter). Lancet, 2(7998):1301, 1976.

186. Posman CL, Morawa LG: Vascular injury from intrapelvic migration of a threaded pin. J Bone Joint Surg, 67A:804–806, 1985.

187. Pugh WL: A self-adjusting nail-plate for fractures about the hip joint. J Bone Joint Surg, 37A:1085–1093, 1955.

188. Rae JF, Banzon MT, Weiss AB, Rayhack J: Treatment of unstable intertrochanteric fracture with anatomic reduction and compression hip screw fixation. Clin Orthop, 175:65–71, 1983.

189. Raugstad TS, et al.: Treatment of pertrochanteric and subtrochanteric fractures of the femur by the Ender method. Clin Orthop, 138:231–237, 1979.

190. Regazzoni P, Reud T, Winguest R, Allgower M: The Dynamic Hip Screw Implant System. New York, Springer Verlag, pp. 1–51, 1985.

191. Rennie W, Mitchell N: Compression fixation of peritrochanteric fractures and early weight bearing. Clin Orthop, 121:157–162, 1976.

192. Richmond JC, Kazes JA, MacAusland WR: An evaluation of three current techniques of interal fixation for intertrochanteric and subtrochanteric fractures of the hip. Orthopaedics, 4:895–898, 1981.

193. Ring PA: Treatment of trochanteric fractures of the femur. Br Med J, 1:654–656, 1963.

194. Riska EB: Trochanteric Fractures of the Femur. Acta Orthop Scand, 42:268–280, 1971.

195. Roberts A, et al.: A comparison of the functional results of anatomic and medial displacement valgus nailing of intertrochanteric fractures of the femur. J Trauma, 12:341–346, 1972.

196. Rosenfeld RT, Schwartz DR, Alter AH: Prosthetic replacement for trochanteric fractures of the femur. J Bone Joint Surg, 55A:420, 1973.

197. Rothermel JE, Garcia A: Treatment of hip fractures in patients with Parkinson's syndrome on levodopa therapy. J Bone Joint Surg, 54A:1251–1254, 1972.

198. Rowe CR: The management of fractures in elderly patients is different. J Bone Joint Surg, 47A:1043–1059, 1965.

199. Ruff MF, Lubbers LM: Treatment of subtrochanteric fracture with a sliding screw plate device. J Trauma, 26:75–80, 1986.

200. Russin LA, Sonni A: Treatment of intertrochanteric and subtrochanteric fractures with Ender's intramedullary rods. Clin Orthop, 148:203–212, 1980.

201. Sahlstrand T: The Richards compression and sliding hip screw system in the treatment of intertrochanteric fractures. Acta Orthop Scand, 45:213–219, 1974.

202. Salzman EW, Harris WH: Prevention of venous thromboembolism in orthopaedic patients. J Bone Joint Surg, 58A:903–913, 1976.

203. Sangeorzan BJ, Ryan JR, Salciccioli GG: Prophylactic femoral stabilization with the Zickel nail by closed technique. J Bone Joint Surg, 68A:991–999, 1986.

204. Sarmiento A: Intertrochanteric fractures of the femur: 150 degree angle nail plate fixation and early rehabilitation: a preliminary report of 100 cases. J Bone Joint Surg, 45A:706–722, 1963.

205. Sarmiento A: Avoidance of complications of internal fixation of intertrochanteric fractures. Clin Orthop, 53:47–59, 1967.

206. Sarmiento A: Unstable intertrochanteric fractures of the femur. Clin Orthop, 92:77–85, 1973.

207. Sarmiento A, Williams EM: The unstable intertrochanteric

fracture: treatment with a valgus osteotomy and I-beam nail-plate. J Bone Joint Surg, 52A:1309–1318, 1970.
208. Sartoris DJ, Kerr R, Goergen T, Resnick D: Sliding screw plate fixation of proximal femur fracture: radiographic assessment. (40)
209. Schatzker J, Waddell JP: Subtrochanteric fractures of the femur. Orthop Clin North Am, 11:539–554, 1980.
210. Schneider M: Hip fractures in elderly patients. JAMA 239:106–107, 1978.
211. Schultz RJ: The lesser trochanter as a guide for the operative fixation of hip fractures. Orthop Clin North Am, 5:529–532, 1974.
212. Schumpelick W, Jantzen PM: A new principle in the operative treatment of trochanteric fractures of the femur. J Bone Joint Surg, 37A:693–698, 1955.
213. Seinsheimer F III: Subtrochanteric fractures of the femur. J Bone Joint Surg, 62A:635–645, 1980.
214. Shaftan GW, Herbsman H, Pavlides C: Selective conservatism in hip fractures. Surgery, 61:524–527, 1967.
215. Sherk HH, Crouse FR, Probst C: The treatment of hip fractures in institutionalized patients. Orthop Clin North Am, 5:543–550, 1974.
216. Sherk HH, Foster MD: Hip fracture: condylocephalic rod vs. compression screw. Clin Orthop, 192:255–259, 1985.
217. Siler VE, Caldwell JA: Treatment of intertrochanteric fractures of the femur by modification of Russell balanced traction. Am J Surg, 47:431–442, 1940.
218. Singh M, Nagrath AR, Maini PS: Changes in trabecular pattern of the upper end of the femur as an index of osteoporosis. J Bone Joint Surg, 52A:457–467, 1970.
219. Sisk TD: Fracture of the hip and pelvis. In Crenshaw AH (ed): Campbell's Operative Orthopaedics, 7th ed. St. Louis, Mosby, 1987.
220. Snook GA, Chrisman OD, Wilson TC: Thormboembolism after surgical treatment of hip fracture. Clin Orthop, 155:21–24, 1981.
221. Soballe K, Christensa F: Laceration of the superficial femoral artery by an intertrochanteric fracture fragment. J Bone Joint Surg, 69A:781–782, 1987.
222. Sorenson VK: Comminuted intertrochanteric fracture of the femoral neck. Acta Orthop Scand, 46:651–653, 1975.
223. Speed K: Treatment of fracture of the femur. Arch Surg, 2:45–91, 1921.
224. Stambough JL, Balderston RA, Booth RE, Cohn JC: Conversion total hip replacement: a review of 140 hips over six years follow up. J Arthroplasty, 1:261–269, 1986.
225. Steinberg GG, Desai SS, Kornwitz NA, Sullivan, TJ: The intertrochanteric hip fracture: a retrospective analysis. Orthop 11:265–273, 1988.
226. Stern MB, Goldstein TB: The use of the Leinbach prosthesis in intertrochanteric fractures of the hip. Clin Orthop, 128:325–331, 1977.
227. Stevens DB: Method of operative treatment for intertrochanteric fractures of the femur. Curr Pract Orthop Surg, 7:56–77, 1977.
228. Stover CN, Fish JB, Heap WR: Open reduction of trochanteric fracture. NY State J Med, 71:2173–2181, 1971.
229. Sullivan PE, Markos PD, Minor MAD: An Integrated Approach to Therapeutic Exercise: Theory and Clinical Application. Reston, VA, Reston Publishing, pp 1–100, 1982.
230. Svend-Hansen H, Bremerskov V, Gtrik J, Ostri P:Low dose heparin in proximal femoral fractures: failure to prevent deep-vein thrombosis. Acta Orthop Scand, 52:77–80, 1981.

231. Taylor GM, Neufeld AJ, Nickel VL: Complications and failures in the operative treatment of intertrochanteric fractures of the femur. J Bone Joint Surg, 37A:306–316, 1955.
232. Taylor JC, Russell TA, LaVelle DG, Calandruccia RA: Clinical results in 100 femoral shaft fractures treated with Russell-Taylor interlocking nail system. Proc 54th Annu meet AAOS, San Francisco, p 155, 1987.
233. Tengve B, Kjellander J: Antibiotic prophylaxis in operations on trochanteric femoral fractures. J Bone Joint Surg, 60A:97–99, 1978.
234. Thornton L: The treatment of trochanteric fractures of the femur: two new methods. Piedmont Hosp Bull 10:21, 1937.
235. Tobin WJ: The internal architecture of the femur and its clinical significance. J Bone Joint Surg, 37A:57–72, 1955.
236. Tronzo RG: Hip nails for all occasions. Orthop Clin North Am, 5:479–491, 1974.
237. Tronzo RG: Use of an extramedullary guide pin for fractures of the upper end of the femur. Orthop Clin North Am, 5:525–527, 1974.
238. Tronzo RG: Special considerations in management. Orthop Clin North Am, 5:571–583, 1974.
239. Velasco RU, Comfort TH: Analysis of treatment problems in subtrochanteric fractures of the femur. J Trauma, 18:513–523, 1978.
240. Waddell JP, Czitiom A, Simmons EH: Ender nailing in fractures of the proximal femur. J Trauma, 27:911–916, 1987.
241. Waddell EN: The prevention of deformity in intertrochanteric fractures of the femur. Postgrad Med J, 43:385–399, 1967.
242. Weeden R, Rosenthal H, Miller P: Mortality statistics on fractured hips (1935–1955). J Bone Joint Surgery, 39A:1218, 1957.
243. Weiss NS, et al.: Decreased risk of fractures of the hip and lower forearm with postmenopausal use of estrogen. N Engl J Med, 303:1195–1198, 1980.
244. Weissman SL, Salama R: Trochanteric fractures of the femur. Clin Orthop, 67:143–150, 1969.
245. Wellin DE, Galloni L, Gelb RI: Ipsilateral, intertrochanteric and displaced femoral fractures. Clin Orthop, 183:71–75, 1984.
246. Wilson HJ, et al.: Treatment of intertrochanteric fractures with Jewett nail: experience with 1,015 cases. Clin Orthop, 148:186–191, 1980.
247. Wilson-MacDonald J: Subcapital fracture complication intertrochanteric fracture. Clin Orthop, 201:147–150, 1985.
248. Wolfgang GL, Bryant MH, O'Neill JP: Treatment of intertrochanteric fracture of the femur using sliding screw plate fixation. Clin Orthop, 163:148–158, 1982.
249. Wright LT: Oblique subcervical (reverse intertrochanteric) fractures of the femur. J Bone Joint Surg, 29:707–710, 1947.
250. Zickel RE: An intramedullary fixation device for the proximal part of the femur. J Bone Joint Surg, 58A:866–872, 1976.
251. Zickel RE: Subtrochanteric femoral fractures. Orthop Clin North Am, 11:555–568, 1980.
252. Zickel RE, Mouradian WJ: Intramedullary fixation of pathologic fracture and lesions of the subtrochantic region of the femur. J Bone Joint Surg, 58A:1061–1066, 1976.
253. Zukor DJ, Miller BJ, Hadjipavlou AJ, Lander P: Hip pinning past & present: Richard's compression screw fixation vs. Ender's nailing. Can J Surg 28:391–395, 1985.

PART IV

Clinical Syndromes

Clinical Presentation of Degenerative Joint Disease, Rheumatoid Arthritis, and Avascular Necrosis of the Hip

DAN M. GURBA

The patient who presents for evaluation with a destructive process of the hip joint generally has classic symptoms and physical findings. These classic findings usually are not specific for the underlying cause of the hip disease. Conversely, the associated radiographic changes may provide specific clues regarding the patient's primary problem. This chapter attempts to delineate those points of the patient's evaluation that are common to, and those that are specific for, osteoarthritis, rheumatoid arthritis, and avascular necrosis of the hip.[25]

The most consistent finding in the clinical history of the patient with hip disease is pain. Specifics regarding the location, referral, causative factors, and character of pain may be sufficient for the physician to establish an accurate diagnosis. What a patient describes as "a painful hip," may mean something entirely different to the physician. Every practicing orthopedist understands the axiom "hip pain is back pain until proven otherwise."

The character of the pain may be described by the patient as stabbing, sharp, burning, or simply as a dull deep aching pain. Almost every patient has occasions, either when changing positions or initiating ambulation,[4] that the pain is intense and knife-like.

The tissues about the hip joint that are potential sites of origin for the pain include the synovial membrane, capsule and ligaments; periosteum; and subchondral bone. Normal articular cartilage does not contain innervation throughout its depth. Patients who describe some of the most severe pain include those with an acute inflammatory process such as septic arthritis or those with one of the inflammatory arthropathies. The inflammatory diseases affecting the hip most often include rheumatoid arthritis, juvenile rheumatoid arthritis, ankylosing spondylitis, and psoriatic arthritis. A rapid change in the intensity of the pain may result from the occurrence of the subchondral fracture in avascular necrosis of the femoral head, or the collapse of large osteoarthritic cysts. Any arthritic process that causes an effusion and distention of the joint irritates synovial, capsular, and ligamentous nerve endings. Mechanical events that cause bony collapse or grating of bone more likely irritate periosteal and subchondral nerve endings.

Even more important than the character of the pain is the location of pain about the hip. Accurate identification of the location of the patient's maximal discomfort may be instrumental in determining the correct diagnosis and possibly helping the patient to avoid unnecessary diagnostic studies and therapeutic trials. Certainly, unusual presentations of pain are possible with any pathologic process. Generally, however, a detailed history and careful questioning regarding the location of the patient's pain, combined with the physical examination results in a high probability of correct diagnosis.[28]

Classically, pain originating in the hip joint is located in the groin. The most common referral pattern of this pain is into the anterior and medial aspect of the thigh, to the level of the knee. Pain originating in the hip joint rarely, if ever, extends below the level of the knee. Pain in the area of the buttock and lateral hip only occasionally originates from the hip joint, and that diagnosis should be made only with exclusion of the more common causes of that pain. The actual location of the patient's perceived hip pain may be determined to be in the gluteal area over the ischial tuberosity or at the sacrosciatic notch and secondary to inflammatory processes at those points. If the pain is slightly more lateral in the gluteal area, it may be localized directly at the insertion of the short external rotator muscles, which can be a point of localized tendinitis. The pain may be located laterally over the greater trochanter, and if associated with localized tenderness, usually is secondary to bursitis. Often the patient points to the area of his perceived hip pain directly over the sacroiliac joint. This is rarely a referral point of pain from the hip joint and more likely secondary to musculoligamentous back strain or a referral point of pain from the lumbar annulus. Although knee pain in the area of the adductor tubercle is a common referral site for hip joint disorders, secondary to the course of the obturator nerve, peripatellar, lateral, and medial joint line knee pains are more likely secondary to localized knee disorders. Finally, buttock pain that radiates into the posterior aspect of the thigh, posterolateral aspect of the calf and into the ankle or foot indicates true sciatica of nerve root origin. Although possible, it would be highly unusual for this type of pain to be secondary to sciatic nerve irritation at the level of the hip joint. One other point worth mention, although rare, is that of intense groin pain associated with abdominal symptoms. Involvement of the iliopsoas muscle in intraabdominal or intrapelvic tumors or infection classically refers pain to the groin.

Typically, the motionless and nonweight-bearing hip does not produce pain unless significant inflammation is present. Distension of the hip joint capsule from inflammation is most relieved when the hip joint capsule is at maximal relaxation. This occurs with the hip slightly flexed, abducted, and externally rotated. Passive internal rotation, especially in extension, by decreasing the joint space available and increasing the tension on stretched synovium and capsule, increases pain primarily in the groin region. Any motion that produces tension on the synovium produces discomfort. Pain with standing, walking, and in particular, initiating ambulation, grows in intensity as the hip joint disease progresses. The endstage arthritic hip may produce pain at rest, including awakening the patient from sleep.

Occasionally, because of a high pain threshold, the patient complains more of functional loss of the hip rather than pain. This patient may complain more of "just not being able to walk," but it may be nearly impossible to extract a significant pain history. Routine activities of daily living are usually affected as the disease process progresses. This includes putting on shoes and socks, cutting toenails, and arising from low seated chairs or the bathtub. The patient may have resorted to some type of ambulatory aid, such as a cane, even though he may not have brought it with him at the time of the interview.[2] If the patient's activities of daily

living or ambulation have been significantly affected, the patient still may be a candidate for surgical intervention even though pain may not be the primary complaint.

Finally, a history of substance use or abuse because of hip pain may be significant. Whether the substance is prescription or nonprescription analgesics or alcohol, the ultimate toll on the patient's overall health from these medications can be severe. Even nonprescription analgesic and antiinflammatory medication can cause severe gastric symptoms ultimately requiring further medication, hospitalization, or surgery.

Physical examination of the patient with hip pain begins with the patient walking down the hall to the examining room. In many cases this results in a gait pattern that better resembles the patient's "normal," gait, rather than that performed by the patient when specifically asked by the physician to ambulate in the room. If the patient, in fact, has pain of hip joint origin, he will ambulate with an "antalgic" gait.

The hallmark of an antalgic limp is decreased standing time on the affected limb. To accomplish this, the time that the contralateral leg spends in the swing phase is decreased.[34] One should not be misled by the quick stride of the normal leg as an indication of pain on that side. Conversely, the swing phase of the painful extremity will be slower and shorter. The patient may attempt to ambulate more on the forefoot rather than on the flat foot because of a flexion contracture or because of a subconscious attempt to reduce pain by tightening all muscles of the extremity. In normal ambulation, the pelvis rotates forward on the hip of the extremity in the stance phase approximately 40°. The stiff or painful hip will not allow this normal rotation even though the contralateral normal leg is attempting to take a longer than normal stride during its swing phase. Finally, the painful and weakened hip may demonstrate a positive Trendelenburg sign during stance phase. A positive Trendelenburg sign is demonstrated by the unsupported normal hip dropping below the horizontal during the stance phase on the affected side.[1] This may or may not be compensated for by varying degrees of shift of the upper body toward the affected side during the stance phase. This "abductor lurch" is a subconscious attempt to shift the center of gravity over the affected hip joint, thus reducing the body weight lever arm.[10,24]

The actual physical examination of the patient's hip begins with inspection. Simple observation of the skin may reveal a surgical incision from a previous procedure that the patient has failed to mention. While the patient stands, view the front and rear. The pelvis should be assessed for obliquity secondary to leg length discrepancy. Observation from the side is useful in assessing the degree of lumbar lordosis. An abnormally flat lumbar spine may be secondary to paravertebral muscle spasm from underlying spinal disease. An exaggerated lumbar lordosis, however, may be secondary to a fixed flexion contracture of the hip. The elderly patient with an arthritic hip often is the same patient with degenerative changes of the posterior facet joints of the lumbar spine and spinal stenosis symptoms. A common situation is that of a patient with pain referrable to an arthritic hip and spinal stenosis. The question always arises, "will one operation take care of all components of the pain." The obvious answer is no, however, a hip replacement may partially relieve spinal stenosis symptoms by eliminating the hip flexion contracture that secondarily causes increased lordosis or hyperextension of the lumbar spine. Hyperextension of the lumbar spine usually increases the symptoms of spinal stenosis.

Palpation of the hip joint should be gentle, and as always, proceed from normal to painful areas. Palpation of bony landmarks about the hip with the patient standing should include the anterior superior iliac spine and the iliac crests. This provides yet a more accurate estimation of pelvic obliquity. Likewise, palpation of the greater trochanters with the patient standing should reveal a horizontal and level alignment. A congenital dislocation or proximal femoral disorder may alter this. From posterior, the posterior superior iliac spines are subcutaneous and easily palpable. The ischial tuberosity is somewhat difficult to palpate with the hip in extension, but with flexion, the gluteus maximus moves upward and the tuberosity is easily identifiable. Although the sacroiliac joint is not directly palpable, its center, being at approximately S2, is crossed by a horizontal line connecting the posterior superior iliac spines. A horizontal line connecting the iliac crests identifies the L4-L5 interspinous space.

Soft tissue structures that are palpable about the hip anteriorly include the adductor tendons and the sartorius muscle ridge bordering the femoral triangle. Proximally the inguinal ligament can be palpated between the anterior superior spine and the pubic tubercle. Within the femoral triangle, the femoral artery can be palpated and used as a landmark to identify the location of the femoral nerve laterally and the femoral vein medially. The most medial portion of the femoral triangle should be assessed for enlarged lymph nodes.

Palpation laterally about the hip should always be performed to identify tenderness associated with trochanteric bursitis. Some patients may demonstrate a palpable or audible snapping sensation about the lateral aspect of the hip, generally secondary to a snapping fascia lata. The snapping sensation may or may not be associated with pain, but is often of concern to the patient.

Posteriorly, the sciatic nerve may be palpable midway between the greater trochanter and the ischial tuberosity with the hip flexed. Tenderness of the nerve with gentle palpation may be caused by lumbar disc disease, piriformis, tendinitis, or direct injury to the nerve, such as a contusion from a fall or an injection. Occasionally patients may have tenderness directly over the ischial tuberosity secondary to bursitis in that area.

Passive range of motion should be assessed with the patient in the supine position. If possible, the range of motion should first be examined on the uninvolved side in an effort to determine what is normal for the patient. The Thomas test is useful for identifying fixed flexion contractures of the hip. With the normal hip maximally flexed, lumbar lordosis is eliminated, as is any pelvic tilt that allows a diseased hip to appear to be in full extension. The diseased hip with a fixed flexion deformity will be elevated from the examining table, and the degree of fixed flexion deformity can be estimated by observation from the side of the patient.[16] Normal flexion of the hip should be further possible to 120°. With the patient supine and the hip in extension, abduction should be possible to 50°. With slight flexion of the hip, adduction can be measured in the same position and should be possible to approximately 25°. All measurements should be made with one hand on the pelvis to assure that the motion is not being produced in the lumbar spine. Approximately 35° of internal rotation and 45° of external rotation should be possible with the hip in extension, as well as in 90° of flexion. In extension, this estimation is made by observing the position of the patella, and in flexion, by observing the direction of the tibial shaft with reference to the neutral position. Regardless of the cause of hip joint disease, the motions most and earliest affected are that of internal rotation and abduction.

An attempt should be made to assess the strength of the flexor, extensor, abductor, and adductor muscle groups about the hip, even though they may be significantly limited by pain. The iliopsoas, as the primary hip flexor, is innervated by the femoral nerve and lumbar nerve roots 1 through 3. The primary hip extensor is the gluteus maximus muscle, which is innervated by the inferior gluteal nerve from the first sacral nerve root. The gluteus medius muscle is the primary abductor and is innervated by the superior gluteal nerve of L5 nerve root origin. Although there are many adductors of the hip, the adductor longus is the primary muscle and is innervated by the obturator nerve from the second through fourth lumbar nerve roots.

Sensory testing about the hip and thigh may be useful for identifying a dermatome loss indicating spinal nerve root disease. Likewise, numbness or pain in the distribution of the lateral femoral cutaneous nerve may be secondary to meralgia paresthetica and no underlying hip joint pathology.

Reflex and muscle strength evaluation, as well as pulse examination of the remainder of the extremity, are critical in identifying underlying neurologic or vascular abnormalities.

Abnormalities in other bones or joints of the affected limb, should be assessed. The patient with an awkward gait secondary to a painful hallux valgus can certainly present with lateral hip pain because of tendinitis and bursitis about the greater trochanter.

An estimation of the patient's leg lengths can be made by observing pelvic obliquity with the patient standing, but if any length discrepancy is perceived, a measurement of the true leg lengths from the anterior superior iliac spines to the medial malleoli should be made.

To assess whether the patient with the diseased hip is a candidate for hip joint replacement surgery, all of the above historic and physical data, as well as radiographic findings are pertinent. The Medicare program has recently established precertification review criteria for performance of total hip replacement. The indications for surgery include: (1) A reasonable surgical risk and reasonable expectation for improvement (The procedure should allow for improvement in quality of life for the patient by at least a reduction in pain if not an increase in the patient's activity level. The ideal situation is when the patient's activity can be increased to the point that he can remain independent and out of long-term care facilities). (2) The patient's history should include chronic pain for at least 6 months duration and a failure of conservative treatment during that time. The conservative treatment can include the use of ambulatory aids, such as a cane, medication, injection, and physical therapy. Bracing is mentioned as a conservative treatment, although not particularly useful at the hip joint. (3) Has the hip disease produced disability or incapacity causing significant interference with the performance of activities of daily living, such as arising from a chair, dressing, or personal hygiene?

(4) The physical examination of the patient should demonstrate a limitation of motion in the hip joint, and the patient should have an observable limp. (5) The patient should demonstrate radiographic evidence of significant hip joint narrowing or irregularity with osteophyte, sclerotic subchondral bone, or cystic formation.

To this point, the clinical history and physical examination of the patient with a painful hip have been discussed without regard to specific cause. Specific clinical and radiographic findings in osteoarthritis, rheumatoid arthritis, and avascular necrosis are addressed in the following sections.

The pattern of pain in the patient with osteoarthritis of the hip is that of a gradual increase in both the intensity and duration of repeated attacks.[20] It is not unusual for the patient at his or her baseline activity to remain relatively pain free, but to initiate an "attack" of pain by overuse. The amount of "overuse" necessary to produce the "attack" obviously decreases with progression of the disease. Even in the relatively pain free state, most patients complain of a stiffness about the hip that "loosens up" with a short period of walking. In the ensuing months to years, pain initially increases, but may actually decrease late in the disease process as motion becomes severely restricted.[21] The pain of the osteoarthritic hip can be located anteriorly, laterally, or posteriorly, and is commonly referred along the anterior and medial aspect of the thigh toward the inner aspect of the knee.[1] It nearly always is aggravated by walking and movement to the extremes of motion.[22] Nearly all patients with osteoarthritic hips are atuned to weather changes, thus the term "barometric joint." After an acute attack of pain secondary to overuse, most patients improve by rest, moist heat, and anti-inflammatory medication.

Many patients complain of a "crackling" or "creaking" sensation about the hip that may be reproduced at the time of physical examination.[22] This crepitation is usually associated with some degree of pain.

As significant changes begin to occur in the hip joint, patients begin to notice a gait disturbance in themselves. Typically, it may be noticed first with walking on uneven terrain or attempting to walk with increased speed. As previously mentioned, the limp and associated decreased walking endurance may be of more concern to the patient than the actual pain. Although the patient may "put up with the pain," the decreased walking ability may threaten the patient's primary form of exercise and potentially his independence. The elderly patient who becomes unable to walk to the grocery store, get up from a chair without assistance, or put on his own socks and shoes faces the possibility of institutionalization (Fig. 12–1).

At the time of physical examination, muscle spasm and tenderness about the hip joint may be difficult to elicit, but loss in motion can nearly always be demonstrated. The hip commonly is held in flexion, adduction, and external rotation at the time of examination. A hip flexion contracture may be identified by the Thomas test as previously described. Loss of internal rotation is essentially always present early in the disease process, and attempted internal rotation, at the time of physical examination, usually causes groin pain. A leg length discrepancy may or may not be present, depending on the degree of disease at the joint.

It may be difficult to correlate the degree of the patient's pain with the radiographic appearance of the hip. Loss of range of motion is better correlated with the degree of osteocartilaginous destruction on the x-ray. The patient that presents relatively early with minor pain and minimal radiographic changes often asks about the quickness of the disease's progression. The rate of progression of the clinical and radiographic findings in osteoarthritis of the hip are extremely variable. Furthermore, preventative measures to slow the rate of progression, such as anti-inflammatory medication and curtailment of activity, have not been shown to be effective. Limitation of weight-bearing on the hip, by either weight reduction or the use of a cane in the contralateral hand, are at least beneficial in relieving symptoms. Weight reduction in the obese patient empirically seems to prolong the arthritic hip, although hard data is not available to support this.

Osteoarthritis of the hip may be primary, or secondary to an underlying cause as listed in Table 12–1.[27,12,33] The radiographic findings in secondary forms of osteoarthritis are too lengthy to discuss at this juncture, and the reader is referred to other sources.[30]

In primary osteoarthritis (Figs. 12–2 to 12–4), joint space narrowing and subchondral sclerosis appear concomitantly and early. Often this occurs first inferior medially, but may occur superiorly in the weight-bearing area. Marginal osteophytes occur early at the inferior portion of the femoral head. As the disease progresses and the joint space continues to narrow superiorly, collapse of subchondral bone may occur without the appearance of the subchondral fracture line of osteonecrosis. As the femoral head flattens, cysts may develop within the subchondral bone of the femoral head and the acetabulum, primarily in the weight-bearing areas.

The clinical presentation of rheumatoid arthritis of the hip usually follows previous diagnosis of the disease process. The vast majority of patients develop the initial symptoms of rheumatoid arthritis insidiously over weeks to months. The initial symptoms may be systemic or articular. Systemic symptoms include fatigue, malaise, or a diffuse musculoskeletal pain. The articular presentation is classically symmetric. Morning stiffness is a classic complaint and probably associated with the accumulation of edema within the inflamed tissue at sleep. Weakness in activities of daily living secondary to muscle atrophy around affected joints may be noticed by the patient.[29] Up to one-third of patients with rheumatoid arthritis may develop symptoms more rapidly. Even so, rarely can a patient pinpoint a specific time when his pain developed, as can some patients with osteonecrosis.

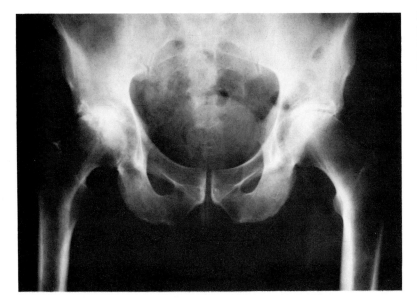

FIG. 12–1. Superomedial osteoarthritis in a 71-year-old male with classic pain distribution, stiffness, and a limp. The bilateral "pistol-grip" deformities are most likely secondary to mild unrecognized slipped capital femoral epiphyses.

TABLE 12–1. *Causes of Secondary Osteoarthritis*

Systemic metabolic diseases
   Hemachromatosis
   Wilson's disease
   Ochronosis
   Gaucher's disease
Hemoglobinopathies
   Sickle cell disease
   Thalassemia
Endocrine diseases
   Acromegaly
   Hyperparathyroidism
Bone dysplasias
   Multiple epiphyseal dysplasia
   Spondyloepiphyseal dysplasia
   Osteopetrosis
   Engelmann's disease
Crystal deposition diseases
   Pseudogout
   Apatite crystal deposition disease
Inflammatory diseases
   Rheumatoid arthritis
   Juvenile rheumatoid arthritis
   Ankylosing spondylitis
   Psoriatic arthritis
   Reiter's syndrome
   Pigmented villonodular synovitis
Miscellaneous
   Hemophilic arthropathy
   Neuropathic arthropathy
   Poliomyelitis
   Intra-articular labrum
   Femoral anteversion
   Paget's disease
   Osteonecrosis (systemic lupus erythematosus)
Local Disorders
   Pyogenic arthritis
   Tuberculosis arthritis
   Metastatic disease
   Traumatic arthritis
   Congenital dislocated hip
   Legg-Calve-Perthes disease
   Slipped capital femoral epiphysis
   Congenital dysplasia
"Pistol-grip" deformity

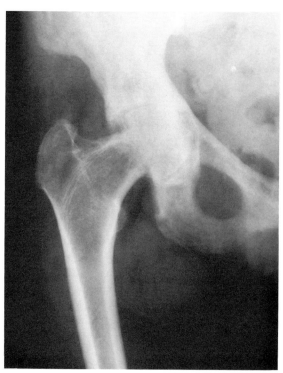

FIG. 12–2. A 65-year-old female with a pagetoid hemipelvis, coxa vara, medial osteoarthritis, and developing protrusio acetabuli.

The joints most commonly involved in rheumatoid arthritis are the metacarpal phalangeal joints, proximal interphalangeal joints, and the wrists. In general, larger joints become symptomatic after smaller joints. For this reason, most patients that present to the orthopedist with rheumatoid arthritis of the hip have previously been medically evaluated and have met the criteria for establishing the diagnosis of rheumatoid arthritis.[18]

When the patient with rheumatoid arthritis does develop hip involvement, the pain and functional limitations can be severe. A radiographic study of seropositive rheumatoid arthritis patients has shown hip disease in approximately 50%.[5] The location of pain classically is in the groin and may extend into the anteromedial thigh. With any significant involvement, the limitation of motion of the hip joint in rheumatoid arthritis is usually more severe than that found in other disease processes. Specifically, flexion and adduction contractures can be so severe that personal hygiene is impossible. Because of multiple joint involvement, the classic antalgic gait of hip joint disease may not be apparent (Fig. 12–5).

Radiographic findings in rheumatoid arthritis of the hip classically demonstrate concentric narrowing of the articular cartilage with less subchondral sclerosis and more juxta-articular osteopenia. Cystic formation in the subchondral area of the femoral head and the acetabulum are classic in rheumatoid disease and all forms of inflammatory arthritis. As in osteoarthritis, progression of the radiographic changes may be rapid or slow.[13] Occasionally, the patient presents with complete destruction of the joint space and superior portion of the femoral head in a short period of time.[3] This may result from a combination of the rheumatoid process and osteonecrosis secondary to steroid therapy (Fig. 12–6).

In summary, the diagnosis of rheumatoid arthritis is rarely made in a patient at the time of presentation for hip pain only. When the patient with rheumatoid arthritis does present with hip joint disorders, the overall evaluation of the patient with regard to systemic and multiple joint involvement

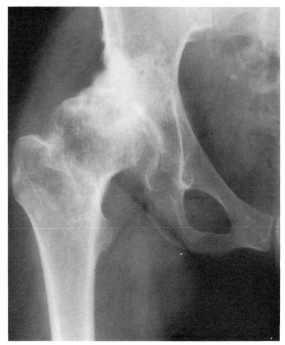

FIG. 12–3. A 35-year-old female with known Legg-Perthes disease and resultant coxa magna, a shortened femoral neck, and superolateral arthritis. The patient has developed not only groin pain, but also lateral hip and gluteal pain, possibly caused by the subluxation.

is critical when discussing treatment options. Evaluation of the stability of the cervical spine is important when considering anesthesia. When considering surgical replacement of the hip, the status of the upper extremities is critical in the postoperative period for protected weight-bearing. The range of motion and function of the knees, ankles, feet, and contralateral hip are critical to the postopera-

tive rehabilitation in the patient with the arthritic hip.

The patient with osteonecrosis of the hip usually presents with nonspecific clinical signs and symptoms.[7,31] Occasionally, the diagnosis may be made while the patient remains totally asymptomatic. More commonly, as in most causes of hip disease, the initial complaint usually is pain. Even when the primary complaint of the patient is pain at the time of presentation, radiographic changes on plain x-rays may not be present. The initial onset of pain without radiographic changes may be secondary to tissue ischemia, increased osseous pressure, or microfractures within the avascular area.[8,9] Radiographic changes may lag the onset of pain by up to 6 months.

Patients with osteonecrosis of the hip generally present in their thirties or forties. Given a predisposing factor, presentations in younger and older age groups also are common. Seventy percent of patients are male and over 50% will develop bilateral disease by 2 years. The most common predisposing factors are a history of relatively high dose steroid administration or alcohol ingestion (Fig. 12–7).[19] Other less common conditions associated with osteonecrosis of the femoral head are listed in Table 12–2.[15,17]

The physical findings in the patient with osteonecrosis, like the description of pain, are generally nonspecific. Very early in the course of the disease, motion may be preserved, unlike the early osteoarthritic hip, in which decreased motion is an early finding. A limp and decreased range of motion generally develop late in the disease process as joint destruction occurs.

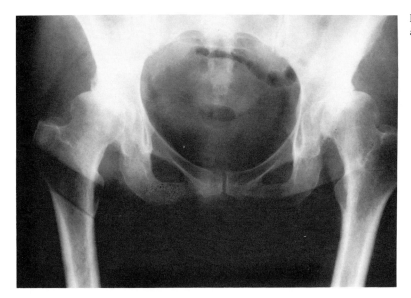

FIG. 12–4. A 62-year-old female with dysplastic acetabuli and superolateral osteoarthritis.

FIG. 12–5. A 25-year-old female with juvenile rheumatoid arthritis and incapacitating groin and knee pain. Upper extremities, ankles, and feet have been spared.

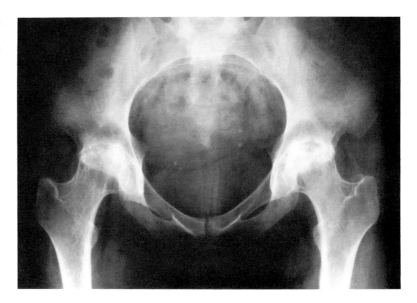

The patient with osteonecrosis usually develops symptoms insidiously, but occasionally may be able to remember a specific time when his or her hip pain began. This is in contrast to the osteoarthritic or rheumatoid patient whose histories are routinely of an insidious onset. The acute onset of pain may represent the actual avascular event, the development of a subchondral fracture line, or the collapse of subchondral bone into an avascular area. If the patient presents with an acute onset of true groin pain, but the plain radiographs are unremarkable, osteonecrosis of the femoral head must be

TABLE 12–2. *Conditions Less Commonly Associated with Osteonecrosis of the Femoral Head*

1. Chronic liver disease
2. Renal transplantation
3. Collagen vascular disorders
4. Sickle cell disease
5. Pancreatitis
6. Metabollic bone disease
7. Hyperlipidemias
8. Pregnancy
9. Gaucher's disease
10. Radiation
11. Ileitis and colitis

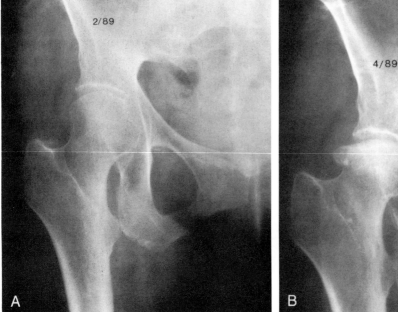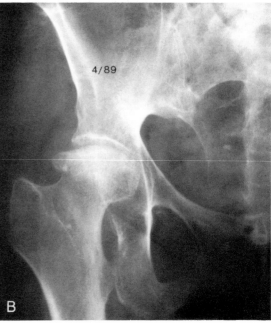

FIG. 12–6A,B. A 52-year-old patient with severe rheumatoid arthritis and a long history of steroid use. The femoral head underwent rapid and severe collapse of an avascular area of porotic bone.

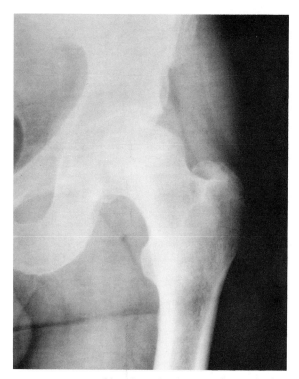

Fɪɢ. **12–7.** A 61-year-old male with a history of steroid administration for lymphoma. Pain developed at the time of collapse in the groin and anterior thigh.

ruled out with either a bone scan or MRI scan.[14,26] When the patient with an acute onset of groin pain presents with obvious early radiographic evidence of osteonecrosis, protected weight-bearing becomes important not only for pain relief, but also for potential prevention of collapse. A complete discussion of treatment options for the various stages of osteonecrosis is not within the scope of this chapter. A recognition of the clinical and radiographic

staging is important, however, in the patient's clinical presentation.

The two most commonly used clinical and radiographic staging systems for avascular necrosis of the femoral head are those proposed by Ficat and Steinberg (Tables 12–3 and 12–4).[6,32] As noted in the previous staging systems, one of the earliest radiographic changes is that of increased density in the superior lateral portion of the femoral head. This sclerosis is partially because of disuse osteoporosis of the adjacent vascularized bone in the femoral neck region. A portion of the sclerosis also is caused by the healing process, in which new living bone is layed down on avascular trabeculae. Only slightly later in the same stage of the disease, large areas of segmental collapse may lead to mechanically compressed and radiographically more dense bone. Depending on the amount of collapse, a cyst will develop and may be large. Within this radiolucent or "cystic area" will be found granulation tissue with active bone resorption and deposition (Fig. 12–8).

In Stage III, as defined by the Steinberg system, the femoral head remains spherical, but a radiolucent line (crescent sign) is noted immediately below the subchondral bone of the avascular area. Whether or not the patient has been symptomatic to this point, the collapse of dead cancellous bone and development of the subchondral fracture may initiate or exacerbate symptoms (Fig. 12–9).

Although it is possible at this point for the femoral head to undergo a perfect healing response, the usual course is that for progression to Stages IV through VI. Specifically, the superior weight-bearing surface collapses into the necrotic area. Although early after the collapse, the articular cartilage is un-

TABLE **12–3.** *Ficat Staging System*

Stage	Clinical Features	Radiographic Signs	Haemodynamics	Scintigram	Diagnosis Without Core Biopsy
Early					
0 Preclinical	0	0	+	Reduced uptake?	Impossible
I Preradiographic	+	0	+ +	Increased uptake	Impossible
II Before flattening of head or sequestrum formation	+	Diffuse perosis, sclerosis, or cysts	+ +	+	Probable
Transition		Flattening Crescent sign			
Late					
III Collapse	+ +	Broken contour of head Sequestrum Joint space normal	+ or normal	+	Certain
IV Osteoarthritis	+ + +	Flattened contour Decreased joint space Collapse of head	+	+	Arthritis

Tᴀʙʟᴇ 12–4. *Steinberg Staging System*

Stage 0	Normal roentgenogram, normal bone scan
Stage I	Normal roentgenogram, abnormal bone scan
Stage II	Sclerosis and/or cyst formation in femoral head
	A. Mild (less than 20%)
	B. Moderate (20 to 40%)
	C. Severe (greater than 40%)
Stage III	Subchondral collapse (crescent sign) without flattening
	A. Mild (less than 15%)
	B. Moderate (15 to 30%)
	C. Severe (greater than 30%)
Stage IV	Flattening of head without joint narrowing or acetabular involvement
	A. Mild (less than 15% of surface and less than 2 mm. depression)
	B. Moderate (15 to 30% of surface or 2 to 4 mm depression)
	C. Severe (greater than 30% of surface or greater than 4 mm depression)
Stage V	Flattening of head with joint narrowing or acetabular involvement
	A. Mild (determined as above plus estimate of acetabular involvement)
	B. Moderate
	C. Severe
Stage VI	Advanced degenerative changes

involved, the irregularity of subchondral bone ultimately leads to joint space destruction and advancing osteoarthritis. As in any disease process, the history and physical examination are critical in establishing a correct diagnosis of the cause of hip pain. An accurate description of the exact location of the pain by the patient generally determines if, in fact, the pain originates in the hip joint. Although not as definitive, a description of the quality of the pain and its mode of onset may be useful in delineating the cause of the hip disease. Radiographic evaluation will then confirm the presence of hip joint disease which, in most cases, has already been established by the clinical presentation. The radiographic evaluation is more useful in delineating the exact cause, i.e., degenerative joint

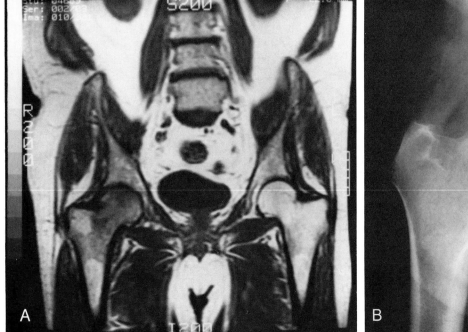
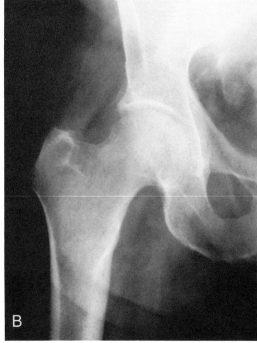

Fɪɢ. 12–8A,B. A 53-year-old male with right groin, anterior thigh, and knee pain of acute onset. Despite minimal changes on the plain radiograph, the MRI demonstrates dramatically decreased signal intensity in the right femoral head.

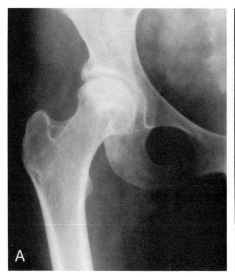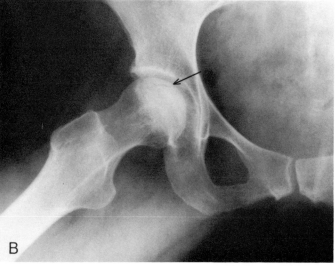

Fɪɢ. 12–9A,B. A 38-year-old female with osteonecrosis and a large cystic area. Pain was temporarily relieved by core decompression and the lucent area is denser. Pain redeveloped when the subchondral fracture developed six months later and showed no signs of healing.

disease, rheumatoid arthritis, or avascular necrosis. Only after the presence of hip disease is established and the cause determined, can an appropriate treatment be recommended based on the patient's level of disability.

References

1. Aᴍsᴛᴜᴛᴢ HC, Kɪᴍ WC: Osteoarthritis of the hip. *In* Moskowitz RW, Howell DS, Goldberg VM, Mankin HJ (eds.): Osteoarthritis: Diagnosis and Management. Philadelphia, Saunders, pp. 423–442, 1984.
2. Bʟᴏᴜɴᴛ WP: Don't throw away the cane. J Bone Joint Surg, 38A:695, 1956.
3. Cᴏʟᴛᴏɴ C, Dᴀʀʙʏ A: Giant granulomatous lesions of the femoral head and neck in rheumatoid arthritis. Ann Rheum Dis, 29:626, 1970.
4. Cᴏᴏᴋᴇ TD, Dᴡᴏsʜ IL: Clinical features of osteoarthritis in the elderly. Clin Rheum Dis, 12:155, 1986.
5. Dᴜᴛʜɪᴇ R, Hᴀʀʀɪs C: A radiographic and clinical survey of the hip joints in sero-positive rheumatoid arthritis. Acta Orthop Scand, 40:346, 1969.
6. Fɪᴄᴀᴛ RP: Idiopathic bone necrosis of the femoral head. J Bone Joint Surg, 67B:3, 1985.
7. Gʟɪᴍᴄʜᴇʀ JJ, Kᴇɴᴢᴏʀᴀ JE: Osteonecrosis: the pathobiology, clinical manifestations, therapeutic dilemmas, instructional course 103. Annual Meeting, American Academy of Orthopaedic Surgeons, Atlanta, 1980.
8. Gʟɪᴍᴄʜᴇʀ MJ, Kᴇɴᴢᴏʀᴀ JE: The biology of osteonecrosis of the human femoral head and its clinical implications. II. The pathological changes in the femoral head as an organ and in the hip joint. Clin Orthop, 139:283, 1979.
9. Gʟɪᴍᴄʜᴇʀ JJ, Kᴇɴᴢᴏʀᴀ JE: The biology of osteonecrosis of the human femoral head and its clinical implications. III. Discussion of the etiology and genesis of the pathological sequelae, comments on treatment. Clin Orthop, 140:273, 1979.
10. Gʀᴇᴇɴᴡᴀʟᴅ AS, Nᴇʟsᴏɴ CL: Biomechanics of the reconstructed hip. Orthop Clin North Am, 4:435, 1973.
11. Gʀᴜᴇʙᴇʟ Lᴇᴇ DM: Disorders of the Hip. Philadelphia, Lippincott, 1983.
12. Hᴀʀʀɪs WH: Etiology of osteoarthritis of the hip. Clin Orthop, 213:20, 1986.
13. Hᴀsᴛɪɴɢs DE, Pᴀʀᴋᴇʀ SM: Protrusio acetabuli in rheumatoid arthritis. Clin Orthop, 108:76, 1975.
14. Hᴀᴜᴢᴇᴜʀ JP, et al.: The diagnostic value of magnetic resonance imaging in non-traumatic osteonecrosis of the femoral head. J Bone Joint Surg, 71A #5:641. June, 1989.
15. Hᴇʀɴᴅᴏɴ JH, Aᴜғʀᴀɴᴄ OE: Avascular necrosis of the head: a review of its incidence in a variety of conditions. Clin Orthop, 86:43–62, 1972.
16. Hᴏᴘᴘᴇɴғᴇʟᴅ A: Physical examination of the hip and pelvis. *In* Hoppenfeld S (ed): Physical Examination of the Spine and Extremities. New York, Appleton-Century-Crofts, 1976.
17. Hᴜɴɢᴇʀғᴏʀᴅ DS (ᴇᴅ): Ischemia and Necrosis of Bone. Baltimore, Williams & Wilkins, 1980.
18. Hᴜʀᴅ ER: Estra-articular manifestations of arthritis. Semin Arthritis Rheum, 8:151–176, 1979.
19. Iᴛᴀʏ S, Hᴏʀᴏᴢᴏᴡsᴋɪ H, Isʀᴀᴇʟɪ A: Corticosteroid induced osteonecrosis of femoral head. Orthop Rev, 13:59–65, 1984.
20. Lᴀᴡʀᴇɴᴄᴇ JS, Bʀᴇᴍɴᴇʀ JM, Bɪᴇʀ F: Osteoarthrosis: prevalence in the population and relationship between symptoms and x-ray changes. Ann Rheum Dis, 25:1, 1966.
21. Mᴀᴄʏs JR, Bᴜʟʟᴏᴜɢʜ PG, Wɪʟsᴏɴ PD Jʀ: Coxarthrosis: a study of the natural history based on correlation of clinical, radiographic, and pathologic findings. Semin Arthritis Rheum, 10:66–80, 1980.
22. Mᴏsᴋᴏᴡɪᴛᴢ RW: Osteoarthritis—signs and symptoms. *In* Moskowitz RW, Howell DS, Goldberg VM, Mankin HJ (eds): Osteoarthritis: Diagnosis and Management. Philadelphia, Saunders, pp. 149–154, 1984.
23. Nɪʟssᴏ BE, Dᴀɴɪᴇʟssᴏɴ LB, Hᴇʀɴʙᴏʀɢ SA: Clinical features and natural course of coxarthrosis and gonarthrosis. Scand J Rheumatol, 43:12, 1982.
24. Pᴀᴜᴡᴇʟs R: Biomechanics of the Normal and Diseased Hip. Berlin, Springer-Verlag, 1976.
25. Pᴏʟʟᴇʏ HF, Hᴜɴᴅᴇʀ GG: Rheumatologic Interviewing and

Physical Examination of Joints. Philadelphia, Saunders, 1978.

26. Robinson HJ Jr, Hartleen P, Lund G, Schreiman J: Evaluation of magnetic resonance imaging in diagnosis of osteonecrosis of the femoral head. J Bone Joint Surg, 71A:650, 1989.

27. Schumacher HR: Secondary osteoarthritis. *In* Moskowitz RW, Howell DS, Goldberg VM, Mankin HJ (eds): Osteoarthritis: Diagnosis and Management. Philadelphia, Saunders, pp. 235–264, 1984.

28. Sculco TP: Hip pain. *In* Beary JF, Christian CL, Sculco TP (eds): Manual of Rheumatology and Outpatient Orthopedic Disorders. Boston, Little, Brown, 1981.

29. Short CL, Bauer W, Reynolds WS: Rheumatoid Arthritis. Cambridge, Harvard University Press, 1957.

30. Solomon L: Patterns of osteoarthritis of the hip. J Bone Joint Surg, 58(B):176–185, 1976.

31. Steinberg ME: Avascular necrosis of the femoral head. *In* Tronzo RG (ed): Surgery of the Hip Joint, Vol. 2. New York, Springer-Verlag, pp. 1–20, 1987.

32. Steinberg ME, et al.: Treatment of avascular necrosis of the femoral head by a combination of bone grafting, decompression, and electrical stimulation. Clin Ortho, 186:137, 1984.

33. Stulberg SD: The etiology and natural course of osteoarthritis of the hip (coxarthritis). *In* Moskowitz, RW, Howell DS, Goldberg VM, Mankin HJ (eds): Osteoarthritis: Diagnosis and Management. Philadelphia, Saunders, pp. 265–274, 1984.

34. Waters RL et al.: The energy cost of walking with arthritis of the hip and knee. Clin Orthop, 214:278, 1987.

CHAPTER THIRTEEN

Hip Fracture

ERIC L. HUME

Scope of the Problem

With the aging of the American population, metabolic bone disease is and will continue to be important to our patients and to our socioeconomic system. By age 75, one-fourth of Caucasion women will have osteoporosis as determined by measurement of bone density.

Osteoporosis is classified by location of fracture. Osteoporotic spinal compression fractures have the highest incidence in postmenopausal women and cause significant morbidity. The economic cost, however, is limited because most of these patients can be managed as outpatients or with a short hospitalization followed by return to the home.

In absolute numbers, hip fractures have a lower incidence; morbidity, mortality, and cost of the hip fracture care is huge. Holbrook[26] states, that in 1984, hip fracture care cost $7.2 billion; 4 billion dollars, of which was nursing home costs. The aging of our population will increase these costs. Phillips[45] quotes estimates of 29.2 million people age 65 or older in the United States with projections up to 34.9 million by the year 2000. Kreiger[32] shows an annual fracture incidence of approximately five fractures per 1000 for people 70 to 74 years old, and over 30 fractures per 1000 in those over 85. Caucasian women over the age of 50 have approximately 15% lifetime risk of hip fractures. Patients who suffer hip fractures have a 12 to 20% increased risk of death in the first year after hip fracture, and another 15 to 25% of these patients remain in long-term care facilities for at least one year after the fracture. Phillips,[45] in 1986, showed that for women with only hip fractures accounted for 83,000 nursing home stays, representing approximately 74% of all stays.

In a recent study,[74] 241 hip fracture patients were followed for 2 years, with a 21.6% mortality rate for the overall group, 8% mortality rate for the low risk group, and 49.5% mortality rate for those at high risk. This average mortality of high risk patients was six times the risk for the elderly population. After the first year post hip fracture, the mortality rate went back to that of the age-matched population. A higher standard mortality ratio correlated with more severe osteoporosis as measured by the Singh grading, and with an ASA (American Society of Anesthesia) Class 3 or 4 (high risk). Although hip fractures make up the overall smaller percentage of the fractures of osteoporosis, they represent a serious risk to the patient and a high cost to society. It is the significant morbidity and mortality which makes this fracture a tremendously important issue.[62]

Risk Factors

Several basic issues can be identified as risk factors for hip fracture. Epidemiologic studies show the difficulty of assessing hip fracture risk.[72] First, bone substance loss undoubtedly makes bones weaker. Bone loss, called osteoporosis, has been recognized since the 1940s when Albright first described the osteopenia occurring with the loss of ovarian function. Second, bone quality can vary. Dense bone does not equate with strong bone. The classic example is Paget's disease. In Paget's disease, unusually dense bone may be fragile and susceptible to pathologic fracture. Some concern exists that sodium fluoride treatment, used for spinal osteoporosis, may contribute to cortical bone fragility and may increase the incidence of long bone fractures. Third, neuromuscular coordination and muscle conditioning are important factors in the incidence in falls and the rate of fracture from a fall. Decreased neuromuscular coordination increases the likelihood of a fall. Further, poor coordination and strength interfere with a patient's ability to safely absorb the energy of a fall and protect long bones from fractures.

Bone Density

Mechanical testing has evaluated the effect of bone loss on fracture strength of the hip. The absolute amount of bone predicts the in vitro hip fracture strength and energy. Accurate in vivo bone densitometry methods exist, which are potentially clinically useful for screening. If these in vivo bone density measurements correlate well with in vitro measurements, screening could be used to recommend treatment. Unfortunately, bone density measurements predict patient fracture rates with less accuracy[38] than in vitro measurements predict hip fracture force and energy.

In 1955, W.J. Tobin[70] summarized the historic background of the osteology of the upper end of the femur. He defined the primary and secondary compression and tension trabecula and quoted Wards description of the Wards triangle. Singh[63] observed decreasing the number of trabecula in osteoporosis and advanced a roentgenographic classification based on the primary and secondary compression and tension trabecula. Singh described a system that ranges from 1 for severe bone loss to 6 for normal trabecula. He discussed the difficulties of accurately measuring the amount of osteoporosis. This system continues to be used to describe severity of hip bone loss. Cooper reported the good correlation of Singh index and hip fracture risk for a population less than 75 years of age. He believes the poor correlation among older patients implies the risk of falls and falling becomes the critical issue.[9] Dequeker[15] pointed out the difficulty of using the Singh system to predict spine fractures. In his series of 14 femoral neck fractures, all patients were 3 years old or less. There was only a 50% incidence of a low Singh grade associated with a vertebral collapse.

Dolen,[16] in 1976, measured mechanical strength and x-ray spectrophotometry of 61 autopsied femoral neck specimens. The coefficient of correlation was 0.89 comparing the bone mineral content of the femoral neck with the ultimate fracture force. Leichter[35] measured bone mineral density by commercial bone photometer, Compton's scattering, and Singh index, and correlated these densities to strength. Bone mineral and strength gave a regression coefficient of 0.68. Singh index and strength was significant, but with regression coefficient of 0.49. None of the bone mass measurements agreed with the fracture energy. This study found a strong correlation between ultimate strength and cancellous bone density, as measured by Compton's scattering. Carter and Hayes[7] also showed the compressive behavior of bone as a two-phase structure to be function of density.

Studies continue to look for noninvasive methods of predicting a fracture risk. Dual energy radiography and quantitative CT have been evaluated.

In a cadaver study Sartoris[60] showed a correlation of 0.54 for femoral neck fracture force and density. When he studied a clinical population, he showed decreased femoral neck mineral content with increased age, increased femoral neck mineral content in taller and heavier subjects, and no relationship between femoral neck mineral content and spinal compression fractures or Singh index.

Lotz and Hayes[37] studied 12 cadavers by quantitative computer tomography (QCT) and mechanical testing. They showed an excellent correlation of fracture load with total bone in the intertrochanteric area ($R^2 = 0.93$). However, they noted that the cadaver hip fracture work was one-tenth the energy available during a nontraumatic fall, typical of falls around the home. Although they demonstrated excellent correlation of bone strength and QCT measurement, they point out that the risk of falling and inability to break the fall may be more important than osteoporosis.

Correlation between bone density and fracture rate also has been investigated. Elsasser[17] compared 32 fracture patients with 28 age-matched controls and found the best correlation via the trabecula bone of the distal radius. Methods that measure bone distribution rather than mass may be the most accurate for predicting fracture rate. Portigliatti-Barbos[47] used polarized light microscopy to demonstrate the relative ratio of transverse to longitudinal lamellae. This method proved to be a useful way to evaluate trabecular alignment.

Fazzalari[18] did a histologic analysis of trabecular bone in surgical specimens from hip arthroplasties done for osteoarthritis and for femoral neck fractures. The bone mineral content of the osteoarthritic patients and fractured neck patients was equal. Trabeculae were thinner in the fractured patients. However, trabecular spacing in the fractured patients was more like the controls than the large spacing of the osteoarthritic patients. The effect of disuse may affect the results in the femoral neck in arthritic patients because of pain. The fractured hips showed no significance for thickness compared to controls. Cornell,[11] et al., compared consecutive hip fracture patients with the age-matched control and found no correlation between dual photon absorptiometry and histology.

Cummings[13] reviewed 15 controlled case studies. He concluded that most vigorous studies demonstrated less bone mass in the hip fracture patients, but in this review the differences were small and two populations overlapping. He also concluded from this review that tendency to fall may be more important than bone mass in predicting risk for hip fractures.

Ross[50] reviewed new papers as well as the papers that Cummings reviewed. He concluded that reduced bone mass is associated with increased risk of fracture. He pointed out that the cross-sectional study was affected by the subject selection or by postfracture bone loss caused by disuse. He recommended reliance on the results of prospective studies with care for subject selection. Ross calculated risk ratios for hip fractures and found increased risk for hip fracture based on wrist and hip bone mass. His analysis included an article by Cummings,[12] who studied prospectively 9703 women age 65 and older with a 1.6 year followup. These patients had 53 fractures. Fracture risk was inversely related to bone density measurements of the calcaneus, distal radius, and proximal radius; the risk of hip fracture doubled in each decade. Bone loss was associated with fracture risk, but other factors were clearly operative in the risk of hip fractures in elderly women.

Bone Quality

Bone quality is related to a fracture. The most obvious clinical example is fracture of bones in Paget's disease. Patients with Paget's disease who have significantly increased pathologic bone density undergo fractures with relatively minor trauma. Paget's disease is an extreme example of the difficulty in predicting fracture risk based on bone mass alone. This example demonstrates the concept that the quality of bone affects bone strength, and may help explain the disparity in prediction value between in vitro and in vivo mineral content studies of femoral fracture strength.

This bone quality concept becomes especially critical in evaluating bone density results of treatment protocols. Noninvasive bone mineral measurements are embraced for assessing treatment efficacy based on the good theoretical background described above and on the ease of data collection. If treatment generates increased bone mass with pathologic bone fragility, then studies relying on density determination may offer erroneous clinical results.

Hedlund[23] and Riggs[53] worried about an increased incidence of hip fracture in osteoporotic women treated with sodium fluoride. Riggs,[54] et al., demonstrated a 10 to 12% increased in bone density of the femoral neck and other sites in fluoride-treated patients in a 4 year randomized prospective study. Fluoride-treated patients had 3.2 times the number of nonvertebral fractures compared to placebo patients. Seven hip fractures occurred in the fluoride-treated patients and three hip fractures in the placebo groups. This trend in hip fractures was not statistically significant. The two deaths, one in the fluoride group and one in the placebo group, were partially attributable to hip fracture. Riggs' prospective study used a higher dosage of sodium fluoride (75 mg/day) compared to other centers. The increased incidence of long bone fracture despite increased bone mass may be caused by increased amounts of pathologic bone.[36]

Risk of Falling and of Falls

Melton and Riggs stated that with bone strength, the risk of falling and the risk of injury in each fall define the risk of fracture.[40] Prevention of falls, therefore, is an important goal. Tinetti and Speechley reviewed risk factors for falling and prevention steps to avoid falls.[69]

Data described by Lotz and Hayes[37] show that during a simple nontraumatic fall ten times the amount of energy required to fracture a normal hip in vitro is available. This information makes one wonder why bones do not fracture more commonly. A structure that absorbs energy must be able to produce high forces over relatively long distances because the energy absorbed is the product of force and elongation. Muscle mass is directly proportional to the amount of energy that the muscle is able to absorb. Further, to be effective, the muscle force must be applied in a coordinated fashion to break a fall without breaking bones. It becomes clear then that the huge excess of energy available requires muscle mass and coordination to break a fall. These mechanisms play an important part in the risk of falling and the risk of fracturing during a fall. These factors may explain the poor correlation between bone mineral density and fracture incidence, especially in older patients.[9]

Some evidence suggests that bone mineral mass and muscle mass may correlate.[3,5,14,21,46,59,66] This correlation may be responsible for some of the correlation that exists between fracture incidence and bone density.

This evidence suggests a mechanism whereby exercise and fitness may be valuable. Currently, no clinical data clearly demonstrates fracture prevention. On the basis of the increased neuromuscular coordination and the increased muscle mass related to exercise, a fit patient should be better able to absorb the energy of a fall and may have stronger bones than an unfit patient. Exercise and fitness, therefore, can be recommended on the basis of the theoretical benefit.

Osteoporosis Types

Osteoporosis can be classified into type I and type II. A good classification scheme identifies cause, predicts risks, and allows treatment recommendations. At present, osteoporosis classification has limited use. The osteoporosis classification proposed by Riggs and Melton[57] describes the typical patient by age and sex.

Type I

Type I osteoporosis, also called postmenopausal osteoporosis, implies menopausal loss of ovarian function as the cause. Type I osteoporosis patients, typically Caucasian women approximately 15 to 20 years after the loss of ovarian function, develop progressive spinal compression fractures in the thoracic and thoracolumbar regions of the spine.[48] The cause of type I osteoporosis is supported by the prevention efficacy of estrogen replacement therapy (ERT) in blunting spine bone loss and lowering the fracture rate. Cessation of ovarian function is not the only cause. Two facts suggest other etiologic contributions: (1) men in this age group have spinal compression fractures, but at a much lower rate than women, and (2) ERT does not absolutely prevent the disease occurrence.

Type I osteoporosis, numerically, is more important than type II osteoporosis. Type I causes significant pain, alteration of lifestyle, and financial costs for treatment. Considering the larger number of patients and the lower cost of treatment, type I is an important, but less pressing, social and economic issue than type II osteoporosis.

Type II

The effects of type II osteoporosis are felt most profoundly by patients over 70 years of age. More than 90% of hip fractures occur in individuals over the age of 70. Fractures occur in the proximal femur, proximal tibia, proximal humerus, and distal radius.

The ratio of hip fracture in male and female patients is approximately two females to one male. This sex distribution suggests that the cause of type II osteoporosis is less a function of ovarian hormones and more a function of other age-related factors, although estrogen is a cause.[2] Biopsy of hip fracture patients shows 31% normal bone, 12% osteomalacia, and 32% decreased bone volume.[24] Type II osteoporosis may be caused by age-related decrease of one hydroxylation of vitamin D to active 1,25 dihydroxyvitamin D.[64,71] These patients often have a secondary increase in parathyroid hormone. The type II patient with these vitamin D changes may represent only a subset of patients with the mild renal osteomalacia. Reduction of osteoblast function associated with age may contribute to hip fracture risk.[9] It is probable that other metabolic changes in the elderly conspire to generate the mixed group we know as type II osteoporosis. Further definition of these causes will improve classification and treatment.[52]

Screening

Bone density measurements can be made safely, precisely, and inexpensively. These are necessary characteristics for a useful screening test. Probably, the most important characteristic for useful screening test is predictive value. As discussed, prediction is problematic. Bone density correlates well with fracture risk. However, overlap of the fracture and nonfracture data and the high percentage of elderly patients with bone mass below the fracture threshold limit the value of screening.[39] Early screening efforts were directed toward the type I osteoporosis patients.

The task force of the National Osteoporosis Foundation[30] describes clinical indications for bone mass measurement. This group summarizes the issues discussed above and recommends that bone mass measurements be indicated for four groups of patients: (1) estrogen deficient women who have enough bone loss to recommend estrogen replacement therapy, (2) patients with x-ray sufficient evidence of vertebral fracture or osteopenia to recommend treatment, (3) patients who require corticosteroid therapy, and, (4) patients with asymptomatic primary hyperparathyroid disease. The task force does not recommend widespread screening.

Safe, effective ERT can be used to prevent coronary artery disease and bone loss in ovarian sufficient women, especially after surgical menopause. Recommendation of ERT does not require screening for patient selection. Another problem with bone density screening is that preventive therapy is more effective before bone loss occurs. If bone loss progresses to the point that the bone density determination measures the loss, the chance to prevent bone loss has been missed. The decision to recommend ERT, diet supplements, and exercise is based on risk ratios with and without preventive therapy at a time before bone loss has occurred.

Several bone measurement techniques are available. Dual photon absorptiometry (DPA) of the femoral neck accounts for 75 to 85% of the variance of ultimate fracture strength. The technique is precise and relatively inexpensive with low radiation dosage. Its accuracy is affected by overlying calcified tissue. DPA has an accuracy rate of 3 to 6%. The radiation dosage is approximately 5 millirems.

Quantitative CT (QCT) can be done on standard CT equipment with appropriate software and phantoms. The accuracy of a QCT is approximately 5 to 10% with an exposure of 100 to 300 millirems.

Dual energy x-ray photometry is a technique that recently has evolved. Short-term precision is 0.05 to 1% with the long-term precision that has yet to be defined. Radiation exposure is relatively low.

Prevention and Treatment

The terms prevention and treatment have specific, well defined definitions. When discussing osteoporosis, the distinction between the two can start to become blurred, as does the definition of osteoporosis. For immediately perimenopausal women who have normal bone density, calcium, vitamin D, and ERT, preventive therapy would consist of exercise. However, is the same program prevention treatment for 20-year postmenopausal women? Drugs such as calcitonin, fluoride, etidronate, calcitriol, phosphate, and parathyroid hormone, are used only to treat established disease. Is an established disease simply defined by lower bone density with noninvasive testing, or by the onset of symptomatic disease, i.e., fractures? Osteoporosis prevention, as with many diseases, is the better and more predictable goal.

Prevention

Calcium

Calcium supplementation has been much discussed. At present, patients should avoid a chronic calcium deficiency,[6] which is typical of the modern American diet from the time when adolescents and young adults switch from milk to other nondairy beverages. NIH Consensus Conferences[42] on osteoporosis suggest the calcium minimum daily requirement to be 1000mg/day for women before menopause and for all men. Minimum daily requirement implies that recommended amount would be adequate for 95% of the population. With that definition, many require less calcium in a day. One thousand milligrams is equivalent of three to four dairy servings. The American population does not get this, especially with concerns for cholesterol and weight control.

The postmenopausal period is marked by decreased calcium absorption, possibly secondary to decreased serum PTH and the associated decreased calcitriol.[56] The period of bone loss in the postmenopausal period may be partially related to this decrease in calcium absorption. The NIH Consensus Conference[42] has recommended calcium supplementation resulting in a dietary intake of 1500 milligrams of calcium daily. This is equivalent to five or six dairy servings daily; most postmenopausal women do not reach this level.

Dairy foods can cause problems. Lactose intolerance is present in a significant portion of this population. These people could use calcium supplementation or low lactose dairy products such as yogurt and enyzme-treated milk. However, low-fat yogurt, if used to meet the minimum daily requirement of calcium, would also supply between 1500 to 2000 calories/day. Although the resulting obesity is a protective of bone loss, it is not to be encouraged. Calcium supplement has not been implicated in urinary lithiasis if the patient has not had a prior episode of stones. Calcium balance can be measured, but is inaccurate and requires hospitalization with a restrictive regimen.

At the present time, it is recommended that patients avoid calcium deficiencies by starting supplements at the time that adults or adolescents switch from dairy products as the beverage. There is no evidence that calcium intake above that needed for neutral calcium balance prevents osteoporosis.

Vitamin D

Vitamin D supplementation is a similar philosophy to that of calcium supplementation, as described above. Deficiency should be avoided.[6] Vitamin D usually does not require daily supplementation as calcium does, because vitamin D is a fat soluble hormone and is stored in significant amounts in the liver. Vitamin D concentrations vary slowly over long periods of time. The kidney is able to aggressively activate vitamin D even when faced with low amounts of the stored forms of vitamin D. Vitamin D deficiency is rarely seen in the industrialized countries. Vitamin D is not found naturally in any food other than liver. Dairy products have been supplemented with vitamin D in many industrialized countries. Four hundred units of vitamin D is the minimum daily requirement for all adults, and has been recommended by the NIH Consensus Conferences.[42] The other source of vitamin D is sunlight. One hour per week of direct sunlight will supply adequate amounts of endogenous vitamin D from skin exposure to ultraviolet light. In the northern part of North America, the indirect sunlight is of no value for much of the year.

Although 50,000 units of vitamin D a week has been suggested, this level is not recommended.[49] On a chronic basis, this high dosage of vitamin D puts the patient at significant risk for vitamin D toxicity. Vitamin D toxicity causes serum calcium elevation at the expense of bone loss.

Vitamin D has potential for prevention for the postmenopausal and elderly patient. Osteomalacia is found in 12% of hip fracture patients.[25] After menopause, calcium absorption decreases, in part because of a secondary decrease of activated vitamin D, calcitriol.[64,71] The elderly patient may have a primary decrease of activated vitamin D because of mild renal impairment. Low level chronic disease has been operating for a significant period when these levels are abnormal. Ideally, treatment could be initiated before the severe chemical abnormality exists. Vitamin D abnormalities can cause loss of hip bone density. Slovak[64] and Tsai[71] both saw blunted rates of renal vitamin D one alpha hydroxylation in response to parathyroid hormone infusion in elderly patients. Tsai[71] found that the hip fracture patients had less vitamin D activation after PTH than the average elderly patient. These findings suggest that decreased activation of vitamin D in the aging kidney is a risk factor for hip fracture. This evidence suggests the potential utility in both osteoporosis populations for calcitriol to improve overall calcium metabolism. Calcitriol use has not yet been proven and has serious potential toxicity.

Patient screening remains an issue. At the present time, patients who would benefit from calcitriol treatment demonstrate low normal serum calcium, low serum phosphate, and elevated serum alkaline phosphatase typical of mild osteomalacia. Patients who have these serum chemistry changes should be further evaluated with serum 25 hydroxy vitamin D, 1,25 dihydroxyvitamin D, parathyroid hormone, and renal functions. If parathyroid hormone is high, 1,25 dihydroxyvitamin D is low normal or low, 25 hydroxy vitamin D is normal and phosphate is normal or low, and calcitriol could be useful. These chemistry changes are typical of renal osteomalacia for which calcitriol is the drug of choice. Often these patients have mild renal dysfunction without uremia. Creatinine clearances of

20 to 40 ml/min are typical. Frequently these patients present with stress fractures.

If 25 hydroxy vitamin D also is low, the diagnosis is vitamin D deficiency. Vitamin D should be given until the values show an adequate chemical response.

Estrogen

Estrogen replacement therapy (ERT) is the single most important preventive and therapeutic option in postmenopausal women. Data show risk of hip fracture associated with menopause[2,31,43] and bone density.[8,41] Specific application of estrogen supplementation continues to be controversial.[67] Recent data demonstrating the beneficial effect of ERT on coronary artery disease have caused the medical community to regain confidence of its use. ERT should be considered after natural menopause and especially after an early surgical menopause. The controversial aspects of ERT are: (1) what type of estrogen should be used; (2) should progesterone be used with estrogen; (3) how long should they be prescribed; (4) what is the risk of breast cancer associated with ERT; and (5) what patients should have ERT offered to them?

Premarin at 0.625 mg/day, cycled with 10 mg of progesterone on a monthly basis, is effective to prevent the loss of bone mass. Low dosages of estrogen cycled with progesterone have prevented the endometria carcinoma that was described in the late 1970s. This regimen of 0.625 mg of Premarin on days 1 to 25 with 10 mg of progesterone on days 16 to 25, cycled on a monthly basis, has been the most prescribed method of estrogen replacement for postmenopausal women during the 1980s. A concern is that the progestin induced partial reversal of the beneficial changes in serum lipids that the estrogen induced. The beneficial effect on serum lipid of estrogen is also thought to cause the decreased risk of coronary artery disease in menopausal women and especially in surgical menopausal women treated with estrogen replacement therapy.

Estradiol skin patches release estrogen into the peripheral circulation without first passing through the liver, as with oral estrogen absorbed through the portal circulation. Estradiol is natural in human women; Premarin is a congregated equine estrogen isolated from the urine of pregnant horses. Estradiol may be a more physiologic stimulus and more appropriate estrogen replacement although experience with Premarin has been good.

Aspects of timing of the estrogen therapy are controversial. However, there is no controversy regarding when it should be started. If started when estrogen deficiency begins, ERT prevents bone loss. Estrogen started late protects against further bone loss, although, significant bone loss may already have occurred. Late discontinuation of ERT ten years after the menopause allows bone loss and delays menopausal changes. With more data suggesting that estrogen is effective at preventing coronary heart disease, estrogen therapy will probably be pursued by the elderly population.

The major concern about ERT is breast carcinoma. For many women the emotional concern over breast carcinoma is more compelling than the concern over the higher rates of coronary artery disease and osteoporosis morbidity and mortality. The literature is split between articles describing no effect and those describing increased breast carcinoma rate with ERT. Bergkvist[4] suggested that the risk of breast carcinoma may be increased by progestins offering another reason to reconsider using this agent. Considering the rates of breast carcinoma, heart disease, and osteoporosis, NIH recommends ERT for women at risk of osteoporosis.[42]

Kiel[31] published the Framingham data on postmenopausal use of estrogen and the risk of hip fracture in 2873 women. He found the hip fracture was inversely related to weight, regardless of age. Estrogen was preventive if taken anytime after menopause, but the recent use of estrogen appeared to be protective in women under the age of 75. Jensen[29] published a double blind placebo control study in 70-year-old women and found a protective effect against further bone loss. Moore[41] demonstrated the vertebral bone mineral benefit associated with long-term estrogen use.

Paganini-Hill[43] did a case-matched control study looking at 91 hip fracture patients. They showed a risk ratio of 0.42 for estrogen usage of more than 5 years, with improved risk ratios against hip fracture with duration beyond 5 years. They found this effect to be most significant in surgically menopausal women. Diabetes, low weight, low physical activity, corticosteroids, early menopause, heavy cigarette smoking, and low sunlight exposure all were risk factors for hip fractures; none of them interfered with the protective effect offered by estrogen against hip fracture.

Exercise

Exercise can potentially lower fracture risk by maintaining bone mass, strength, and neuromuscular coordination. In premenopausal and early postmenopausal women exercise has little risk. Benefi-

cial effects include blood pressure control and coronary artery disease protection. Immobilization causes bone loss; inactivity is a risk factor for hip fracture. Is the contrary true? Will increased activity further increase bone density or strength for a patient with an appropriate activity level?

Another area of controversy is the type of exercise to be performed. Weight bearing activity is thought by some to be necessary to increase bone density and strength. Probably low repetition, high load exercise locally increases bone mineral density and strength. Rubin and Lanyon[58] demonstrated the importance of high load bone stimulus opposing disuse of the bone. Further, they found high loads required only 18 repetitions. A low repetition, high load, site specific regimen may be any activity that uses body weight or significant muscle loads across the specific bony sites.

Human data correlate muscle mass[3,5,14,21,46,59,66] and fitness[1,61] with bone mass. Low load, high repetition exercises, such as running, raise a potential adverse effect of exercise for premenopausal women. Elite young women athletes often have amenorrhea related to their level of exercise. The estrogen deficiency in these women is apparently a more powerful adverse effect on bone mass than the potential beneficial effect of exercise. Evaluation of women college students[28] demonstrated amenorrheic long distant runners have lower bone mass than their eumenorrheic sedentary classmates; the amenorrheic runners had better bone density than classmates who are amenorrheic for other reasons. Potential confounding variables, including body habitus, athletic preselection, and nutrition, are difficult to control. The concern raised is that the exercise-induced ovarian dysfunction may be more important to bone mass than exercise itself.

Hume[27] found a similar result in sexually mature female Sprague Dawley rats, with or without oophorectomy and with or without exercise. Exercise blunted the bone mineral and strength loss associated with oophorectomy, but did not prevent it.

Exercise cannot prevent the effects of menopause, but it can be a valuable adjunct in women regardless of ERT usage. Exercise prevents bone loss that results from disuse and may increase bone strength and mass. Exercise improves neuromuscular coordination and muscle mass and may, therefore, lower the risk of falling.

Treatment

Treatment protocols for hip fracture have offered little data, especially compared to the spine. Spine protocols may offer little for hip fracture risk. This important area demands investigation.[53]

Sodium Fluoride

Sodium fluoride has been used to treat symptomatic spine osteoporosis. Riggs[55] and Lane[33] retrospectively studied treated patients using the patient's prior fracture history as the control. They found an increase of bone mineral density and a decreased fracture rate in the lumbar spine in response to sodium fluoride treatment.

Concerns have been raised that long bone fracture risk may be increased with fluoride treatment.[53] A prospective randomized study at the Mayo Clinic was designed and published by Riggs.[54] Patients received 75 mg of sodium fluoride per day. Sixty-six women who were treated for 4 years gained bone density of 35% in the lumbar spine and approximately 12% in the femoral neck compared to the matched placebo group. Despite increased bone density, the treated group had no change in vertebral fracture rate, but had a significantly *higher* rate of nonvertebral fractures. The fluoride group sustained seven hip fractures and the placebo group three hip fractures, statistically not a significant difference. This data has caused serious doubt regarding the use of sodium fluoride. Riggs did not quote the serum fluoride levels of his patients.

Pak[44] used a lower dosage of slow release sodium fluoride. About 15 mg of sodium fluoride given per day resulted in fasting serum fluoride levels of 5 to 10 micromoles per liter during treatment. His prospective study did not include a placebo group; the fluoride patients alone had a significant fracture rate reduction starting after 1 year of treatment compared to pretreatment. Twenty-one patients on the fluoride treatment had no hip fractures; 23 patients on phosphate and fluoride had one hip fracture. Although Pak's study is smaller than Riggs' and did not include a placebo control, Pak's study used low dosages of slow release sodium fluoride with apparent safety and good vertebral fracture effect.

Certainly increased bone mass in the spine and femoral neck would be interpreted as a benefit of the sodium fluoride. Because Riggs described a high nonvertebral fracture rate with fluoride treatment, other fluoride dosing must be evaluated before fluoride can be widely embraced.[22]

Etidronate

A pair of studies demonstrate etidronate to be effective treatment of type I postmenopausal osteoporosis. Both articles demonstrated just under 2% yearly increase in spine bone mass with a significant decrease of spine compression fracture rate after the first year of treatment. Storm[68] did not measure bone mineral content in the proximal femur. Each of the two study groups contained 33 patients. Two hip fractures occurred in the placebo group and one hip fracture in the etidronate group. Ten nonvertebral fractures occurred in six placebo patients and six nonvertebral fractures in five etidronate patients. All the nonvertebral fractures in the treated group occurred in the first year of treatment; no further fractures occurred thereafter. Watts[73] measured the bone mineral content of the proximal femur. The femoral neck density was not affected. This placebo group had no hip fractures and the etidronate group had one hip fracture over a two-year study, with just under 100 patients in the two study groups. These two prospective studies suggest that etidronate appears to effectively lower the spine fracture rate, apparently by increasing the bone mass. The femoral neck bone density and fracture rate did not change in these small, prospective studies. Hodsman, in a smaller study, cycled the etidronate with phosphate, also with a lowered fracture rate.[24]

Thiazide

LaCroix[34] prospectively evaluated just under 10,000 men and women, 65 years of age and older, in three different communities. This population had 242 hip fractures in four years. Thiazide use lowered the hip fracture risk by one-third. This beneficial effect of thiazide was independent of sex, age, disability, body mass, smoking, and other antihypertensive drugs. The agent may be beneficial because it decreases urinary calcium excretion and may prevent the chronic calcium deficiency by blocking urinary calcium excretion. Felson,[19] published a retrospective case control analysis of the Framingham cohort that evaluated thiazide use. Recent treatment with thiazide alone was protective of hip fracture, but combination drugs were not.

Calcitonin

Calcitonin is the only FDA-approved drug for the management of postmenopausal osteoporosis. The literature is based on lumbar bone density results.

Calcitonin has not been shown to affect hip fracture rate.

ADFR

The utility of cycled drugs has been proposed by Frost.[20] The theory suggests activation of bone remodeling, followed by depression of osteoclast activity, and a free period before repeating. Hodsman,[24] as just mentioned, and Slovik,[65] with PTH and calcitriol, have published ADFR protocols with no hip data.

Other Osteopenic Conditions

A variety of other conditions are common causes of osteopenia and pathologic fracture. The population characteristics described for osteoporosis are: type I, women 15 to 20 years after the loss of ovarian functions, and type II, elderly men and women. Patients who do not fit into these populations defined by age and sex, *probably* have a pathologic condition other than osteoporosis. Patients who fit this age and sex category *may* have other conditions. These other diagnoses must be considered before the diagnostic assumption of osteoporosis.

Metastatic Disease and Multiple Myeloma

Marrow packing neoplastic disease can occur with diffuse osteopenia, or with local lytic or blastic bone disease. The localized lesions of these diseases lead the physician to suspect the neoplastic process and begin an appropriate workup. The diffuse osteopenic presentation may be overlooked, especially in postmenopausal women or elderly patients. History, physical examination, and simple laboratory values are effective screening tools. The peak age of occurrence for a multiple myeloma is the sixth decade, but may be seen as early as the fourth decade.

Patients with multiple myeloma may present with anemia, renal disease, hypercalcemia, or fractures. Lytic bone lesions are frequently absent despite the fact that these patients have osteopenia. Osteopenia occurs because osteoplastic activating factors (OAF) are often secreted by the multiple myeloma. OAF is also responsible for the hypercalcemia seen in 20 to 30% of the patients. Multiple myeloma occurs with an incidence of three out of 100,000 (men more frequently than women), and

also represents approximately 1% of cancers. Physical examination frequently is not specific.

Laboratory evaluations show anemia, hypercalcemia, elevated creatinine, elevated sedimentation rate, and serum and urine proteins abnormalities. A large majority of patients will have at least one of these abnormalities at the time of presentation. If appropriate, further laboratory evaluation includes serum and urine protein electrophoresis and immunophoresis. Proteinuria may be myeloma proteins or albumin from early renal failure. Myeloma proteins demonstrate the monoclonal spike that characterizes the type of disease. Sixty percent of patients will have a positive serum electrophoresis and 20% will have positive urine electrophoresis only. Twenty percent of patients will have positive serum and urine electrophoresis. Some percentage of patients has normal serum and urine proteins and may require random bone marrow biopsy. The diagnosis of multiple myeloma is made when two of the following three characteristics are present: (1) typical lytic lesion, (2) typical electrophoresis and immunophoresis patterns, and (3) widespread infiltration with malignant plasma cells on bone marrow aspirate. Bone scans may miss aggressive lesions. X-rays are valuable only if the specific lytic lesions are seen. Typical x-ray findings on skull films have multiple punched out lesions.

Breast carcinoma increases until incidence menopause. From menopause there is a constant increase, up to the peak of age 65. The effect of estrogen is still controversial. Physical examinations and mammography are mainstays of diagnosis and are part of the evaluation of the patient with the osteopenia, pathologic fracture, hypercalcemia, or anemia.

Lung carcinoma continues to be the most common form of malignancy in men, and peaks between the fifth and seventh decades. Smoking represents a major risk factor. Those who smoke one and one-half to two packs of cigarettes per day have 10 times the rate of lung cancer than nonsmokers. Lung cancer accounts for one-fourth of male cancer deaths. The increased incidence of smoking in women has been followed by increased incidence of lung carcinoma in women. Secondary smoking is implicated in a significant number of lung tumors, adding to the risk of exposure to ionizing radiation such as radon and risk from other air pollutants. Lung carcinomas can cause hypercalcemia and osteopenia because of increased parathyroid, a hormone-like substance, but any metastatic tumors to bone, including breast, prostate, and thyroid, may cause hypercalcemia and diffuse bone disease. Lung carcinoma can occur with metastatic disease to bone and fracture from localized lesions or from diffused osteopenia from the parathyroid-like response. The aggressive nature of lung disease makes bone scans less precise. Chest x-rays and skeletal survey radiographs aimed at looking for other lytic metastatic areas should be ordered for a patient with a smoking history. Septum for cytology may be helpful.

Prostate cancer represents approximately 10% of cancer deaths among males. The incidence rises with increasing age. Autopsy studies show incidence as high as 60% in the eighth decade of life. Fewer than one-sixth of these are clinically apparent prior to death. Routine rectal exam is critical to routine screening. One-fifth of patients with prostate cancer present with symptoms from metastatic disease and may require biopsy for a histologic diagnosis. Acid phosphatase is frequently elevated after metastatic disease to bone. Biopsy of lesions or blind biopsy of the ilium may be useful. X-ray and bone scans are reliable to evaluate metastatic disease to bone.

Common locations of metastatic diseases from hypernephroma are the hip, pelvis, lumbar spine and thoracic spine. Lumbar spine compression fractures should raise concern about a metastatic process because the osteoporotic fractures initially are localized to the lower thoracic spine and thoracolumbar junction.

Hyperparathyroidism

Because multichannel serum screening is part of routine health care, primary hyperparathyroid disease now presents as asymptomatic hypercalcemia, not as the classic "stones, groans, and bones." Primary hyperparathyroid patients may be followed by serial calcium determinations, adequate hydration to avoid renal lithiasis, and bone mineral determination to look for advancement of bone disease. Serial bone density determination is recommended by the Scientific Advisory Board of the National Osteoporosis Foundation.[30] Parathyroidectomy is recommended if bone density value falls below one standard deviation in asymptomatic patients. Symptomatic hypercalcemia, renal lithiasis, or fracture also require surgical parathyroidectomy. Typically, these patients are older than 50 years, and 60 to 80% are women; the incidence is 42 per 100,000 population. The diagnosis of primary hyperparathyroid disease requires elevated serum calcium.

Hypercalcemia is evaluated by measuring serum parathyroid hormones. The diagnosis of primary hyperparathyroidism is made by positive radioim-

munoassay for PTH in a hypercalcemic patient. Biologic PTH assays would demonstrate positive results in some of the malignant lesions described because these lesions may secrete a substance with parathyroid-like activity.

Secondary Hyperparathyroidism

Secondary hyperparathyroidism is the appropriate parathyroid response to either low serum calcium or elevated serum phosphate.

Renal Disease

Serum calcium control depends on coordination between the parathyroid function and vitamin D metabolism; the kidney plays a central role in this coordination. Active 1,25 dihydroxyvitamin D, is pathologically regulated in parathyroid disease and in renal disease. Renal bone disease is caused by inadequate vitamin D activation, i.e., renal osteomalacia, or serum phosphate elevation, i.e., renal osteodystrophy. Bone disease at end-stage renal disease is a mixture of both renal osteomalacia and renal osteodystrophy. The most common cause of secondary hyperparathyroidism in the United States is renal disease.

If the renal tubular function falls, the decreased rate of 1-alpha hydroxylation of 25 hydroxy vitamin D causes low levels of 1,25 dihydroxy D (active vitamin D). The stored form, 25 hydroxy vitamin D, can be measured and is normal, but the active 1,25 dihydroxy D is inappropriately low. When the active vitamin D concentration falls, intestine absorption and kidney reabsorption of calcium falls and serum calcium concentration drifts down. The secondary parathyroid response supports the falling serum calcium level. This disease process is treated by giving calcitriol, the active form of 1,25 dihydroxy D. Calcitriol should be started only after serum phosphate abnormality is treated. Raising serum calcium in the face of an elevated serum phosphate level causes metastatic soft tissue calcification. When low serum calcium causes a secondary hyperparathyroidism in renal disease it is known as renal osteomalacia. As discussed, the elderly may have a mild form of type II osteoporosis with asymptomatic renal disease. Depression of 1,25 dihydroxyvitamin D formation may be one of the important etiologic factors in hip fractures.

The other syndrome of renal secondary hyperparathyroidism is renal osteodystrophy. Decreased rate of glomerular filtration elevates serum phosphate levels. Elevated serum phosphate levels stimulate secondary hyperparathyroidism. If renal tubular function is maintained, the serum calcium concentration is supported by vitamin D activation in response to the elevated PTH. These elevated phosphate levels and normal or elevated calcium levels cause the classic picture of metastatic soft tissue calcification with a calcification of the small digital vessel in the hands and feet. Osteolysis occurs at the phalanges on the radial surface, distal end of the clavicles, and symphysis pubis. The treatment is phosphate binder given orally to lower the serum phosphate levels. This must be done before considering vitamin D treatment.

Most patients with renal disease have a mixture of renal osteomalacia and renal osteodystrophy. Careful management of renal parathyroid disease requires attention to serum calcium and phosphate levels. Phosphate binders, calcium supplements, and oral doses of 1,25 dihydroxyvitamin D can effectively blunt osteolysis and allow for normal bone matrix mineralization. Despite careful attention to serum calcium and phosphate levels, serum parathyroid hormone measured by radioimmunoassay remains elevated, at least in part, because small amounts of PTH peptides are excreted in the kidney.

Tertiary hyperparathyroidism occurs in late end-stage renal disease when the parathyroid begins autonomous secretions without control by serum calcium and phosphorous levels. Careful attention to phosphate and calcium levels has decreased the incidence of this disease. Tertiary hyperparathyroidism remains the only indication for parathyroidectomy in renal disease. Appropriate parathyroid function is necessary for serum calcium maintenance and bone healing because intestine and bone can continue to respond appropriately to PTH in renal disease. Bone turnover initiated by parathyroid hormone osteoclast stimulation is necessary to allow bone healing. Absence of this osteoclastic activation makes the bone inactive and unable to heal.

Vitamin D Deficiency

Vitamin D deficiency causes the syndromes of rickets in skeletally immature patients and osteomalacia in skeletally mature patients. The major difference between the two is disruption of calcification of actively functioning growth plate. These diseases occur when storage levels of vitamin D are inadequate because of dietary deficiency or because of inadequate skin exposure to ultraviolet light. Serum calcium levels then fall. Parathyroid hormone responds appropriately to maintain serum calcium levels at the cost of bone destruction. The elevated parathyroid hormone level causes normal kidneys to dump phosphate. Therefore, in early vitamin D deficiency phosphate is significantly low, calcium is normal, and alkaline phosphatase is increased. With a severe vitamin D deficiency, the serum calcium level drops. Vitamin D deficiency can be treated by large dosages. Looser's line, pseudofractures, and stress fractures around the hip are not uncommon.

Corticosteroids

Oral corticosteroids have improved treatment of rheumatoid arthritis, asthma, inflammatory bowel disease, and organ transplantation. Corticosteroids, given either iatrogenically or as the primary or secondary hypercorticolism of adrenal or pituitary disease, cause significant bone disease. Corticosteroids interfere with intestinal absorption and renal reabsorption of calcium and cause general catabolic effect on the connective tissue through decreased collagen synthesis. The risk of bone disease is a function of both dosage and duration of corticosteroid treatment. Prevention of bone disease requires the lowest dosage of steroids that is consistent with the primary disease, oral calcium supplementations, and adequate vitamin D. Bisphosphonates may be important in prevention of glucocortical-induced osteoporosis.[51]

References

1. BALLARD JE, MCKEOWN BC, GRAHAM HM, ZINKGRAF SA: The effect of high level physical activity (8.5 METs or greater) and estrogen replacement therapy upon bone mass in postmenopausal females, aged 50-68 years. Int J Sports Med, II:208–214, 1990.
2. BEARD CM, et al.: Ascertainment of risk factors for osteoporosis: comparison of interview data with medical record review. J Bone Miner Res, 5(7):691–699, 1990.
3. BELL NH, et al.: The effects of muscle-building exercise on vitamin D and mineral metabolism. J Bone Miner Res, 3(4):369–373, 1988.
4. BERGKVIST L, et al.: The risk of breast cancer after estrogen and estrogen-progestin replacement. N Engl J Med, 321(5):293–297, 1989.
5. BEVIER WC, et al.: Relationship of body composition, muscle strength, and aerobic capacity to bone mineral density in older men and women. J Bone Miner Res, 4(3):421–432, 1989.
6. BURNELL JM, BAYLINK DJ, CHESTNUT CH, TEUBNER EJ: The role of skeletal calcium deficiency in postmenopausal osteoporosis. Calcif Tissue Int, 38:187–192, 1986.
7. CARTER DR, HAYES WC: The compressive behavior of bone as a two-phase porous structure. J Bone Joint Surg, 59(A):954–962, 1977.
8. CAULEY JA, et al.: Endogenous estrogen levels and calcium in-

takes in postmenopausal women. JAMA, 260(21): 3150–3155, 1988.

9. COOPER C, BARKER DJP, MORRIS J, BRIGGS RSJ: Osteoporosis, falls, and age in fracture of the proximal femur. Br Med Bull, 295:13–15, 1987.

10. COOPER C, et al.: Indices of calcium metabolism in women with hip fractures. Bone Miner, 5:193–200, 1989.

11. CORNELL CN, et al.: Quantification of osteopenia in hip fracture patients. 34th Annu Meet, Orthop Res Soc, 370, 1988.

12. CUMMINGS SR, et al.: Appendicular bone density and age predict hip fracture in women. JAMA, 264:665–668, 1990.

13. CUMMINGS, SR: Are patients with hip fractures more osteoporotic? Review of the evidence. Am J Med, 78:487–494, 1985.

14. DALSKY GP: Effect of exercise on bone: permissive influence of estrogen and calcium. Med Sci Sports Exerc, 22(3):281–285, 1990.

15. DEQUEKER J, GAUTAMA K, ROH YS: Femoral trabecular patterns in asymptomatic spinal osteoporosis and femoral neck fracture. Clin Radiol, 25:243–246, 1974.

16. DALEN N, HELLSTROM LG, JACOBSON B: Bone mineral content and mechanical strength of the femoral neck. Acta Orthop Scand, 47:503–508, 1976.

17. ELSASSER U, HESP R, KLENERMAN L, WOOTTON R: Deficit of trabecular and cortical bone in elderly women with fracture of the femoral neck. Clin Sci, 59:393–395, 1980.

18. FAZZALARI NL, DARRACOTT J, VERNON-ROBERTS B: Histomorphometric changes in the trabecular structure of a selected stress region in the femur in patients with osteoarthritis and fracture of the femoral neck. Bone, 6:125–133, 1985.

19. FELSON DT, et al: Thiazide diuretics and the risk of hip fracture. JAMA, 265(3):370–373, 1991.

20. FROST HM: Treatment of osteoporosis by manipulation of coherent bone cell populations. Clin Orthop, 143:227–244, 1979.

21. GLEESON PB, et al.: Effects of weight lifting on bone mineral density in premenopausal women. J Bone Miner Res, 5(2):153–158, 1990.

22. HARRISON JE: Fluoride treatment for osteoporosis. Calcif Tissue Int, 46:287–288, 1990.

23. HEDLUND LR, GALLAGHER JC: Increased incidence of hip fracture in osteoporotic women treated with sodium fluoride. J Bone Miner Res, 4(2):223–225, 1989.

24. HODSMAN AB: Effects of cyclical therapy for osteoporosis using an oral regimen of inorganic phosphate and sodium etidronate: a clinical and bone histomorphometric study. Bone Miner, 5:201–212, 1989.

25. HORDON LD, PEACOCK M: Osteomalacia and osteoporosis in femoral neck fracture. Bone Miner, 11:247–259, 1990.

26. HOLBROOK TL, GRAZIER K, KELSEY JL, STAUFFER RN: The frequency of occurrence, impact and cost of selected musculoskeletal conditions in the United States. Chicago, American Academy of Orthopaedic Surgeons, 1984.

27. HUME EL, et al.: Normalized bone mass and strength in exercising oophorectomized and sham operated rats. 35th Annu Meet, Orthop Res Soc, Las Vegas, NV.

28. JACOBSON PC, et al.: Bone density in women: college athletes and older athletic women. J Orthop Res, 2:328–332, 1984.

29. JENSEN GF, CHRISTIANSEN C, TRANSBL I: Treatment of postmenopausal osteoporosis: a controlled therapeutic trial comparing estrogen/gestagen, 1,25-dihydroxy-vitamin D3 and calcium. Clin Endocrinol, 16:515–524, 1982.

30. JOHNSTON CC, MELTON LJ, LINDSAY R, EDDY DM: Clinical indications for bone mass measurements. J Bone Miner Res, 4 (Suppl 2), 1989.

31. KIEL DP, et al.: Hip fracture and the use of estrogens in postmenopausal women: the Framingham Study. N Engl J Med, 317(19):1169–1174, 1987.

32. KREIGER N, et al: Epidemiological study of hip fracture in postmenopausal women. Am J Epidemiol, 116:141–148, 1982.

33. LANE JM, et al.: Treatment of osteoporosis with sodium fluoride and calcium: effects on vertebral fracture incidence and bone histomorphometry. Orthop Clin North Am, 15:729–745, 1984.

34. LACROIX AZ, et al.: Thiazide diuretic agents and the incidence of hip fracture. N Engl J Med, 322(5):286–290, 1990.

35. LEICHTER I, et al.: The relationship between bone density, mineral content, and mechanical strength in the femoral neck. Clin Orthop, 163:272–281, 1982.

36. LINDSAY R: Fluoride and bone—quantity versus quality. N Engl J Med, 322(12):845–846, 1990.

37. LOTZ JC, HAYES WC: The use of quantitative computed tomography to estimate risk of fracture of the hip from falls. J Bone Joint Surg, 72(A):689–700, 1990.

38. MAKIN M: Osteoporosis and proximal femoral fractures in the female elderly of Jerusalem. Clin Orthop, 218:19–23, 1987.

39. MELTON LJ, EDDY DM, JOHNSTON CC: Screening for osteoporosis. Ann Int Med, 112:516–528, 1990.

40. MELTON LJ, RIGGS BL: Risk factors for injury after a fall. Clin Geriatr Med, 1:525–539, 1985.

41. MOORE M, et al.: Long-term estrogen replacement therapy in postmenopausal women sustains vertebral bone mineral density. J Bone Miner Res, 5(6):659–664, 1990.

42. NATIONAL INSTITUTES OF HEALTH CONSENSUS DEVELOPMENT PANEL: Osteoporosis. NIH Consensus Development Conference Statement, 5, 1984.

43. PAGANINI-HILL A, et al.: Menopausal estrogen therapy and hip fractures. Ann Int Med, 95(1):28–31, 1981.

44. PAK CYC, et al.: Safe and effective treatment of osteoporosis with intermittent slow release sodium fluoride: Augmentation of vertebral bone mass and inhibition of fractures. J Clin Endocrinol Metab, 68(1):150–159, 1989.

45. PHILLIPS S, FOX N, JACOBS J, WRIGHT WE: The direct medical costs of osteoporosis for american women aged 45 and older, 1986. Bone, 9:271–279, 1988.

46. POCOCK N, et al.: Muscle strength, physical fitness, and weight but not age predict femoral neck bone mass. J Bone Miner Res, 4(3):441–448, 1989.

47. PORTIGLIATTI-BARBOS M, CARANDO S, ASCENZI A, BOYDE A: On the structural symmetry of human femurs. Bone, 8:165–169, 1987.

48. PRIOR JC, VIGNA YM, SCHECHTER MT, BURGESS AE: Spinal bone loss and ovulatory disturbances. N Engl J Med, 323(18):1221–1227, 1990.

49. RAPIN CH, et al.: Biochemical findings in blood of aged patients with femoral neck fractures: a contribution to the detection of occult osteomalacia. Calcif Tissue Int, 34:465–469, 1982.

50. ROSS PD, DAVIS JW, VOGEL JM, WASNICH RD: A critical review of bone mass and the risk of fractures in osteoporosis. Calcif Tissue Int, 46:149–161, 1990.

51. REID IR, SCHOOLER BA, STEWART AW: Prevention of glucocorticoid-induced osteoporosis. J Bone Miner Res, 5(6):619–623, 1990.

52. RESNICK NM, GREENSPAN SL: "Senile" osteoporosis reconsidered. JAMA, 261(7):1025–1029, 1989.

53. RIGGS BL, et al.: Incidence of hip fractures in osteoporotic women treated with sodium fluoride. J Bone Miner Res, 2(2):123–126, 1987.

54. Riggs BL, et al.: Effect of fluoride treatment on the fracture rate in postmenopausal women with osteoporosis. N Engl J Med, 322(12):802–809, 1990.

55. Riggs BL, et al.: Effect of the fluoride/calcium regimen on vertebral fracture occurrence in postmenopausal osteoporosis: comparison with conventional therapy. N Engl J Med, 306:446–550, 1980.

56. Riggs BL: Pathogenesis of osteoporosis. Am J Obstet Gynecol, 156(5):1342–1346, 1987.

57. Riggs BL, Melton LJ: Involutional osteoporosis. N Engl J Med, 314:1676–1677, 1986.

58. Rubin CT, Lanyon LE: Kappa Delta Award paper: osteoregulatory nature of mechanical stimuli: function as a determinant for adaptive remodeling in bone. J Orthop Res 5:300–310, 1987.

59. Sandler RB: Muscle strength assessment and the prevention of osteoporosis. J Am Geriatr Soc, 37:1192–1197, 1989.

60. Sartoris DJ, et al.: Dual-energy projection radiography in the evaluation of femoral neck strength, density, and mineralization. Invest radiol, 20:476–485, 1985.

61. Schapira D: Aerobics and postmenopausal osteoporosis. Stress Med, 6:157–163, 1990.

62. Sexson SB, Lehner JT: Factors affecting hip fracture mortality. J Orthop Trauma, 1(4):298–305, 1988.

63. Singh M, Nagrath AR, Maini PS, Haryana R: Changes in trabecular pattern of the upper end of the femur as an index of osteoporosis. J Bone Joint Surg. 52(A):457–467, 1970.

64. Slovik DM, et al.:Deficient production of 1,25-dihydroxyvitamin D in elderly osteoporotic patients. N Engl J Med, 305:372–374, 1981.

65. Slovik DM, et al.:Restoration of spinal bone in osteoporotic men by treatment with human parathyroid hormone (1–34) and 1,25 dihydroxyvitamin D. J Bone Miner Res, 1(4):377–381, 1986.

66. Snow-Harter C, et al.:Muscle strength as a predictor of bone mineral density in young women. J Bone Miner Res, 5(6):589–595, 1990.

67. Specht EE: Hip fracture, skeletal fragility, osteoporosis and hormonal deprivation in elderly women. West J Med, 133:297–303, 1980.

68. Storm T, et al.: Effect of intermittent cyclical etidronate therapy on bone mass and fracture rate in women with postmenopausal osteoporosis. N Engl J Med, 322:1265–1271, 1990.

69. Tinetti ME, Speechley M: Prevention of falls among the elderly. Med Intel 320(16):1055–1059, 1989.

70. Tobin WJ: The internal architecture of the femur and its clinical significance. J Bone Joint Surg, 37(A):57–71, 1955.

71. Tsai KS, Heath H, Kumar R, Riggs BL: Impaired vitamin D metabolism with aging in women. J Clin Invest, 73:1668–672, 1984.

72. van Hemert AM, Vandenbroucke JP, Birkenhager JC, Valkenburg HA: Prediction of osteoporotic fractures in the general population by a fracture risk score. Am J Epidemiol 132(1):135–123, 1990.

73. Watts NB, et al: Intermittent cyclical etidronate treatment of postmenopausal osteoporosis. N Engl J Med, 323(2):73–79, 1990.

74. White BL, Fisher WD, Laurin CA: Rate of mortality for elderly patients after fracture of the hip in the 1980s. J Bone Joint Surg, 69:1335–1340, 1987.

CHAPTER FOURTEEN

Treatment for Tumors About the Hip

RICHARD LACKMAN

Musculoskeletal neoplasms present a tremendous challenge to the hip surgeon. The proper diagnosis may be much less obvious than with other hip disorders and frequently requires a high index of suspicion in order to be given sufficient consideration. Once a neoplasm is suspected, the proper initial assessment is essential so that a valid impression of the type and extent of the problem is obtained. Biopsy techniques are likewise critical and the definitive surgical treatment is often extensive and demanding.

In order to establish a thorough approach to the patient with a neoplasm, a methodical and comprehensive thought process on the part of the surgeon is required. It is this clinical approach to the problem that this chapter strives to present.

Natural History

In order to develop a clinical approach to neoplastic processes, some understanding of tumor biology is required. The basic parameters of tumor growth relate to the histologic type of tumor, the histologic grading and the anatomic site.[4] Most lesions tend to grow centripetally as an ever enlarging sphere. This growth process is altered both by the active reaction of host tissues as well as by the passive ability of host tissues to inhibit tumor penetration. In the majority of tumors, host reaction may help to separate the lesion itself from the surrounding tissues. This area of separation is termed the capsule of the lesion. It usually consists of compressed tumor and normal tissue and frequently contains an immature fibrous layer as in the case of a latent lesion.

Benign lesions typically are completely separated from the surrounding tissues by their capsule. One exception to this is the benign aggressive lesion (e.g., giant cell tumor, desmoid tumor) which may penetrate the surrounding tissues in accordance with its aggressive growth characteristics. All ma-

lignant lesions stream beyond the gross limits of the tumor itself into the surrounding tissues. In this situation, the capsule fails to contain the lesion and is termed a "pseudocapsule." The clinical importance of understanding the presence or absence of a true capsule about a lesion is that this determines the type of surgical margin required to remove the lesion, as discussed later. Although the capsule may completely or incompletely separate a lesion from surrounding normal tissues, it can almost never prevent the continued growth of an active lesion.

Some appreciation for the natural history of tumor growth is also helpful in predicting the course of a lesion in an individual. Many lesions in the skeletally immature may, at some point, cease to grow and then spontaneously heal. The most commonly occurring example of this is the nonossifying fibroma or metaphyseal fibrous defect. Other lesions frequently attain a latent status and may remain stable for many years. Common examples of this behavior include enchondromas, eosinophilic granuloma, and osteoblastoma in bone and desmoid tumors, fibromas, lipomas, and hemangiomas in soft tissue. Unlike benign tumors, malignant lesions usually pursue a course of continued, steady, and often rapid growth. This is not always the case, however, and one cannot rule out a lesion being malignant based on the amount of time the lesion has been present at a stable size.

The histology of a malignant lesion is the most important prognosticating factor regarding the lesion's ability to metastasize.[8] The natural history of all high grade sarcomas is fairly similar regardless of the cell type and whether they occur in bone or soft tissue. In all of these high grade lesions, the majority already have at least microscopic distant metastases at presentation as exhibited by the high tendency to develop clinically apparent metastases without effective systemic treatment. Low grade sarcomas, likewise, share the basic behavioral tenet of prolonged local growth prior to the development of metastatic disease.[2] Both high and low grade lesions share essentially the same local growth characteristics. In all of these lesions, whether they occur in bone or soft tissue, tumor extends microscopically beyond the confines of the lesion itself and into the surrounding tissues. Although all malignant lesions stream malignant cells beyond the limits of their pseudocapsules, these capsular structures are frequently obvious clinically and often confuse the surgeon who supposes that all clinically encapsulated lesions are benign. Even very high grade lesions such as synovial sarcoma and malignant fibrous histiocytoma often have clear plains along their pseudocapsules and can be easily shelled out. The ability to shell out a lesion, however, has no bearing on histologic grade and never constitutes adequate surgery for a malignant lesion.

Natural Barriers To Tumor Penetration

In order to have a proper understanding of tumor growth and behavior, one must also have an appreciation of the natural physical barriers that exist in the body and how their presence affects the growth of tumors in various settings. Remember that tumors without further constraint, tend to grow as an ever enlarging sphere. When one area of the sphere contacts a tissue plain that is difficult to penetrate the tumor accommodates to this and continues to enlarge along the paths of least resistance. It would be optimal if one could define for each type of tissue a numerical grade defining its ability to restrict tumor penetration when compared to an assigned norm, say skeletal muscle. This would greatly aid the surgeon in deciding how much tissue to resect around the lesion to yield the same relative value in each case. Unfortunately, no such mathematical figures exist but one can at least grade in relative terms the ability to retard tumor penetration. Table 14–1 illustrates the relative values of various tissues regarding tumor penetration. Again, this is not a strictly defined relationship but rather a relative

TABLE 14–1. *Relative Ability of Tissues to Inhibit Tumor Penetration*

Most Resistant	Thick Fascia
	Cortical Bone
	Tendon
	Ligament
	Fat
Least Resistant	Skeletal muscle
	Cancellous bone

scale that is helpful to the surgeon in deciding how widely to resect around the lesion when performing resection surgery. Accordingly, a 3 mm margin through dense fascia may be the equivalent of a 3 cm margin through skeletal muscle. Likewise, a 5 mm margin through cortical bone may have the same ability to inhibit tumor penetration as a 5 cm margin through cancellous bone or loose connective tissue.

Preoperative Evaluation

The clinical approach to a patient with a suspected tumor is of critical importance. Proper prebiopsy studies are imperative to adequately delineate the nature of the mass and its anatomic setting. The first study to be obtained following an adequate history and physical is a plain x-ray. This should always be the first study performed because it is inexpensive, safe, and yields considerable information. The plain x-ray differentiates bony from soft tissue masses and shows the extent of bone involvement as well as the nature of the lesion's border, which reflects on its biologic potential. Even in the case of soft tissue lesions, plain x-rays often give a good clue regarding location of a lesion and may show soft tissue calcification suggestive of either a benign or a malignant lesion.

In years past, the arteriogram was the next study in line and was really the gold standard in terms of information relative to the anatomic setting. Now with the availability of CT scans and MRI scans, the arteriogram is of little diagnostic value in the preoperative workup of extremity lesions. Arteriography can be used therapeutically when highly vascularized lesions can be embolized prior to definitive resection but this is almost never indicated prior to biopsy. For example, in the case of a known cell type that tends to be highly vascular, metastatic hypernephroma, embolization may well be worthwhile prior to resection, especially for lesions about the hip and pelvis where the use of a tourniquet is not possible.

CT scans and MRI scans are invaluable in the preoperative assessment of musculoskeletal lesions.[1] CT scans delineate very well the anatomic setting of a tumor but, for the most part, give little information regarding the nature of the lesion. One notable exception to this is the benign lipoma. One can reliably diagnose a benign lipoma on CT scan when one encounters a lesion of uniform black fat density with only occasional interstitial stranding. This is a much different picture than is noted with even a very low grade liposarcoma, which tends to have a sandy appearance. The MRI scan gives considerable information about bone or soft tissue lesions as well. Typically, CAT scans are better for evaluating cortical involvement; MRI scans excel in delineating both the extraosseous and marrow involvement of bone tumors and the extent of soft tissue tumors.

Finally, the technetium-99 bone scan is also helpful in assessing the nature of the lesion and its present behavior. A calcified lesion showing no increased uptake on bone scan is almost always quiescent. Lytic lesions such as myeloma occasionally may not show up as hot spots but most lytic lesions do. In most cases then, the preoperative assessment of a musculoskeletal lesion includes a plain x-ray. If there is any question about the lesion being a primary musculoskeletal neoplasm then a CT scan and MRI scan and bone scan are valuable. Once a preoperative assessment has been made, a biopsy is needed to elucidate the pathologic nature of the lesion. Chapter 20 covers the treatment of biopsy of musculoskeletal lesions.

Surgical Treatment Alternatives

One of the great challenges of musculoskeletal tumor surgery is that each case is somewhat different and individual. Each has its own combination of tumor grade, cell type, and clinical setting. In spite of this myriad of situations that confront the surgeon, one only has a limited number of choices in terms of surgical alternatives.

Basically stated, the nature and setting of a lesion determine its treatment. Integral with this is the concept that the treatment should not be more harsh than the disease. As such, it is the responsibility of the tumor surgeon to select the treatment that adequately deals with the disorder at hand while tailoring the surgery and adjunctive treatments to minimize functional and cosmetic deficits.

Intralesional Surgery

Benign lesions in bone offer the surgeon an opportunity to perform procedures with little or no morbidity and at the same time achieve a high rate of local control, which translates as cure in the context of many of these lesions.[10]

The rationale behind intralesional surgery is that a benign tumor is basically contained within the limits of the gross lesion and does not stream into the surrounding cancellous bone. Removing the lesion totally should therefore not leave behind residual tumor that could cause a recurrence. Those lesions in bone most commonly treated in this fashion include osteoid osteoma, osteoblastoma, enchondroma, chrondromyxoid fibroma, chondroblastoma, eosinophilic granuloma, giant cell tumor, and aneurysmal bone cyst. For whatever lesion encountered, intralesional surgery should be performed in a similar fashion. In order to do this properly, several steps to the procedure must be followed:

1. Adequate soft tissue exposure
2. Complete unroofing of the lesion
3. Curettage
4. Burring to extend the curettage
5. Cautery (phenol, liquid nitrogen)
6. Irrigation
7. Bone graft or bone cement

Adequate soft tissue exposure is essential with intralesional surgery as with any surgical procedure. Overlapping soft tissues obscure one's view and increase the risk of soft tissue seeding. Whenever possible the soft tissues should be shielded with sponges or towels so that contamination of these tissues with neoplastic particles is minimized. This is especially important for any cartilage tumor because cartilage can readily seed into almost any surrounding tissue.

Complete unroofing of the lesion is the next step and the one most frequently skimped on by the occasional tumor surgeon. As shown in Figure 14–1

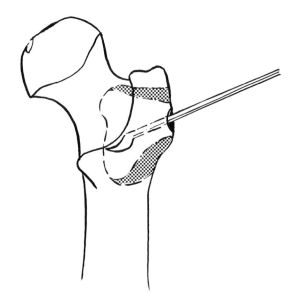

Fig. **14–1.** Successful intralesional surgery depends on one's ability to see the entire surface of a tumor-bearing cavity.

successful intralesional surgery depends on one's ability to see the entire contents of a tumor-bearing cavity. This necessitates complete unroofing of the lesion so that every square millimeter of the tumor cavity is visible. This prevents the surgeon from inadvertently leaving behind gross tumor, which could continue to grow and cause local recurrence.

Curettage of the lesion is best done with a large curette followed by progressively smaller curettes so that all visible cavities are evacuated. Many lesions include sclerotic septae within the lesion. These must be removed, usually with a burr or rongeur, so that no tumor-bearing nooks remain.

The burr is then used to extend the curettage beyond the rim of the curetted cavity. Many of the lesions for which intralesional surgery is indicated have an irregular border with crests and undulations as shown in Figure 14–2. Simple curettage will not remove the fingers of tumor contained within this transitional zone. Careful use of a burr will allow the surgeon to excise all tissues of this zone of transition back to normal tissue. Careful and intelligent use of the burr can greatly aid in reducing local recurrence while not increasing the associated morbidity. Care should be taken to preserve articular cartilage whenever possible when dealing with juxta-articular lesions.

Once the tumor has been burred, it is reasonable to attempt some form of cauterization of the interior of the lesion so that none of the evacuated tissues can reimplant into the wall of the cavity. Several options are available to the surgeon in this regard. Liquid nitrogen may be applied to create a repeated freeze-thaw cycle. This can be effective but is difficult to apply and contain. Some authors have advocated extensive electrocautery of the cavity though few studies of this technique have been published. The author's preferred technique is to carefully shield the soft tissues around the cavity and then paint the cavity carefully with 90% phenol solution. Great care must be taken not to allow the phenol to contact any of the soft tissues around the wound or any part of the operating team's gowns, gloves, or drape. After application, the phenol can be flushed away with sterile ethyl alcohol followed by copious irrigation with a water pick device.

Once the cavity preparation is complete some form of filler is usually indicated. The principal choices here are autograft or allograft cancellous bone or bone cement. Autogenous cancellous bone is the most desirable filler in most cases. It rapidly incorporates and carries no risk of transmissable diseases such as hepatitis or AIDS. Bone cement is, however, useful especially when support for the articular surface has been lost. In this situation, filling the defect with bone cement provides good support for the articular surface and can maintain the congruity of the joint. Because cement is a stress sharing substance, the surrounding bone will usu-

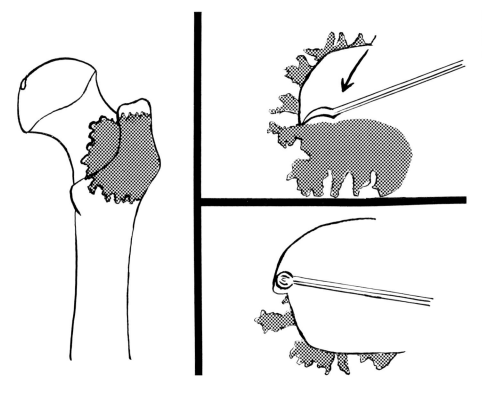

FIG. **14–2.** After thorough curretage, a burr is used to resect the interdigitating margin between tumor and bone.

ally hypertrophy and become stronger with time and gradually progressive weight-bearing.

Limb Salvage Surgery

Historical Perspective

In recent years limb salvage surgery has surfaced as a viable alternative to amputation.[3] Although there was initial concern regarding its safety, limb salvage has been shown to be as safe as an amputation when performed in accordance with the basic tenets of oncologic surgery. Several factors have emerged to enable the surgeon to perform adequate tumor ablation without the need for limb removal. Among the most important of these factors was the development of viable reconstructive techniques especially in the context of bone sarcomas. Several reconstructive options now exist for bone defects. These include articular and intercallery prostheses and allografts as well as vascularized or nonvascularized autografts. Improvement in internal fixation techniques during the past decade also has aided greatly in this regard.

All available reconstructive techniques pose advantages and disadvantages. Prostheses often can be relied on for short-term results with good active range of motion of the involved joint and the ability to begin early weight-bearing. This makes them especially well suited to the elderly or those whose disease indicates a short predicted survival. When used in the context of younger patients, however, or those with a longer life expectancy problems with fracture and loosening can be expected. Nonvascularized autografts are readily available and are permanent once incorporated. They do suffer, however, from a prolonged period to incorporation and a fair incidence of nonunion and stress fracture.

Vascularized bone grafts are a valuable and fairly recent addition to the surgeon's armamentarium.[5,7] Although they possess the good qualities of ready availability and rapid incorporation, they add significantly to the length of the operative procedure and may be associated with difficulty in internal fixation. Also, if the vascularity of the graft fails, incorporation may be relatively slower than with a nonvascularized transfer because of an inhibition of vascular penetration by the soft tissues surrounding the graft.

Allografts have gained increasing popularity during the past 5 years especially as studies showing good short- to medium-term results have become available.[9] Those factors in favor of allografts include their ready availability and their permanent nature once incorporated. The essential problems associated with allograft use include a long period to incorporation, a high risk of early and late infection, and a high rate of nonunion. One must also consider the potential for fracture and, in the case of osteoarticular grafts, ligamentous instability and accelerated degenerative disease of the involved joint. All present reconstructive options therefore, offer particular advantages and disadvantages. Careful consideration of these factors should precede the use of any of these techniques.

Also important in contributing to modern limb salvage techniques has been the development of effective adjunctive treatments, specifically radiation therapy and chemotherapy. Radiation therapy is a local modality that can help decrease tumor size and viability when given preoperatively.[14] The one major drawback with preoperative radiation is a significant increase in wound complications that can be expected when performing extensive operations through large fields of tissues previously subjected to 4000 or more rads of external beam radiation. In spite of this, radiation given preoperatively can increase resectability of radiosensitive lesions that are otherwise difficult to resect. For the most part, this excludes chondrosarcoma and osteosarcoma, which are relatively radioresistant.

Because postoperative radiation usually is not given until 2 to 3 weeks following surgery, it has a lesser effect on wound healing. Given postoperatively to a well planned field, external beam radiation can significantly decrease the local recurrence rate of radiosensitive lesions following wide resection. Several large series have shown that for radiosensitive lesions (i.e., soft tissue sarcomas) postoperative radiation following a well planned wide resection can give local control values approaching those gained with wide amputation.[12]

The surgeon can help to optimize radiation therapy by marking the periphery of the operative field with four to six small hemaclips. It is also possible to mark any area of questionable tumor margin with clips so that these areas can receive special attention by the radiation therapists in planning a coned-down field. Without this type of information, planning a radiation field is much more difficult and usually forces the radiation therapist to expose a larger volume of tissue than would otherwise be necessary. This is to be avoided because the morbidity from radiation increases with increasing field size.

Chemotherapy as an adjunct offers several advantages. When given preoperatively it can effectively debulk tumors while also providing systemic treatment at that time in the course of the disease when the systemic tumor burden is at its smallest. Also, unlike preoperative radiation, preoperative chemotherapy does not adversely affect the vascularity of tissues and so is not associated with an increased wound complication rate. When given postoperatively, chemotherapy can increase the disease-free survival for some lesions, notably adolescent osteosarcoma.[6]

Current treatment recommendations for sarcomas are outlined in Table 14–2. Low grade radioresistant lesions require a wide surgical margin and this alone usually constitutes adequate treatment. Included in this category are chondrosarcoma, chordoma, and adamantinoma. Low grade radiosensitive lesions basically encompass the low grade soft tissue sarcomas. Wide margin surgery done for these lesions is associated with a high local recurrence rate and so requires adjunctive radiation therapy. This combination provides a high rate of local control.

High grade radioresistant lesions, namely osteosarcoma, require wide margin surgery for local control. Good local control, however, has little effect on disease-free survival, which requires chemotherapy to counter the systemic spread of tumor. High grade soft tissue sarcoma are likewise a systemic disease in most patients by the time of presentation of the primary tumor. Local control for these lesions is obtained in the same fashion as with the low grade soft tissue sarcomas by combining wide margin surgery with adequate radiation. Ideally, these patients also should receive systemic chemotherapy in order to counter the systemic spread of the tumor. Unfortunately, data showing a positive effect of chemotherapy on disease-free survival in patients with high grade soft tissue sarcomas are scant at present.[11]

Resection For Pelvic Sarcomas

Pelvic sarcomas present a broad spectrum of tumor location, size, and extraosseous extension , all of which combine to determine the amount of resection necessary. The easiest lesions to deal with are those in the iliac wing. Those tumors that are

TABLE 14–2. *Sarcoma Treatment*

Radio resistant	Radio sensitive
Low Grade	
Surgery	Surgery and Radiation
Chondrosarcoma	
Chordoma	Soft tissue sarcomas
Adamantioma	
High Grade	
Surgery and Chemotherapy	Surgery, Radiation, and Chemotherapy
Osteosarcoma	Soft tissue sarcomas

reasonable in size, especially the low grade lesions, frequently can be treated by *en block* excision of the wing of the ilium. This is followed by fixation of the supra-acetabular area directly to the sacroiliac region by pivoting the involved hemipelvis about the pubic symphysis. This causes minor shortening of the involved leg but otherwise little morbidity. Unfortunately, these lesions are less common than those involving the acetabular region or the pubis.

For lesions in the difficult acetabular and pubic locations, two basic options exist. These include standard hemipelvectomy (Fig. 14–4) and internal hemipelvectomy, which preserves the lower limb. Pubic lesions close to the symphysis occasionally can be resected with preservation of the hip joints in which case no reconstruction is necessary. When acetabular involvement is noted, extra-articular resection of the hip joint may be necessary if real concern about seeding of the hip joint is present.

Resection for these periacetabular lesions is begun with the patient positioned for a typical hemipelvectomy. This is usually the lateral decubitus position with the leg prepared free and the trunk supported loosely so that it can be rolled forward and backward on the table. A Foley catheter and central venous and arterial monitors are essential. A rigid stent placed cystoscopically into the ureter on the involved side also is helpful in delineating the location of this structure because the stent can be palpated intrapelvicly.

A typical internal hemipelvectomy incision begins at the posterior iliac spine and runs anteriorly above the wing of the ilium and over the inguinal ligament almost to the pubic symphysis. This incision is transected by a second incision starting laterally and extending distally over the greater trochanter and along the proximal femur. The gluteus maximus muscle forms the bulk of this large posterior flap and should be protected along with its blood supply from the inferior gluteal artery. For the same reason it is desirable not to ligate the hypogastric artery for fear of devascularizing the gluteus flap. The other principal structures that must be identified and protected are the sciatic nerve as it exits the greater sciatic notch and the femoral neurovascular bundle as it runs distal to the inguinal ligament. Again, the location and extent of the lesion dictate the amount of resection.

Reconstruction following internal hemipelvectomy is possible in some cases. Hemipelvis allografts have been performed but should be considered experimental. The most common method of reconstruction is the iliofemoral fusion. This is possible only in those patients with a fair amount

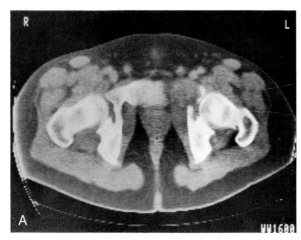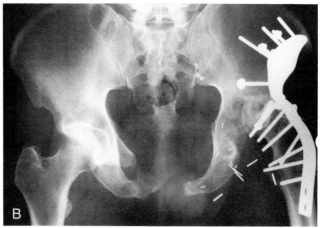

Fig. **14–3A.** Preoperative CAT scan showing a sarcoma involving the left pubis and acetabulum. **B.** Postoperative x-ray of the same patient after partial internal hemipelvectomy and iliofemoral fusion.

of ilium remaining to which the femur can be fixed. Use of a large cobra plate permits rigid fixation. Once fusion is complete, usually within three months, these patients have essentially the same gait as those undergoing other hip fusions, however the leg shortening is more pronounced (Fig. 14–3).

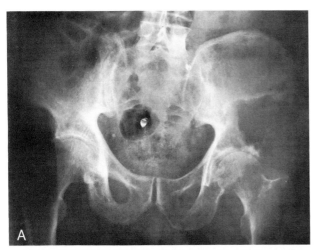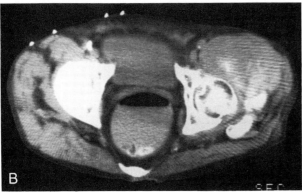

Fig. **14–4.** Not all lesions are candidates for limb salvage surgery. This high-grade malignant fibrous histiocytoma required standard hemipelvectomy for local control.

In many cases, internal hemipelvectomy requires removal of such a large portion of the hemipelvis that no boney reconstruction or fusion is possible. These patients can still bear weight on the involved extremity, which articulates against the soft tissues of the pelvis. The function following this procedure can be compared to that following a Girdlestone pseudoarthrosis but with greater leg pistoning and less active motion[13] (Fig. 14–4).

Resection of proximal femoral tumors and reconstruction with proximal femoral replacement prostheses has emerged as a viable treatment option for lesions in this location. This is described in Chapter 25.

References

1. BLAND KI, McCoy M, KINARD RE, COPELAND EM: Application of magnetic resonance imaging and computerized tomography as an adjunct to the surgical management of soft tissue sarcomas. Ann Surg, 205:473–481, 1987.
2. DEVEREAUX DF, et al.: Surgical treatment of low grade soft tissue sarcomas. Am J Surg, 143:490–495, 1982.
3. EILBER FR, et al.: Is amputation necessary for sarcomas? A seven year experience with limb salvage. Ann Surg, 192:431–437, 1980.
4. ENNEKING WF, SPANIER SS, GOODMAN MA: A system for the surgical staging of musculoskeletal sarcomas. Clin Orthop, 153:106–120, 1980.
5. GOLDBERG VM, et al.: Biology of vascularized bone grafts. Orthop Clin North Am, 18:197–205, 1987.
6. GOORIN AM, ABELSON HT, FREI E: Osteosarcoma: fifteen years later. N Eng J Med, 313:1637–1643, 1985.
7. JUPITER JB, et al.: The reconstruction of defects in the femoral shaft with vascularized transfers of fibular bone. J Bone Joint Surg, 69:365–374, 1987.
8. LAWRENCE W, et al.: Adult soft tissue sarcomas. Ann Surg, 205:349–359, 1987.
9. MANKIN HJ, DOPPELT S, TOMFORD W: Clinical experience with

allograft implantation: the first ten years. CORR, 174:69–86, 1983.

10. McDonald DJ, et al.: Giant cell tumor of bone. J Bone Joint Surg, 68:235–242, 1986.

11. Rosenberg SA: Prospective randomized trials demonstrating the efficacy of adjustment chemotherapy in adult patients with soft tissue sarcomas. Cancer Treat Reports 68:1067–78, 1984.

12. Shire MH, et al.: Control of locally advanced extremity soft tissue sarcomas by function-saving resection and brachy-therapy. Cancer, 53:1385–92, 1984.

13. Steel HH: Partial or complete resection of the hemipelvis: an alternative to hindquarter amputation for peri-acetabular chondrosarcoma of the pelvis. J Bone Joint Surg, 60:719–730, 1978.

14. Suit HD, et al.: Treatment of the patient with stage M_0 soft tissue sarcoma. J Clin Oncology, 6:854–862, 1988.

CHAPTER FIFTEEN

Septic Arthritis of the Hip

R. MICHAEL BUCKLEY
STEPHEN J. GLUCKMAN

Septic arthritis of the hip is a serious and challenging problem for the clinician. This continues to be the case despite the advent of new diagnostic modalities and multiple potent antimicrobials. The typical constellation of symptoms and signs may be absent, and the diagnosis is often delayed. Because early recognition and therapy is directly related to morbidity and mortality, it is essential for physicians who may care for these patients to be familiar with typical and atypical presentations, etiologic agents, the utility of diagnostic tests, and the array of therapeutic agents available.

Although other causes will be mentioned, this chapter concentrates primarily on bacterial arthritis of the hip in the adult. We have excluded postsurgical infections.

Incidence

The true incidence of nonsurgical septic arthritis of the hip is difficult to determine. Reports from the 1950s suggested that bacterial arthritis was a major feature of illness in only .02% of hospital admissions.[36] However, gonococcal infections have commonly been under-reported, and joints are not routinely examined at autopsy. Kelly, et al., reviewed the experience at the Mayo Clinic of adult bacterial arthritis of the hip and found 26 patients in 20 years.[14] Of 59 patients seen with septic arthritis at Boston City Hospital between 1965 and 1972, 5 had infections of the hip.[8] In a review from Oxford, England, from 1945 to 1975, septic arthritis of the hip and knee was more common than septic arthritis of other joints, but septic arthritis of the knee had become relatively more common than of the hip by the 1960s. Over the 30 year period there were 29 hip infections in patients over 15 years of age.[25] Thus nonsurgical septic arthritis of the hip is an unusual occurrence, further challenging the diagnostic skills of the clinician.

Predisposing Factors

Certain host factors that predispose patients to develop septic arthritis are found consistently in all the series cited previously. The most common factor is concurrent extra-articular infection. Because nearly all cases of nonsurgical septic arthritis are considered to be hematogenous in origin, a primary focus of such sepsis can often be identified. Blood cultures are positive only in approximately 50% of cases, however, many patients have a positive bacterial culture from another site such as urine, skin, or sputum.[8] The site obviously varies with the bacteria involved (e.g., a carbuncle with staphylococcus and a urinary tract infection with gram negative organisms). A more recent cause of nosocomial sepsis, infected intravenous catheters, may become another important predisposing and associated infection.

In the past decade the infectious complications of IV drug use have become well known. Although septic arthritis in these patients often involves the sternoclavicular joint, hips too can become infected. Finally, septic arthritis of the hip may complicate disseminated gonococcal infection.[31]

Prior arthritis of the infected joint is another important association. Bacterial arthritis can complicate many forms of joint disease including gout, pseudogout, lupus, osteoarthritis, and avascular necrosis of the femoral head.[9,10,28,34] Rheumatoid arthritis, however, seems to be the major joint disease predisposing to septic arthritis.[13,21] This is particularly important to keep in mind because pyarthrosis complicating rheumatoid arthritis may be difficult to diagnose. Patients may only complain of a minimal increase in pain over their previous joint discomfort, and their steroid therapy may suppress fever.

Serious chronic illness such as diabetes mellitus and cirrhosis may predispose to infections of joints, as may malignancy and immunosuppressive therapy. Prior antibiotic therapy has recently been found as an association with septic arthritis. Whether it truly predisposes to joint infection or simply changes the bacteria involved is speculative.[8]

Steroid injections into joints has often been mentioned as an iatrogenic factor in septic arthritis. Hollander, et al., found 14 episodes of septic arthritis in 4000 patients receiving over 100,000 intrasynovial injections.[2] This is probably more infections than chance alone, and a history of joint injection should always be sought when evaluating a patient suspected of having septic arthritis.

Clinical Presentation

The classic symptoms in septic arthritis of the hip are fever, joint pain, joint tenderness and swelling, and decreased range of motion on examination. However, these classic symptoms are not always present as evidenced by the fact that a delay in diagnosis of up to 3 weeks was commonly found in one large series.[14] Fever is not always present, and it can be transient and low grade. Only 25% of patients have a shaking chill, and septic shock associated with bacterial arthritis is rare.[8] Hip pain from known prior arthritis further complicates the picture. The clinician's index of suspicion must therefore be high. Low grade fever in the setting of hip pain should suggest sepsis, as should any increase in pain on flexion or adduction of the hip over that previously noted. If any of the predisposing factors discussed in the previous section are also present, especially concurrent extra-articular infection, suspicion should be further heightened. Because delay in recognition is associated with worse prognosis, prompt steps should be taken to make a rapid diagnosis.

Bacteria Associated With Septic Arthritis

Although it is important to have working knowledge of the organisms associated with septic arthritis in some order of frequency, it is essential to make a specific diagnosis in individual cases by culture of synovial fluid as well as appropriate extra-articular sites.

The gonococcus, the most common cause of bacterial arthritis in most large series, rarely infects the hip.[31] When it does infect the hip the clinical presentation is similar to other forms of bacterial arthritis. It is not generally seen as part of the disseminated gonococcal infection syndrome, which is

Table 15–1. *Bacteria Causing Septic Arthritis*

Gonococcus—Approximately 50%*
Staphylococcus aureus—25 to 50%
Methicillin Resistant Staphylococcus Aureus—0 to 25%+
Pneumococcus—0 to 10%
Haemophilus—approximately 1%
Streptococcus pyogenes—0 to 10%
Anaerobic streptococci—0 to 10%
Gram negative bacilli—5 to 30%
   pseudomonas+
   Escherichia coli
   proteus
   serratia+

*Rarely causes hip infection
+Mostly in IV drug users

characterized by skin rash, migratory polyarthritis or arthralgias, and tenosynovitis. Rather it presents as a monarthritis after the skin lesions and other signs of the bacteremic phase have passed.[31] Bacteria that cause nongonococcal septic arthritis of the hip are similar to those that cause septic arthritis of other joints. In Kelly's series of 26 patients Staphylococcus aureus infected 16, Pseudomonas 3, Proteus species, Streptococcus pyogenes, and anaerobic streptococcus, 2 each, and Escherichia coli, 1.[14] Other series have similar relative frequencies with the pneumococcus and Haemophilus influenzae also occasional pathogens (Table 15–1). Gram negative organisms have been more frequent pathogens in the last 15 years, and in drug addicts methicillin resistant Staphylococcus aureus is being seen with alarming frequency.[2]

The virulence of the infecting bacteria has some bearing on prognosis. In general, gram negative rods carry a higher mortality and morbidity in septic arthritis. Of the gram positive organisms staphylococci produce more residual joint disability than do the streptococci. Still, the single most important prognostic factor that the clinician has an influence over is the rapidity and accuracy of the diagnosis, and the prompt institution of appropriate therapy.

Tuberculous and Fungal Septic Arthritis

Mycobacteria and fungi are rare causes of hip infection. Joint involvement now occurs in less than 1% of patients with tuberculosis. It occurs as a chronic monarticular arthritis of a weight-bearing joint in the presence of a positive purified protein derivative. Diagnosis is best achieved by examination of both synovial fluid and tissue. Histologic examination and culture tests of synovium has the highest yield. Early diagnosis is again important for optimal functional results with therapy.[36]

Mycotic joint infections are rare. The characteristics, the organisms involved, and the outcome of such infections depend primarily on the associated underlying disease.[36] Again, diagnosis is best established by histologic examination and culture tests of both synovium and synovial fluid.

Diagnosis

A combination of the historical features, physical examination findings, and synovial fluid analysis usually results in the proper diagnosis of septic arthritis. Further, these features often give the clinician an indication of the likely pathogen. Additional testing is rarely indicated and rarely helpful. Though atypical presentations do occur, a story of the subacute or acute onset of pain, swelling and warmth in a single joint, or uncommonly several joints, associated with the physical findings of fever, joint inflammation, and significantly decreased joint motion should suggest the diagnosis of septic arthritis.

When the clinical setting suggests an infected joint it is essential to aspirate the joint. Analysis of the synovial fluid is the single most important test in the diagnosis of septic arthritis. Fluoroscopic guidance may be needed for hip aspiration: it is crucial to be sure that the joint has been sampled. Fluid should be placed in a heparinized tube. Several key tests include white blood cell count in the fluid, gram stain, culture, and analysis for crystals in a polarizing microscope. Culture tests should generally be performed on the routine aerobic and anaerobic media. Thayer-Martin media is not necessary for a normally sterile fluid, and the antibiotics in this medium may interfere with the isolation of some sensitive gonococci.

There is some overlap with other causes of acute inflammation, nonetheless, the WBC count in the synovial fluid is of value in the diagnosis of an infected joint. Although WBC counts in the fluid have been reported to be as low as 6800/mm in acute nongonococcal septic arthritis,[8] Krey, et al.,[16] in a series of 310 patients with culture-proven disease found 70% to have a count of more than 50,000/mm. An elevation to this degree was seen in only 10% of patients with crystal-induced disease, and 4% with acute rheumatoid arthritis. Rosenthal, et al., described a series of 71 patients with nongonococcal septic arthritis in which the average WBC count was 132,000/mm. Although a relatively low WBC count can be seen with septic arthritis, the higher the count the more likely that infection is the cause of the joint inflammation.

Gram stain tests of the fluid are positive in one-half to two-thirds of the cases.[7,8,25] When positive it not only proves the infectious nature of the inflammation, but also gives the clinician a good idea of the exact pathogen.

Crystal-induced arthritis and septic arthritis can occur in the same joint and they can be difficult to differentiate clinically. Therefore, crystals should be looked for in all infected joints and all synovial fluids with crystals should nonetheless be cultured.

The joint fluid viscosity, protein content, and glucose level are not sensitive enough tests to be useful in distinguishing the causes of an acutely inflamed joint; they add nothing to the above laboratory evaluation.

Recent work has suggested that the synovial fluid lactic acid level may help distinguish non-gonococcal pyogenic arthritis from other causes of inflammation; it was reported by Brook, et al., to be elevated only in the former situation.[4] Counterimmunoelectrophoresis to detect soluble bacterial antigens has limited value, but occasionally may be useful when the patient has received antibiotics prior to joint aspiration.

Synovial biopsy is not necessary for pyogenic infections, but often is required for the diagnosis of tuberculous arthritis.

Blood cultures should always be performed. They can be expected to be positive in 35 to 50% of patients with nongonococcal septic arthritis. Culture tests of the cervix, throat, and rectum for gonococci are important in the evaluation of arthritis when that organism is suspected.

Additional laboratory testing is rarely useful. Erythrocyte sedimentation rate usually is elevated, but is not specific enough to be beneficial. The peripheral WBC count is variable.[8,25,30]

X-ray is not generally a helpful test in this setting. It will confirm soft tissue swelling, and often show an increase in the joint space caused by fluid. Neither are specific findings. Later changes include joint space narrowing as the cartilage is destroyed and periarticular osteopenia.

Radionucleotide scanning is sensitive for joint inflammation, but not specific enough to help distinguish the cause. These techniques occasionally may be useful in distinguishing an overlying cellulitis from septic arthritis when the preferred procedure of joint aspiration is not feasible.[17] Similarly CT scanning is unlikely to add to joint aspiration in the evaluation of an acutely inflamed joint.

The differential diagnosis includes crystal-induced arthritis, acute rheumatoid arthritis, acute Reiter's syndrome, and acute hemarthrosis. In addition, a number of viruses are associated with acute joint inflammation, most common among these are rubella and hepatitis B.

Cellulitis in the region of a joint can be a differential diagnostic concern. It usually can be distinguished when joint movement is not as dramatically limited as in an infected joint. Aspiration of the joint through an uninvolved area is the definitive test.

Septic bursitis occurs in the olecranon and prepatellar bursae. It is associated with periarticular inflammation but joint motion is relatively preserved. This can be diagnosed by aspiration of the bursa.

Treatment

Recommendations for treatment are based primarily on clinical experience rather than on prospective controlled trials. It is generally agreed that optimal treatment should begin promptly and that it should include antimicrobial agents, drainage, and physical therapy. Because initiating therapy is urgent, it is usually started before the definitive microbiology is known, but after the joint has been tapped and specimens sent for analysis.

Appropriate initial antibiotic therapy depends on the results of the gram stain and on the clinical setting (Table 15–2). Antibiotics have proliferated greatly in the last decade. This has resulted in many acceptable empiric regimens: Table 15–2 suggests some reasonable options but many others also are appropriate. If gram negative diplococci are seen on the gram stain, then one can presume that the infecting organism is Neisseria gonorrhea. Be-

cause increasing numbers of these strains are now resistant to penicillin, ceftriaxone should be used until the results of sensitivity tests are known. Gram positive cocci are likely to be staphylococcus aureus and occasionally streptococci. Unless the setting suggests Methicillin-resistant organisms (MRSA), a semisynthetic penicillin such as nafcillin is suggested. Vancomycin is an alternative when there is a possibility of MRSA or of penicillin allergy. Less commonly, gram negative bacilli are seen on the gram stain. In an otherwise normal host these usually are members of the Enterobacteriaceae such as *Escherichia coli* or Klebsiella from a urinary source, however, coverage should include more resistant organisms such as *Pseudomonas aeruginosa*. A drug with an extended gram negative spectrum such as ceftizoxime or ticarcillin is prudent. If the patient has a penicillin allergy, aztreonam is a reasonable alternative.

A negative gram stain represents a little more of a challenge. Nonetheless, on usually can predict the likely bacteria involved. If the patient is otherwise healthy with no unusual predisposing factors, then Neisseria gonorrhea or Staphylococcus aureus are the major concerns. These are covered with ceftriaxone. If the patient is penicillin allergic, then spectinomycin plus nafcillin can be substituted. As above, if MRSA is a possibility, then vancomycin should be used instead of nafcillin.

Immunosuppressed patients or parenteral drug abusers can be infected with any bacteria. Therefore, the coverage must be broad until the culture and sensitivity test results are known. Vancomycin plus ceftizoxime or ticarcillin is a suggested option. If the patient is penicillin allergic, aztreonam can be substituted as above.

Parenteral administration is the standard route of therapy. Though the need for intra-articular antibiotics has frequently been suggested, essentially all

TABLE 15–2. *Initial Treatment Recommendations*

Gram Stain	Likely Pathogen(s)	Antibiotic(s)	Alternative
1. Gram (negative) diplococci	Neisseria gonorrhoeae	Ceftriaxone	Spectinomycin
2. Gram (positive) cocci	Staphylococcus aureus Streptococci	Nalcillin	Vancomycin
3. Gram (negative) bacilli	Enterobacteriaceae Pseudomonas aeruginosa	Ceftazidime or Ticarcillin	Aztreonam
4. No organisms seen			
a. Normal adult	Neisseria gonorrhoeae Staphlococcus aureus	Ceftriaxone	Spectinomycin plus Vancomycin
b. Immunosuppressed intravenous drug abuser	Any bacteria	Ceftazidime or Mezlocillin plus Vancomycin	Aztreonam plus Vancomycin

antibiotics studied give adequate synovial fluid levels with parenteral administration.[6,11,23,26,27] There is no benefit from intra-articular administration of antibiotics and there is some concern that such instillation may occasionally produce joint inflammation. Some clinicians like to use 2 to 6 weeks of oral antibiotics after a completed course of parenteral therapy, however, the necessity and the efficacy of such additional therapy is unproven.

There are several pediatric series using only oral therapy. This has been administered under carefully monitored conditions to ensure gastrointestinal absorption and compliance.[15,24,35] This route cannot be recommended at the present time for adults though the recent introduction of oral quinolone antibiotics such as ciprofloxacin may eventually make this a realistic option.

The duration of therapy has not been well established, however, for gonococcal joint infection several days of intravenous therapy followed by 10 days of oral therapy is generally curative. For non-gonococcal septic arthritis duration should be between 2 to 4 weeks in most circumstances, the longer course for organisms that are more difficult to cure, such as Staphylococcus aureus and gram negative bacilli.

As with all closed space infections, adequate drainage is mandatory for a successful outcome. Not only is it harder to sterilize an undrained joint, but emergent drainage is necessary to minimize joint injury. Undrained pus in a joint destroys the joint cartilage by a number of mechanisms including ischemic damage resulting from increased pressure, and the direct effects of proteolytic enzymes and superoxide radicals released from the leukocytes. Though there is considerable debate about the relative merits of needle drainage versus arthrotomy for other joints, with the exception of gonococcal infections a septic hip needs opened drainage. Effective needle drainage of this joint is difficult to achieve. Ingress and egress catheters are of no proven value, and are unlikely to add to thorough opened drainage. In addition, they pose a risk for superinfection of the joint.

Rehabilitation is the third component to successful therapy of a septic hip. Early in the therapy the joint should be kept at rest to decrease the pain. After several days passive range of motion can be instituted. Eventually active range of motion to restore as much joint mobility as possible is critical.

Experience with tuberculous infection of a hip joint is less extensive than pyogenic infection. Antimicrobial therapy should be the same as in other active tuberculosis with administration of rifampin, isoniazid, and pyrazinamide for 6 months.

The need for opened drainage is more controversial, because the infection is often more indolent most patients improve without it.[1] The more acute the onset and the higher the joint WBC count, the greater the concern about joint cartilage destruction without adequate drainage.

The only common fungus to infect a hip is Candida. This occurs in the setting of an infected subclavian catheter or an immunosuppressed patient. Presentation is similar to pyogenic bacteria. Amphotericin B, opened drainage, and rehabilitation is the therapy.

Outcome

The prognosis for a septic hip depends on the underlying disease, the microorganism involved, and the duration of time from the onset of symptoms to the initiation of therapy.[11] There are no statistics on hip infections alone, but in general the mortality associated with septic arthritis is between 8 to 15%.[8,25,30] Patients with underlying rheumatoid arthritis seem to do particularly badly.[8,12] The long term outcome for joint function is guarded.

Summary

Infection in the hip joint is most likely to be engrafted upon a previously damaged joint. It is most commonly caused by gonococci and Staphylcoccus aureus, but is occasionally caused by gram negative bacilli and other organisms. Diagnosis is based upon recognition of the clinical presentation and analysis of the synovial fluid. Therapy should be initiated promptly. Empiric antibiotics should be instituted based on the clinical situation and the results of the gram stain. With the exception of gonococcal infections, an arthrotomy should be performed for adequate drainage. Duration of therapy is by convention between 2 to 4 weeks.

References

1. Alvarez S, McCabe WR: Extrapulmonary tuberculosis revisited: a review of experience at Boston City and other hospitals. Medicine, 63:25–55, 1984.
2. Ang-Fonte G, Rozboril M: Changes in gonococcal septic arthritis: drug abuse and methicillin resistance staphylococcus aureus. Arthritis Rheum, 28:210, 1985.
3. Bayer AS, et al.: Gram-negative bacillary septic arthritis:

Clinical, radiologic, therapeutic, and prognostic features. Sem Arthritis Rheum, 7:123, 1977.

4. Brook I, et al.:Synovial fluid lactic acid: a diagnostic test for septic arthritis. Arthritis Rheum, 21:774–779, 1978.

5. Flatman JG: Hip disease with referral pain to the knee. JAMA, 234:967, 1975.

6. Fraser GL: Treatment of nongonoccocal bacterial septic arthritis. Drug Intell Clin Pharm, 15:531, 1981.

7. Garcia-Kutzbach A, Masi AT: Acute infectious agent arthritis: a detailed comparison of proved gonococcal and other blood-borne bacterial arthritis. J Rheumatol, 1:93, 1974.

8. Goldenberg DL, Cohen AS: Acute infectious arthritis. Am J Med, 60:369, 1976.

9. Habermann ET, Friedenthal RB: Septic arthritis associated with avascular necrosis of the femoral head. Clin Orthop, 134:325, 1978.

10. Hess RJ, Martin JH: Pyarthrosis complicating gout. JAMA, 218:592, 1971.

11. Ho G, Toder JS, Zimmerman B: An overview of septic arthritis and septic bursitis. Orthopedics, 7:1571, 1984.

12. Karten I: Septic arthritis complicating rheumatoid arthritis. Ann Intern Med, 70:1147, 1969.

13. Kellgren JH, Ball J, Fairbrother R, et al.: Suppurative arthritis complicating rheumatoid arthritis. Br Med J, 1:1193, 1958.

14. Kelly PJ, Martin WJ, Coventry MB: Bacterial arthritis of the hip in the adult. J Bone Joint Surg, 47(A):1005, 1965.

15. Kolyvas E, et al.: Oral antibiotic therapy of skeletal infections in children. Pediatrics, 65:867, 1980.

16. Krey PR, Bailen DA: Synovial fluid leucocytosis. Am J Med, 67:436–442, 1979.

17. Lisbona R, Rosenthal L: Observations on the sequential use of 99mTC phosphate complex and 67Ga imaging in osteomyelitis, cellulitis, and septic arthritis. Radiology, 123:123, 1977.

18. Manshady BM, Thompson JJ: Septic arthritis in a general hospital 1966–1977. J Rheumatol, 7(4):523, 1980.

19. McCord CW, et al.: Acute venereal arthritis: comparative study of acute Reiter's syndrome and acute gonococcal arthritis. Arch Intern Med, 137:858, 1977.

20. Myers AR, Lane JM: Septic arthritis caused by bacteria. In Kelley WN, et al. (eds): Textbook of Rheumatology, Philadelphia, Saunders, p. 1551, 1981.

21. Myers AR, Miller LM, Pinals RS: Pyarthrosis complicating rheumatoid arthritis. Lancet, 2:714, 1969.

22. Namey TC, Halla JT: Radiographic and nucleographic techniques in the diagnosis of septic arthritis and osteomyelitis. Clin Rheumatol Dis, 4:95, 1978.

23. Nelson JD: Antibiotic concentrations in septic joint effusions. N Eng J Med, 284:349–353, 1971.

24. Nelson JD, Howard JB, Shelton S: Oral antibiotic therapy for skeletal infections of children. I. Antibiotic concentrations in suppurative synovial fluid. J Pediatr, 92:131, 1978.

25. Newman, JH: Review of septic arthritis throughout the antibiotic era. Ann Rheum Dis, 35:198, 1976.

26. Pancoast SJ: Neu HC Antibiotic levels in human bone and synovial fluid. Orthop Rev, 9:49, 1980.

27. Parker RH, Schmid FR: Antibacterial activity of synovial fluid during therapy of septic arthritis. Arthritis Rheum, 14:96, 1971.

28. Quismorio FP, Dubois EL: Septic arthritis in systemic lupus erythematosus. J Rheumatol, 2:73, 1975.

29. Resnik CS, Amman AM, Walsh JW: Chronic septic arthritis of the adult hip: computed tomographic features. Skeletal Radiol 16:513–516, 1987.

30. Rosenthal J, Bole GG, Robman WD: Acute nongonococcal infectious arthritis. Arthritis Rheum, 23:889–897, 1980.

31. Rubinow A: Septic arthritis of the hip caused by neisseria gonorrhea. Clin Orthop, 181:115, 1983.

32. Schmid FR: Principles of diagnosis and treatment of infectious arthritis. In McCarty, DJ (ed): Arthritis and Allied Conditions, 9th ed., Philadelphia, Lea & Febiger, p. 1335, 1979.

33. Schumaker HR: Synovial fluid analysis. In Kelley WN, et al. (eds): Textbook of Rheumatology, Philadelphia, Saunders, p. 568, 1981.

34. Smith JR, Phelps P: Septic arthritis, gout, and osteoarthritis in the knee of a patient with multiple myeloma. Arthritis Rheum, 15:89, 1972.

35. Tetzlaff TR, McCracken GH, Nelson JD: Oral antibiotic therapy for skeletal infections of children. II. Therapy of osteomyelitis and suppurative arthritis. J Pediatr, 92:485, 1978.

36. Ward JR, Atcheson SG: Infectious arthritis. Med Clin North Am, 61:313, 1977.

CHAPTER SIXTEEN

Evaluation of the Patient with Hip Pain

JAMES C. COHEN

Although an estimated 100,000 total hip arthroplasties are performed each year in the United States, most patients seeking initial evaluation for "hip pain" do not have pain emanating from the hip joint. The primary goal of the evaluation is, therefore, to ascertain if the pain is indeed resulting from the hip. In the patient who is considered a possible candidate for hip arthroplasty, the second goal of the encounter is to determine the severity of the patient's symptoms and his functional needs. Because the outcome of hip arthroplasty depends not only on the hip involvement, but also on the patient's age, weight, activity level, accompanying diseases, and emotional status, these also must be carefully evaluated. The third goal of the patient evaluation is to ensure that the patient's expectations of treatment are equivalent to the surgeon's expectations. Both the patient and the surgeon must have a clear understanding of the anticipated rate of success and the associated risk of failure before proceeding. At stake are not only the patient's future comfort, but also his ability to ambulate and function independently. Frequently, a patient is seen after a failed hip replacement futilely requesting that he be "put back to the same condition" that he was in before the surgery. "Surgical implantation of a hip prosthesis is a one way street, whose direction cannot be reversed."[1]

Although most of the information can be gathered in checklist fashion, the orthopedic history should be obtained in such a way that the patient is allowed and encouraged to tell "his story." It is easy to put words in a patient's mouth in the course of a busy office session, and this must be avoided so that a true picture of what is most disturbing to the individual patient becomes apparent. Age is an important bit of information that, although it does not separate one cause from another, it does set the tone for the remainder of the interview. Essentially, the younger the patient, the more intensely the evaluator should look for subjective

and objective manifestations of severe disease. The onset of the pain is important for both medical and legal reasons, and any precipitating events or trauma must be documented.

The location of the hip pain is the key historic factor in determining if, indeed, the pain is originating in the hip joint. In a general orthopaedic practice when the patient is asked to localize the area of pain, frequently an area will be identified in the iliolumbar, sacroiliac, posterolateral thigh, or trochanteric region. Although pain in these areas may originate from the hip, frequently it does not. Patients with an arthritic hip frequently localize their pain by pointing to the hip joint either anteriorly or posteriorly or from all directions and say that the pain is in their buttock or groin. The hip joint receives sensory branches from branches of the femoral, obturator, and also from the nerve to the quadratus femoris muscle. Classically, the patient has pain referred down the anterior thigh to the knee. Pain in the hip region can emanate from a wide variety of anatomic sources other than the hip joint. The differential diagnosis includes inguinal hernias; neurologic problems, such as herniated discs; spinal stenosis; diabetic neuropathy; occlusive vascular disease; and retroperitoneal tumors. Stress fractures, tendinitis, and trochanteric bursitis or metastatic lesions also may occur with a similar pattern of pain as a degenerative hip (Table 16–1). An attempt to differentiate these conditions by history is frequently unrewarding, and a careful examination is required. The duration and progression of a patient's symptoms should be determined. A history of variable but progressive pain over a period of years that has become significantly more severe over several months is reassuring when evaluating a patient with osteoarthritis for hip arthroplasty. Acute, severe pain, regardless of the radiographic picture, should make the physician question the cause.

The differentiation between hip disease and spi-

TABLE 16–1. *Differential Diagnosis of Hip Arthritis*

Spinal stenosis
Herniated disc
Diabetic neuropathy
Inguinal hernia
Occlusive vascular disease
Retroperitoneal tumor
Stress fracture
Metastasis to femur or pelvis
Trochanteric bursitis
Synovitis

nal stenosis is an important one. Patients with true sciatica usually have pain that radiates below the level of the knee, especially into the posterior and lateral calf. Hip disorders may produce pain that radiates too, but usually not below the knee. Patients with spinal stenosis typically do not have disability with respect to the use of a stationary bicycle, whereas patients with vascular disease may develop significant claudication with nonweight-bearing exertion.

Next, a series of questions are asked that are directed at assessing the degree of pain and the consequent limitation of function. An attempt to rate the intensity of pain is made. The patient is asked to classify his perception of his overall degree of pain as either mild, moderate, severe, or intolerable. This is a useful piece of information, and can be repeated at future evaluations to help gauge the progression of the symptoms. Gathering this type of information may not be adequate for statistical comparison, but this information combined with the patient's functional age determines the direction of treatment in a majority of patients with degenerative hips. While trying to avoid a cookbook mentality, patients under the age of 65 should be scrutinized to determine if the pain is in the severe to intolerable range before considering operative intervention. Also important in these younger patients is observing objective signs of significant pain during the examination. Another parameter that is useful is the patient's degree of walking tolerance. This is frequently listed in the number of blocks that a patient can walk both with and without pain. The presence of pain at rest and pain at night is determined. Frequently, in hip arthritis, the patient's symptoms are aggravated by walking and relieved by rest. The symptoms of vascular and neurologic claudication also present in a similar manner. Pain in a degenerative hip is especially severe at the initiation of ambulation, as well as after walking certain distances. Tumors, infections, and neurologic disorders can produce significant pain at rest and at night. Nevertheless, night pain is most useful as another parameter to sequentially moni-

tor the progression and severity of the pain. Other factors that serve to estimate the degree of pain are the use of walking aids and the amount of pain medication used. To get a fuller picture of the patient's functional limitation and general mobility, it should be ascertained whether the patient is able to reach his foot for dressing and hygienic purposes. Does he have difficulty in climbing stairs or getting into and out of a car?

Both the indications and conditions for surgery must be met before proceeding with hip arthroplasty. As with any surgical candidate, a careful medical history is essential to estimate the perioperative risks. In the patient who is under consideration for hip arthroplasty, an additional focus is necessary. Of all the possible complications of hip arthroplasty, infection may be the most devastating. Therefore, a careful history exploring possible foci for infection is sought. Specifically, the patient is questioned regarding carious teeth or periodontal disease. Have there been recent urinary tract infections or symptoms of prostatism? If a treatable problem exists, it should be treated well in advance of the hip operation.

Now that autologous blood transfusion is commonplace, specific questions regarding hemoglobinopathies are essential. The presence of a hemoglobinopathy is important, not because of its role as a possible cause of avascular necrosis, but rather because of the possible disastrous outcome that results from the reinfusion of SC thalasemic blood. Factors predisposing to thrombophlebitis and pulmonary emboli substantially increase the patient's risk and must be reviewed so that proper precautions can be taken.

A complete history of medications used is important. Anti-inflammatory drugs should be stopped 7 days before surgery so that platelet dysfunction can be avoided. Obviously, the use of steroids must be known so that adrenal insufficiency can be similarly avoided. Allergies to various medications should be listed. At the preoperative evaluation, all patients should be questioned concerning risk factors for infection with the human immunodeficiency virus so that patients who are at risk can be tested for the human immunodeficiency virus antibody. This information should benefit both the patient and the surgeon.

The hip examination is directed at determining if the patient's hip pain originates from the hip joint. Gentle rotation of an arthritic hip usually reproduces the patient's symptoms and guarding will be felt by the examiner. Charnley[2] taught that almost any patient over 65 can be accepted for a total hip replacement on grounds of pain alone, whereas in younger patients the objective assessment was most important. The assessment includes: the use of a walking aid, gait without an aid, range of motion of the hips, and objective signs of pain associated with movement. If the history is unclear regarding the source of the patient's pain, frequently this portion of the examination also is equivocal. An intense examination is therefore needed to look for other sources of pain that present as "hip pain."

A careful neurologic examination is necessary to look for signs of spinal stenosis or discogenic pain. Even if the patient's symptoms are primarily caused by hip arthritis, any degree of spinal stenosis will compromise the result of surgery. If any of the signs of spinal stenosis are found, both the physician's and the patient's expectations need to be adjusted accordingly. Physical signs of spinal stenosis are unusual, but may include diminution of reflexes either unilaterally or bilaterally and occasionally motor weakness primarily of the dorsiflexors of the ankle and great toe. The vascular examination rarely discloses significant information that changes the direction of treatment, but when it does, it does so dramatically. Not only must distal pulses be palpated to rule out vascular claudication as the source of pain, the femoral artery must be palpated for the possibility that an aneurysm is the source of the patient's hip pain. The abdomen must be palpated in all patients to rule out abdominal aortic aneurysm, a condition that is relatively common in the elderly. One of the easiest diagnoses to make is that of trochanteric bursitis because the patient's pain is easily reproduced by palpation over the greater trochanter. Similarly, the other bony landmarks, including the iliac spines, saroiliac joints, ischial tuberosities, and pubis also are palpated, looking for occult sources of pain. Evaluation of the other joints and the strength of the upper and lower extremities also is important in anticipating the patient's rehabilitation requirements. Leg lengths should also be measured preoperatively.

Plain radiographic evaluation is primarily helpful in simply confirming the impression that the pain was or was not originating from the hip joint. More frequently, a discrepancy exists between the severity of the radiographic findings and the severity of the symptoms.

Computerized axial tomography or magnetic resonance imaging studies of the abdomen and pelvis may be the only means to rule out a retroperitoneal tumor as the cause of the patient's symptoms.

Charnley[2] wrote that patients over the age of 65 are accepted for hip arthroplasty on their "subjective sensations and the objective scrutiny of the surgeon relates mainly to the patient's psychological state." In the evaluation of younger patients, he emphasized that "physical signs must take precedence over subjective sensations."

In summary, the patient with significant hip arthritis does not present a diagnostic challenge. However, if a clear picture does not emerge from the evaluation of hip pain, it must be realized that a diagnostic challenge does indeed exist and definitive answers must be found before proceeding on the "one way street" of hip arthroplasty.

Bibliography

1. BOOTH RE, et al.: Total Hip Arthroplasty. Philadelphia, Saunders, p. 58, 1988.
2. CHARNLEY J: Low Friction Arthroplasty of the Hip; Theory in Practice. New York, Springer-Verlag, 1979.

PART V

Surgical Techniques

CHAPTER SEVENTEEN

Hip Arthroscopy

RICHARD A. BALDERSTON

M.S. Burman[3] is considered the pioneer of arthroscopy in this country. His 1931 publication was the earliest reference to arthroscopy in the English language. He described a series of new instruments and presented information on what he termed "direct visualization of the knee, hip, shoulder, wrist, elbow, and ankle joints." He credited Bircher,[1] however, with the first description of arthroscopy in 1922. Burman noted that it was not difficult to see into the hip joint, but he alluded to the problem of obtaining complete visualization because of difficulty with distention and with placing instruments deep into the hip joint.

The development of the field of arthroscopic surgery has vastly improved the management of intra-articular pathologic processes. Advances in fiberoptic and camera technology and in the fabrication of a variety of small handheld and motorized instruments are largely responsible for improved diagnostic accuracy and for new surgical techniques and innovative treatment alternatives. Because of the easy accessibility, most of this technology has been applied to the knee and, more recently, the shoulder, ankle, wrist, and elbow.

The hip joint remains a frontier for arthroscopists. It is the largest joint in the body but it is also covered by deep muscular layers. The spherical contour of the deeply seated ball and socket and the depth of its location make it difficult to easily access the joint with arthroscopic surgical instruments and to maneuver instruments once placed inside the joint. Until recently, distraction of the joint while maintaining the ability to alter hip joint position has not been easy to accomplish. A number of important applications of hip arthroscopy have been described (see below), but as a result of the limitations noted, this particular aspect of arthroscopic surgery remains in its earliest stages of development.

Anatomy

An in-depth understanding of the surface and three dimensional anatomy of the hip is essential prior to considering arthroscopy of this joint. The anatomy of the hip joint and capsule are described in Chapter 1, but this section discusses some relevant anatomic points with respect to arthroscopy. The joint capsule is thickened or reinforced in areas corresponding to attachment of fibers from the femur to the pelvis. These structures are the iliofemoral, ischiofemoral, and pubofemoral ligaments. These ligaments become taut and lax depending on joint position, with the anterior fibers comprising the iliofemoral ligament (ligament of Bigelow) taut in extension and the ischiofemoral ligaments taut in flexion. The capsular attachments are from the acetabular rim to the femoral neck. The lateral and posterior capsule insert more proximally on the neck, thus effectively decreasing the size of the working space in this area for arthroscopy as compared to the more distal attachment of the anterior capsular structures (see Figure 1–6).

A number of muscles are directly adjacent to the hip joint. These anatomic relationships have been described in Chapter 1. The rectus femoris lies anteriorly with the reflected head intimately adherent to the capsule. More medially are the iliopsoas and the pectineus. The posterior musculature adjacent to the capsule includes the gemelli, pyriformis, and the quadratus femoris. The gluteus minimus lies laterally.

The acetabular socket is lined by a horseshoe-shaped articular cartilage surface termed the lunate surface (Fig. 17–1). This is easily visible upon initial entry into the joint. The acetabular rim is also lined and deepened circumferentially by a triangular-shaped condensation of fibrocartilage, called the acetabular labrum. The junction of the labrum with the articular cartilage is sometimes not easily differentiated in arthroscopic evaluation except in the

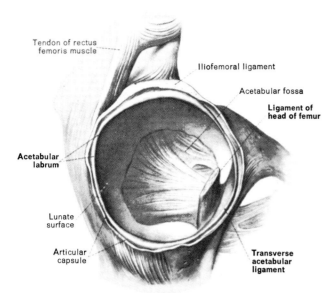

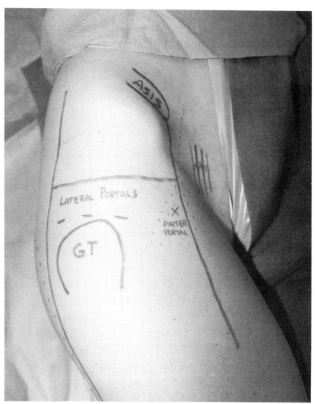

Fig. 17–1. Diagram of right hip showing pertinent gross anatomy that can be viewed arthroscopically. (From Clemente CD: Anatomy: A Regional Atlas of the Human Body, 3rd ed. Baltimore, Urban & Schwarzenberg, 1987.)

Fig. 17–2. Surface landmarks of the hip area: anterior superior iliac spine (ASIS), greater trochanter, neurovascular bundle. Safe region is demarcated by vertical line through the ASIS and along posterior border of the greater trochanter. Note the lateral femoral cutaneous nerve anteriorly and sciatic nerve posteriorly (dotted lines). Lateral portal sites are depicted along the superior edge of the greater trochanter. Anterolateral portal site is depicted.

case of abnormality or defect in this structure.[10] The central and medial aspect of the socket is comprised of the ligamentum teres and is characteristically surrounded by adipose tissue lining the acetabular fossa. The transverse acetabular ligament lies medially and inferiorly bridging the acetabular notch. The fibers of this structure are difficult to visualize because they are usually covered with the synovium.

The surface anatomy of the hip is most important in establishing safe zones for placement of the arthroscopic instruments and fluid ingress and egress cannulas. The important landmarks include the anterior superior iliac spine, the tip of the greater trochanter, the posterior border of the greater trochanter, and the neurovascular bundle in the femoral triangle (Fig. 17–2). The safe region is located between a vertical line drawn down from the anterior superior iliac spine and another line drawn vertically at the posterior border of the greater trochanter. The inferior border is identified by a horizontal line drawn at the level of the greater trochanter perpendicular to the long axis of the femur. The superior border is marked by a horizontal line parallel to this line and 3 cm proximal, which demarcates the superior extent of the acetabulum.

Care must be taken to avoid penetration posterior to the border of the greater trochanter to avoid injury to the sciatic nerve and deeper posterior structures. Care must also be taken when guiding instruments anteriorly to keep them parallel to the neck of the femur and to avoid excessive medial ex-

cursion into the soft tissues of the femoral triangle adjacent to the anterior capsule. Furthermore, the femoral artery should be identified and palpated prior to violating the skin with needles or instruments.

The lateral femoral cutaneous nerve crosses the inguinal ligament 1 to 2 cm medial to the anterior superior iliac spine and crosses over the sartorius 2 to 3 cm below the anterior superior iliac spine as it arborizes onto the anterolateral thigh (Figs. 17–2, 17–3). Placement of instruments via anterolateral portals must take this into account. It is recommended that prior to placing the sharp trocar and sheath in this area, blunt dissection be performed into deeper tissues to avoid injury to this nerve.

Surgical Technique

In general, standard arthroscopic equipment can be used for hip arthroscopy. The instrumentation necessary for hip arthroscopy includes the follow-

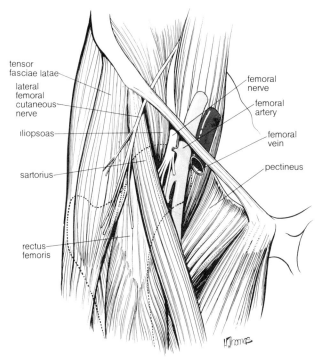

FIG. 17–3. Muscles and neurovascular structures about the anterior aspect of the hip. Note the arborization of the lateral femoral cutaneous nerve. (From Parisien JS (ed): Arthroscopic Surgery. New York, McGraw Hill, 1988.)

ing: a standard arthroscopic camera; 0,30, and 70° 4.5-mm arthroscopes with standard sheaths and trocars, preferably without a bridge on the arthroscope because a bridge effectively shortens the scope; several cannulas with blunt and sharp obturators capable of accepting the arthroscope, preferably with diaphragms to prevent fluid egress when the obturator is removed; standard arthroscopic

punches or graspers; a motorized shaver system; arthroscopic pump system; C-arm fluoroscopy; and a mechanism for applying traction to the limb. Extra long arthroscopes, shavers, and hand instruments are now available and greatly facilitate the procedure in obese or extremely muscular individuals. Also available are cannulated obturators to facilitate placement of the arthroscope sheath and working cannula (Fig. 17–4).

The issue of adequate traction for joint distraction is a critical one. Without ample distraction, thorough evaluation of the joint is difficult with current instrumentation. A single report, however, describes a technique that uses changes in hip position without application of traction.[12] Distraction of the hip joint has been achieved by a variety of techniques including skeletal traction, skin traction,[6,7] and traction via a fracture table with a peroneal post.[2,4,5,11,13,18,20] In an experimental study of hip distention, Ericksson, et al.,[4] identified three forces that resist distraction: active muscle resistance, vacuum within the joint, and passive resistance of the soft tissues. The study identified that 300 to 400 N was sufficient to distract the joint 10 mm in an anesthetized patient.

Recently, a hip distraction device that permits adjustment and mobilization of the extremity during surgery and provides good fixation and control of the extremity while allowing monitoring of hip distraction force has been introduced.[8,16] This device, the hip distractor (Arthronix, New City, NY), greatly facilitates thorough arthroscopic inspection of the joint because adequate distraction is routinely achieved and the joint position can be adjusted throughout the surgical procedure ensuring

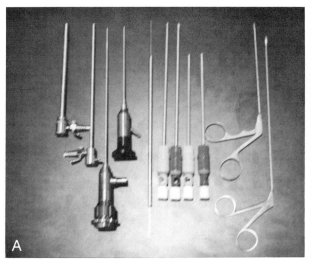
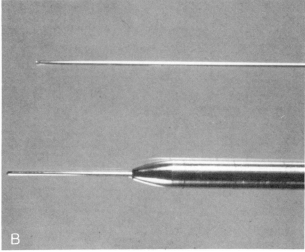

FIG. 17–4. **A.** Standard and extra-long arthroscopes, shavers, and graspers (Dyonics, Andover, MA). **B.** Cannulated obturator to facilitate placement of arthroscope sheath and working cannulas (Dyonics, Andover, MA).

complete visualization. The device is applied with the patient in the lateral decubitus position stabilized on a bean bag or with posts. A well padded peroneal post is placed with the pressure directed laterally on the hip joint. Longitudinal traction is then applied with a boot fixed to the foot and the amount of traction can be monitored via a strain gauge. The net force vector is approximately down the axis of the femoral neck. Initial traction is adjusted to approximately 50 pounds. After 5 to 10 minutes, the soft tissue relaxation results in a net reduction in force to 35 to 40 lb and joint distraction of at least 10 mm is achieved. Some patients with early degenerative joint disease or other causes of stiffness may require more traction to achieve adequate distraction (Fig. 17–5).

Several surgical approaches have been used for arthroscopic evaluation of adult hips. Burman,[3] in 1931, advocated the anterior paratrochanteric puncture and to date, most authors have used the anterolateral approach.[2,4,5,13,15,20] This technique involves placing the patient supine on the fracture table. Traction is applied via a traction apparatus on the fracture table. The landmarks noted above are established. Parisien[15] describes the point of insertion of a spinal needle at the intersection of the

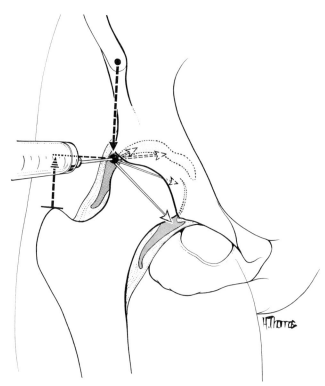

FIG. 17–6. Area of needle insertion for anterolateral approach described by Parsien. (From Parisien JS (ed): Arthroscopic Surgery. New York, McGraw-Hill, 1988.)

vertical line from the anterosuperior iliac spine and the horizontal line 3-cm proximal to the greater trochanter (Fig. 17-6). The spinal needle is then directed 45° medially and posteriorly into the joint. Additional portals can be created on the horizontal line anterior and posterior to this point.

Glick[6–8] has recently popularized the lateral approach for arthroscopic evaluation of the hip. He believes that this approach provides better access to the entire hip joint, most notably, posteriorly. It is also the opinion of this author that this is a useful and safe approach especially in conjunction with the hip distractor described above. The patient is placed on the operating table in the lateral decubitis position and securely positioned with a bean bag after anesthesia is administered. Anesthetic choice is important because some types of anesthetics do not provide complete relaxation and this is imperative for good joint distraction. General anesthesia with maximum muscle relaxation is preferable although spinal anesthesia may also be used. Fluoroscopy is necessary to verify joint distraction and to facilitate instrument placement. The C-arm should be draped and positioned to obtain an anteroposterior image (Fig. 17–7). The lower extremity is placed in the hip distractor and 50 lb of traction are applied with the hip initially in 30° of abduction and 15° of flexion (Fig. 17–8). The hip area is then

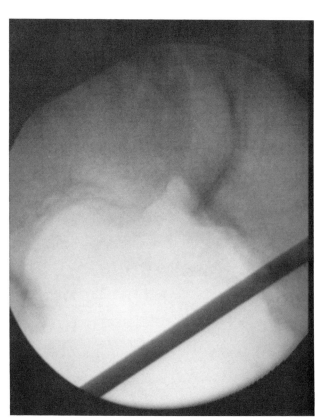

FIG. 17–5. Fluoroscopic view of distraction achieved by 40 lb of traction on a mildly arthritic hip.

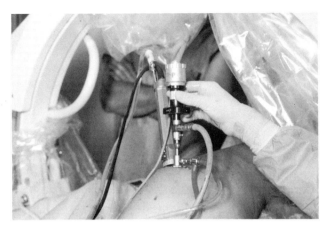

FIG. 17–7. C-arm positioned to provide anteroposterior image.

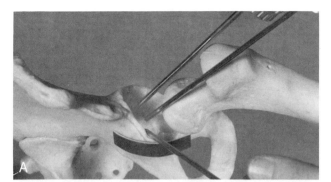

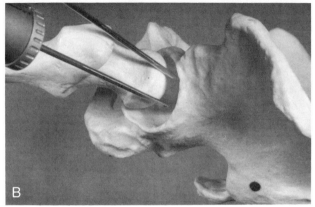

FIG. 17–9. **A.** Placement of arthroscope and shaver in lateral portal along the femoral neck and eggress cannula via anterolateral portal. **B.** Posterior view of hip joint with arthroscope and shaver along the femoral neck.

prepped in the routine fashion. Draping should allow exposure anteriorly to the pubic symphisis and posteriorly to the sacroiliac joint in order not to obscure surface landmarks and to permit access as necessary. The surface landmarks are then outlined as described above.

Three potential portal sites are identified just superior to the superior edge of the greater trochanter, one in the middle, one 3 cm anterior at the anterior edge, and one, if necessary, 3 cm posterior at the posterior edge of the greater trochanter (see Fig. 17–2). When placing instruments in the most anterior of the lateral portals, it is necessary to ensure that excursion of the obturator does not approach the femoral neurovascular bundle (Fig. 17-9A). Posterior instrument placement must be directly along the posterior neck to avoid injury to the sciatic nerve (Fig. 17-9B). An additional anterolateral portal may be marked at the intersection of the vertical line drawn from the anterior superior iliac spine and a horizontal line drawn at the level of the supe-

rior edge of the greater trochanter (see Fig. 17–2.) Again, care must be taken not to injure the lateral femoral cutaneous nerve in this region. A small skin incision followed by blunt dissection into the deeper tissues will prevent injury to this superficial nerve.

An 18 gauge spinal needle and trocar is advanced into the joint through the central lateral portal un-

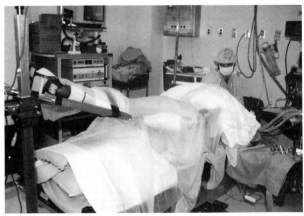

FIG. 17–8. Hip distractor (Arthronix, New City, NY) applied to a patient on a standard table in the lateral decubitus position. Note the well padded perineal post.

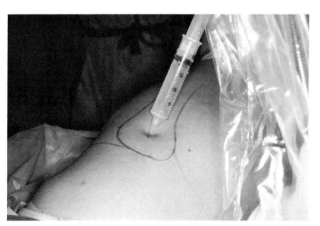

FIG. 17–10. Spinal needle is advanced into hip joint under fluoroscopic control, then the joint is distended. Outline of the femoral head is depicted.

der direct fluoroscopic visualization (Fig. 17–10). Twenty to 30 mm of a 50:50 mixture of 0.5% Bupivacaine with 1:1,000,000 Epinephrine and 1% Lidocaine with 1:1,000,000 Epinephrine is then injected into the joint. Intra-articular positioning is verified by fluid backflow through the needle. A skin incision is made immediately adjacent to the spinal needle and a 5.5 arthroscopic sheath and sharp cannula are advanced under image control to the joint edge just piercing the capsule. The capsule must be entered using the sharp trocar because it is a substantial structure and it is difficult to penetrate with a blunt trocar. The arthroscopic sheath can then be advanced into the joint using the blunt trocar. Glick[7,8] has noted that a definite "give" is perceived as the instrument enters the joint. At this time, in addition to fluoroscopic imaging, injection of fluid through the sheath and visualization of back flow is necessary to verify intra-articular placement. The trocar may glance off the lip of the acetabulum and pass superior to the hip joint. In this case, no give is felt. Fluoroscopic guidance will prevent excessive aberrant excursion of the instruments. An 18-gauge needle can then be placed in the posterior or anterior portal to permit fluid egress. Alternatively, the anterolateral portal can be used exclusively for fluid egress. The accessory portals can be created with cannulas with diaphragms to permit establishment of pressure in the joint while allowing easy access for instruments and the arthroscope. If such cannulas are not readily available, a diaphragm can be fashioned over a standard cannula using a simple rubber cap from a red top tube. A cross cut in the cap will permit easy placement of instruments.

As with all joints, the inspection should be carried out systematically and in an organized fashion. Initially, the anterior and anteromedial aspect of the joint is visualized using the 30°-arthroscope. Additional flexion aides in visualization anteriorly; the labrum and femoral and acetabular cartilage are then inspected. The interval between the labrum and articular cartilage is not always easily identified but this region should be inspected carefully for possible lesions.[10] A 70°-arthroscope is then used to better visualize the fovea and ligamentum teres. Visualization of the most medial and inferior aspect of the capsule may require placement of the arthroscope in the more anterior portal. Recall that the posterior capsule inserts higher on the neck than the anterior capsule. Placing the hip in neutral position or 5 to 10° of extension facilitates posterior visualization. In all positions, rotation of the hip will improve visualization.

Indications

One of the most common applications for diagnostic hip arthroscopy has been as the final step in the evaluation of long-standing unresolved hip pain unresponsive to conservative treatment.[4,5,7,8,15] In many cases, direct intra-articular visualization has yielded diagnostic information not available through noninvasive means. The standard diagnostic workup generally includes standard x-rays followed by a bone scan and possibly an MRI scan. If there is a history of trauma, a CT scan may be useful to evaluate the possibility of a free fragment in the joint. Pain about the hip and groin can also be a manifestation of extra-articular processes not visible on diagnostic imaging such as a snapping iliopsoas tendon or neurologic, gynecologic, or abdominal processes. A hip aspiration or arthrogram is an important part of the evaluation. This permits a standard assessment of the joint fluid and also yields information regarding the articular surfaces and significant capsular defects. It also provides the opportunity to perform a Lidocaine injection test. A positive response to direct intra-articular injection of Lidocaine, namely, complete or nearly complete resolution of symptoms, in the face of previously negative diagnostic studies, is an indication for diagnostic arthroscopy. Other diagnostic applications for hip arthroscopy include synovial biopsy for suspected pigmented villonodular synovitis,[11] rheumatoid arthritis,[5] or infection. The technique also permits evaluation of the joint surface in avascular necrosis,[5,15] osteochondritis,[2] or in cases of penetration of internal fixation devices.[7]

Although the scope of operative intervention remains limited primarily because of limitations of instrumentation, hip arthroscopy has been used in the treatment of loose bodies,[5,6] tears of the acetabular labrum,[10,18] chondromatosis,[14,20] plica resection between the femoral head and acetabulum,[5] and joint debridement for degenerative joint disease.[4,15] This author, in addition, has successfully applied the technology to the resection of a thickened and torn ligamentum teres in a competitive athlete and in the treatment of chondrolysis of the femoral head in a patient with normal x-rays. (See case reports.) In total hip arthroplasty, there are several descriptions of arthroscopic removal of entrapped material in the joint[13,19] and one case describes the manipulation of a 1-cm fragment of cement out of the acetabular component.[16] Others have described the extraction of a bullet from within the hip joint using a posterior approach with a limited incision through the short external rotators to protect adjacent structures.[9]

Case Reports

1. A 64-year-old woman presented with a history of 6 months of progressive right hip pain radiating into the groin and buttock with associated decreased hip motion. She had no history of trauma and no other pertinent past medical history.

On physical examination, she had 100° of hip flexion and a 15° loss of internal and external rotation as compared to the contralateral side as well as a 25° loss of abduction with pain on the extremes of rotation. The contralateral hip was asymptomatic.

Radiographic examination of the right hip demonstrated slight narrowing of the joint space with minimal osteophyte formation and cystic changes in the acetabulum suggestive of possible chronic synovitis or pigmented villonodular synovitis.

Arthroscopy was performed to obtain synovial tissue for diagnosis. This revealed evidence of chondrolysis. This chondrolysis was associated with a loose fragment of cartilage (Fig. 17–11). The predominant surface of the acetabulum and femoral head were normal, but the acetabulum had some chondromalacia on the superior surface. The free fragment was excised, the acetabular roof was debrided, and the patient was placed on crutches with toe-touch weight-bearing for 6 weeks.

At the 6 month follow-up, the patient noted significant reduction of painful symptoms and no longer required the use of an assistive device. Physical examination demonstrated absence of pain at the extremes of rotation and 15° improvement in abduction.

2. A 24-year-old elite-level woman's softball player developed right hip pain insidiously over 6 months prior to presentation. She noted a snapping sensation in the hip and sense of grinding with exertional activities. The pain was aggravated with exercise and relieved with rest. She had a prolonged use of anti-inflammatory drugs without relief. She localized the pain to the groin area anteriorly.

Physical examination demonstrated that the hip had full symmetrical motion as compared to the contralateral side. Active extension with the hip in a maximally flexed position produced an audible and painful clicking sensation. There was some pain at the extremes of rotation with the hip flexed.

Initial x-ray evaluation did not demonstrate bony abnormalities. A CAT scan did not reveal obvious bony abnormalities of the femoral head or acetabulum. Likewise, an MRI scan and a three-phase bone scan were negative.

The patient underwent an aspiration arthrogram followed by injection of Lidocaine. The aspiration did not yield diagnostic information but intra-articular Lidocaine completely eliminated her symptoms. At that point, the patient was administered an intra-articular injection of Betamethasone, which provided only transient symptomatic relief.

She underwent a diagnostic hip arthroscopy that revealed evidence of a hypertrophied ligamentum teres and chondromalacia of the adjacent articular cartilage of the acetabulum. The labrum was noted to be intact. There was mild synovitis present in the anterior aspect of the joint (Fig. 19–12). The patient underwent debridement of the ligamentum teres and gentle debridement of the adjacent articular cartilage on the lunate surface.

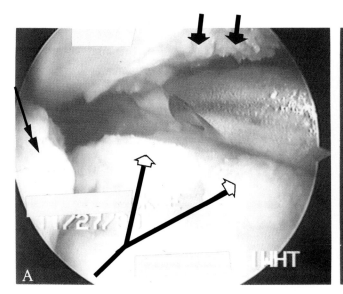
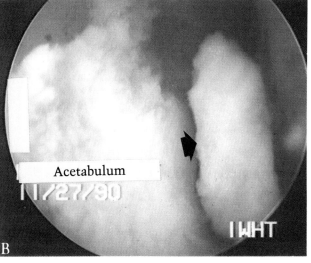

Fig. 17–11. A. Cartilage erosion with advanced chondromalacia of the acetabulum (solid arrow) and cartilage blisters on the femoral head (open arrow). Free fragment is depicted (double arrow). **B.** Free cartilage fragment in hip joint (arrow).

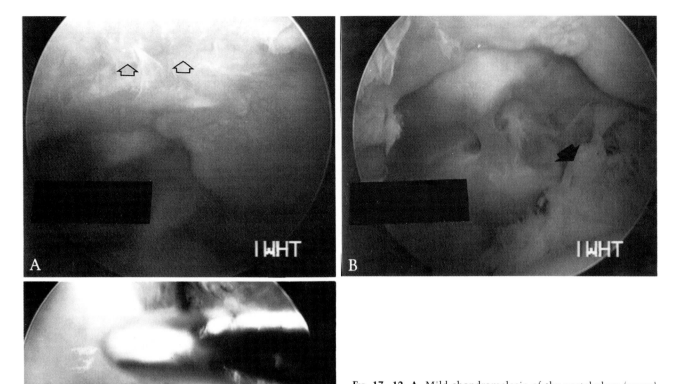

Fig. 17–12. **A.** Mild chondromalacia of the acetabulum (arrow). **B.** Hypertrophied and torn ligamentum teres (arrow). **C.** Labrum intact (open arrow). Synovitis anteriorly (solid arrow).

She was placed on crutches for 6 weeks postoperatively and at her 7 month follow-up, she noted resolution of the snapping sensation and significant improvement in her symptoms without subjective weakness or pain. She has elected not to pursue her softball career.

Complications

There have been relatively few complications reported after hip arthroscopy. No deep infections have been reported but transient traction neurapraxias,[7,8,17] scrotal pressure wound,[4] injury to the lateral femoral cutaneous nerve,[4,5] and instrument breakage[6] have been reported.

Surgical technique with respect to the experience of the operating surgeon as well as the attention to detail of anatomic landmarks, set-up, and proper instrument usage have a significant impact on the complication rate. All vital neurovascular structures should be well out of the way of the instruments. Position of the hip joint during instrument placement is important to note. If the hip is flexed, the sciatic nerve is more closely applied to the posterior structures and would be at increased risk for injury when attempting placement through the posterior portal. Likewise, if the hip is extended, placement anteriorly would be associated with greater risk. The joint space is relatively narrow and the arc of curvature of the joint is such that care must be taken to avoid damage to the joint surfaces of the femoral head and acetabulum upon penetration of the capsule and with insertion and reinsertion of instruments. Movement of instruments inside the joint is restricted and must be performed slowly and deliberately under direct arthroscopic visualization if possible.

The traction device that has been described has

the potential to place significant stress on the neurovascular structures of the affected limb. As with arthroscopic procedures in other joints requiring distraction, care must be taken to avoid excessive traction or excessive duration of traction. Traction should be limited to 1.5 to 2 hours, with an interval of 10 to 15 min prior to reapplication of force. A maximum force of 60 lb. has been recommended,[17] but higher forces have been used. Careful application of appropriate padding to the perineal post and the foot is also required to prevent traction injury into these areas.

Summary

Arthroscopic surgical techniques have been successfully applied in the treatment of a variety of disorders of the hip joint. Indications for diagnostic arthroscopy have been clearly established. The continued development of new surgical instrumentation will expand the indications for operative arthroscopy of the hip and facilitate surgical treatment of a variety of hip disorders.

References

1. BIRCHER E: Beitrag zur Pathologie (arthritis Deformans) und diagnose der meniscus-Verletzungen (Arthroendoscopie). Bruns' Beitr. z. Klin. Chir., CXXVII, 239, 1922.
2. BOWEN JR, KUMAR VP, JOYCE JJ, BOWEN JC: Osteochondritis dissecans following Perthes disease: arthroscopic-operative treatment. Clin Orthop 209:49-56, 1986.
3. BURMAN MS: Arthroscopy or direct visualization of joints. An experimental cadaver study. J Bone Joint Surg 13A:669-695, 1931.
4. ERIKSSON E, ARVIDSSON I, ARVIDSSON H: Diagnostic and operative arthroscopy of the hip. Orthopaedics 9:169-176, 1986.
5. FRICH LH, LAURITZEN J, JUHL M: Arthroscopy in diagnosis and treatment of hip disorders. Orthopaedics 12:389-392, 1989.
6. GLICK JM: Hip arthroscopy using the lateral approach. AAOS Instructional Course Lectures 37:223-231, 1988.
7. GLICK JM, et al.: Hip arthroscopy by the lateral approach. Arthroscopy 3:4-12, 1987.
8. GLICK JM: Hip arthroscopy in operative arthroscopy (JB McGinty, et al., (editors). New York, Raven Press, 1991.
9. GOLDMAN A, MINKOFF J, PRICE A, KRINICK R: A posterior arthroscopic approach to bullet extraction from the hip. J Trauma 27:1294-1300, 1987.
10. IKEDA T, et al.: Torn acetabular labrum in young patients. Arthroscopic diagnosis and management. J Bone Joint Surg 70B:13-16, 1988.
11. JANSSENS X, et al.: Diagnostic arthroscopy of the hip joint in pigmented villonodular synovitis. Arthroscopy 3:283-287, 1987.
12. KLAPPER RC, SILVER DM: Hip arthroscopy without traction. Contemp Orthop 18:687-693, 1989.
13. NORDT W, GIANGARRA CE, LEVY IM, HABERMANN ET: Arthroscopic removal of entrapped debris following dislocation of a total hip arthroplasty. Arthroscopy 3:196-198, 1987.
14. OKADA Y, et al.: Arthroscopic surgery for synovial chondromatosis of the hip. J Bone Joint Surg 71B:198-199, 1989.
15. PARISIEN JS (ed): Arthroscopic Surgery. New York McGraw Hill, 1988.
16. SHIFRIN LZ, REIS ND: Arthroscopy of a dislocated hip replacement: a case report. Clin Orthop 146:213-214, 1980.
17. STONE JW, GUHL JF, FEDER KS: Technique for hip arthroscopy perspectives in orthopaedic surgery. 1:73-82, 1990.
18. SUZUKI S, et al.: Arthroscopic diagnosis of ruptured acetabular labrum. Acta Orthop Scand 57:513-515, 1986.
19. VAKILI F, SALVATI EA, WARREN RD: Entrapped foreign body within the acetabular cup in total hip replacement. Clin Orthop 150:159-162, 1980.
20. WITWITY T, UHLMANN RD, FISCHER J: Arthroscopic management of chondromatosis of the hip joint. Arthroscopy 4:55-56, 1988.

CHAPTER EIGHTEEN

Arthrodesis of the Hip Joint

ANTHONY F. DEPALMA

Fred Albee performed the first hip fusion in America in 1908. According to Nove-Josser and Husener, Lampugnani and Albert performed the operation in 1884 for old congenital dislocations of the hip. During the first half of the twentieth century, hip fusion was considered one of the most effective orthopaedic operations provided it was successful, because it eradicates the disease, relieves the pain, and restores the patient to an acceptable way of life. The operation, however, is formidable and in the early years of this century its failure rate was high, and the complications resulting from long periods of immobilization of the body and unaffected joints were many. The elderly, in particular, tolerated the operation poorly. Over the years, as the indications for the operation were better defined and the skills of orthopaedic surgeons improved, a steady decline in the rates of nonunions occurred. In 1950 Stinchfield and Cavallaro reported a nonunion rate of 23%; Lipscomb and Mc-Caslin in 1961, 22%; Watson-Jones and Robinson in 1956, 6%; DePalma and Fenlin in 1966, 7%; and Barmada, Abraham, and Ray in 1976, 0%.

Nevertheless, the advent of total hip replacement with its promise of a painless, free-moving joint, and the false impression held by many orthopaedic surgeons that the operation, over the years, caused disabling deterioration of the back, ipsilateral knee, and contralateral knee have made hip arthrodesis a less desirable operation, one to be avoided and performed only as a salvage procedure.

These concepts, however, now need a second look. The roseate promises of total hip replacement have not materialized: the rates of loosening of the components of a total hip are too high both in young and elderly patients; the rates of failure following revision of failed prostheses are too high. And, as noted later in this chapter, of all the salvage procedures available to the patient following failure of the total hip, especially in the young active patient, hip fusion offers the best chance for returning the patient to an acceptable and productive way of life. This is particularly true today because

the modern methods of achieving a fusion—by using internal fixation and central compression—eliminate or minimize the use of plaster immobilization with its horrendous complications, and reduce the rate of nonunion to almost zero.

Over the years many operative techniques of arthrodesis of the hip have been described and used, but in general they fall into three categories: (1) intra-articular arthrodesis, (2) extra-articular arthrodesis and (3) combined intra-extra-articular arthrodesis. Many of the combined intra-extra-articular arthrodeses also use some type of internal fixation such as Knowles pins, long Smith-Petersen nails, intramedullary splines, compression plates, and compression screws to induce rapid fusion. And, if the one and one-half plaster spica is used, to permit its early removal.

Essentially the extra-articular fusions use some type of bone graft extending from the femur across the joint space to the ilium. Such a graft is used in the operation described by Badgly, Chandler, Hibbs, Henderson, Gromley, and Wilson. Davis and Ranawat used a muscle pedicle bone graft removed from the crest of the ilium. The operation described by Brittain and that described by Trumble are true extra-articular procedures.

Within the past few years still another category of operations has evolved. In this category the denuded femoral head and neck of the femur are displaced centrally either through a hole in the medial wall of the acetabulum large enough to accomodate the femoral head as described by Charnley or by displacing the femoral head centrally through a hinged trap made of the medial wall of the acetabulum, or by doing an osteotomy of the pelvis and displacing the lower segment centrally as described by Schneider and Barmada, Abraham, and Ray.

No single operation is suitable for all patients who would benefit from arthrodesis. But the age of the patient, the nature of the disease, the existing deformity of the limb, and the goals of the surgeon dictate the type of operation selected. Nevertheless, long years of experience have crystallized principles that must be observed to avoid serious complications and to achieve a successful fusion: (1) An extra-articular arthrodesis is rarely indicated. It should be used only when a situation exists that severely alters the normal anatomy and the normal mechanics of the hip. (2) Internal fixation of the hip with Knowles pins or a Smith-Petersen nail without denuding the cartilage of the femoral head and of the acetabulum results in a high rate of nonunion and failure of the internal fixation device. (3) In children, internal fixation should be avoided. (4) Combined intra-extra-articular procedures provide the highest fusion rates. (5) The addition of internal fixation, when not contraindicated, assures rigid immobilization of the joint—a condition essential to produce a solid bony fusion. (6) Compression of the prepared femoral head against the prepared acetabulum promotes rapid and solid arthrodesis of the joint such as that achieved by the cobra plate compression or the Harris compression bolts.

Position of Arthrodesis

Ewald, et al., as the result of a biological study, concluded that the optimum position for a fused limb is 30° of flexion, neutral position in abduction-adduction, and five° of external rotation. This study revealed that normal subjects immobilized with the hip in 30° of flexion expended normal amounts of energy when walking at a comfortable speed; however, when the hip was immobilized in full extension or in 60° degrees of flexion they expended greater amounts of energy. These findings were comparable to the findings noted in patients with an arthrodesis of the hip at approximately 30° of flexion when walking at a comfortable speed; the energy consumed was within the normal range. But whether the limb is fused in a patient at 30° of flexion or immobilized in a normal subject at 30 degrees of flexion, the comfortable speed for both is slower than normal.

Many clinical studies reveal great variance in the position of the limbs after arthrodesis. Sponseller and McBeath in a study of 53 fused hips noted the following average values for position of the extremity: flexion, 38° (10 to 60°); abduction, 4° (−10 to 30°); rotation, 0° (13° internal to 30° external rotation). Yet, most of these patients had a satisfactory and often an active lifestyle on an average of 38 years after fusion of the hip. Many orthopaedic surgeons believe that adduction in a fused limb of children increases with growth until skeletal maturity. This opinion was confirmed by Fulkerson's study

of 13 patients, 9 were available at the followup study. The age at the time of fusion ranged from 7 to 18 years; all were skeletally immature. The average time between fusion and the study was 9 years. All patients showed a tendency for the fused hip to adduct after the plaster cast was removed. One hip was refused after skeletal maturity; it did not increase in adduction.

Most patients perform satisfactorily with hips fused in 20 to 40° of flexion, although more flexion for sedentary and older persons may be more desirable. Certainly hips fused in slight adduction function satisfactorily. All of the patients in Fulkerson's study had hips fused in slight adduction and all functioned satisfactorily, including sports. All had an acceptable gait. Stinchfield and Cavallaro also noted the desirability of slight adduction in fused hips. Hips fused in abduction over 5° function less satisfactorily and are more prone to cause degenerative changes in the contralateral hip and in the lumbar spine.

It is difficult to attain the desired position of flexion on the operating table. Thompson's method of positioning the patient on the fracture table after operation and before applying the plaster cast allows the hip to fuse in 20° of flexion (Fig. 18–1).

Price points out that immobilizing the limb in neutral rotation, neutral abduction, and slight ele-

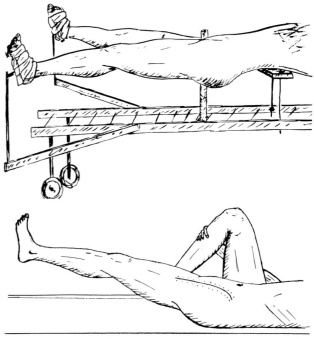

Fig. 18–1. With the affected extremity positioned parallel to the floor when a single spica is applied after operation, the hip fuses in 20° of flexion, as seen when the lumbar curve is flattened. (From Thompson FR: Combined hip fusion and subtrochanteric osteotomy. J Bone Joint Surg, 38:19, 1956.)

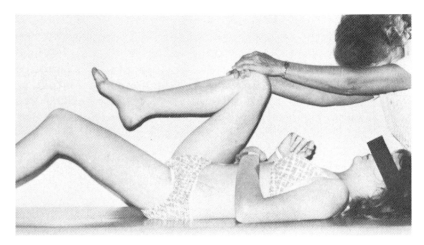

Fɪɢ. 18–2. The Thomas test. With the curve of the lumbar spine flattened this hip is fused in 30° of flexion. (From Price, CT, Lovell WW: Thompson arthrodesis of the hip in children. J Bone Joint Surg, 62:1120, 1980.)

vation (10°) above the horizontal allows fusion to occur with the limb flexed 30° when the lumbar lordosis is obliterated (Fig. 18–2).

There is general agreement that the slightly adducted position or the neutral position of the fused limb will produce an acceptable gait provided the extremities are of equal length. In the face of shortening of the fused limb, some abduction is mandatory. Stinchfield and Cavallaro found the most acceptable gait in patients with slight adduction and no shortening of the fused limb, an acceptable gait in patients with neutral abduction-adduction, and no shortening of the fused limb and a poor gait in patients with abduction and no shortening of the fused limb.

Osteotomy

Farakas, in 1939, described the use of subtrochanteric osteotomy with medial displacement of the lower fragment to treat tuberculous hips both in children and adults. The operation was designed to eliminate all motion at the hip joint, particularly motion caused by the action of the adductor muscles and the iliopsoas muscle while the patient was in a plaster cast. He believed that total and uninterrupted rest was required to heal the tuberculosis of the joint.

Osteotomy was not generally used to induce fusion of nontuberculous hips. Thompson was the first to use subtrochanteric osteotomy for this purpose in nontuberculous hips. The principle of the operation is to prevent the long lever arm of the femur from producing motion at the site of arthrodesis. Thompson pointed out that after fusion of the hip joint the femur with the center of its head acting as a fulcrum generates a lever action of 23 to 1,

the femur being 35 cm and the radius of the femoral about 1.5 cm. This 23 to 1 ratio converts minor thigh movements of a thigh in a plaster cast to movements of considerable significance, and if the knee is extended in the cast the ratio rises to 55 to 1.

The osteotomy eliminates this lever action at the fusion site during the early postoperative weeks. And most likely, the lever action is not operative again until union occurs at the osteotomy site— usually about 7 weeks (Fig. 18–3). Price and Lovell have reported the use of the Thompson operation with a subtrochanteric osteotomy in 14 patients with nontuberculous, nonparalytic conditions. Thirteen of the patients attained a solid, bony fusion and one a painless fibrous pseudoarthrosis (Fig. 18–4).

Another advantage of subtrochanteric osteotomy is that it permits positioning the limb in the de-

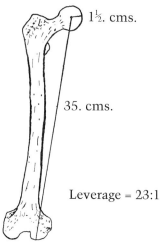

Fɪɢ. 18–3. The normal lever action at the hip joint is 23 to 1; with the limb extended it can rise to 55 to 1. (From Thompson FR: Combined hip fusion and subtrochanteric osteotomy. J Bone Joint Surg, 38:14, 1956.)

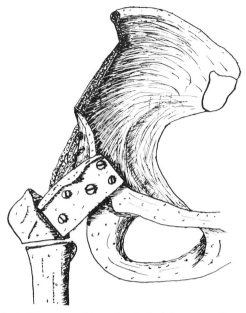

Fig. 18–4. Thompson hip arthrodesis. The subtrochanteric osteotomy eliminates all leverage at the hip joint. The proximal fragment of the femur is immobilized to the pelvis by a bone graft fixed with five screws. (From Thompson FR: Combined hip fusion with subtrochanteric osteotomy allowing early ambulation. J Bone Joint Surg, 38:15, 1956.)

sired position and correcting any deformity not corrected by the fusion operation. But it should be remembered that occasionally union at the subtrochanteric area may be delayed requiring immobilization long after the hip is solidly fused.

Postoperative Management

The type of operation performed determines the postoperative management of the patient. In general, if no rigid internal fixation is used, or if a subtrochanteric or intertrochanteric osteotomy is made, external immobilization is mandatory. A plaster cast is applied from the nipple line to the toes on the operated side and to just above the knee on the unaffected side. Every eight weeks the cast is removed and the fusion is evaluated roentgenographically. After fusion is well advanced a single walking spica is applied and protected weight-bearing using crutches is started, or, depending on the status of the fusion, a short, single spica is applied. Immobilization is continued until the fusion is solid. Fusion is rarely achieved before 4 months, and it may take longer. Solid fusion occurs earlier in adults than in children. After all immobilization is discarded, the orthopaedic surgeon should check the adult patient at regular intervals of 3 to 6

months for 1 or 2 years. And he should keep children under observation until they are skeletally matured because a deformity of the limb may develop as the result of abnormal growth of the proximal femoral epiphysis or contracture of the flexor and adductor muscles.

If no osteotomy is done and the hip has been rigidly fixed by internal fixation, such as a compression plate, Harris bolts or an intramedullary spline, a cast may not be necessary and the patient is allowed to bear weight with crutches a few days or a week after surgery, or in these patients a single, short leg spica is applied and the patient is permitted to bear weight immediately with crutches.

Gait With a Fused Hip

The orthopaedic surgeon should understand the mechanism of gait in a patient with a fused hip, and the difference between the gait in a person with a fused hip and the gait in a person with normal hips. The knowledge not only allows the surgeon to explain to the patient what kind of gait he can expect with a fused hip, but also he can clarify the goals of the persons involved in the postoperative management and rehabilitation of the patient.

Gore, et al., studied the gait characteristics of 28 men with a fused hip on one side and 28 men with normal hips. The men in both groups were of similar age and height. These workers noted that the gait in the men with a fused hip is slower because the cadence is slower and the step length is shorter; also they walk with a wider-based gait. Whereas in normal walking the stance and swing phases of the right and left limb are practically the same and produce a rhythmic gait, in persons with hip fusions the stance phase of the fused side is shorter than on the normal side and the swing phase on the fused side is longer than on the sound side producing an arrhythmical gait.

To achieve a satisfactory, comfortable gait some alteration must occur in the normal motions of the uninvolved joints; these are really compensatory motions increasing the excursion of the limb both on the fused and the normal side. The most pronounced alteration is the increased anteroposterior tilt produced by movement in the lumbar spine. This observation makes obvious the need of a freely moving, pain free lumbosacral spine in persons with a fused hip. Also, increased transverse rotation of the pelvis occurs, which increases step length. On the normal side, during stance, this ro-

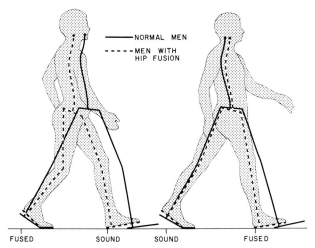

Fɪɢ. 18–5. Stick figures showing the position of the lower limbs and trunk at the instant of heel-strike in patients with unilateral hip fusion compared with normal men. The differences between men with a fused hip and men with normal hips are exaggerated slightly in this figure. (From Gore DR, et al.: Walking patterns of men with unilateral hip fusion. J Bone Joint Surg, 57:763, 1975.)

tation occurs in the hip; on the fused side, during stance, pelvic rotation occurs through the knee and to a lesser degree through the ankle and foot. To allow this rotation on the fused side, the knee flexes slightly during the stance phase. A fully extended knee (the position that the knee normally assumes in the stance phase) allows little or no rotation. The final compensatory motion permitting increased step length of both limbs is an increased flexion-extension range of the sound hip. By means of these compensating alterations a person with a fused hip can walk with a gait that is functionally and cosmetically acceptable (Fig. 18–5).

Arthrodesis of the Hip in Children

During the early decades of this century and prior to the advent of antibacterial therapy for tuberculosis, tuberculosis of the hip was a common and devastating disease in children. Dobson, as late as 1951, reporting on the prognosis of tuberculosis of the hip, based his observations on 320 patients of which 47.5% were under the age of 10 years. During these early years, rest was the only facet in the treatment of tuberculosis of the hip on which there was universal agreement. And "the rest" must be complete, uninterrupted, and prolonged. But there was no agreement as to how to achieve this "rest." Those who believed that conservative therapy was the treatment of choice in order to promote healing of both the primary lesion and the secondary lesion

(the hip joint) before surgical arthrodesis was performed had to live with the horrendous complications that resulted from total immobilization of the whole body and the limb. One of the most distressing complications in children was shortening of the limb on the affected side. In 1947, McCarrol and Heath reported on 72 children with hip tuberculosis treated by prolonged immobilization and inactivity, then followed by either an intra-articular or an extra-articular arthrodesis. Seventy-five percent attained a successful fusion; however, all the limbs of these children were atrophied and many centimeters shorter than the normal limb, and the knees were so relaxed that lateral motion often was equal to the degree of flexion and extension. Other common deformities of the limbs were genu valgum and medial and anterior bowing of the tibia. In 28 out of the 42 patients immobilized for 2 to 8 years, shortening of the limb ranged from 5 to 17.5 centimeters; 24 patients immobilized 3 years or longer revealed an average shortening of 8.3 centimeters.

These were some of the problems that faced the orthopaedic surgeon at this time period, and these unsolved problems led to a desperate and urgent desire to overcome them. The results of the efforts and courage of these surgeons include concepts in the treatment of hip joint disease and operative procedures that we today take for granted. In 1944, G. Gill found the reason why so much shortening occurred in the limbs of children following prolonged periods of immobilization and inactivity: the lower femoral epiphysis and the upper tibial epiphysis closed prematurely. Gill's observations were later confirmed by McCarrol and Heath. Brittain and Trumble evolved true extra-articular arthrodeses that were primarily designed to achieve a fusion without entering the joint and also prevent the formation of sinuses. On the other hand, Hibbs believed that the best treatment for tuberculosis of the hip was early and complete debridement of the joint, removing all necrotic and granulomatous tissue, early fusion of the joint, early weight-bearing in the cast, and early mobilization of the patient. This approach to the problem was followed by many new intra-articular and intra-extra-articular operations: Hibbs, Wilson, Ghormley, Henderson, Chander, and Badgely. Obturator neurectomy was added as a preliminary procedure to hip arthrodesis to prevent flexion and adduction contractures of the limb. And, the first subtrochanteric osteotomy was performed by Farkas. It was first performed without hip fusion to eliminate the action of the adductors and the iliopsoas on the tuberculous hip while the patient was immobilized in plaster. Later

Thompson added the procedure to fusion of nontuberculous hips.

Today, tuberculosis as a systemic or local disease is practically nonexistent, yet the occasional case still occurs in the United States, and in the underdeveloped countries the disease is still prevalent. Antibiotic therapy has altered the orthopaedic surgeon's approach to the problem. Nevertheless, even if the patient's response is favorable to antibiotic therapy, if the joint shows evidence of bone destruction, fusion of the joint is indicated in order to prevent serious deformities of the limb and leg length discrepancies. Today, treatment of tuberculosis of the hip or any other joint should be a joint responsibility of both the orthopaedic surgeon and the internist knowledgeable in the treatment of infectious diseases.

The usual uncomplicated result of tuberculosis of a joint is fibrous ankylosis. And it was hoped that antibiotic therapy would result in a mobile joint and eliminate fibrous ankylosis in uncomplicated joints. This goal, however, has not materialized in many instances because the nature of the disease may preclude invasion of the affected tissues—bone and cartilage—by the antibiotics. Also, the diagnosis may be made after destruction of bone and cartilage has occurred.

The studies of Stevenson reveal that as the result of antibiotic therapy healing of tuberculosis of the hip and knee has occurred more rapidly than in the era before the advent of antibiotics, and also a higher percentage of mobile joints has followed specific antibiotic therapy. Nevertheless, some of these mobile joints have sustained sufficient intraarticular damage that disability may arise in the future and require some form of surgical intervention.

Indications for Arthrodesis of the Hip

Indications in the Immature Person

Many diseases can produce a painful and disabling hip in skeletally immature persons. Many of these can be treated by arthrodesis which, if successful, relieves pain, eradicates the disease, , permits a functional and acceptable gait, and returns the patient to an active and productive lifestyle. The following disorders fit into this category: tuberculosis, septic arthritis, degenerative changes caused by slipped capital femoral epiphysis, con-

genital coxa vara, aseptic necrosis of the femoral head, fractures of the neck of the femur, Perthes disease, congenital dislocation of the hip, Otto pelvis, and trauma.

It is important at this time, when optimism sweeps the public on the merits of total hip replacement, that the results of this procedure be critically scrutinized. The reports that are appearing in the literature on end result studies disclose that although total hip replacement has found its place in the elderly and the young rheumatoid patients, it is unwise in skeletally immature patients with a painful, disabling hip who are otherwise in good health and active. The alternatives for these patients are: cup arthroplasty, femoral or pelvic osteotomy, endoprosthesis, and arthrodesis. The results of cup arthroplasty recorded in the literature speak for themselves: the operation is now obsolete. Of the rest of the alternatives, arthrodesis is the operation that returns the patient to an active, acceptable lifestyle for many years. Many end result studies confirm this opinion. Also, as noted by White, the type of arthrodesis performed in these patients should be done with an eye on the future. It is generally known that with an arthrodesis the patient may enjoy many years of active living and may never want or need conversion of the arthrodesis to a total hip replacement. But, if for some reason conversion should be desirable, the procedure can be performed provided the anatomy of the area is not grossly altered.

The study of Fulkerson emphasizes the worthiness of arthrodesis of the hip in immature persons with disabling hip pain. Nine patients were studied. At the time of operation the age ranged from 7 to 18 years. The average time between fusion and the last followup study was 9 years. Four nonunions occurred requiring a second operation to achieve fusion. At the last followup visit all the patients had an excellent functional result and all enjoyed a full childhood lifestyle being engaged in sports and productive occupations. No patient desired or needed conversion to total hip arthroplasty.

Indications in the Young Adult

For young, active adults with a disabling, painful hip, regardless of the cause, arthrodesis of the hip is the operative procedure that will assure them of a painless hip and an active life. Arthrodesis should take precedence over femoral or pelvic osteotomies because these operations distort the normal anatomy of the hip joint and may make conversion to a total hip replacement at a later time difficult or impossible. The study of Sponseller, McBeath, and Perpick discloses some interesting observations that favor arthrodesis of the hip in young, active adults. These workers evaluated the results of arthrodesis in 53 patients who had a successful hip fusion at least 20 years ago (average 38 years). At the time of the fusion, all the patients were under 35 years of age; the average age was 14 years, the range was from 3 to 35 years. At followup evaluation the average age was 52 years, the range was from 20 to 54 years.

Subjectively, 78% of the patients were satisfied with the operation, 11% were uncertain and 11% were dissatisfied. More women (87%) were satisfied than men (70%). Of the 53 patients, 45 were employed outside the home and 18% of those were doing heavy labor; only 14% were doing sedentary work. Thirty-four percent believed they had no significant limitations. Although there were obvious limitations in competitive sports, all the patients had been able to participate in sports activities to some degree in their younger years. Sixteen of the 23 women were married and had children. Only 1 woman thought the arthrodesis caused difficulty with the sex act. Of the 53 patients, only 13 had had a conversion to total hip replacement. From these observations it becomes obvious that arthrodesis in young, active adults is the operation of choice and not a salvage operation.

The causes for hip disability in this age group are many; most of them are extensions of a disease process acquired in childhood or adolescence, and some are acquired after skeletal maturity, such as trauma, osteonecrosis of the femoral head, and osteoarthritis.

In the selection of patients for arthrodesis it is important to rule out any disorder in the contralateral hip joint, particularly in the patient with osteonecrosis of the femoral head. For acquisition of an acceptable gait with a fused hip, the contralateral knee also must function normally.

Stewart and Coker and Watson-Jones observed that back pain does not rule out a hip arthrodesis. In fact, they noted that back pain was relieved in some of their patients following arthrodesis of the hip. Nevertheless, patients with back pain and pain in the ipsilateral knee have a less favorable result after arthrodesis than those patients with no knee pain and a mobile, painless lumbar spine. Like the lumbar spine, the ipsilateral knee is essential in the mechanics of an acceptable and functional gait in patients with a fused hip.

As in skeletally immature persons, young adults with unilateral hip disease have these alternatives

to arthrodesis: cup arthroplasty, endoprosthesis, resurfacing procedures, femoral or pelvic osteotomy, and total hip replacement. The failure rate of cup arthroplasty is too high to consider it a suitable operation. Chandler, et al., and Lang, et al., report a failure rate of 28 to 50% within the first decade following the operation. The same is true of total hip arthroplasty. Chandler, et al., reported a rate of 57% of actual or potential loosening of the components of this procedure in patients under 30 years of age. Dorr, et al., report a failure rate of 28% in patients under 45 years of age. Resurfacing procedures in young patients give no better end results. Jolley, et al., and Head reported failure rates of 13 to 34% at the end of a 2 to 3 year followup study.

In view of these observations, hip arthrodesis with its long-term functional capability becomes the operation of choice in young, active adults with unilateral hip disease.

Many orthopaedic surgeons believe that arthrodesis of the hip has a deleterious effect on the back, contralateral and ipsilateral knee, and on the contralateral hip. The observations made in some long-term studies should dispel these beliefs. Callaghan, et al., in a retrospective study reported the end results on 28 patients who underwent an arthrodesis 17 to 53 years earlier (average 35 years). They noted that 60% of the patients had pain in the ipsilateral knee, however, the average time of onset after arthrodesis was 23 years. Likewise 60% of the patients had back pain but the average time of onset after the arthrodesis was 25 years. Pain occurred in the contralateral hip in approximately 25% of the patients, and its onset was on an average of 20 years after the arthrodesis was performed. Only one patient of the 28 was unemployed because of pain in the back and knee. Seventy percent of the patients could walk a mile and the same number could sit comfortably for 2 hours.

The findings in the knee joint were of particular significance: anteroposterior laxity in the ipsilateral knee was noted in 75% and mediolateral laxity in 80%. Patients with a fused hip in abduction had pain in the back and ipsilateral knee more frequently than the patients with a hip fused in adduction. Also, they had more degenerative changes in the ipsilateral knee than the patients with the hip fused in adduction or in the neutral position. Because of pain in the back or in the ipsilateral knee or pain in both back and knee 6 patients had a total hip replacement. All 6 patients were relieved of the back pain but only 2 of the 4 who had pain in the ipsilateral knee were relieved by the total hip arthroplasty.

Arthrodesis for Failed Arthroplasty

The most frequent causes for failure of arthroplasties are infection and mechanical failure. After a failed arthroplasty caused by infection, the rates of failure after reinsertion of a total hip are between 25% and 73%. And, the revisions following mechanical failure are just as disappointing. Charnley reported a failure rate of 40%. As a salvage procedure, Clegg pointed out that the Girdlestone operation has proven to be unsuccessful: it does not relieve pain in most patients and from a functional viewpoint it fails to provide an acceptable lifestyle. Almost all patients must have some form of support in order to ambulate. As pointed out by Kostwik, et al., the answer to this problem is arthrodesis of the hip joint in patients under 50 years of age and revision in patients over 50 years of age provided that the patient has not had previous multiple operations. In such instances, arthrodesis has much more to offer the patient in the relief of pain and improved function. The choice of operation in these patients is important because these patients do not look ahead for a movable hip. The procedure should be definitive, effective, and successful. The answer to this problem as shown by Kostwik, et al., is a modification of the A-O technique for hip arthrodesis, using the cobra plate.

Surgical Technique of Arthrodesis of the Hip Joint

Incisions

The incisions most frequently used to fuse a hip joint are: (1) the anterior iliofemoral incision or one of its modifications, (2) the lateral thigh incision, and (3) the posterior curved gluteal incision. The anterior iliofemoral incision is used in intra-articular and combined intra-extra-articular arthrodesis (Fig. 18–6). The lateral incision is used in extra-articular arthrodesis with or without a subtrochanteric or intertrochanteric osteotomy (Fig. 18–7). The posterior curved gluteal incision is used for extra-articular fusions such as the ischiofemoral arthrodesis (Fig. 18–8).

Intra-articular Arthrodesis

An intra-articular arthrodesis is rarely used because the area of contact between the femoral head denuded of its cartilage and the denuded acetabulum is not large enough to ensure a solid bony fusion. This type of fusion done alone results in a high rate of nonunion. Nevertheless, when this operation is used in combination with extra-articular bone grafts or some metallic device to establish rigid internal fixation, it plays an important role in the attainment of high rates of successful arthrodesis.

Technique

Expose the capsule of the joint through an anterior iliofemoral incision and incise the capsule to expose the femoral head and neck. By externally rotating the limb, dislocate the femoral head and expose the acetabulum. Using long curettes and gouges denude the femoral head and the acetabulum of all cartilage down to raw, bleeding bone. If there is any necrotic tissue in the joint, remove it. If it is a tubercular joint do a complete synovectomy. Reduce the dislocation and approximate the raw head to the raw acetabulum. In some instances, the pathologic process in the joint has destroyed much of the head and neck of the femur and also the inner walls of the acetabulum so that after removal of the necrotic tissue a wide gap remains between the head and the acetabulum. This problem is best solved by denuding the superior surface of the greater trochanter and displacing it medially into the acetabulum so that its superior raw surface makes contact with the roof of the acetabulum. It may be necessary to remove the lesser trochanter if it impinges on the ischium and prevents sufficient medial displacement of the femur. Also, the limb may have to be placed in wide abduction to adequately seat the trochanter in the acetabulum. In such a situation do a subtrochanteric osteotomy and bring the limb into the desired neutral position. After closure of the wound apply a one and one-half plaster spica.

Combined Intra-articular and Extra-articular Arthrodesis

The essential feature of this operation is the addition of an iliofemoral graft or a muscle pedicle graft to the intra-articular operation. The procedure is used in both tuberculous and nontuberculous hips. Some procedures add internal fixation devices to ensure rigid fixation. As a rule metallic internal fixation devices are not used in children; however, Thompson has reported the use of metallic lag screws to secure a bone graft to the femur and the pubic ramus in skeletally immature patients. Five of these patients had septic arthritis. By this

Fig. 18–6. Anterior Iliofemoral Incision. **A.** Begin the incision on the iliac crest 7.5 cm behind the anterior superior iliac spine and extend it down from the spine for 15 cm. **B.** Mobilize the skin flaps and retract them up and down; divide fascia over the iliac crest and develop the interval between the fascia lata and the sartorius muscle. **C.** Deepen the incision over the crest down to bone and, by subperiosteal dissection, strip the fascia lata, gluteus medius, and gluteus minimus muscles off the wing of the ilium. Extend the dissection into the thigh developing the interval between the fascia lata and the sartorius and rectus femoris. Ligate the ascending branch of the lateral circumflex artery which traverses the wound.

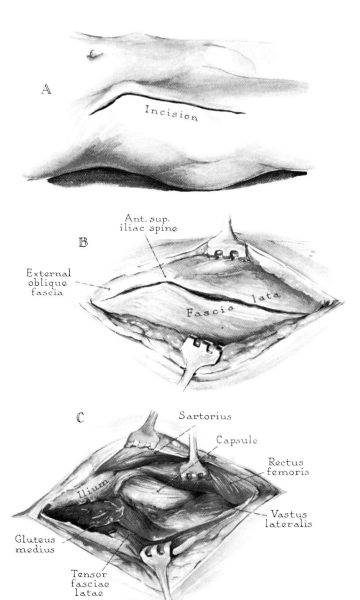

A

Incision

B

Ant. sup. iliac spine

External oblique fascia

Fascia lata

C

Sartorius

Capsule

Rectus femoris

Vastus lateralis

Ilium

Gluteus medius

Tensor fasciae latae

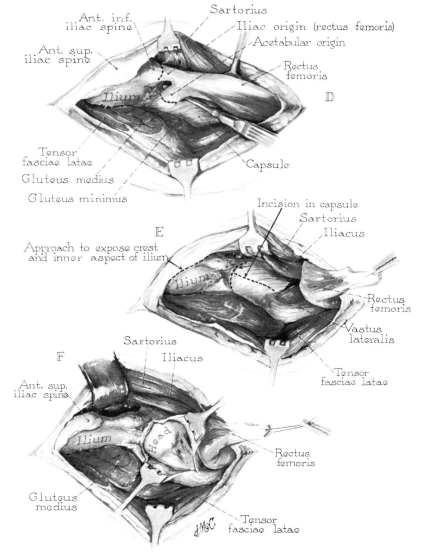

FIG. **18–6** *(continued)*. **D.** Expose the two heads of the rectus femoris muscle. **E.** Divide the heads of origin of the rectus femoris and retract the muscle downward. **F.** Expose both sides of the wing of the ilium by sharp subperiosteal dissection. Separate the sartorius from the anterior-superior iliac spine and retract it medially with the abdominal and iliopsoas muscles. Open the hip joint with a T-shaped incision in the capsule. (From Banks SW, Laufman H: An Atlas of Surgical Exposures of the Extremities. Philadelphia, WB Saunders, 1954.)

FIG. 18–7. Exposure of the hip joint and subtrochanteric region of the femur through a lateral hip and thigh incision. **A.** Begin the incision at the iliac crest in line with the center of the greater trochanter and extend it distally for 20 cm over the lateral aspect of the thigh, ending 7.5 cm below the greater trochanter. **B.** Divide the fascia lata in the line of the skin incision. Identify the tensor fascia latae, mobilize it, and retract it medially. **C.** Mobilize the gluteus medius muscle in the upper part of the incision and retract it posteriorly exposing the capsule of the hip joint. **D.** Make an appropriate incision in the capsule exposing the hip joint. In the distal part of the wound mobilize the intermuscular septum and retract it with the fascia lata posteriorly. By subperiosteal dissection, separate the vastus lateralis from the subtrochanteric area of the femur and retract it distally. (From Banks SW, Laufman H: An Atlas of Surgical Exposures of the Extremities. Philadelphia, WB Saunders, 1953.)

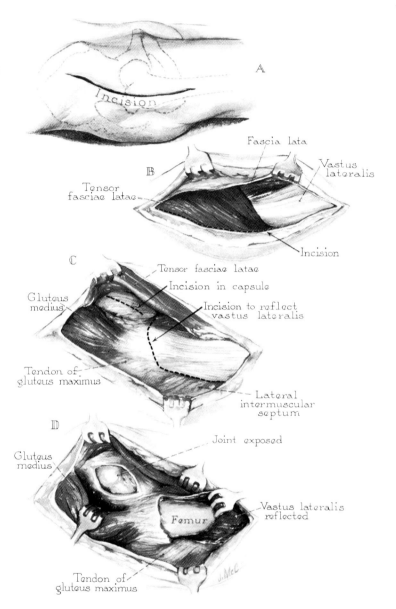

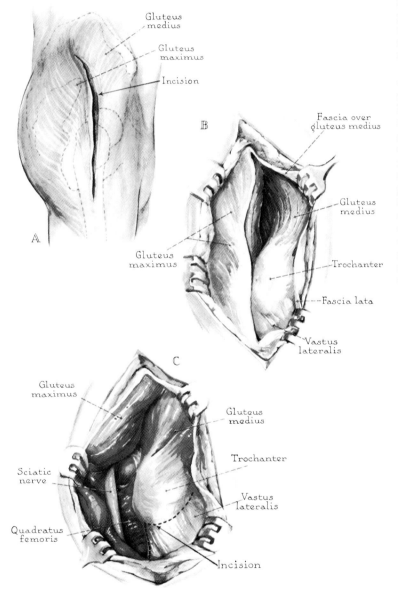

Gluteus medius

Gluteus maximus

Incision

A

Fascia over gluteus medius

B

Gluteus medius

Gluteus maximus

Trochanter

Fascia lata

Vastus lateralis

C

Gluteus maximus

Gluteus medius

Trochanter

Sciatic nerve

Vastus lateralis

Quadratus femoris

Incision

FIG. 18–8. Posterior curved gluteal incision exposing the subtrochanteric area and the ischial tuberosity. **A.** Begin the distal limb of the incision at the top of the greater trochanter and extend it distally along the shaft of the femur for 12.5 cm. Begin the upper limb of the incision at the top of the greater trochanter and extend it upward and backward for 10 cm in the interval between the gluteus maximus and the gluteus medius. **B.** Develop the interval between the gluteus maximus and gluteus medius, extending distally between the fascia lata and the gluteus maximus and beyond to expose the vastus lateralis. **C.** Mobilize the gluteus maximus from the gluteus medius and the greater trochanter and retract it upward and medially. Identify the insertion of the gluteus medius into the greater trochanter and the sciatic nerve under the gluteus maximus. Identify the quadratus femoris as it runs transversely across the field from the ischial tuberosity to its insertion into the intertrochanteric crest of the femur.

Fɪɢ. 18–8 *(continued)*. Posterior curved gluteal incision exposing the subtrochanteric area and the ischial tuberosity. **D.** By subperiosteal dissection detach the quadratus femoris from the ischial tuberosity and the intertrochanteric region of the femur and retract it upward. **E.** By subperiosteal dissection detach the upper portion of the vastus lateralis from the femur and retract it distally. The tuberosity of the ischium is further exposed by subperiosteal stripping of tissue attached to it. (From Banks SW, Laufman H: An Atlas of Surgical Exposures of the Extremities. Philadelphia, WB Saunders, 1953.)

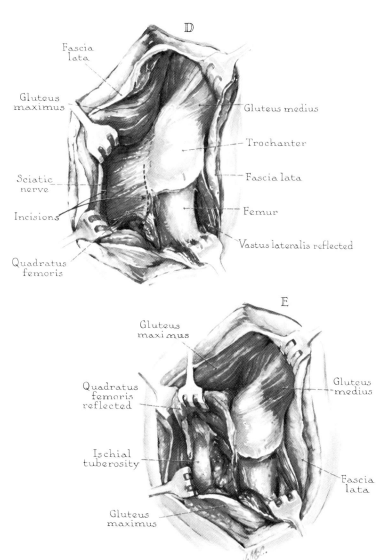

method he attained a solid fusion in thirteen hips and a fibrous union in one.

The literature reveals that many operations of this type have been performed. All were based on the same principles, and all, if meticulously performed, were successful in eradicating the disease and attaining a high rate of solid bony fusions. To describe all these operations would be needless repetition, however, some of the more effective ones and those that are still used today will be described (Fig. 18–9).

Hibbs Hip Arthrodesis

Begin the incision over the anterior iliac crest 5 to 7 cm posterior to the anterosuperior spine. Continue the incision distally over the center of the greater trochanter and along the lateral aspect of the femur for 8 to 10 cm distal to the base of the greater trochanter. After splitting the deep fascia in the line of the incision, develop by blunt dissection the interval between the tensor fasciae latae muscle laterally and the gluteus medius and minimus muscles medially exposing the capsule. Next, incise the periosteum at the base of the trochanter and reflect it distally. With a broad osteotome or an electric saw detach the anterior three-fourths of the trochanter together with about 5 cm of the cortex of the femur. You now have a pedunculated bone graft with the proximal end retaining its muscle and periosteal attachments and its distal end consisting of about 5 cm of the outer cortex of the femur. Divide the capsule and with an osteotome denude the superior surface of the neck of the femur down to cancellous bone. Cut a trough in the ilium just above the acetabular rim large enough to accept the graft. Rotate the graft and lay it on the

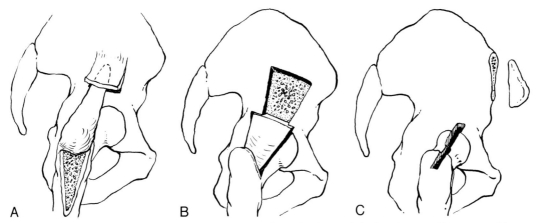

FIG. 18–9. Principal techniques of intra-articular and extra-articular arthrodesis of the hip. (From Abbott LC, Hibbs RA, Henderson MS, Ghormley RK, Lucas DB: Arthrodesis of the hip in wide abduction. J Bone Joint Surg, 36:1130–1131, 1954.)

bared superior surface of the neck of the femur and wedge its distal end into the trough in the ilium. Anchor the graft with sutures through the periosteum of the graft and through the periosteum immediately above the trough in the ilium, and through the periosteum of the femur below. The amount of abduction of the limb to bring it to the desired postoperative position usually is enough to impact the graft into the iliac trough (Fig. 18–9A).

Henderson Hip Arthrodesis

Expose the hip joint by the anterior iliofemoral incision, divide the capsule, and dislocate the joint. Denude the femoral head and the acetabulum of all its articular cartilage. If the joint is tubercular remove all necrotic bone and other joint debris and do a complete synovectomy. Next decorticate the superior surface of the neck of the femur exposing bleeding cancellous bone. Remove enough of the medial portion of the femoral head so that on reduction of the joint the raw surface of the femoral head abuts tightly against the medial wall of the acetabulum. On the medial aspect of the greater trochanter at the juncture of the trochanter and the neck of the femur, cut out a deep and wide cleft. From the side of the ilium cut out a graft large enough to fit firmly in the cleft in the trochanter, span the superior surface of the femoral neck and lie on the side of the ilium when the limb is in the adducted position. Next, elevate a bone flap just above the acetabulum which will firmly seat the proximal end of the graft when the limb is brought from the adducted position to the desired position. Finally, harvest some cancellous bone grafts from the side of the ilium and pack them tightly against the length of the graft (Fig. 18–9B).

Ghormley Hip Arthrodesis

Begin the incision on the iliac crest approximately 9 to 10 cm posterior to the anterosuperior spine of the ilium and extend it distally to just below the tip of the greater trochanter. Then extend it anteriorly to about 12 to 15 cm below the anterosuperior spine of the ilium. Reflect the skin flaps anteriorly, exposing the muscles attached to the wing of the ilium. Divide the muscle attachments to the crest of the ilium and, by sharp subperiosteal dissection, strip the gluteus medius and gluteus minimus from the crest and the side of the ilium exposing the anterior iliac crest and the anterosuperior spine. With a thin, sharp osteotome remove a graft approximately 9 to 10 cm long consisting of the iliac crest and the anterosuperior spine of the ilium. Next, incise the capsule from the ilium to the base of the trochanter exposing the head and neck. Cut out a deep trough extending from the superior aspect of the acetabulum through the head and neck of the femur and deep into the greater trochanter. Shape the graft to fit the trough and impact it in the trough (Fig. 18–9C).

Ranawat, Jordan, Wilson Jr., Hip Arthrodesis

The operation described by Ranawat, et al., does not differ from that described by Davis. Both use a large muscle pedicle graft taken from the iliac crest, both dislocate the femoral head in order to denude the femoral head and the acetabulum of their cartilage (although in the joints that have very little motion Ranawat, et al., did not dislocate the head), and both perform a subtrochanteric osteotomy, if it is deemed necessary. The Ranawat and Davis operations differ from the Hibbs and Warren operations in that the grafts are not twisted on their pedicles when the grafts are seated in their beds. Although Davis in his original description of the operation did not use internal fixation across the joint, other surgeons using the technique have supplemented it with rigid internal fixation such as Knowles pins or a long Smith-Petersen nail.

Technique

The patient is positioned on a fracture table, lying on the unaffected side. A modification of the anterior iliofemoral incision is used. Begin the incision at the highest point on the iliac crest, extend it along the crest, across the anterosuperior superior spine and continue it distally on the front of the thigh to the level of the greater trochanter. If an osteotomy of the femur is to be done, extend the incision over the lateral surface of the thigh. Identify the lateral femoral cutaneous nerve and preserve it, then divide the fascia just medial to the sartorius muscle. Next, detach the inguinal ligament from the anterosuperior iliac spine and, by sharp subperiosteal dissection, detach the 3 abdominal muscles from the iliac crest and also detach the iliacus muscle from the iliac fossa and retract it medially exposing its juncture with the iliopsoas tendon. Retract the tendon medially to protect the femoral vessels and nerve. At the completion of this dissection the inner surface of the ilium including the il-

iac crest, the anterosuperior iliac spine, anteroinferior iliac spine and the pubic portion of the acetabular rim are clearly visualized. Now, on the inner side of the ilium, using sharp straight and curved osteotomes, outline the muscle pedicle graft, which consists of both the anterosuperior and anteroinferior iliac spines and the adjacent bone. Begin the cut in the ilium 4 cm medial to the anterosuperior spine, extend it downward through the inner table of the ilium and parallel to its anterior border and into the roof of the acetabulum penetrating the entire thickness of the acetabular roof. Using sharp curved osteotomes divide the outer table of the ilium from inside out.

Next, reflect the graft downward and outward and develop a plane in the gluteus medius and gluteus minimus muscles on the outer aspect of the ilium and adjacent to the line of the osteotomy (Fig. 18–10). The graft has attached to it part of the origin of the gluteus medius, the gluteus minimus, and the entire origin of the tensor fasciae latae, sartorius, and rectus femoris muscles. By retracting the pedicle muscle graft laterally the anterior aspect of the hip joint comes into view. Excise enough of the anterior capsule to expose the rim of the acetabulum and the anterior surface of the head and neck of the femur. At this time, if an intraarticular arthrodesis is contemplated, the femoral head is dislocated and the cartilage of the head and acetabulum is removed. Next, fix the femur in the acetabulum using either Knowles pins or a long

Fig. 18–10. The osteotomy through the outer surface of the ilium has been completed, the graft is free with the attached muscle. Note that the lower end of the graft enters the acetabulum. (From Ranawat CS, Jordan LR, Wilson PD Jr: Technique of muscle pedicle bone graft in hip arthrodesis. J Bone Joint Surg, 53:927, 1971.)

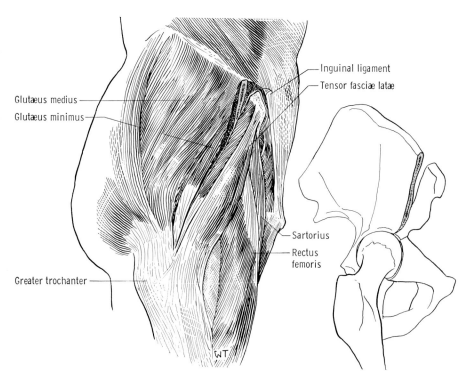

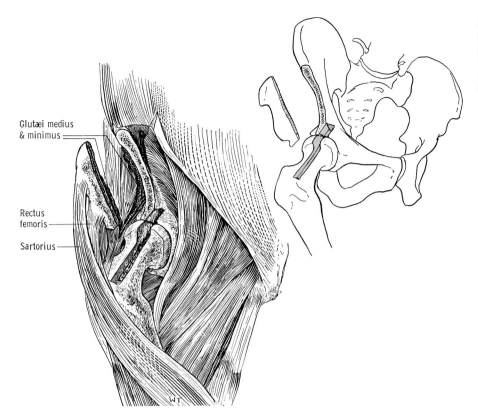

Glutæi medius
& minimus

Rectus
femoris

Sartorius

Smith-Petersen nail. This may be followed by a subtrochanteric osteotomy. (Note: An osteotomy is not performed in all patients, and if done, internal fixation of the osteotomy may be used in some operations and not in others.) Make a slot across the hip joint beginning in the ilium and extending across the femoral head and femoral neck to the intertrochanteric line 1.5 cm deep and wide enough to receive the graft (Fig. 18–11). Insert the graft in the slot so that its acetabular end is next to the intertrochanteric line (Fig. 18–12). Anchor the graft with two screws, one penetrating the ilium, the other penetrating the femoral head.

After closure of the wound, a one and one-half plaster spica cast is applied.

Thompson Arthrodesis

This procedure combines the advantages of an intra-articular fusion, an extra-articular fusion using a bone graft bridging the pelvis and the femur, and a subtrochanteric osteotomy, which eliminates movement at the joint and permits positioning the limb in the desired position. Price and Lovell used this operation in 15 children with nontuberculous, nonparalytic conditions. All hips fused solidly except 1, which developed a fibrous pseudoarthrosis. There were no delayed unions.

Technique

Use the anterior iliofemoral incision (Fig. 18–6) to expose the joint. Split the iliac apophysis along the crest of the ilium and elevate the periosteum from both on the medial and lateral sides of the ilium. Divide the origins of the sartorius and rectus femoris muscle and retract them medially exposing the iliopsoas muscle. Reflect the iliopsoas from the anterior aspect of the hip joint and the pubic ramus. With sharp, thin osteotomes remove from the anterior 6 cm of the iliac wing and crest a broad bone graft consisting of both cortices. Next, excise the superior and anterior portions of the capsule, dislocate the head, and denude the head and the acetabulum of all cartilage. Reduce the dislocation and prepare a flat bed for the graft by trimming the anterior inferior spine or any other bony prominences. Place the graft against the pelvis and the head and neck of the femur and anchor it to its bed by 5 lag screws. The middle screw passes through the head of the femur and into the posterior wall of the acetabulum (Fig. 18–13).

After the graft is firmly fixed, retract the soft tissues distally and divide the femur just above the level of the lesser trochanter.

Apply a one and one-half plaster spica while the affected limb is held in neutral rotation, neutral abduction, and slight elevation (10°) from the horizon-

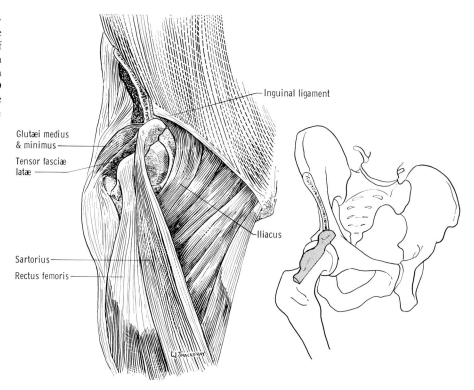

FIG. 18–12. The graft with the attached muscle is seated in the trough on the anterior surface of the hip joint. The inset outlines, in shaded area, the graft in situ. (From Ranawat CS, Jordan LR, Wilson PD Jr: Technique of muscle pedicle bone graft in hip arthrodesis. J Bone Joint Surg 53:928, 1971.)

Inguinal ligament

Glutæi medius & minimus

Tensor fasciæ latæ

Iliacus

Sartorius

Rectus femoris

tal plane. This position allows the hip to fuse in 30° of flexion when the lumbar spine is flat.

Ischiofemoral Arthrodesis

This operation was first described and used by Trumble in 1932, and he reported another series of

operations in 1937. It is an operation designed to attain an ischiofemoral fusion without invading the joint. The operation was primarily designed to fuse tubercular hip joints. The results of the operations discussed in the 1937 report reveal that the tibial grafts he employed were wide and moderate to short in length. Of the 5 operations he had one failure of fusion. Stratford, in 1953, reviewed his own

FIG. 18–13. Thompson arthrodesis. The femoral head and acetabulum are denuded of cartilage. A large iliac graft is anchored with five screws across the front of the joint. Finally an intertrochanteric osteotomy is performed. (From Price CT, Lowell WW: Thompson arthrodesis of the hip. J Bone Joint Surg, 62:1119, 1980.)

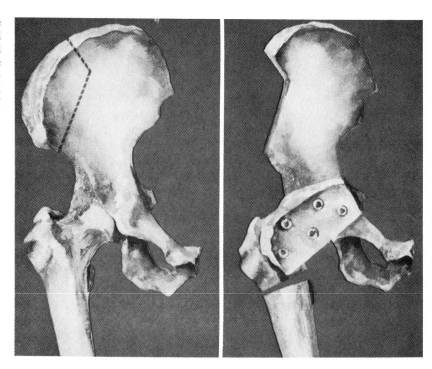

Trumble operations performed for tubercular hips. He reported a failure rate of 33% (13 of 36 fusions failed). He concluded that the short wide graft placed horizontally between the ischium and the femur gives the best result, whereas a long obliquely positioned graft is less satisfactory and tends to fracture or go on to nonunion.

Brittain described his operation in 1941. The operation, like Trumble's operation, is an extra-articular arthrodesis. This operation, however, is performed blindly through the lateral side of the limb. It does take advantage, however, of the benefits of a subtrochanteric osteotomy. It is a difficult operation to perform and it carries great risks, such as severance of the sciatic nerve or large blood vessels. Nevertheless, in Brittain's hands these complications did not occur. He pointed out certain features of the operation that must be observed if failure of fusion and injury to the sciatic nerve and blood vessels are to be averted: the tibial graft must be wide, the slot in the ischium must not be made in the tuber ischii but at the bifurcation of the pelvic rami below the acetabulum to avoid injury to the sciatic nerve, the posterior edge of the osteotome must be in front of the posterior margin of the greater trochanter and the osteotome must be held at all times horizontally and must not be directed posteriorly. After the osteotomy the shaft of the femur must be displaced medially so that it abuts against the ischium and lies in contact with the endosteal surface of the tibial graft. Finally, involvement of the ischium by the tubercular process is a contraindication for an ischiofemoral fusion.

Because the Brittain operation is done blindly it is technically difficult to perform and, aside from the potential danger to the sciatic nerve and large blood vessels, the chief cause of failure is improper insertion of the graft and insufficient medial displacement of the femoral shaft. Visely reported a 20% failure rate; Chan and Shin reported 12% failures; and Brittain, in 1948, reported the results of the operation in 95 patients who received 105 operations. The operation was performed in 38 patients with tuberculosis of the hip, 52 patients with osteoarthritis of the hip, and five patients with infective arthritis of the hip. Brittain reported a successful fusion rate of only 80%.

Kirkaldy-Willis described his operation in 1950. The operation is really a combined intra-articular and extra-articular operation. It is a modification of the Brittain operation done through an anterior approach. He pointed out that his operation has the same mechanical principles of the Brittain operation and also these advantages: the operation is easier to perform through an anterior incision; the

graft between the ischium and the femur cannot slip, the anterior approach does not endanger the sciatic nerve, the use of cancellous bone chips in addition to the strut graft enhances the fusion process, an intra-articular procedure can be done if deemed desirable, and a solid bony fusion occurs in 3 to 4 months, whereas in the Brittain operation fusion is never seen in less than 6 months and the patient is often immobilized for 12 months.

It becomes apparent that today the effectiveness of antibiotic therapy has practically eradicated joint tuberculosis and has made operations of the ischiofemoral design almost obsolete. Yet, the occasion may arise when an ischiofemoral arthrodesis is indicated. Moreover, the current methods of arthrodesis of the hip using the principles of compression, central displacement of the head of the femur, and rigid fixation have a low rate of failure (some studies report no failures) and reduce the indications for ischiofemoral arthrodesis to an insignificant level.

Technique of Trumble Arthrodesis

Expose the posterior aspect of the hip joint by a posterior curved gluteal incision beginning at the posterior aspect of the greater trochanter. Extend it distally and across the posterior aspect of the thigh to the level of the middle of the gluteal fold. Develop the interval between the gluteus maximus and gluteus medius. Divide the insertion of the gluteus maximus and retract it toward the midline exposing the sciatic nerve, the quadratus femoris and the greater tuberosity. Divide the attachments of the quadratus femoris into the intertrochanteric portion of the femur and the ischial tuberosity. Retract the muscle upward exposing the tuberosity of the ischium (Fig. 18-8).

With a sharp, fine osteotome cut a deep notch in the posterior part of the tuberosity of the ischium. Next, by subperiosteal dissection, expose an area just below the lesser trochanter on the posteromedial aspect of the femur and elevate, with a sharp osteotome, a three-sided flap of bone still attached by periosteum on its fourth side. Next, remove a wide graft of proper length from the tibia and insert it between the ischium and the femur. The clefts in the ischium and femur should be so placed that when the graft is in place it will be horizontally between the femur and the ischium (Fig. 18-14). Stratford estimated that a short graft was less than 6.5 cm; a moderate length graft was 6.5 to 9 cm, and a long graft over 9 cm. In width, a narrow graft measured less than 1.3 cm and a wide graft measured more than 1.3 cm.

FIG. 18–14. Left. Roentgenograph taken postoperatively; the graft is short and wide. Right. Same patient. Roentgenograph taken after fusion is completed; note hypertrophy of graft. (From Stratford B: The Trumble graft. J Bone Joint Surg, 35:251, 1953.)

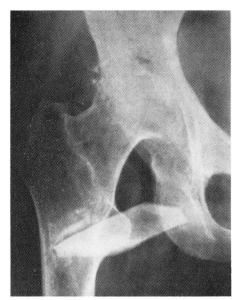 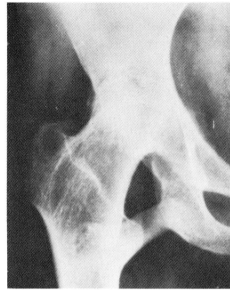

Postoperative Management

After operation the patient is immobilized in a plaster cast for 3 months.

Technique of Brittain Arthrodesis

Brittain performed the operation with the patient on an orthopaedic table with both feet attached to the foot plates and with slight traction on the limbs. Today one places the patient on a fracture table as for a hip nailing, avoiding any pressure from behind that might displace the sciatic nerve anteriorly against the neck of the femur. Through a lateral incision expose the upper end of the femur and identify the abductor ridge on the lateral aspect of the femur (Fig. 18–7). Under radiographic control position a guide pin at the level of the abductor ridge, direct it proximally at an angle of 45° to the lateral surface of the femur and parallel to the floor, advance the pin through the femur and into the ischium just below the acetabulum at the bifurcation of the pelvic rami for a distance of 2.5 to 3 cm. With a sharp, wide osteotome divide the femur in the line of the guide pin. Advance the osteotome into the ischium dividing both cortices. While dividing the femur hold the osteotome at all times in the horizontal plane. It must not be directed posteriorly and its posterior edge must be in front of the posterior surface of the greater tuberosity. Now remove the guide pin and, by moving the osteotome up and down, open up a V-shaped slot in the ischium. The slot in the ischium should be wider than the graft it is to receive. Next, remove a wide cortical graft from the same limb. The graft should be long enough to span the distance from just inside the inner cortex of the ischium to the outer surface of the femur at the site of the osteotomy. Now shape one end of the graft like a chisel (do this with the electric saw). Place the graft on the osteotome with its endosteal surface facing downward and drive the graft across the femur until it abuts against the ischium. Next dislodge and pull out the osteotome and drive the graft into the slot in the ischium. Finally, displace the upper end of the femur medially so that it abuts against the ischium and hold it there by slight abduction of the limb. After closure of the wound apply a double plaster spica (Fig. 18–15).

Technique of Kirkaldy-Willis Arthrodesis

Expose the hip joint through an anterior iliofemoral incision (Fig. 18–6). Split the deep fascia in line with the outer margin of the sartorius. Detach the sartorius from its origin and retract it medially exposing the rectus femoris muscle. Develop the interval between the rectus femoris and the iliopsoas. Next, reflect the iliopsoas muscle from the pubic ramus and from the medial aspect of the joint capsule down to its insertion into the lesser tuberosity. Divide the tendon of the iliopsoas close to its insertion and retract the muscle medially. Just distal and posterior to the lesser trochanter, by subperiosteal dissection, strip off the fibers of insertion of the pectineus and adductor magnus muscles for 3 to 4 cm. This brings into view the obturator externus lying between the joint capsule above and the pectineus and adductor magnus below. Now push a Bennett retractor through the fibers of the obtura-

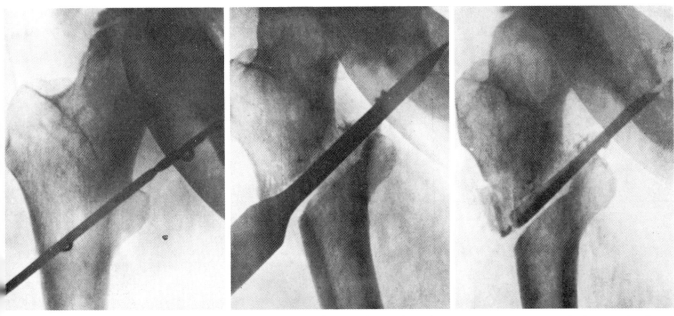

FIG. 18–15. Left. Roentgenograph showing drill through the femur and into the ischium. Center. Roentgenograph showing chisels in situ penetrating the ischium. Right. Roentgenograph showing graft in situ; the shaft of the femur has been displaced medially. (From Brittain HA: Ischiofemoral arthrodesis. J Bone Joint Surg, 30:643, 1948.)

tor internus muscle and into the obturator foramen. Position the tip of the retractor behind the ramus of the ischium and pull on the handle of the retractor medially retracting the sartorius, iliopsoas, pectineus and adductor magnus muscles and exposing the interval between the lesser trochanter and the obturator foramen. At this point insert a box retractor obliquely medially and posteriorly, now the obturator externus is clearly seen. With a sharp periosteal elevator strip the obturator muscle off the ischium and roughen the surface of the bone. Divide the ischium. If the lower margin of the acetabulum is diseased the line of division in the bone is at the level of the obturator foramen and the bone should be divided completely. Otherwise the line of division is above the level of the obturator foramen and the osteotome penetrates the bone for 3 to 4 cm. Divide the origins of the vasti muscles into the lateral and proximal end of the femur. Strip them from the bone and retract them laterally exposing the anterolateral surface of the femur at the level of the lesser tuberosity. Make a drill hole through the femur directed inward and backward toward the ischium: the diameter of the hole is just less than half the diameter of the femur.

Cut from the iliac crest a whole thickness bone graft measuring about 3 cm wide and 8 to 10 cm long. Place the wide end of the graft in the cleft in the ischium, then abduct the limb and place the outer pointed end of the graft opposite the hole in the femur and adduct the limb to lock firmly the

bone graft in its new bed. The graft may have to be tailored to fit the hole in the femur and the slot in the ischium or the hole and the slot may have to be contoured to attain a firm fit with the limb in the desired position. With the graft in place, roughen the neck of the femur with a sharp osteotome from below the lesser trochanter to the lower margin of the acetabulum and pack small cancellous bone chips between the femoral neck and the graft and between the femur and the ischium below the graft (Fig. 18–16).

Postoperative Management

A double hip spica is applied holding the affected limb in the neutral position and the opposite limb slightly abducted.

Rigid Internal Fixation in Arthrodesis of the Hip Joint

It was previously recorded that rigid internal fixation was added to the combined intra-extra-articular arthrodesis in order to permit early mobilization of the patient, and if possible, to eliminate the use of plaster casts. Many techniques using different metallic devices have been described, but essentially the principles on which the operations are based are the same. A few illustrative techniques will be described.

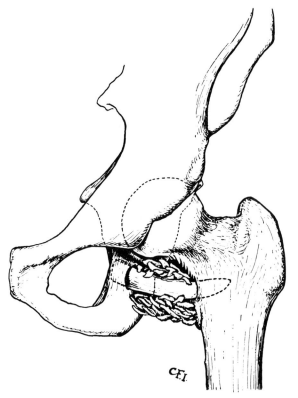

Fig. 18–16. Kirkaldy-Willis arthrodesis of the hip. A large graft extends from the ischium to the ilium. The inferior surface of the femoral neck and the surface of the ischium are roughened. Cancellous bone is packed above and below the graft. (From Stewart M: Arthrodesis. *In* Campbell's Operative Orthopaedics, 6th ed. Edited by AS Edmonson and AH Crenshaw. St Louis, CV Mosby, 1980.)

Arthrodesis With Rigid Internal Fixation

Watson-Jones-Robinson Arthrodesis Technique

The patient lies supine on a fracture table. Expose the hip by an iliofemoral incision (Fig. 18–6). Excise the capsule and dislocate the joint by rotating the limb externally at least 90°. Now the acetabulum comes into view. Remove all cartilage from the femoral head and acetabulum. Make a small incision over the lateral aspect of the femur just below the greater trochanter. Insert a guide wire and pass it through the femoral neck through the upper part of the femoral head until it protrudes from the femoral head. Reduce the hip and select a Smith-Petersen nail of proper length; it should extend 2.5 cm beyond the femoral head. But before inserting the nail the limb must be fixed in the desired position of arthrodesis. This is accomplished by foot plates which are sterilized and screwed into place at the end of the table and the patient's feet are tied to the plates with sterile bandages. First the total apparent limb is corrected by pushing on the

sound limb and pulling on the affected one until the malleoli are level. In doing this take care to achieve apparent equality of leg lengths by tilting the pelvis and not by distracting the affected joint.

With the hip reduced the limb should be in neutral rotation, in no more abduction than is required to correct the shortening, which is seldom over 10 to 15°. There must be no flexion of the limb. As the patient lies on the table the lordosis of the lumbar spine is sufficient to permit fusion of the hip with the limb in 30° of flexion.

Now pass the guide wire into the pelvis and punch the nail over it and impact the femur firmly against the acetabulum. From the dorsum of the ilium cut a full thickness graft slightly wedge-shaped and drive the narrow end into a slot cut in the bone just above the acetabulum. Pack cancellous bone chips from the ilium tightly around the graft, femoral neck, and femoral head (Fig. 18–17).

Postoperative Management. Apply a plaster spica to the toes on the affected side and to above the knee on the sound side and maintain this immobilization for not less than 4 months. Shorter periods of immobilization increase the rate of nonunion. In 1956, Watson-Jones and Robinson reported on a series of 120 patients ranging in age from 10 to 70 years, all afflicted by osteoarthritis. Failure of arthrodesis occurred in 6%.

Lam Arthrodesis Technique

Lam reported his experience with a long Smith-Petersen nail in 1968. His series comprised 69 patients. Fifty-eight patients received an arthrodesis as described by Watson-Jones and Robinson. In 4 patients a central dislocation as described by Charnley was performed and supplemented with a long Smith-Petersen nail and in 7 patients the arthrodesis was done without dislocation of the hip joint. The nature of the disease in the hip joint precluded dislocation of the joint. These patients had severe protrusio acetabuli. In these, the joint was fixed in the desired position by a long Smith-Petersen nail, then a large wedge was cut from the lateral side of the joint and the space was filled with iliac bone. In addition a large iliac corticocancellous graft was slotted across the joint space (Fig. 18–18). The hips were fused in 15° of flexion, neutral rotation, and without unnecessary abduction or adduction.

Postoperative Management. No cast was applied. The patients began to ambulate on crutches after a mean period of 3.2 weeks. Union was attained in 87% of the patients. Thirteen percent failed to

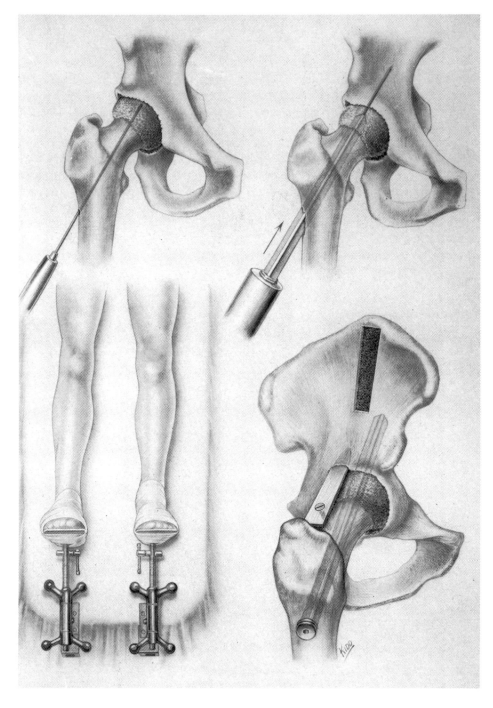

Fig. 18–17. Watson-Jones arthrodesis of the hip. After denuding the cartilage from the femoral head and neck, a guide wire is passed through the neck and upper part of the femoral head. Then, by using the foot clamps, the desired position of the limb is attained. Next drive a long nail over the wire into the pelvis. Finally, a bone graft is slotted into the acetabulum and anchored to the femoral neck with one screw. (From Watson-Jones R, Robinson WC: Arthrodesis of the osteoarthritic hip. J Bone Joint Surg, 38:363, 1956.)

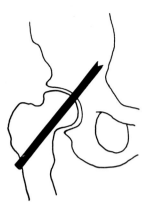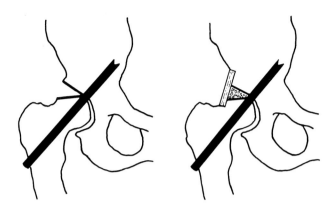

FIG. 18–18. Left. The hip, in the neutral position, is transfixed with a long nail. Center. A wedge of bone is cut from the lateral aspect of the joint. Right. The space is packed with cancellous bone chips and a large full-thickness graft is slotted across the lateral aspect of the joint. (From Lam SJS: Arthrodesis of the hip. J Bone Joint Surg, 50:15, 1968.)

show a bony fusion (9 patients), but only 3 of these patients complained of severe symptoms. This again confirms the findings of others that a firm fibrous union is painless and does provide the needed stability for which the fusion was originally performed. Three patients sustained fractures of the upper femoral shaft at the site of the entry of the nail. All healed following treatment—one by applying a 5 hole plate to the femur and 2 by plaster immobilization.

Stewart and Coker Arthrodesis

First perform a Henderson arthrodesis using an extra-articular Henderson type graft (see Fig. 18–9B). Supplement the fusion with a long Smith-Petersen nail and multiple Knowles pin fixation. No external support is used and the patient starts ambulation in one to two weeks (Fig. 18–19).

DePalma Arthrodesis

With the patient in the supine position, expose the hip joint by an anterior iliofemoral incision and strip, by subperiosteal dissection, the muscles from the outer and inner walls of the ilium as far as the brim of the superior acetabulum (Fig. 18–20). Excise the capsule and dislocate the head of the femur by external rotation of the limb (Fig. 18–21A). Resect about three-fifths of the head of the femur, then round it off with a rasp. Next, denude the acetabulum of all cartilage down to subchondral bone (Fig. 18–21B). Displace the remaining portion of the head and the neck into the acetabulum. At this time do whatever tailoring of the head and neck is necessary to ensure good contact between the femoral head and neck and the undersurface of the acetabulum. Enough of the head should be removed so that when it is displaced centrally the greater trochanter abuts against the acetabular rim. Next, redislocate the femoral head and divide the abductor

muscles close to their insertion into the greater trochanter and expose the outer and superior aspects of the trochanter (Fig. 18–21C).

The specially designed intramedullary spline is 25 cm long and 12 mm wide tapering at the distal end. On the inner surface of the distal 18 cm is a centrally placed vertical fin to prevent rotation of the limb (Fig. 18–22). With the patient's pelvis level on the table, place the head of the femur in

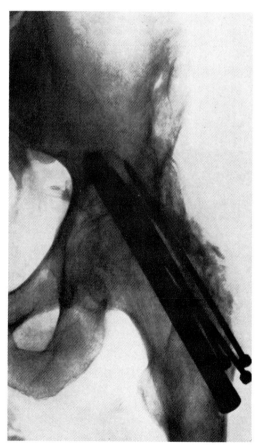

FIG. 18–19. Roentgenograph of a Henderson hip arthrodesis supplemented with a long Smith-Petersen nail and four Knowles pins. Patient was ambulated with external support two weeks after surgery. (From Stewart MJ, Coker TP: Arthrodesis of the hip. Clin Orthop, 62:146, 1969.)

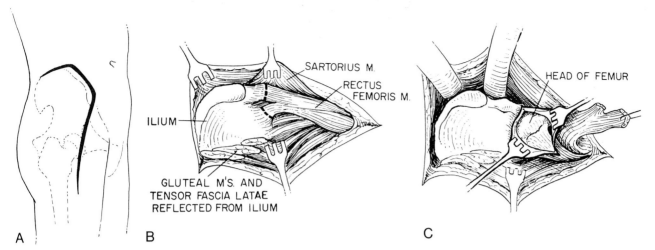

FIG. 18–20. Approach to the ilium and the hip joint. (From DePalma AF, Fenlin JM Jr: Arthrodesis of the hip with intramedullary fixation. Clin Orthop, 48:192–195, 1966.)

the acetabulum and displace it centrally. The femur is rotated to the neutral position and the end of the spline is placed at its site of insertion at the juncture of the greater trochanter and the femoral

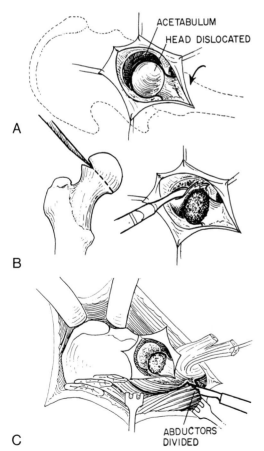

FIG. 18–21. Preparation of intra-articular fusion and division of the abductors. (From DePalma AF, Fenlin JM Jr: Arthrodesis of the hip with intramedullary fixation. Clin Orthop, 48:192–195, 1966.)

neck (Fig. 18–23). It may be necessary to notch the cortex with an osteotome to start the spline at this point. Rotate the spline so that its surface is parallel with the surface of the ilium. Drive the spline into the medullary canal of the femur until only 5 or 6 mm of the central fin projects above the surface of the neck. Now let the leg lie flat on the table with the patella straight up. This position will allow the limb to fuse in about 20° of flexion (Fig. 18–24). Finally, place the limb in neutral abduction-adduction and bend the spline to conform to this position when opposed against the side of the ilium (Fig. 18–25). With a special clamp hold the spline against the side of the ilium in the desired position and bolt it against the side of the ilium with three bolts with beveled washers that conform to the inner surface of the ilium (Fig. 18–26).

Finally, remove long strips and chips of cancellous bone from the side of the ilium. Pack the chips in any area of incongruity remaining in the acetabulum and tuck the long strips under an osteoperiosteal flap raised on the trochanter and lay them against the ilium adjacent to the spline (Fig. 18–27).

This procedure can be adapted with only minor modifications in the absence of a head and neck (Fig. 18–28). In these cases the trochanter must be displaced medially inside the acetabulum so that its superior surface is in contact with the roof of the acetabulum. It may be necessary to remove the lesser trochanter if it impinges on the ischium and prevents the desired medial displacement of the femur. Also it may be necessary to abduct the limb in order to maintain the desired contact between the greater trochanter and the roof of the acetabulum. In such cases, a subtrochanteric osteotomy

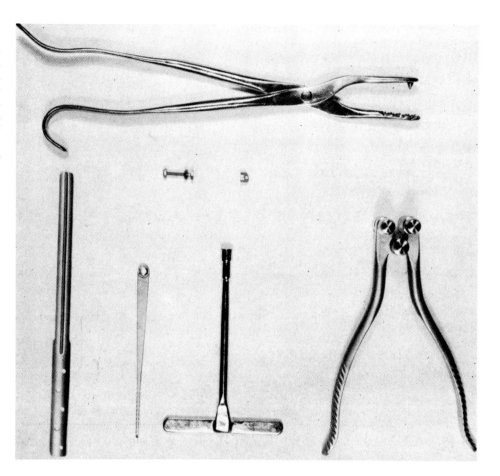

Fɪɢ. 18–22. Special instruments required for intra-articular fusion: clamp to hold the spline against the ilium, spline with a central fin, bolt with nut and special washer, instrument to hold screw, special wrench, and bending iron. (From DePalma AF, Fenlin JM Jr: Arthrodesis of the hip with intramedullary fixation. Clin Orthop, 48:192–195, 1966.)

will be necessary to bring the limb into the desired position for arthrodesis. In these cases, drive the spline through the trochanter (Fig. 18–28).

Postoperative Management. After 7 to 10 days a walking plaster spica extending to above the knee on the affected side is applied and the sound limb is free. In 2 to 3 weeks permit partial weight-bearing with crutches. The cast is changed every 6 to 8 weeks until the fusion is solid. The average time to reach this point was 17 weeks. This technique pro-

vided a successful fusion in 93% of the 44 cases with a minimum followup of 1 year.

White Arthrodesis of the Hip

Essentially this is another procedure which combines intra- and extra-articular fusion supplemented by rigid fixation and compression. But the arthrodesis differs significantly from most of the

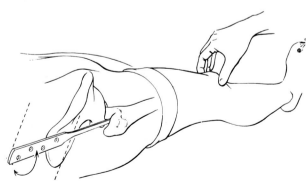

Fɪɢ. 18–23. Determination of rotation before insertion of spline. (From DePalma AF, Fenlin JM Jr: Arthrodesis of the hip with intramedullary fixation. Clin Orthop, 48:192–195, 1966.)

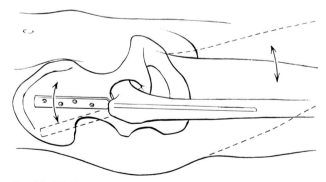

Fɪɢ. 18–24. Determination of flexion before fixation of spline. (From DePalma AF, Fenlin JM Jr: Arthrodesis of the hip with intramedullary fixation. Clin Orthop, 48:192–195, 1966.)

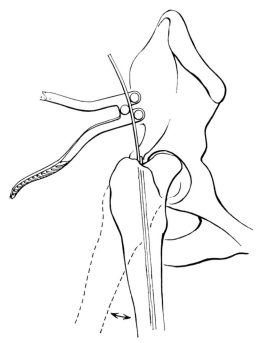

Fig. 18–25. Bending spline to desired position of abduction-adduction. (From DePalma AF, Fenlin JM Jr: Arthrodesis of the hip with intramedullary fixation. Clin Orthop, 48:192–195, 1966.)

procedures already described and from the arthrodeses utilizing central displacement of the femoral head by displacing it through the medial wall of the acetabulum or by doing an osteotomy of the pelvis. These procedures will be subsequently described. Whereas most arthrodeses are designed to achieve a

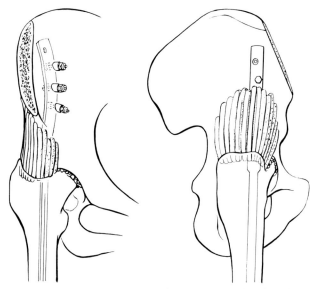

Fig. 18–27. Placement of grafts from ilium to the slotted trochanter. (From DePalma AF, Fenlin JM Jr: Arthrodesis of the hip with intramedullary fixation. Clin Orthop, 48:192–195, 1966.)

high rate of fusion and rapid mobilization of the patient without attempting to preserve the normal anatomy of the hip joint, White strives for the same goals but attempts to maintain the normal anatomy of the hip joint and to minimize the functional and structural shortening of the limb. There is a reason for all this; the reason being that many hips fused in skeletally immature persons and in young, active adults with unilateral hip disorders,

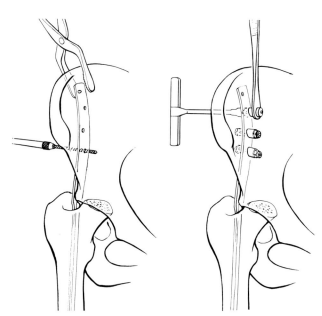

Fig. 18–26. Fixation of spline to the ilium. (From DePalma AF, Fenlin JM Jr: Arthrodesis of the hip with intramedullary fixation. Clin Orthop, 48:192–195, 1966.)

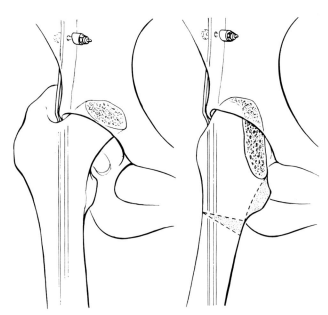

Fig. 18–28. Left. Normal relation of spline to ilium and femur. Right. Modified relation with absence of the head and neck of the femur. (From DePalma AF, Fenlin JM Jr: Arthrodesis of the hip with intramedullary fixation. Clin Orthop, 48:192–195, 1966.)

after many years of service, require conversion to total hip replacement. And if the anatomy of the joint has been severely altered by an arthrodesis done earlier in life, conversion may be difficult and even impossible. The studies of McBeath and Welch support this trend. McBeath reported on 58 skeletally immature patients whose hips were fused at an average age of 14 years; 12 percent of these required conversion to a total hip replacement performed on an average of 38 years after the fusion operations. Welch's study included 42 adult patients fused at an average age of 27 years; 38% of these patients required a conversion operation on an average of thirty-one years following the arthrodesis.

The number of arthrodeses performed on young persons with unilateral hip disease is on the rise because it is now being generally accepted that for the young person, active and otherwise healthy, with unilateral hip disorders, arthrodesis is the operation of choice. And it will remain so until the causes for mechanical failures of hip arthroplasty and surface replacement are identified and resolved. No one knows what the future holds in the development of metal reinforced acetabuli, press fits, and cementless hips. Perhaps the future developments may permit lowering the age at which total hip replacement may be done. But today there is no hip arthroplasty that matches the durability and the functional capacity of a successful arthrodesis in the young, otherwise healthy, person with unilateral hip disease.

And, although today tuberculosis of the hip in the young is not the problem it was in the early decades of this century, traumatic hip disorders are a real concern. As an example, in the Kostwick and Alexander report trauma was the cause of the hip disorder for which an arthroplasty was done and subsequently failed in 11 of the 14 patients, and of the 11 patients 8 were under the age of 50 years.

Technique. Place and immobilize the patient in the lateral decubitus position. Expose the hip joint by a posterolateral incision and divide the capsule at its attachment to the acetabulum. Dislocate the femoral head posteriorly and remove all cartilage and osteonecrotic bone from the femoral head and acetabulum down to bleeding bone. Use an acetabular reamer equal to the diameter of the denuded femoral head to deepen the acetabulum in a superior-medial direction. This increases the contact area, does not violate the medial wall, and does not produce significant shortening (Fig. 18–29). Now reduce the femoral head and seat it firmly in the deepened area. Next, place the limb in the desired

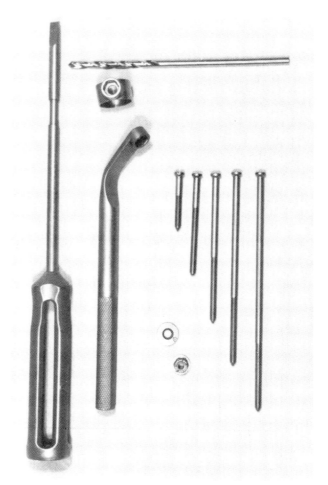

FIG. 18–29. Harris bolt system. The vitallium bolts measure 4.0 mm in diameter and range in length from 20 to 180 mm. A washer fits on the head and a washer-nut assembly fits on the bolt inside the pelvis. Each hole is made with a 4.2 mm drill. Placement of the washer-nut assembly is facilitated by the long-handled carrier. (From White RE Jr: Arthrodesis of the hip. *In* The Hip. Edited by RB Welch. St Louis, CV Mosby, 1984.)

position of fusion and fix it firmly. Use a sterile goniometer to check the desired position.

Make a second incision along the anterior-inferior iliac half of the iliac crest and strip subperiosteally the iliacus exposing a broad area for the placement of the washer-nut combination of the Harris bolts. The length of the vitallium Harris bolts ranges from 20 to 180 mm and the diameter is 4.0 mm. The washer-nut combination fastens on the inside of the pelvis and there is a washer for the head of the bolt. Retract the iliacus medially and make each hole with the 4.2 mm drill bit under direct vision. Use a depth gauge to select the appropriate length bolt (Fig. 18–29). Use at least 4 bolts, and in large patients use 6 bolts. Most bolts traverse the femoral neck and head, some can pass through the greater trochanter above the level of the superior surface of the femur into the iliac

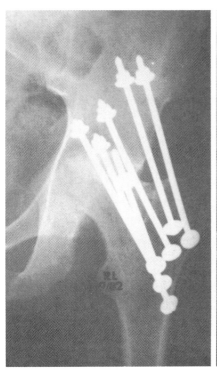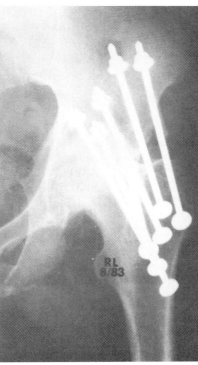

Fɪɢ. **18–30.** Left. Six bolts were used; two pass through the greater trochanter above the surface of the femoral neck. There is good bone contact and rigid internal fixation under compression. Right. A solid bony fusion has been achieved. (From White RE Jr.: Arthrodesis of the hip. *In* The Hip. Edited by RB Welch. St Louis, CV Mosby, 1984.)

wing. Tighten each bolt individually making compression at the contact area between the femoral head and acetabulum. The bolts now provide rigid internal fixation, which is mechanically strong. Without disturbing the attachment of the abductor muscles a large corticocancellous graft and also cancellous bone chips are removed from the inside of the iliac wing. Pack the cancellous bone chips at the site of contact between the head and neck, filling in all spaces. Cut a large slot from the posterior-superior aspect of the acetabulum into the femoral neck and into the trochanter. Tailor the corticocancellous graft to fit into the slot and then anchor it in place with two screws (Fig. 18–30).

Postoperative Management. Apply a single hip spica cast and allow weight-bearing.

Hip Arthrodesis with Pelvic Osteotomy and Compression with the Cobra Head Plate

Schneider combined the use of the cobra head plate with pelvic osteotomy to attain an arthrodesis in young patients with osteoarthritis in whom osteotomy is contraindicated or has failed, and in joints destroyed by bacterial infections including tuberculosis. He reported in 1974, 112 cases fused by this procedure and achieved a successful fusion in 87%; 90% of the patients were partially weight-bearing after 3 weeks without external immobilization. Schneider noted that this operation adhered to some important principles in bone healing: (1) Retention of bone viability and stabilization are condusive to bone formation and consolidation. (2) Stable internal fixation is effective in the treatment of infections of both infected nonunions and infected joints. (3) Stabilization of a vascularized pseudoarthrodesis produces bony union without disturbing the intervening tissue, and this situation is comparable to stabilization of an arthritic joint without dislocation of the joint. And (4) joint dislocation and resection disturbs the circulation of the components of the joint rendering the area less favorable for bone production.

Essentially, the Cobra head plate is an internal fixation device that exerts pressure—it functions as a tensing band, and the pressure it exerts is in direct proportion to its distance from the axis of loading. Because the Cobra head plate is placed on the lateral aspect of the pelvis and femur, it lies as far from the axis of loading as possible, and when the limb bears weight, maximum stability occurs at the site of arthrodesis (Fig. 18–31). In addition, in this position it effectively blocks rotation—an advantage that internal devices lying in the femoral neck and close to the axis of rotation do not have. The transverse extension of the Cobra head plate is really an extension transversely of the straight lateral plate. These transverse extensions permit an-

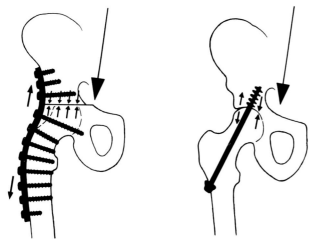

FIG. 18–31. Left. Tension band effect of the cobra headplate. The pressure produced results in interfragmentary friction over the entire contact area. The bone graft seated laterally under the plate is also under pressure. The contact area is large and free of internal fixation devices. Right. With internal fixation devices placed in the femoral neck, loading lateral to the implant tends to distract the fragments. Under these conditions an iliofemoral graft is not under compression. (From Schneider R: Hip arthrodesis with cobra headplate and pelvic osteotomy. Reconstr Surg Traumat 14:5, 1974.)

choring the head of the plate into the stout dense bone at a sufficient distance from the transverse axis of rotation to be effective in stabilizing the forces of flexion and extension that act in the sagittal plane at the site of arthrodesis.

Displacement of the femur medially reduces the dislocating force at the hip joint. This is produced by osteotomizing the pelvis at the level of the roof of the acetabulum and displacing the lower segment of the pelvis medially. An important feature of the pelvic osteotomy is the increase in contact area between the femur and the pelvis. This procedure does not dislocate the femoral head, hence its blood supply remains intact. All these features are conducive to rapid bony fusion.

Schneider Technique of Hip Arthrodesis (Fig. 18–32)

Position the patient in the supine position on the operating table and drape the patient so that the iliac crests are exposed and the limbs are freely movable. By draping the uninvolved extremity, the limb is now readily accessible to the surgeon during the operation when determining leg length. Expose the hip region through a lateral femoral incision beginning three of four finger-breadths above the greater trochanter and extending distally 25 or 30 cm.

With a thin osteotome remove a thin layer of the greater trochanter with the gluteus medius and

minimus attached to it. Retract it upward exposing the joint capsule and the iliac wing. Excise the anterior and superior portions of the capsule. Insert a Hohmann retractor along the posterior wall of the acetabulum and into the sciatic notch to protect the sciatic nerve. Place another Hohmann retractor along the anterior wall. Next, with osteotome and curettes, clear and smooth the bone immediately above the superior iliac brim of the acetabulum and the iliac bone above it making a smooth bed for the head of the plate. If some distortion of the ilium is present, cut out in a slightly posterior direction a bed for the plate so that it lies flat on the bone. Next, perform the osteotomy, starting with the oscillating saw and completing it with an osteotome. Use bone spreaders so that the oscillating saw and the osteotome cut the bone; the depth of the cut should always be visualized and the surgeon should not extend the cut medially beyond the surface of the bone.

The osteotomy starts at the upper border of the hip joint. Direct it medially and parallel to the roof of the acetabulum. In order to prevent the leg from going into abduction when compression is applied, the osteotomy must be either parallel or directed slightly upward and medially, never downward and medially. Now, with the saw, remove two broad pieces of bone from the trochanter; these will be used as grafts: one will be shaped to fit between the plate and the head and neck and the other will bridge a slot anteriorly from the head of the femur to the ilium. Place a broad osteotome in the osteotomy site and lever the lower segment of the pelvis and the femur medially.

Expose the shaft of the femur by retracting the vastus lateralis anteriorly and position the limb in 10° of adduction, neutral rotation, and between 10 and 25° of flexion, depending on the age of the patient. Lay the plate across the joint and examine it for fit. The trochanter may need some tailoring or the plate some bending before the plate fits satisfactorily across the joint.

With the limb in the desired position and the plate fitting satisfactorily so that it lies parallel to the femoral shaft and the central hole of the head lies 5 mm above the joint line in the roof of the acetabulum, drill a hole for the central screw, tap it, and insert the screw. Upon tightening this screw the plate pushes the pelvis and femur medially. Next, clamp the plate to the femur and apply the tensioner and tighten it slightly. This puts the osteotomy site under some pressure.

Check the position of the limb, aim for this position: neutral position between adduction and abduction, 20 to 30° of flexion and neutral rotation.

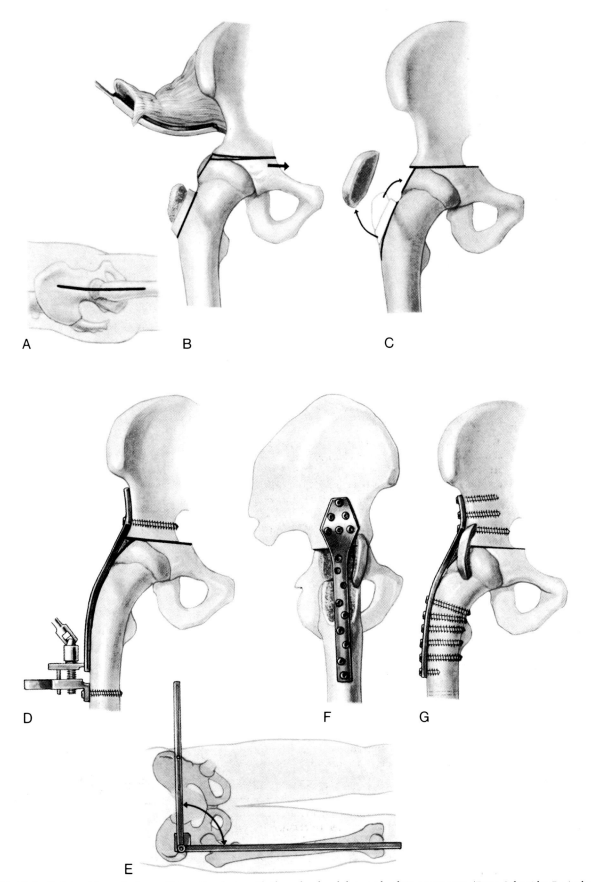

FIG. 18–32 A–E. Schneider technique of hip arthrodesis with the cobra headplate and pelvic osteotomy. (From Schneider R: Arthrodesis of the hip with cobra headplate. *In* Manual of Internal Fixation, 2nd ed. Edited by ME Muller. New York, Springer-Verlag, 1979.)

With the feet placed together the internal malleolus on the affected limb is one centimeter higher than the malleolus on the sound side. If the limb position is satisfactory insert the remaining screws into the head of the plate. Then shape one of the trochanteric bone grafts to fit in the wedge-shaped space on the lateral aspect of the acetabulum between the plate and the prepared surface of the femoral neck. Also, pack bone chips posteriorly and laterally between the head and the acetabular roof. Tighten the tensioner making strong compression between the head and pelvis, and the plate and the bone chips. Insert the remaining screws. Finally, cut a slot in front of the ilium and femoral head and into it impact the shaped second trochanteric graft. In closing the wound bring the abductors and the vastus lateralis over the plate. It should be noted that the first two screws immediately below the head plate usually are 70 mm long cortex screws. These screws take a firm hold on the lower segment of the pelvis. The distal screw in the plate is usually 16 mm long and traverses only one cortex.

Postoperative Management

Usually no cast is applied after surgery. The exceptions are cases of severe osteoporosis and cases with osteolysis associated with infection.

Arthrodesis with Central Dislocation or Displacement of the Femur

These operations have these advantages over most of the arthrodeses previously described: (1) the limb's center of weight-bearing is shifted toward the midline of the body, (2) all movements are blocked—abduction, rotation and adduction, (3) the contact area between the femur and the pelvis is increased, and (4) the abductor medius is no longer essential. But, as was pointed out previously, not all these are desirable in persons who require a conversion later in life. Distortion of the normal anatomy caused by disrupting the medial wall of the acetabulum and the loss of the trochanter and the abductor muscles may make conversion impossible or difficult. Nevertheless, by the addition of rigid internal fixation and the use of compression devices such as the Charnley spring compressor and the Cobra head plate, these operations assure a high rate of successful fusions. Most patients are not immobilized in plaster, and for those that are, the period of immobilization is short.

Charnley Arthrodesis—A Technique Using Central Dislocation of the Hip

Charnley designed this technique to attain immediate stability of the hip, rapid bony fusion, and to permit the patient early mobilization without the use of plaster casts. But his expectations were not realized, for with this operation few patients attained a bony fusion. Yet, the fibrous ankylosis in many patients was painless and even permitted a few degrees of motion. Later, Charnley added the spring compressor to the technique directing compression on the centrally dislocated head. In 1955 he reported the end results on 105 patients followed for 1 to 6 years after the operation. In approximately 50% Charnley used the spring compressor. About half of the hips had a fibrous union and 35% had frank movement—the freer the movement the less satisfactory the result. Five percent developed fatigue fractures of the neck of the femur; however, in three % they were picked up only by routine check radiographs. Five patients required osteotomy of the femur for malposition of the limb. Yet, the fibrous unions gave results as good as bony union, and 15% of the hips with fibrous union went on spontaneously to bony union. He assessed his results as excellent or good in 88% and fair or unchanged in 12%; no patient was made worse.

Many other surgeons reported their results with the Charnley operation, some used the spring compressor (Creganin, Morris) and some did not (Piggott). It seems that there was great variability in the rate of solid fusion: Piggott, 72%; Morris, 76%; Creganin, 86%. Nevertheless, all these workers noted that the fibrous unions were just as effective as the bony unions. Charnley attributes the success of the fibrous ankylosis to the bone block to the adduction that is produced by this operation.

Technique: (Central Dislocation of the Hip)

Position the patient on a fracture table with a sandbag under the loin of the affected side. The assistant flexes the thigh 45° and adducts the limb over the opposite limb. Expose the hip joint through a T-shaped incision. The transverse limb begins over the anterosuperior iliac spine. Extend it backward over the greater tuberosity toward the ischial tuberosity. The longitudinal limb begins over the top of the greater tuberosity and continues over the lateral aspect of the femoral shaft for 15 to 16 cm. Split the fascia lata in the line of the longitudinal incision, divide the insertion of the gluteus maximus into the fascia lata, and extend the cut for 5 cm behind the greater trochanter. Develop the interval between the flaps of the fascia lata and the vastus lateralis. Also, develop the interval between the tensor fascia femoris and the gluteus medius and retract the tensor fascia femoris anteriorly. With a sharp osteotome shave off the greater tuberosity and the insertions of the gluteus medius and minimus as one unit and reflect the muscles upward, stripping them off the superior surface of the capsule until the superior brim of the acetabulum is exposed. Retract the muscles superiorly against the side of the ilium and fix them there with 2 Steinman pins drilled into the side of the ilium.

Expose the hip joint with a T-shaped incision in the capsule and dislocate the hip by rotating it externally until the foot of the rotated limb is over the opposite shoulder of the patient and the femoral neck faces laterally.

Using Charnley's special instruments, tailor the femoral head into a cylinder (Fig. 18–33). First, with a sharp osteotome, remove all osteophytes from the periphery of the femoral head, then pick the trephine that is concentric with the neck of the femur and apply it to the head directing it 45° to the axis of the femoral shaft and in the coronal plane disregarding any anteversion or retroversion.

The coronal plane is perpendicular to the horizontal plane in which the femur and tibia lie, while an assistant holds the knee flexed 90°.

Next, remove the sandbag from under the loin. Now the patient is lying flat on the table with the pelvis level. An assistant applies a sling around the head of the femur and distracts it toward the foot of the table.

You are now ready to drill a hole in the medial wall of the acetabulum. First place the starting drill 1.3 cm anterior to the center of the floor of the acetabulum. Perforate the medial wall and enlarge the hole with successive reamers directed horizontally at an angle of 45° to the long axis of the body. When the desired size of the hole has been reamed, reduce the dislocation and push the head through the hole. By radiographs check the position of the femoral head. If the head has not penetrated the medial wall enough, dislocate the head and trim away some of the posterior and inferior rim of the acetabulum. Also, the opening may be enlarged by reinserting the last reamer while rotating the brace and directing the axis of the reamer in the desired position. The blocked position of the limb when the head is in its final position should be neutral abduction-adduction and neutral rotation.

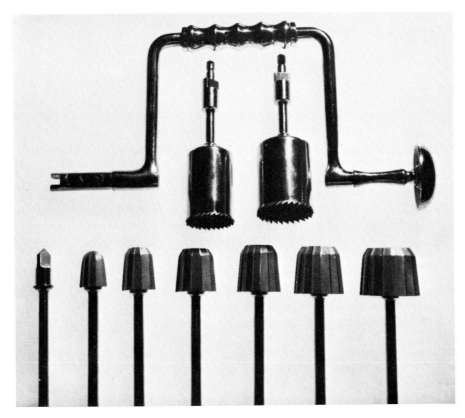

Fig. 18–33. Special tools designed by Charnley and used in the operation for central dislocation of the hip joint. (From Stewart M: Arthrodesis. *In* Campbell's Operative Orthopaedics, 6th ed. Edited by AS Edmonson and AH Crenshaw. St Louis, C.V. Mosby, 1980.)

Postoperative Management

Apply a single hip spica with the foot and ankle free and the knee flexed 20 to 30°. This cast is worn for 4 weeks then the part below the knee is removed. Walking with a cast is started 6 weeks after the operation.

Application of the Spring Compressor (Fig. 18–34)

Perform the same operation as described, but before closing the wound apply the spring compressor. Retract the insertion of the vastus lateralis distally. Position the limb in the desired position for arthrodesis. Select a point 2.5 cm below the insertion of the vastus lateralis and perforate the cortex with a 6.3 mm drill. Now change the direction of the drill and aim it at a point just inside the superior rim of the acetabulum. Hold the drill horizontally and pass it through the bone until it emerges just superior to the neck of the femur at its base. Now replace it with a 4 mm drill and drive it through, piercing the superior rim of the acetabulum and further in until the shoulder of the drill strikes bone. Remove the drill and insert the screw drilling it into the pelvis until only 4 cm of its outer end remains outside the femoral shaft. Now apply the oblique block, the spring, and finally the nut. Tighten the nut until the spring is flat.

Postoperative Management

Apply a single spica for 4 weeks, then cut the cast down to above the knee and remove the entire cast after 2 more weeks.

At a second operation the spring compressor is removed and the patient is permitted weight-bearing usually at the end of the seventh week.

Barmada Arthrodesis (Cobra Plate Compression Technique with Central Dislocation of the Femoral Head)

This is a modification of the cobra plate compression technique for hip fusion; but instead of osteotomizing the pelvis, the head of the femur is dislocated centrally through the medial wall of the acetabulum. According to Barmada, the advantages of this technique over that of pelvic osteotomy with medial displacement of the lower half of the innominate bone are: the technique is simpler to perform, blood loss is reduced, and pelvic distortion is avoided. The technique is highly effective in attaining a successful arthrodesis. Using the cobra plate compressing technique Barmada had no failures in 16 consecutive arthrodeses.

Technique

The patient lies in the supine position on the operating table. Expose the hip joint through a straight lateral incision, 30 cm long and centered over the greater trochanter. Split the tensor fasciae latae in line with the conjuncture of the tensor fasciae latae and the gluteus maximum muscles. Divide the origin of the vastus lateralis and displace the muscle distally and medially. Next, with a sharp osteotome, remove a thin layer of the trochanter with the gluteus medius and minimus attached and retract it upward exposing the joint capsule and the wing of the ilium. Divide the capsule and dislocate the joint. Remove the articular cartilage from the femoral head. Map out a square window on the medial wall of the acetabulum large enough to allow the femoral head through it and drill 4 holes in the acetabulum in such a manner that on opening the window it will swing on a superior hinge (Fig. 18–35). Push the femoral head through the window, which now fits snugly around the head. With medial displacement of the femur the lateral aspect of the acetabulum approximates the superior aspect of the femoral neck. After the bone surfaces are cleared of all soft tissue place the leg in 10° of adduction, 5° of external rotation, and 30° of flexion.

Apply the cobra plate over the lateral surface of the femur and ilium (determine the size of plate to be used depending on the size of the patient; there are three plate sizes). With an osteotome, tailor the surface of the trochanter to permit satisfactory seating of the plate. It may be necessary to bend the plate or even groove the ilium in order to get the desired fit of the plate. Pack the bone chips between the lateral border of the acetabulum, the neck of the femur, and the plate. If more bone chips are needed harvest them from the anterior aspect of the ilium or the greater trochanter.

Fix the plate to the ilium with a single screw passing through the central hole 5 mm above the joint. Next, clamp the plate to the femur and apply the compression device (Fig. 18–36). Apply the compression. As compression develops the limb shifts from the adducted position to neutral, at this point stop compression and insert the remaining

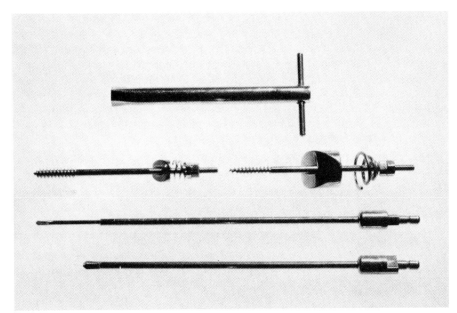

FIG. 18–34. Tools and devices used in Charnley's compression arthrodesis. Beginning at top: wrench or spanner to tighten nut, two complete assemblies, a 4-mm tapping drill, and a 6.3-mm tapping drill. (From Stewart M: Arthrodesis. *In* Campbell's Operative Orthopaedics. 6th ed. Edited by AS Edmonson and AH Crenshaw. St Louis, C.V. Mosby, 1980.)

screws through the plate. Finally, remove the compression device. The plate will accept either cortical or cancellous screws on the ilium.

If the disease process has shortened the head and neck, sufficient medial displacement of the femur is attained by deepening the acetabulum with a reamer. Also, the necessary amounts of cartilage and bone are removed from the femoral head. In cases with complete destruction of the head further medial displacement of the femur may not be necessary if contact between the femur and acetabulum is good. In such instances roughen the bone on the superior aspect of the femoral neck and the adjacent acetabulum and pack bone chips in this area before applying the cobra plate.

Postoperative Management

In most instances no external immobilization is needed, however, occasionally as security against falling, a single hip spica cast is applied about 2 weeks after operation and is worn for 6 weeks. On the third week after surgery the patient begins par-

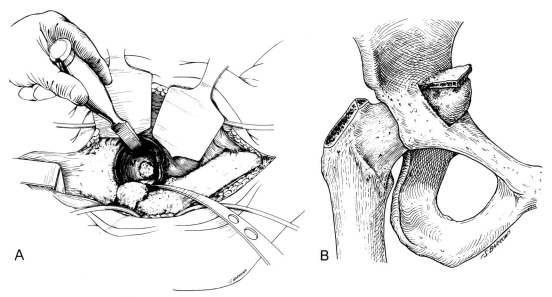

FIG. 18–35. A. Trap door has been cut in the medial wall of the acetabulum. **B.** Femoral head is dislocated centrally. (From Barmada R, Abraham E, Ray RD: Hip fusion utilizing the cobra headplate. J Bone Joint Surg, 58:542, 1976.

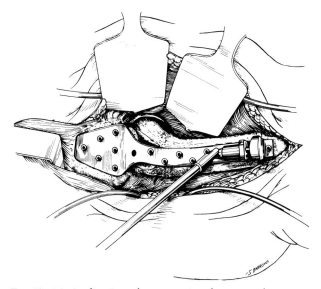

Fɪɢ. 18–36. Application of compression device to obtain compression. (From Barmada R, Abraham C, Ray RD: Hip fusion utilizing, the cobra headplate. J Bone Joint Surg, 58:543, 1976.)

tial weight-bearing; after 2 more months the patient bears full weight on the operated limb.

Arthrodesis Using Muscle Tension as a Compressive Force—The Abduction Principle

Prior to the time of internal fixation capable of producing dynamic compression to stimulate bone production several ingenious operations were designed to induce solid bony arthrodesis. All of these operations used muscle tension to provide the compression force (Fig. 18–37). These techniques were used in the most difficult cases: usually in tuberculous hips with secondary pyogenic infections and draining sinuses and with massive destruction of the head and neck; and in patients with destruction of the head and neck from other causes such as aseptic necrosis of the femoral head following nonunion of the femoral neck, sepsis following cup arthroplasty, old irreducible dislocations of the hip, and failed arthrodeses and arthroplasties.

In 1931 Abbott and Fischer described a technique they called "arthrodesis of the hip in wide abduction." In 1954 Abbott and Lucas again described the technique with the modifications they had made. Essentially the earlier operation was done in three stages: (1) correction of any deformities about the hip, (2) fusion of the hip in wide abduction, and (3) reduction of the abducted limb by subtrochanteric osteotomy (Fig. 18–38). The common deformities

to be corrected were adduction, flexion, and shortening. This was accomplished by traction to the extremity, gradually bringing it into wide abduction. If the greater trochanter was fixed to the side of the ilium, the limb was first mobilized by excision of the scar tissue then traction was applied. When the greater trochanter was opposite the acetabulum the second stage of the operation was performed: through an anterior iliofemoral incision the acetabulum and the upper end of the femoral shaft were exposed and the acetabulum was denuded of all debris and cartilage down to bleeding cancellous bone. Also, any remaining part of the femoral neck was removed and the trochanter and adjacent femoral shaft were denuded of cortical bone. Then the greater trochanter was placed in the acetabulum and the limb abducted 30 to 90 degrees depending on the angle providing optimal contact. A double spica was applied holding the abducted position of the limb. Usually, a bony fusion was attained in 5 to 6 months. At this time, the third stage of the operation was done: a subtrochanteric osteotomy was performed but the position of the limb was not changed. Two weeks later, if the roentgenographs showed abundant callus at the osteotomy site, the cast was removed and skin traction was applied to both extremities. The abduction on the operated side was reduced gradually, slowly bending the callus. After about 10 days the desired position of the extremity was reached. A spica plaster cast was then applied until union at the osteotomy site was solid.

The modifications reported by Abbott and Lucas were: (1) The stage one operation was eliminated. They found that the deformities could be eradicated at the time of the surgery during stage two. (2) Following placement of the trochanter in the acetabulum with the limb in wide abduction the time for osteotomy of the femur was reduced to 4 to 8 weeks depending upon the amount of consolidation at the fusion site as demonstrated by the roentgenographs. (3) At the time of osteotomy the limb was brought down to its desired position and the gradual reduction of abduction by slowly bending the callus was eliminated.

Technique—Arthrodesis of the Hip in Wide Abduction

Expose the hip joint by an anterior iliofemoral incision (Fig. 18–6), excise the superior and anterior capsule, and expose the intracapsular structures. Thoroughly debride the joint, especially in tubercular and septic hips and remove all cartilage from

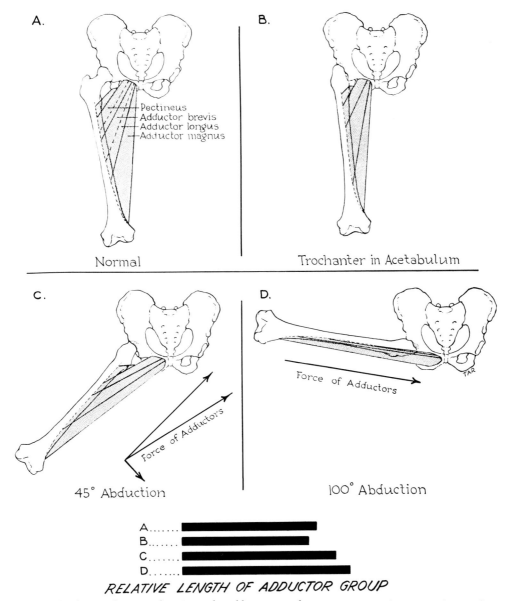

FIG. 18–37. **A.** When the limb is in the neutral position the adductor muscles are at rest exerting no passive tension on the leg. **B-C.** After excision of head and neck and placement of the trochanter in the acetabulum, abduction of the limb causes the adductors to exert passive tension on the leg, pushing the trochanter into the acetabulum. (From Abbott LC, Lucas DB: Arthrodesis of the hip in wide abduction. J Bone Joint Surg, 36:1133, 1954.)

the acetabulum including the subchondral bone down to bleeding cancellous bone. Resect any remnants of the femoral neck at its base and strip off the gluteal insertions from the greater trochanter. Deepen the roof of the acetabulum to allow better seating of the trochanter. Next, denude the greater trochanter of all cortical bone and place it in the acetabulum. Holding the limb externally rotated 5 to 10° and the thigh flexed 35° slowly abduct the limb until the adductors tighten. The tightness of the adductors will determine the amount of abduction. At least 45° of abduction is required to impact firmly the trochanter in the acetabulum. The fit

should be snug; pack cancellous bone chips in any open spaces between the trochanter and the acetabulum. While the limb is held in the desired position of abduction (a sterile instrument stand with an adapted gutter attachment serves this purpose well) close the wound and apply a bilateral hip spica extending to the toes on the affected side and to the knee on the sound side.

After 6 to 8 weeks, remove the cast and clinically and by roentgenographs determine the state of the fusion. If the fusion is solid, expose the femur through the lower limb of the iliofemoral incision. Divide the femur 5 cm distal to the lesser trochan-

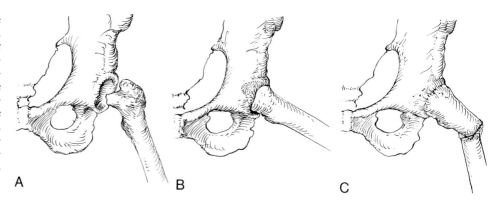

Fig. 18–38. Three stages of the arthrodesis of Abbott and Lucas. **A.** Preoperatively the greater trochanter lies opposite the acetabulum. **B.** Position of the tailored greater trochanter inside the acetabulum. **C.** Subtrochanteric osteotomy to place the limb in the desired position. (From Abbott LC, Lucas DB: Arthrodesis of the hip in wide abduction. J Bone Joint Surg, 36:1129, 1954.)

ter, the cut traverses the femur three-quarters of its diameter, and fracture the medial cortex. Adduct the distal shaft and displace it slightly inward so that the medial cortex of the upper fragment drops into the medullary canal of the lower fragment (Fig. 18–39). Place the limb in the desired position of arthrodesis and apply a bilateral hip spica cast. Maintain cast immobilization until the osteotomy is healed and then begin protected weight-bearing.

Femoroischial Transplantation

David Bosworth developed this operation for patients with tuberculosis of the hip with massive destruction of the upper end of the femur and acetabulum. He reasoned that if the femur was severed below the sclerosis caused by the tuberculosis and inserted into the ischium, which has good osteogenic properties, a successful fusion would result. He performed the first operation in 1936, and in 1942 reported on the end results in 9 patients with

femoroischial transplantation. If successful, femoroischial transplantation gives the same cosmetic, weight-bearing, and functional result as arthrodesis of the hip. The procedure also can be used in instances of old suppurative arthritis of the hip, aseptic necrosis, and nonunited traumatic lesions in which ankylosis is desirable but difficult to achieve.

The patients operated on in this study ranged in age from 12 to 52 years, averaging 30 years. In all patients the onset of the tuberculous process started in childhood. Many surgical procedures had been done on these patients. In 4 patients sinuses drained continuously—in one patient for 50 years.

Of the 9 patients operated on, 2 died before the ankylosis could be expected to occur. Five of the remaining 7 achieved a solid fusion, and 1 other operated on 3 months earlier appeared to have roentgenographic evidence of union. In the other patient the operation was a failure; this patient had multiple sinuses before the operation and 1 sinus still persisted after the operation.

Four of the 5 in whom ankylosis was attained

Fig. 18–39. **A.** Cut made from roentgenograms of a normal hip showing the amount of shortness of the limb after removal of the head and neck and placement of the trochanter in the acetabulum. **B.** Amount of shortening after a subtrochanteric osteotomy was performed. (From Abbott LC, Lucas DB: Arthrodesis of the hip in wide abduction. J Bone Joint Surg, 36:1136, 1954.)

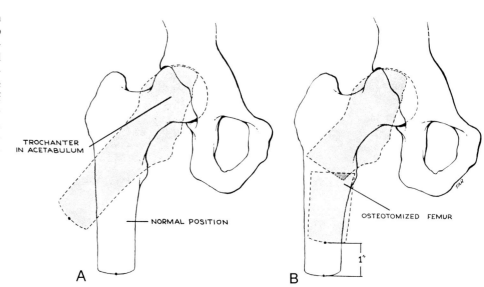

were fully rehabilitated as far as weight-bearing was concerned. These patients achieved full weight-bearing in 4 to 12 months.

Technique

The first stage of the operation is only done when there are draining sinuses. The purpose of the operation is to thoroughly debride the diseased trochanteric portion of the femur, remnants of the femoral neck, and other infected granulomatous tissue. Approach the area through a lateral thigh incision and, just above the level of the tuberosity, perform an oblique osteotomy of the femur; the pointed end of the distal fragment points upward and inward. Next, by sharp periosteal dissection, remove the trochanteric mass, fibrous tissue, and granulomatous tissue to the level of the acetabulum and lateral surface of the ilium. (Bosworth left the wound open and treated it by the Orr method, carbolizing the tissues at each dressing).

The femoroischial transplant, the second stage of the operation, can be done without the first stage if no sinuses are present and may be done in the other patients when healing has followed the first stage.

Use a lateral thigh incision, extending it from the level of the trochanter to well down on the femur.

Divide the fascia lata and vastus lateralis in the line of the skin incision exposing the femoral shaft. Expose the shaft of the femur by subperiosteal dissection as far as just above the level of the tuberosity of the ischium. At this point divide the femoral shaft in an oblique manner upward and inward making a pointed end of the distal shaft pointing upward and inward. Now retract the distal end of the femur and by blunt dissection expose the distal and lateral surfaces of the tuberosity of the ischium. This part can be done by visualizing the ischium by retraction of the soft tissues and the femur or it can be done blindly. Next, gouge out of the surface of the ischium, using a sharp, large curette, creating a hole large enough to accommodate the end of the femur. (To some degree the leg length can be increased by cutting the shaft of the femur long. Furthermore cutting the bone long increases the compressive forces at the site of contact between the femur and the ischium.)

Place a large bone skid in the hole in the ischium, flex the thigh 90° and lever the end of the femur into the hole. Lower the limb to 150° making marked compression at the contact area by increasing the tension of the fasciae and muscles of the thigh. Now the end of the femur is also covered by a cuff of ischial periosteum and fibrous tissue as it enters the defect in the ischium. Place the limb in

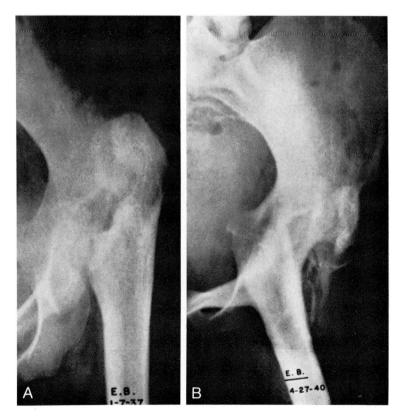

Fɪɢ. **18–40. A.** A 21-year-old patient with a tubercular hip of sixteen years duration. **B.** Femoroischial transplantation in same patient, in one stage. It was solid after 8 months, permitting weight-bearing. (From Bosworth DM: Femoroischial transplantation. J Bone Joint Surg, 24:40, 1942.)

the desired position and after closure of the wound apply a double hip spica. After several weeks free the sound limb without changing the cast, which is worn for at least 3 months. Roentgenographic evidence of bony union determines when the patient is taken out of plaster and weight-bearing started (Fig. 18–40).

References

1. ABBOTT LC, FISCHER FJ: Arthrodesis of the hip, with special reference to the method of securing ankylosis in massive destruction of joint. Surg Gynecol Obstet, 52:863, 1931.
2. ABBOTT LC, LUCAS DB: Arthrodesis of the hip in wide abduction. J Bone Joint Surg, 36A:1129, 1954.
3. ALBEE FH: Arthritis deformans of the hip: a preliminary report of a new operation. JAMA, 1:1977, 1908.
4. ALHBACK S, LINDAHL O: Hip arthrodesis: the connection between function and position. Acta Orthop Scand, 37:77, 1966.
5. ALTCHEK M: Arthrodesis of the hip by central dislocation and ilio-femoral nailing. J Bone Joint Surg, 47B:694, 1965.
6. ALVIK I: Arthrodesis of the hip: a method allowing weight-bearing and walking postoperatively. Acta Orthop Scand, 32:451, 1962.
7. ALVIK I: Arthrodesis and arthroplasty of the hip joint. Acta Orthop Scand, 33:253, 1963.
8. AMSTUTZ HC, SAKAI DN: Total joint replacement for ankylosed hips. J Bone Joint Surg, 57A:619, 1975.
9. AMSTUTZ HC, MA SM, JINNAH RH, MAI L: Revision of aseptic loose total hip arthroplasties. Clin Orthop, 170:21–33, 1982.
10. BADGLEY C: Personal communication, 1947.
11. BARMADA R, ABRAHAM E, RAY RD: Hip fusion utilizing the cobra plate. J Bone Joint Surg, 58A:541, 1976.
12. BECKENBAUGH RD, ILSTRUP DM: Total hip arthroplasty: a review of three hundred and thirty-three cases. J Bone Joint Surg, 60A:306, 1978.
13. BOSWORTH DM: Femoro-ischial transplantation. J Bone Joint Surg, 24:38, 1942.
14. BREWSTER RC, COVENTRY MB, JOHNSON EW JR: Conversion of the arthrodesed hip to a total hip arthroplasty. J Bone Joint Surg, 57A:27, 1975.
15. BRITTAIN HA: Ischio-femoral arthrodesis. J Bone Joint Surg, 30B:642, 1948.
16. BUCKHOLZ HW, GARTMANN HD: Infektion-sprophylaxa und operative behandlund der schleichenden tiefen infektion der totalen endoprothese. Chirurg, 43:446, 1972.
17. BURNS BH: Fixation of the osteo-arthritic hip. Guy's Hosp Rep, 103:13, 1954.
18. CARNESALE PG: Arthrodesis of the hip: a long-term study. Orthop Digest, pp. 12–14, Oct. 1976.
19. CARTER PJ, WICKSTROM J: Arthrodesis of the hip: an assessment of results in one hundred patients. South Med J, 64:451, 1971.
20. CHAN KP, SHIN JS: Brittain ischio-femoral arthrodesis for tuberculosis of the hip: an analysis of seventy-six cases. J Bone Joint Surg, 50-A:1341, 1968.
21. CHANDLER FA: Hip-fusion operation. J Bone Joint Surg, 15:947, 1933.
22. CHANDLER HP, SCHMIDT EW, AUFRANC OE: Vitallium-mold arthroplasty in patients under the age of twenty-one. In Proceedings of the American Orthopaedic Association. J Bone Joint Surg, 50A:1496–1497, 1968.
23. CHANDLER HP, REINECK FT, WIXSON RL, McCARTHY JC: Total hip replacement in patients younger than thirty years old: a five-year follow-up study. J Bone Joint Surg, 63B:1426–1434, 1981.
24. CHAPPELL GE JR: Current trends in the treatment of the young adult with disabling hip disease. Clin Orthop 106:35, 1975.
25. CHARNLEY J: Stabilisation of the hip by central dislocation. In Proceedings of the British Orthopaedic Association, May, 1955, (abstract). J Bone Joint Surg, 37B:514, 1955.
26. CHARNLEY J: Compression arthrodesis. Edinburgh, England, Livingstone, 1953.
27. CHOLMELEY JA: Femoral osteotomy in extra-articular arthrodesis of the tuberculous hip. J Bone Joint Surg, 33B:342, 1956.
28. CHOLMELEY JA, NANGLE EJ: Ischiofemoral arthrodesis by the posterior approach. J Bone Joint Surg, 33B:365, 1951.
29. COCKIN J: Osteotomy of the hip. Orthop Clin North Am, 2:75, 1971.
30. COLLIS DK: Cemented total hip replacement in patients who are less than fifty years old. J Bone Joint Surg, 66A:353–359, 1984.
31. COMPERE EL, THOMPSON RG: Arthrodesis of the hip in children. Q Bull Northwestern Univ Med School, 29:335, 1955.
32. CREGAN JC: Cerntral dislocation stabilization of the hip: a review of 140 cases. Clin Orthop, 55:165, 1967.
33. CRENSHAW AH: Muscle pedicle bone graft in arthrodesis of the hip. South Med J, 50:169, 1957.
34. DAVIS JB: The muscle pedicle bone graft in hip fusion. J Bone Joint Surg, 36A:790, 1954.
35. DEPALMA AF, FENLIN JM JR: Arthrodesis of the hip with intramedullary fixation. Clin Orthop, 48:191, 1966.
36. DOBSON J: Ischio-femoral arthrodesis for tuberculous arthritis in children. J Bone Joint Surg, 34B:525, 1952.
37. DOBSON J: Arthrodesis in tuberculosis of the hip joint: an analysis of fifty cases. J Bone Joint Surg, 30B:95–105, 1948.
38. EFTEKHAR NS: Indications and contra-indications for total hip replacement. In Eftekhar NS (ed): Principles of Total Hip Arthroplasty. St. Louis, Mosby, p. 223, 1978.
39. EFTEKHAR NS, STINCHFIELD FE: Experience with low friction arthroplasty. Clin Orthop, 95:60, 1973.
40. EVARTS CM, KENDRICK JI: Cup arthroplasty. Orthop Clin North Am, 2:93, 1971.
41. EWALD BA, LUCAS DB, RALSTON HJ: Effect of immobilization of the hip on energy expenditure during level walking. Technical Report No. 44, Biomechanics Laboratory, University of California, San Francisco and Berkeley, 1961.
42. FREIBERG JA: Experiences with the Brittain ischio-femoral arthrodesis. J Bone Joint Surg, 28:501, 1946.
43. FREMONT-SMITH P: Antibiotic management of septic total hip replacement: A therapeutic trial. In Harris WH (ed): The Hip: Proceedings of the Second Open Scientific Meeting of the Hip Society. St. Louis, Mosby, 1974.
44. FRYMOYER JW, ET AL.: Epidemiologic studies of low back pain. Spine 5:419, 1980.
45. FULKERSON JP: Arthrodesis for disabling hip pain in children and adolescents. Clin Orthop, 128:296–302, 1977.
46. GARDINER TB: Nail and graft arthrodesis of the hip. J Bone Joint Surg, 44B:588, 1962.
47. GHORMLEY RK: Use of the anterior superior spine and crest of ilium in surgery of the hip joint. J Bone Joint Surg, 13:784, 1931.

48. Gore DR, Murray MP, Sepic SB, Gardiner GM: Walking patterns of men with unilateral surgical hip fusion. J Bone Joint Surg, 57A:759, 1975.

49. Hahn D: Ischio-femoral arthrodesis for tuberculosis of the hip. J Bone Joint Surg, 45B:477, 1963.

50. Hardinge K, Williams D, Etienne A, MacKenzie D, Charnley, J: Conversion of fused hips to low friction arthroplasty. J Bone Joint Surg, 59B:385–392, 1977.

51. Harris WH, McCarthy JC Jr, O'Neill DA: Femoral component loosening using contemporary techniques of femoral cement fixation. J Bone Joint Surg, 64A:1063–1067, 1982.

52. Harris WH, White RE: Resection arthroplasty for nonseptic failure of total hip replacement. Clin Orthop, 176:7, 1983.

53. Head WC: Wagner surface replacement of the hip. J Bone Joint Surg, 63A:420, 1981.

54. Henderson MS: Combined intra-articular and extra-articular arthrodesis for tuberculosis of the hip joint. J Bone Joint Surg, 15:51, 1933.

55. Heusner T: Uber Huftresektion wegen angeborenen Luxation. Arch Klin Chir, 31:666, 1885.

56. Hibbs RA: A preliminary report of twenty cases of hip joint tuberculosis treated by an operation devised to eliminate motion by fusing the joint. J Bone Joint Surg, 8:522, 1926.

57. Hunter G, Welsh R, Cameron H, Bailey W: The results of revision total hip arthroplasty. J Bone Joint Surg, 61B:419, 1979.

58. Jolley MN, Salvati EA, Browb GC: Early results and complications of surface replacement of the hip. J Bone Joint Surg, 64A:366–377, 1982.

59. Kettelkamp DB, Thompson C: Development of a knee scoring scale. Clin Orthop, 107:93, 1975.

60. Kidner FC: End-results of extra-articular fixation of the tuberculous hip in children. JAMA, 91:1865, 1928.

61. King D: Arthrodesis of the adult nontuberculous hip. Stanford Med Bull, 13:381, 1955.

62. Kirkaldy-Willis WH: Ischio-femoral arthrodesis of the hip in tuberculosis: an anterior approach. J Bone Joint Surg, 32B:187, 1950.

63. Kirkaldy-Willis WH, Chaudhri MR, Anderson RJD: Arthrodesis of the hip with staple fixation. J Bone Joint Surg, 40A:114, 1958.

64. Kirkaldy-Willis WH, Mbuthia AS: Abduction arthrodesis of the hip. J Bone Joint Surg, 34B:433, 1952.

65. Lam SJ: Arthrodesis of the hip with special splintage. J Bone Joint Surg, 50B:14, 1968.

66. Lang AG: Cup arthroplasty in children and adolescents. In Proceedings of The American Academy of Orthopaedic Surgeons. J Bone Joint Surg, 57A:1023, 1975.

67. Lang AG, Klassen RA: Cup arthroplasties in teenagers and children. J Bone Joint Surg, 59A:444–450, 1977.

68. Lange M: Arthrodesis of the hip: review of a series of more than five hundred cases. J Inter Coll Surg, 29:638–643, 1958.

69. Liechti R: Hip arthrodesis and associated problems. Berlin, Springer, 1974.

70. Lindahl O: Functional capacity after hip arthrodesis. Acta Orthop Scand, 36:453, 1965.

71. Lindahl O: Determination of hip adduction, especially in arthrodesis. Acta Orthop Scand, 36:280–293, 1965.

72. Lipscomb PR, McCashin FE Jr: Arthrodesis of the hip, review of 371 cases. J Bone Joint Surg, 43A:923, 1961.

73. Lubahn JD, Evarts C McC, Feltner JB: Conversion of ankylosed hips to total hip arthroplasty. Clin Orthop, 153:146–152, 1980.

74. Mayer L: Critique of Brittain operation for fusion of the hip. Bull Hosp Joint Dis, 9:4, 1948.

75. McBeath MD: Hip arthrodesis in young patients: a long-term follow-up study. Presented at the annual meeting of The American Academy of Orthopaedic Surgeons, Anaheim, March, 1983.

76. Morris JB: Charnley compression arthrodesis of the hip. J Bone Joint Surg, 48B:260, 1966.

77. Muller ME, Allgower M, Willenegger H: Manual of internal fixation: Technique recommended by the A-O group. New York, Springer-Verlag, 1970.

78. Pease CN: Fusion of the hip in children: the Chandler method. J Bone Joint Surg, 29:874, 1947.

79. Petty W, Goldsmith S: Resection arthroplasty following infected total hip arthroplasty. J Bone Joint Surg, 62A:889–896, 1980.

80. Piggott J: Charnley stabilization of the hip. J Bone Joint Surg, 42B:476, 1960.

81. Ranawat CS, Jordan LR, Wilson PD Jr: A technique of muscle-pedicle bone graft in hip arthrodesis: a report of its use in ten cases. J Bone Joint Surg, 53A:925–934, 1971.

82. Ranawat CS, Atkinson RE, Salvati EA, Wilson PD Jr: Conventional total hip arthroplasty for degenerative joint disease in patients between the ages of forty and sixty years. J Bone Joint Surg, 66A:745–751, 1984.

83. Root Leon: Hip deformity in cerebral palsy. In Management of Hip Disorders in Children, Edited by JF Katz and RS Siffert. Philadelphia, Lippincott, pp. 183–194, 1983.

84. Salvati EA, Im FC, Aglietti P, Wilson PD Jr: Radiology of total hip replacement. Clin Orthop, 121:74–82, 1976.

85. Schneider R: Hip arthrodesis with the cobra head plate and pelvic osteotomy. Reconst Surg Traumatol, 14:1, 1974.

86. Sharp N, Guhl J, Sorenson RI, Voshell AF: Hip fusion in poliomyelitis in children: a preliminary report. J Bone Joint Surg, 46A:121, 1964.

87. Sponseller PD, McBeath AA, Perpich M: Hip arthrodesis in young patients: a long-term follow-up study. J Bone Joint Surg, 66A:853–859, 1984.

88. Stamm TT: In Brown A: Arthrodesis of the hip. Guy's Hosp Rep, 103:13, 1954.

89. Stewart MJ, Coker TP Jr: Arthrodesis of the hip: a review of 109 patients. Clin Orthop, 62:136, 1969.

90. Stinchfield FE, Cavallero WU: Arthrodesis of the hip joint: a follow-up study. J Bone Joint Surg, 32A:48–58, 1950.

91. Stratford B: The Trumble graft: a review of thirty-six cases. J Bone Joint Surg, 35B:247, 1953.

92. Sutherland CJ, Wilde AH, Borden LS, Marks KE: A ten-year follow-up of one hundred conservative Muller curved-stem total hip replacement arthroplasties. J Bone Joint Surg, 64A:970, 1982.

93. Taitz II: Arthrodesis of a prosthetic hip joint. J Bone Joint Surg, 43A:555, 1961.

94. Thompson FR: Combined hip fusion and subtrochanteric osteotomy allowing early ambulation. J Bone Joint Surg, 38A:13–21, 1956.

95. Trumble HC: A method of fixation of the hip-joint by means of an extra-articular bone graft. Aust NZ J Surg, 1:413, 1932.

96. Trumble HA: Fixation of the hip-joint by means of an extra-articular bone graft: late results. Br J Surg, 24:728, 1937.

97. Van Gorder GW: The Trumble operation for fusion of the hip. J Bone Joint Surg, 31A:717, 1949.

98. Vesely DG: Ischio-femoral arthrodesis: an end-result study of forty-four cases. J Bone Joint Surg, 43A:363, 1961.

99. WATSON-JONES R: Arthrodesis of the osteoarthritic hip. JAMA, 110:278, 1938.

100. WATSON-JONES R, ROBINSON WC: Arthrodesis of the osteoarthritic hip joint. J Bone Joint Surg, 38B:353, 1956.

101. WELCH R: Conversion of hip arthrodesis to a total hip replacement. Presented at the American Orthopaedic Association International Symposium on Frontiers in Total Hip Replacement, Boston, May, 1981.

102. WHITE JW: Smith-Petersen nail fixation in hip surgery. *In* American Academy of Orthopaedic Surgeons: Instructional Course Lectures, Edwards, Vol. 1, Ann Arbor, 1943.

103. WILSON JC: Operative fixation of tuberculous hips in children: end-result study of thirty-three patients from the orthopaedic department of the Children's Hospital. J Bone Joint Surg, 15:22, 1933.

104. WILSON PD: Total hip replacement in management of infected hips. *In* Harris WH (ed): Proceedings of the Second Open Scientific Meeting of the Hip Society. St. Louis, Mosby, pp. 313–318, 1974.

105. WILSON PD, AGLIETTI P, SALVATI EA: Subacute sepsis of the hip treated by antibiotics and cemented prosthesis. J Bone Joint Surg, 56A:879, 1974.

106. WILTSE LL, THOMPSON WAL: Technic for arthrodesis of the hip when the femoral head and neck are absent. Arch Surg, 59:888, 1949.

107. YU HI: Tuberculosis of the hip: a follow-up study of 58 cases with special reference to fusion results in young children. J Bone Joint Surg, 33A:131, 1951.

CHAPTER NINETEEN

Cup Arthroplasty

WILLIAM G. STEWART

Introduction

The cup arthroplasty continues to occupy a place in the spectrum of hip reconstruction. The indications for the use of this procedure have become specific. They include the relief of pain, the correction of deformity, the restoration of motion and the creation of stability. The general aims of this procedure are like those of any hip replacement.

History

Historically, the Vitallium mold arthroplasty represents the basic work of Dr. M.N. Smith-Petersen[17] and the careful observations and developmental changes of the design of the mold, the surgical technique, and the postoperative care of Dr. Otto E. Aufranc. The first glass mold was inserted in 1925. The shape and cup material evolved through the years. Finally, Vitallium was chosen as an inert material and the shape of a hemisphere was chosen as the preferred configuration.[9]

Principle

The principle of the cup arthroplasty involves the interposition of a movable surface prosthesis between two healing bony surfaces. The surfaces of both the femoral head and of the acetabulum are reamed to bleeding cancellous bone (Fig. 19–1). The movable surface prosthesis, the cup, molds the reparative healing process of the bony surfaces from a clot through fibrous reparative tissue into smooth fibrocartilage. In some instances, this final repair appears to be hyaline cartilage (Fig. 19–2). The surface area on both sides of the cup provides a large distribution of pressure as the cup moves within the acetabulum and the head moves within the cup. The cup is made stable by the bony position established at surgery.

Indications

The broad indications for this procedure include those indications for any type of hip reconstruction. The specific indications for a cup arthroplasty, however, are the reason that the procedure maintains its place in the reconstructive spectrum. These are: (1) patient age, (2) bone stock, (3) muscle strength and coordination, and (4) patient cooperation. The ideal candidate is a 25-year-old intelligent patient with a 2-year history of traumatic arthritis secondary to an athletic injury that involves the acetabulum. This patient exemplifies all 4 specific criteria for this operation.

The longevity of a reconstructed hip using either press fit or porous coated components as well as cemented components in the young adult is a concern.[6,8] Aseptic loosening of both the femoral and acetabular components has been well documented by many authors with the use of acrylic cement.[1,12,14] Long-term complications of biologic fixations have not yet been ascertained. Thus, if other conditions are favorable, we would favor the cup arthroplasty for the patient in the age group from 18 to 40. Excellent 20 and 30 year followup reports are available for these patients.[9]

The condition of the bone that makes up the acetabulum and the femoral head is another important, specific consideration for this procedure. The principles of reconstruction of the bony socket are as applicable in cup surgery as they are in total joint replacement. The socket should be located in the normal anatomic position at the confluence of the triradiate cartilage. This is most important in the patient with a complete dislocation of the hip. Bony coverage over the superior aspect of the cup in the deficient acetabulum can be constructed with either homologous bone graft from the patient's ilium or allograft, usually in the form of a femoral head from the bone bank (Fig. 19–3).[10,18]

In cases such as in an Otto pelvis or in a post-

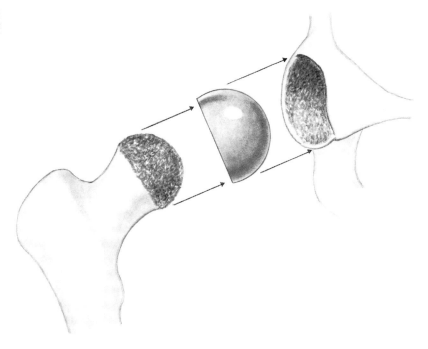

Fɪɢ. **19−1.** The vitallium cup is interposed between the bleeding cancellous surface of the femoral head and acetabulum.

traumatic situation with medial pelvic wall deficiency, a protrusio acetabulum can be grafted with a composite graft (usually from an allograft source) or with morselized bone obtained either from the patient or from an allograft. A large mold that bears its weight on the circumference of the reconstructed socket rather than at the apex of the dome should be used (Fig. 19−4). Incorporation of the graft prevents protrusion of the cup and creates long-term stability. Fibrocartilage between the graft and the cup is formed by motion of the cup as in a primary cup arthroplasty.

One of the major shortcomings of the use of the cup arthroplasty occurs when there is a deficiency in the bone of the femoral head. At the present time, aseptic necrosis, from whatever cause, is a contraindication to this procedure. Removal of all

nonviable bone would necessitate the use of a so-called shaft arthroplasty. Shortening of the involved leg, instability, inconsistent relief of pain, and lack of motion are often complications when a shaft arthroplasty is performed. In spite of the anecdotal exceptions that support the use of a shaft arthroplasty, an alternative procedure should be used when there is a problem with viability of the bone of the femoral head.

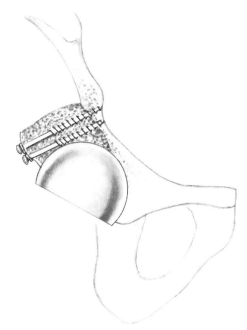

Fɪɢ. **19−3.** Reconstruction of superior aspect of acetabulum using allograft (femoral head).

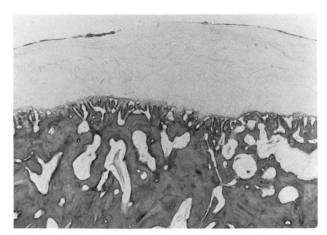

Fɪɢ. **19−2.** Layer of fibrocartilage overlying cancellous bone.

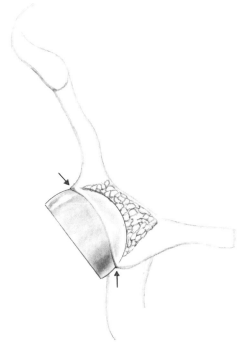

Fɪɢ. **19–4.** Large cup bears weight on the circumference of the socket. Depth of acetabulum is filled with morselized allograft.

Muscle strength and patient cooperation are two specific indications for a mold arthroplasty that have been grouped together. As has been noted previously, the motion of the cup influences the healing process and maturation of scar tissue to fibrocartilage on both sides of the prosthesis. Thus, motion of the hip, and consequently of the cup, has not only a desirable long-term result but also a short-term necessity for completion of the healing process. An uncooperative patient who does not ex-

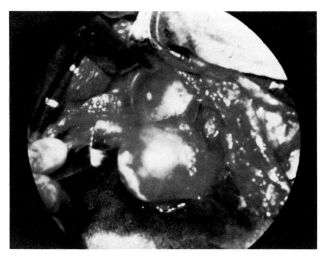

Fɪɢ. **19–5.** Areas of sclerotic bone are seen over the weight-bearing surface of both femoral head and acetabulum. The cup was revised because of pain.

ercise or who does not protect his hip from early weight-bearing may cause compromise in the maturation of the fibrocartilage. This may result in a corn-like formation of sclerotic bone at the weight-bearing surface of either the femoral head or of the acetabulum (Fig. 19–5).[9]

A cup arthroplasty is demanding in its long-term rehabilitation in terms of muscle strength. Stability of the joint as well as range of motion depend on development of muscle strength. This rehabilitation continues intensively for a period of 18 months to 2 years. The patient is urged to exercise his reconstructed joint regularly the remainder of his life. His cooperation is necessary in order to subscribe to this vigorous and lengthy rehabilitation program. The poor success rate in the teenage group underlines this requirement of continued co-operation.[7,13]

Technique

The anterior approach to the hip joint was described by Dr. Smith-Petersen.[16] He advocated this approach when performing a cup arthroplasty. However, over the past two decades, the advantages of the lateral approach to the hip, which involves removal of the greater trochanter, have been described.[16] This approach gives excellent visualization of the acetabulum over its complete circumference. Soft tissue release, debridement of the scar, and a total capsulectomy are easily performed. With this wide three-dimensional exposure, the creation of bony stability is possible. Also, the acetabulum can be reamed to bleeding cancellous bone without destruction of the surrounding muscle.

Additional soft tissue stability is gained by transfer of tendon groups. By advancing the trochanter, the femoral head is directed into the acetabulum. Furthermore, increased strength in abduction thus gained lends stability in gait by reducing the amount of pelvic drop. This reduces muscle fatigue as well as consequent pain.

Transfer of the iliopsoas tendon anteriorly to be a remnant of the anterior hip capsule serves as a "sling" and prevents anterior dislocation (Fig. 19–6). This transfer also reduces the common flexion deformity of the involved hip as well as increasing flexion strength. The lateral approach provides good visualization to allow the psoas transfer.

Femoral head preparation involves removal of all cortical bone. The head is first shaped with a hip gouge and placed in a more valgus attitude (Fig. 19–7). This will prevent the cup from assuming a

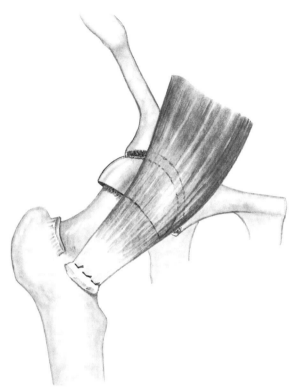

FIG. 19–6. The insertion of the iliopsoas tendon is moved from the lesser trochanter to an anterior position on the femoral neck.

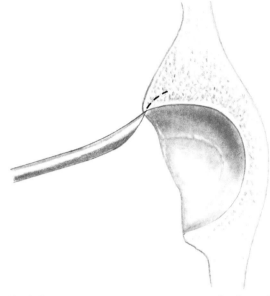

FIG. 19–8. Reverse gouge creates a "containing" lip that will stabilize the cup.

varus position in the postoperative period. The head is then reamed with either hand or power reamers to obtain a bleeding surface.

The preparation of the acetabulum involves creation of bony stability by providing a dome that will accept and retain a cup. When there is a relative lack of acetabular bone stock, a "containing" lip to the reconstructed socket can be most effec-

tively constructed by using the various available hip gouges, i.e., reverse gouge, hip gouge, and acetabular hand gouge (Figs. 19–8, 19–9). The acetabulum is then reamed to provide concentricity as well as to match the size to which the femoral head was reamed. On occasion, a bone graft is necessary to assure lateral stability. In an unstable situation, the leg may be maintained in significant abduction in balanced suspension for a 3 to 4 week period as a pseudocapsule of scar tissue is formed.

It has become apparent that the medial wall of

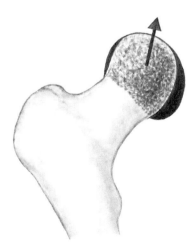

FIG. 19–7. The medial aspect of the femoral head is removed, creating a more valgus attitude than "normal."

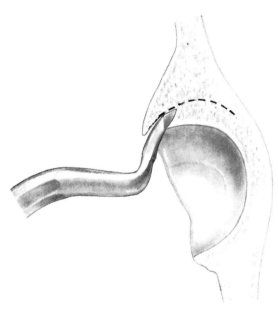

FIG. 19–9. A hip gouge fashions a concentric socket.

the pelvis should not be violated in constructing the acetabulum for a cup arthroplasty. Although the mold itself does not tend to protrude medially in a properly constructed cup arthroplasty, preservation of the medial wall is most necessary if revision to a total hip arthroplasty should become necessary. Thus the lateral graft as previously described should be performed when inadequate bone stock is present to contain the cup.

Postoperative Regimen

The stability of the cup arthroplasty with regard to dislocation is of primary concern during the immediate postoperative period. Prior to wound closure, the hip should be moved through a complete range of motion and the stability of both the cup in the acetabulum and the head in the cup should be visually noted at all extremes of motion. An unstable position can thus be avoided postoperatively. An attitude of flexion and adduction of the leg is the most common position of instability. When this is seen at surgery, the operated leg is maintained in balanced suspension in wide abduction, neutral rotation, and minimal flexion. It is gradually returned to the neutral abduction-adduction position over a 3-week period, which promotes the formation of stability via soft tissue healing. A stable hip is also maintained in balanced suspension for a period of 3 weeks. During this time intensive exercises in all ranges of motion are essential. The passive motion machine has been used on a regular basis beginning on the second or third postoperative day. These exercises mold the reparative tissue response of the bleeding cancellous bone from a clot to stable fibrocartilage.

It is emphasized to the patient that a large percentage of the success of the reconstruction depends on the patient's willingness to participate in the postoperative exercise regimen. This includes a period of 6 months of protected weight-bearing (50%) using axillary crutches. The gradually increasing vigor of the exercise program is aimed at increasing the range of motion and strength of the hip. The patient is routinely started on a stationary bicycle prior to discharge from the hospital. Specific exercises to increase strength are prescribed on an individual basis when the patient is seen in the office for a followup examination. A cane is prescribed after 6 months of crutches. The cane is used until the patient's strength has progressed to a point of no limp in the patient's gait.

Complications

Early complications of the cup arthroplasty include those occurring in the operating room and in the immediate postoperative period. Femoral neck fractures, fractures of the posterior lip of the acetabulum, hemorrhage, and nerve lacerations have been observed during the operation. Other problems that are seen both early and late in this treatment are seen with various other major operations. They include deep and superficial vein thrombosis, myocardial complications, urinary tract infections, hemorrhage, and infection.

Specific early complications involving the patient with a cup arthroplasty are dislocations, nonunion of the trochanter, and heterotopic bone formation. If the patient's operated leg is maintained in wide abduction immediately postoperatively and then is gradually moved to a neutral position over a 3-week period, the incidence of dislocation is reduced to a minimum. A pattern of dislocation of the cup from the acetabulum is more common than the bony head from the cup. If this complication should occur, it can usually be treated by closed reduction and spica cast immobilization for a period of 6 weeks.

Trochanteric osteotomy is recommended to improve the operative exposure, to more appropriately adjust the tension of the abductor muscles, and to lengthen the lever arm by lateral reattachment. Because the hip is protected in balanced suspension and abduction for a longer period of time, trochanteric nonunion is less of a problem in the cup arthroplasty than in total hip replacement. Furthermore, the interposition of cement between trochanter and lateral femoral shaft is not a problem. An upward displacement of the trochanter of less than 3 cm has not been symptomatic. With a vigorous exercise program, the patient usually can eliminate a positive Trendelenburg gait. Further displacement should be repaired surgically. Three weeks of immobilization of the limb in abduction is necessary postoperatively for a displaced trochanter.

The development of heterotopic bone can compromise the long-term result in a patient with a cup arthroplasty. In the age group described, prophylactic radiation even at a dosage of 1000 rads may be inadvisable. The use of Indomethacin in appropriate dosages has been successful in limiting heterotopic ossification in many patients.[5,15]

Late complications of this procedure include soft tissue contractures, aseptic necrosis of the femoral head within the cup, and so-called "corn formation." Patient cooperation in diligent adherence to the postoperative exercise program is most important in avoiding soft tissue contractures. Specific exercises aimed at stretching an early contracture, such as a hip flexion contracture, should be prescribed when the patient is seen during followup office visits. Nonparticipation in the exercise program is often the reason for the poor results of the cup arthroplasty in patients in the early teenage years.[7,13] Obviously, the development of strength around the hip, which eliminates a limp and muscular discomfort, is an important contribution of the postoperative exercise regimen.

Aseptic necrosis of the bone of the femoral head is a complication peculiar to the cup arthroplasty. Preservation of bone is one of the major goals of this procedure. At surgery, the head is shaped with osteotomes and then reamed with either hand or power reamers to a bleeding cancellous surface. It is important to see this bleeding before placing the cup over the head (Fig. 19–10). Protecting the surface with bed rest and exercises followed by partial weight-bearing promotes this revascularization process.

A "corn" under the cup represents a breakdown of the normal healing process. This process has been previously described as proceeding from clot formation, through fibrous reparative tissue to fibrocartilage. A localized area of pressure on either side of the cup involving either the femoral head or the acetabulum may produce an area of sclerotic bone (Fig. 19–11). This phenomenon, or so-called "corn" formation, may cause pain in the reconstructed hip. A revision of the cup may be necessary to diagnose definitely this problem and to remedy it.

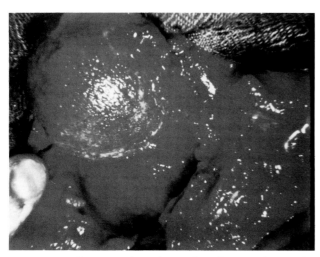

Fig. 19–10. Bleeding surface of cancellous bone is obtained by reaming the femoral head.

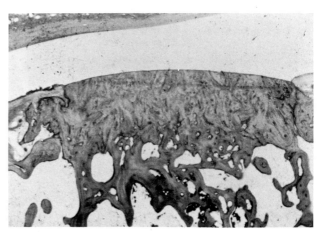

Fig. 19–11. Slide of area of corn formation presenting sclerotic bone rather than fibrocartilage at the surface.

Summary

In our series of 87 cup arthroplasties performed between 1978 and 1983, there were 18 that met the specific indications previously noted. Those indications include the patient's age group between 18 and 40 years, acceptable bone stock on both the acetabular and the femoral sides of the joint, good muscle strength and coordination, and finally good patient cooperation. Using the Harris hip rating scale of those with a 5 year followup, 93% had good to excellent results. One revision was performed elsewhere for reasons unknown.

Of the total 87 cup arthroplasties performed, results were good to excellent in 78%. Seven revisions were performed for reasons primarily involving pain or limitation of motion. Three patients were lost to followup.

Experience indicates that a mold arthroplasty that is properly performed and is properly managed in the convalescent period and is pain free with good motion for 24 months will continue to improve and give the patient a lifetime of serviceable function. This opinion is well documented in the many followup reports of Dr. Otto Aufranc.[2-4] In order to treat this small but important segment of our population with compromised hip function, the cup arthroplasty should be included in the armamentarium of the hip surgeon.

References

1. AMSTUTZ HC, MARKOLF KL, McNEICE GM, GRUEN TA: Loosening of total hip components: cause and prevention. *In* Hip Proceedings of the Fourth Open Scientific Meeting of the Hip Society. St. Louis, Mosby, pp. 102-116, 1976.
2. AUFRANC OE: Constructive hip surgery with mold arthro-

plasty. *In* American Academy of Orthopedic Surgeons: Instructional Course Lectures, Vol. 11. Ann Arbor, Edwards, 1954.

3. AUFRANC OE: Constructive hip surgery with the vitallium mold: a report on 1000 cases of arthroplasty of the hip over a fifteen-year period. J Bone Joint Surg, 39A:237-248, 1957.

4. AUFRANC OE, SWEET EB: Study of patient with hip arthroplasty at Massachusetts General Hospital. JAMA, 170:507-515. 1959.

5. AYERS DC, MCCOLLISTER E, PARKMAN JR: The prevention of heterotopic ossification in high-risk patients by low-dose radiation therapy after total hip arthroplasty. J Bone Joint Surg, 68A:1423-1430, 1986.

6. CHANDLER HP, REINECK FT, WIXSON RL, MCCARTHY JC: Total hip replacement in patients younger than thirty years old: a five-year follow-up study. J Bone Joint Surg, 63A:1426–1434, 1981.

7. CHANDLER HP, SCHMIDT EW, AUFRANC OE: Vitallium-mold arthroplasty in patients under the age of twenty-one. *In* Proceedings of the American Orthopedic Association. J Bone Joint Surg, 50A:1496–1497, 1968.

8. COLLES DK: Cemented total hip replacements in patients who are less than fifty years old. J Bone Joint Surg, 66A:353–359, 1984.

9. AUFRANE OE: Constructive Surgery of the Hip: St. Louis, Mosby, 1962.

10. HARRIS WH, CROTHERS O, OH I: Total hip replacement and femoral head bone grafting for severe acetabular deficiency in adults. J Bone Joint Surg, 59A:752–759, 1977.

11. HARRIS WH: A new lateral approach to the hip joint. J Bone Joint Surg, 49A:891, 1967.

12. IANNOTTI JP, et al.: Aseptic loosening after total hip arthroplasty. J Arthroplasty, 1:99-107, 1986.

13. LONG AG, KLASSEN RA: Cup arthroplasty in teenagers and children. J Bone Joint Surg, 59A:444-450, 1977.

14. PELLICI PM, SALVIETI EA, ROBINSON HJ: Mechanical failure in total hip replacement requiring reoperation. J Bone Joint Surg, 61A:28–36, 1979.

15. RITTER MA, SIEBER JM: Prophylactic Indomethacin for the prevention of heterotopic bone formation following total hip arthroplasty. Clin Orthop, 196:217-225, 1985.

16. SMITH-PETERSEN MN: Approach to and exposure of the hip joint for mold arthroplasty. J Bone Joint Surg, 21A:40, 1949.

17. SMITH-PETERSEN MN: Arthroplasty of the hip: a new method. J Bone Joint Surg, 21:269, 1939.

18. WOOLSON ST, HARRIS WH: Complex total hip replacement for dysplastic or hypoplastic hips using minature or microminature components. 65A:1099-1108, 1983.

CHAPTER TWENTY

Biopsy of Tumors About the Hip

RICHARD LACKMAN

Techniques for the biopsy of musculoskeletal lesions have become more demanding as surgical treatment options for tumors have become more sophisticated. Limb salvage surgery for extremity tumors is now commonplace but leaves little room for error in incision placement. Recent data showing the ill effects of poorly done biopsies[1] combined with the present legal atmosphere in regard to potential malpractice have provided a great impetus for surgeons to refer potential tumors to the treating surgeon for biopsy. Not every lesion can be biopsied at a tertiary center, however. It is mandatory then that all practicing surgeons have an appreciation for the basic tenets of biopsy technique.

Several options exist in regard to type of biopsy. These include open biopsy, fluoroscopic trocar biopsy, and CT scan or ultrasound-directed skinny needle biopsy. Trocar and needle biopsies are mainly advocated in those areas where the lesion is surgically inaccessible or where the disease is likely to be straightforward. CT scan or ultrasound-directed skinny needle biopsy is the least traumatic form of biopsy and is effective in many cases. Metastatic lesions about the acetabulum are especially well suited to this technique.

When the index of suspicion is high that a musculoskeletal lesion may represent a primary tumor, however, limited biopsy techniques then suffer from potentially inadequate and misleading tissue sampling. In most of these cases, a small, well planned open biopsy is probably more effective in providing a correct tissue diagnosis. Open biopsy does have the disadvantage, though, of increased tissue contamination and the restrictions that the biopsy incision places on a subsequent resection incision.

The basic tenets of open biopsy are presented in Table 20–1. Even more than with most other procedures, optimal biopsy incision placement is crucial. The incision should be as small as possible while still allowing adequate exposure for the safe removal of pathologic material. The biopsy incision should be longitudinal on the extremity because

that is the orientation of the anatomic compartments and most resection incisions. Soft tissue retraction should be kept to a minimum to reduce adjacent tissue contamination.

When deciding about incision placement about the pelvis keep in mind that the gluteus maximus muscle is the best flap for coverage following pelvic resections. As such, the gluteus maximus muscle belly should be violated only if absolutely necessary.

Good hemostasis is a must because tumor is carried with wound hematoma spreading from the biopsy incision. Generally, hemostasis is most easily obtained by making only a small entry into the tumor itself, which can then be tightly closed at the conclusion of the procedure. Electrocautery is rarely effective in neoplastic tissues. Defects in bone following open biopsy can be sealed with bone cement or bone wax and thus prevent prolonged oozing and hematoma formation.

Direct exposure of neurovascular bundles is to be avoided because it may necessitate amputation of an otherwise respectable lesion. In general, the biopsy incision is best placed at the point that marks the shortest distance from the skin to the tumor not directly exposing a major neurovascular bundle or violating an important flap structure.

Unlike most orthopedic surgical approaches, when doing a biopsy it is better to go through a single muscle belly than to dissect nicely between two muscles because the latter approach increases the subsequent tissue contamination. It is preferable, for example, to split the vastus lateralis belly to approach the proximal femur rather than to dissect between the vastus lateralis and the lateral intermuscular system.

A frozen section should always be performed when possible prior to incision closure. The object of this is not necessarily to obtain a tissue diagnosis upon which to proceed with definitive surgery but rather to insure that diagnostic material has been obtained. An initial biopsy specimen may be found to be completely necrotic and thus nondiag-

356

TABLE 20–1. *Rules for Biopsy*

1. Make a small incision placed over the lesion (use an image intensifier if necessary).
2. Use a longitudinal incision on extremities, transverse incision on the pelvis.
3. Use a small incision in the capsule of the tumor.
4. Never directly contaminate a neurovascular bundle.
5. Try not to violate major flap structures (gluteus maximus) or functionally important structures (rectus femoris tendon).
6. Ensure minimal retraction.
7. It is better to go through a single muscle belly than to disect between two muscles.
8. Take a frozen section whenever possible.
9. Maintain good hemostasis.
10. If a drain is needed, bring it out just beyond one end of the incision, never adjacent to the middle of the incision.

nostic. It is more convenient for all parties involved if this information is available when the wound still is open so that further specimens can be easily obtained. Also, one can be fooled into biopsying abnormal tissue around a tumor which histologically may show only inflammation and may not yield a diagnosis. Densely calcified specimens such as sclerotic bone may preclude the possibility of frozen section because they are difficult to cut on a microtome without decalcification. The adage that if the scalpel can cut the specimen so can the microtome is probably a good guide.

When biopsying a bone tumor that has extended into the extraosseous tissues, it is usually sufficient to sample the extraosseous material and not further violate the bone itself . This is especially important with lesions that generally can be treated nonsurgically (e.g., Ewings sarcoma). In these cases, extensive sampling of the bone itself may create mechanical weakening and promote later pathologic fracture. Again, the frozen section usually indicates whether or not the tissues sampled are sufficient for pathologic diagnosis. Remember too that infection is the great masquerader. Always send cultures for laboratory analysis if infection is even remotely suspected in the prebiopsy differential diagnosis. The analysis should include aerobic, anaerobic, fungus, and acid fast cultures.

Just as with incision placement, wound closure technique and proper drain placement are essential. The wound should be closed in as many layers as is reasonably possible. Incisions closed sloppily will promote oozing and increase tissue contamination as well as the risk of secondary infection. Drains may be used if indicated. Remember though that any tissues the drain passes through are contaminated with tumor and must be resected *en bloc* with the biopsy tract. Drains brought out alongside the middle of the biopsy incision require a T-shaped incision or extensive soft tissue sacrifice for resection. This greatly increases local morbidity. Ideally, the drain should be brought out through the skin approximately 5 mm from one end of the incision so that the drain tract can be easily excised with the biopsy tract.

Prophylactic antibiotics are a reasonable consideration and always used by the author. Many of these lesions contain in their necrotic tissues fertile ground for the seeding of infection. Deep infection in a tumor, if it does occur, may preclude the use of preoperative chemotherapy because of the risk of sepsis and can lead unnecessarily to amputation. As such, great respect for sterile technique should be maintained at all times while performing a biopsy.

Finally, no lesion should reach the pathology department without the surgeon first reviewing the case with the pathologist. The histology of musculoskeletal lesions can be unnecessarily confusing if one does not consider the microscopic findings in light of the radiographic and clinical setting.

When these basic tenets are followed rarely will a biopsy interfere with definitive treatment. There is no doubt that a biopsy is ideally performed by the same surgeon who will carry out the definitive treatment. This is not always possible, however, and probably more important on a larger scale is the notion that the biopsy should be performed by a surgeon who knows how to do it.

Reference

1. MANKIN HJ, LANGE TA, SPANIER, SS: The hazards of biopsy in patients with malignant primary bone and soft tissue tumors. J Bone Joint Surg, 64:1121–1127, 1982.

CHAPTER TWENTY-ONE

Osteonecrosis of the Femoral Head: Etiology, Pathogenesis, and Treatment

JOSEPH V. VERNACE
RICHARD A. BALDERSTON

Osteonecrosis of the femoral head remains an unsolved and controversial problem. The pediatric orthopedist is constantly faced with the fear of discovering osteonecrosis brought about by treatment of congenital dislocation of the hip or slipped capital femoral epiphysis. A significant amount of orthopaedic research has been directed to Legg-Calve-Perthes disease in an attempt to understand its cause and formulate an ideal management program. Young adults are victims of osteonecrosis as a result of systemic disease or as sequelae of high-energy trauma. The elderly suffer most frequently from osteonecrosis, generally as a result of femoral neck fractures. To this day treatment modalities remain limited in their scope, and a satisfactory long-term result is not assured. The etiology and pathophysiology of this disorder are not completely understood and therefore limit the physician's ability to properly time therapeutic intervention. When the disease is allowed to progress beyond its early stages, salvage procedures, such as total hip arthroplasty, have not had good success in the young active individuals with osteonecrosis.[31,48]

This chapter is limited to a discussion of osteonecrosis of the femoral head in the adult. A review of the etiology and pathogenesis as well as an extensive summary of the treatment modalities available and their success rates in the various stages of the disease is presented.

Historic Perspective

The word "necrosis" first appeared in the English language in 1665 when it was translated from a Latin treatise and defined by Needham as "an inward mortification."[111] This idea that part of a person may die while he is still living, however, was first verbalized by Hippocrates in the section of the Hippocratic corpus "On Fractures." In it, he wrote that in an improperly bandaged foot, "There is risk of necrosis of the heel bone; and if there is necrosis, the malady may last the patient's whole life."[81] Alexander Munro's work in 1738 is probably the earliest true description of avascular or aseptic necrosis of bone.[103] In the mid eighteenth century, Hunter recognized that bone died when separated from its milieu and outlined several criteria for the recognition of dead bone.[88] The gross processes of sequestration and how dead bone serves as a scaffolding for new repair bone, thus enabling entire segments of bone to be reconstituted, were first described by James Russell in his treatise of 1794.[134,135] John Goodsir was the first to apply Lister's acromatic microscope to the study of bone. In 1845, he was able to demonstrate that the repair of dead bone was accomplished by cells.[72] Shortly before this time, Jean Cruveilhier in 1842 first described the gross appearance of late post-traumatic deformation of the femoral head and presumed it to be a result of vascular damage.[93] Franz Konig in 1888 first described the entity of osteochondritis dissecans of the hip in two cases. Although he did not label the condition as such, it is clear from his paper that he was actually describing osteonecrosis of the femoral head, the first such description of its kind.[93,111] Axhausen was the first to use the term "aseptic necrosis" and in 1907 described the microscopic process of repair by which seams of new bone were laid upon dead bone.[8] In 1926, Freund wrote a comprehensive article on idiopathic femoral head necrosis and is given credit for the first detailed description of bilateral disease.[62] An excellent review of the pathology of bone infarction was described by Jaffe and Pomerantz in 1934.[91] Chandler in 1936 composed the concept of osteonecrosis of the femoral head resulting from occlusion or ischemia of specific vessels and coined the phrase "coronary disease of the hip."[29,30] Dallas Phemister and his associates further broadened the understanding of bone necrosis in their reports on necrosis occurring after femoral neck fracture and osteonecrosis associated with Caisson's disease.[94,123,124,126]

Prior to 1962, only 22 cases of idiopathic osteonecrosis of the femoral head could be found in the English literature. In that year, Mankin and Brower added 5 cases of bilateral disease.[106] These past 25 years have subsequently exhibited an explosion of new knowledge in regard to the etiology and pathogenesis of this disease.[27,28,59,60,67,69,85,86,106] Even with the continued research that goes on today, a complete understanding of the mechanism of disease remains obscure. Osteonecrosis of the femoral head is now a well recognized entity that commonly afflicts young individuals and is frequently bilateral. A complete understanding of what is known of its cause, pathogenesis, and long-term outcome of its various treatments is of paramount importance to those who treat adult disorders of the hip.

Etiology

A large group of seemingly unrelated diseases have as a common denominator the occurrence of osteonecrosis of the femoral head (Table 21–1). The distribution and development of the accompanying bony changes in these seemingly unrelated disorders is so consistent, however, that a unifying mechanism of disease is constantly sought. Although each particular instance of osteonecrosis is determined by several interacting factors,[17,69] such as age, underlying disease, mechanical stress, and the persistence of the pathology arising from the causative agent, the cardinal step in its pathogenesis is the establishment of bone ischemia. More precisely, it is a disparity between the oxygen need to the bone cell and the ability of the local circula-

TABLE 21–1. **Orthopaedic Conditions That Lead to Osteonecrosis of the Femoral Head**

Fracture of the femoral neck
Traumatic dislocation of the hip
Trauma to the hip (without fracture or dislocation)
Legg-Calve-Perthes' disease
Slipped capital femoral epiphysis
Hip manipulation (treatment of CDH, SCFE)
Septic arthritis
Reconstructive hip surgery

tion to supply that need. A list of orthopaedic conditions that are associated with femoral head ischemia and subsequent osteonecrosis are listed in Fig. 21–1.

Osteonecrosis is most commonly seen in the bulbous ends of long bones. These areas consist of a honeycomb of cancellous bone covered by a thin shell of cortical bone. The cancellous portion lacks significant hematopoietic tissue and is largely packed with myeloid tissue, fatty marrow, and a sinusoidal network carrying blood to and from the tissues.[149] In the hip, the blood vessels enter this confined cancellous space through periosteal surfaces, along the medullary cavity, and via the ligamentum teres.[27,40,167] Although anastomoses do occur, the blood supply in this region is largely an endarterial system and in the absence of significant collateral circulation, blockage or disruption of these small vessels could rapidly lead to ischemia. The lateral epiphyseal artery is responsible for supplying the superior lateral two-thirds of the femoral head, which is the region most commonly affected in osteonecrosis. Direct insult to this vessel such as might occur with a displaced fracture of the femoral neck, could readily explain subsequent vascular insufficiency. What might not be so readily apparent is that reduced perfusion of the sinusoidal vascular bed can also result from an increase in the contents of the nonexpandable bone compartment, which is one of the proposed mechanisms leading to osteonecrosis in several of the systemic etiologies.[39,59,70,86]

Systemic disorders, such as Gaucher's disease, sickle cell disease, other hemoglobinopathies, and dysbarism have shown a high association with the development of osteonecrosis of the femoral head.[16,35,42,59,74,92,99,139,144,148] Glucocorticoids, alcoholism, gout and hyperuricemia, minor trauma, and collagen vascular disorders also have shown an association.[39,40,49,60,70,84,93] Several authors have grouped these above associations into "definite and possible categories."[59,86] In some cases, none of these associated conditions are readily apparent. This "idiopathic osteonecrosis" group represents a small proportion of the overall population with the diagnosis of osteonecrosis.

Common Etiologies (Table 21–2)
Major Trauma

The most common etiology associated with osteonecrosis of the femoral head is fracture of the neck of the femur.[19,27,149] Both the extraosseous

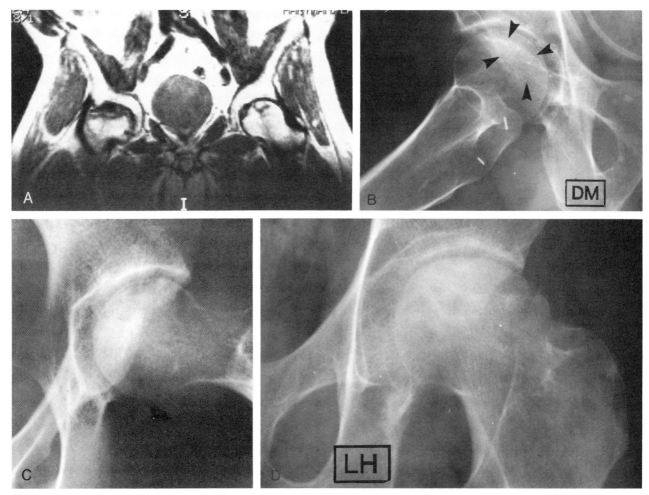

Fɪɢ. 21–1. Correlation of histopathology, radiology, and staging of osteonecrosis of the femoral head. **A.** Stage 1: An initial insult results in ischemia with marrow edema and vacant lacunae evident in 2 to 4 days and eventual osteocyte death and fibrosis. MRI is positive; plain x-rays are negative; bone scan is inconclusive. **B.** Stage 2: Revascularization results in appositional new bone formation at cancellous bone and resorption of subchondral bone, especially at the superolateral aspect. Radiologic signs include early osteopenia, density of the head, and sclerosis. **C.** Stage 3: Subchondral fracture and head collapse result in pseudocyst formation. Radiologic signs include the "crescent sign," femoral head flattening, and preservation of the collapsed joint space. **D.** Stage 4: Joint space narrowing and destruction result in cartilage erosion, bone eburnation, and acetabular degeneration. Radiologic evidence includes gross head collapse with 2° joint destruction.

and the intraosseous blood supply of the femoral head are susceptible to injury with femoral neck fractures.[24,64] The severity of the disruption of the blood supply is usually directly proportional to the displacement of the fracture. The lateral epiphyseal vessels are most susceptible to injury and are com-

Tᴀʙʟᴇ 21–2. *Common Etiologies of Osteonecrosis*

Major trauma
Dysbarism
Hemoglobinopathy (Sickle cell)
Gaucher disease
Irradiation
Glucocorticoids
Alcoholism
Gout and hyperuricemia
Minor injury
Idiopathic

monly torn with varus displacement of the head by a distance of one-half the diameter of the head.[34] With moderate displacement, the medial epiphyseal vessels that course through the ligamentum teres, and less commonly the inferior metaphyseal vessels, may remain intact. As displacement increases, progression from subtotal loss to total loss of blood supply to the femoral head occurs. In addition to arterial insufficiency, significant impairment of venous return has been identified by a number of investigators.[6,59]

If indeed a significant disruption of the blood supply occurs, osteonecrosis is evident histologically within 8 hours from the time of injury.[27] Osteonecrosis is, therefore, an early event following transcervical fracture. Catto found histologic evidence of partial or complete femoral head necrosis in two-thirds of the cases examined in this early postoperative period. In 21 of 24 cases assessed at autopsy Sevitt reported similar findings.[143] Other investigators have reported findings of early histologic osteonecrosis in 65 to 85 percent of cases.[124,145,174]

Several factors play a role in the decreased number of clinically evident cases of osteonecrosis from those that are suggested by histologic evaluation. First, when partial disruption of the blood supply has occurred, there is some degree of revascularization. Second, in most series the diagnosis of posttraumatic osteonecrosis is made by x-ray evaluation. The percentage of cases demonstrating significant radiographic changes represents only a gross evaluation of the disease process. Many authors have correlated the degree of fracture displacement to the incidence of osteonecrosis.[11,12,21,64,90] In addition to increased initial displacement, reduction and fixation in excessive valgus position carries a higher incidence.[24,64,90]

Radiographs rarely show signs of osteonecrosis prior to 4 to 6 months following fracture, but 80 to 90% of cases are evident within the first 2 years. In those fractures that fail to unite, a significant increase in the incidence of osteonecrosis has been noted. Boyd and George in 1947 reported a two-fold increase,[20] whereas other authors have found the rate of osteonecrosis in nonunions to be 4 to 5 times that of united fractures.[19,28,124] In those fractures that do unite, late segmental collapse is seen in nearly 30% of displaced fractures treated by reduction and internal fixation and in approximately 10% of nondisplaced fractures. A significant number of these cases may occur more than 2 years after fracture.[28,59]

Gaucher's Disease

The bone manifestations of Gaucher's disease were first described by Brill in 1904.[59] Both intravascular and extravascular mechanisms have been postulated to explain the development of osteocrosis of the femoral head in this metabolic disorder. A deficiency of betaglucosidase results in an accumulation of glucocerebroside within reticuloendothelial cells.[86] Although found in almost any part of the osseous system, these cerebroside-contained cells most commonly involve the hip.[80] These histiocyte-like cells assume a spindle shape within the marrow of the femoral head. Cushing and Stout, in 1926, believed that this shape is a reflection of increased marrow pressure and resultant cell compression.[42] Continued infiltration of these

Gaucher cells may lead to gradual occlusion of the vasculature with subsequent ischemia and femoral head osteonecrosis.

Pick, in 1925, described the direct invasion of Gaucher cells into the adventitial coat of small blood vessels.[93] Subsequently, Schein and Arken[139] suggested that vascular obstruction and ischemia were caused by the direct intravascular infiltration of vessels by Gaucher cells. Other mechanisms of disease have also been postulated. Masses of Gaucher cells have been found within the lumens of veins. Intraosseous embolization of these cells with resultant ischemia could conceivably account for bone infarction.[93] Jacobs[90] hypothesized that it is the liver involvement with accompanying hyperlipidemia that may be responsible for vascular sludging, thrombosis, and ischemia.

In several studies, a large percentage of cases have demonstrated bilateral involvement.[2,5] In addition, the majority of patients demonstrated femoral shaft involvement as well.[5] Interestingly, healed cases of Gaucher-related osteonecrosis of the femoral head in childhood with subsequent adult recurrence have been reported.[2,95]

Sickle Cell Disease and Other Hemoglobinopathies

Prior to the recognition of osteonecrosis of the femoral head in patients with sickle cell disease by Digs in 1937, radiographic changes were thought to result from osteomyelitis.[80] Osteonecrosis has since been reported in all of the common genetic variants of sickle cell disorder and in rare instances, in those patients with sickle cell trait.[33] Of these variants, osteonecrosis is most commonly seen in sickle cell-hemoglobin C disease (SC), and classic sickle cell anemia (SS).[33,59,129] In those with SC disease, the incidence of osteonecrosis ranges from 20 to 68%. In SS disease, Cockshott,[35] Siegling,[146] and Tanaka[162] reported incidences of 0, 4, and 12%, respectively. Decreased life expectancy in those patients with SS disease has been offered as an explanation for this decreased incidence.

The most commonly accepted mechanism of disease relating osteonecrosis to the S gene is that of intravascular occlusion of the blood supply to the femoral head. As the partial pressure of oxygen in the capillaries falls below 45 mm Hg, the hemoglobin comes out of solution forming liquid crystals that distort the cell envelope; this is known as sickling. The sickle shape leads to increased viscosity of the blood with subsequent stasis and finally thrombosis.[99] This occlusion increases local hypoxia which promotes further sickling and expansion of the area of ischemia and necrosis.

Irradiation

Postradiation osteonecrosis is a well recognized entity.[59] Femoral head osteonecrosis most commonly follows treatment of female genital cancer. Several reports have noted Hodgkin's disease patients at higher risk following radiation therapy. These patients, however, most commonly received combined modalities, including steroids, chemotherapy, and radiation.[53,127] Looney[101] in 1956 followed 80 patients who were radium and luminous dial workers and found 11 cases of osteonecrosis of the femoral head. The average time from contact with radium to the development of hip symptoms was 15 years.

In addition to femoral head osteonecrosis, femoral neck fracture and less commonly so, acetabular osteonecrosis have been reported as well.[44,59] Although radiation induced femoral neck fractures have occurred in patients given doses of less than 1600 rads, the commonly accepted threshold of radiation-induced changes in bone is thought to be 3000 rads with osteocyte death occurring at 5000 rads.[44] Depending on the type of radiation used, bone absorption may be 50 to 100% higher than the surrounding soft tissues because of the greater amount of heavy elemental constituents in bone.

With newer radiation delivery systems, exposure area is decreased and radiation-induced osteonecrosis may be expected to decline in the future.

Dysbaric Osteonecrosis

Osteonecrosis of the femoral head is a known complication of dysbarism.[32,59,86,92,93] The actual incidence of osteonecrosis and bone infarction in those exposed to abnormal pressures varies directly with the degree of pressure, the number of exposures, and the rapidity of decompression. In evaluation of Japanese coastal divers who ignored special decompression procedures, the incidence rose above 50% compared to an incidence of less than 4% in naval divers who followed appropriate decompression schedules.[149] In those cases of osteonecrosis that are juxta-articular, the humeral head is most commonly involved followed by the femoral head, which is involved in approximately half as many cases. In addition to its common associations with caisson workers, deep sea divers and scuba divers, "decompression sickness" and dysbaric osteonecrosis have been described in personnel of high altitude aircraft who go from normal atmospheric pressure to hypobaric conditions.[18,108] Phisiologically, this is similar to moving rapidly from hyperbaric conditions to normal atmospheric pressure.

Several large surveys in both the United States and the United Kingdom failed to reveal any significant correlation between osteonecrosis and actual decompression sickness.[32] In those US navy divers with documented osteonecrosis only 16% reported episodes of decompression sickness. Although the guidelines offered in the newer decompression schedules are considered safe in that they prevent the development of decompression sickness, they may indeed be inadequate in the prevention of dysbaric osteonecrosis. Not only does the incidence of osteonecrosis rise with the number of dysbaric exposures, laboratory studies show that repeated exposures may also shorten the latent period between exposure and the appearance of radiographic findings.[32] Pressures above 17 psi are associated with increased risk of dysbaric osteonecrosis.[92] Experimentally, obesity has been associated with an increased incidence and shortened latent period as well.[32]

The exact mechanism of bone ischemia and subsequent osteonecrosis is still controversial. When subjected to increased pressures, tissues absorb more of the gases in the air than at atmospheric pressures. The oxygen and carbon dioxide, even in excess, are readily transported via the blood stream to the lungs where they are readily expelled. Nitrogen, however, which accounts for 79% of the gases in air, is readily absorbed by the body's tissues. Nitrogen is five times as soluble in fat as in nonfatty tissues such as blood. Thus, a great accumulation of soluble nitrogen is found in the fatty marrow. Several theories have been presented to explain the occurrence of bony ischemia and subsequent necrosis. In addition to the supersaturation that occurs in fatty tissues, gas exchange in the fatty marrow proceeds at a slower rate than in other tissues.[32] With rapid, inadequate decompression, nitrogen bubbles come out of solution, overwhelm the local tissues and cannot be readily cleared from the bloodstream, leading to small vessel occlusion and subsequent bone ischemia. As stated earlier, dysbaric osteonecrosis is not statistically related to episodes of decompression sickness. However, intravascular nitrogen bubbles have been found even after routine asymptomatic decompression. The accumulation of these "silent" embolic bubbles during repeated asymptomatic decompressions has been implicated in the pathogenesis of bone lesions.[92,149]

In addition to an intravascular mechanism, extravascular gas bubbles released during "adequate" decompression may accumulate within the rigid confines of the osseous tissues and lead to increased intramedullary pressure and subsequent occlusion of intraosseous vessels. Histopathological examination of femoral heads that exhibit dysbaric osteonecrosis show areas of platelet aggregation, red cell slugging, and scattered venous thrombi. A disturbance in venous outflow may be an important factor in this extravascular mechanism.[96] In addition, persistence of nitrogen gases in the marrow caused by the slow gas exchange could result in toxic effect of the fat cell membrane with subsequent swelling of these cells, increased pressure, and decreased sinusoidal blood flow.[149]

Glucocorticoids

Although Ficat and Arlet[59] placed glucocorticoids in the probable association category, many authors now feel that enough evidence is present to suggest a direct association between steroid use and the development of osteonecrosis.[39,69,172] This relationship is evident particularly for cases of renal transplantation and systemic lupus erythematosus (SLE).[40,59,86,89] Modification of postoperative renal transplantation protocols have significantly reduced the incidence of osteonecrosis from 17 to 1% in a large series.[97] Zizic[175] reported a prospective study of 54 patients with SLE of whom 52% developed osteonecrosis. Those patients demonstrating bony abnormalities were much more commonly cushingoid than patients without osteonecrosis. Although most associations of steroid-induced osteonecrosis deal with long-term exposure to the glucocorticoids, there are several reports of osteonecrosis following short-term steroid therapy.

Other authors, however, feel that the association between glucocorticoids and the development of osteonecrosis is more complex. Glimcher and Kenzora[68,69] expressed the hypothesis that steroid exposure is but one factor in the development of osteonecrosis in an already compromised host. Cruess[41] reported on 122 patients with steroid induced osteonecrosis and felt that an alteration in fat metabolism was the most likely cause of the condition. Fisher[60] also hypothesized an alteration in fat metabolism, and believed that terminal vascular obstruction in bone via systemic fat emboli were the cause of ischemia and osteocyte death. In addition to systemic fat emboli, it has been shown that the average diameter of the marrow fat cells in the femoral head under the influence of corticosteroids increase significantly in size. This increase in volume might be significant enough to increase marrow pressure resulting from the closed chamber effect in the femoral head. This then may result in diminished perfusion with ensuing ischemia and osteonecrosis. Wang[171] documented an increase in femoral head intramedullary pressure in rabbits following the administration of corticosteroids. In addition, subsequent core decompression performed unilaterally returned this pressure to within normal limits.[172]

Although it seems that alteration in fat metabolism in some way may initiate the onset of osteonecrosis, the exact mechanism of disease in this group has not been defined. Most commonly the osteonecrosis occurs in patients who have had chronic treatment and have other underlying disease processes. Although it is possible that the reports of osteonecrosis following short-term steroid treatment are coincidental and in fact represent cases of idiopathic disease, it appears that in susceptible individuals, even short-term, moderate dose steroid therapy may induce the disorder.

Alcoholism

The history of alcohol abuse among patients with osteonecrosis is common. In 1962, Mankin[106] reviewed the world literature and added five cases to the existing 22 cases of "idiopathic avascular necrosis." Three of his five patients with bilateral disease had a history of alcoholism. Patterson's large series from the Mayo Clinic demonstrated 17% of the patients with a history of alcoholism.[121] Thibodeau's review of 27 patients with avascular necrosis in 1968 revealed the majority to have an association with alcohol.[163]

Current reports substantiate this apparent association of alcohol and osteonecrosis, some citing an incidence as high as 70% excess alcohol intake in their patients.[87] In an attempt to further define this apparent association, Matsuo, et al.,[109] conducted a controlled epidemiologic study comparing 112 patients with "idiopathic" osteonecrosis of the femoral head with 168 matched controls. Patients who consumed more than 400 ml of alcohol per week, had an 11-fold greater risk than nondrinkers for osteonecrosis. In addition, regardless of the presence or absence of liver dysfunction, a clear dose-response relationship was noted for increasing levels of alcohol consumption.[109] The incidence of osteonecrosis among groups of alcoholics who have been studied ranges from 1 to 2%.

The mechanism by which excess alcohol intake

leads to osteonecrosis is not well understood. The most popular current theory is that the pathogenesis is similar to that seen with corticosteroid osteonecrosis. Fatty infiltration, fat cell hypertrophy, and subsequent increased intramedullary pressure have been experimentally induced in rats who are fed an alcohol enriched diet.[149] With the increased pressure, sinusoidal occlusion may then occur, resulting in ischemia. In addition, associated liver dysfunction, pancreatic dysfunction, and hyperlipidemia may lead to intravascular sludging, thrombosis, or fat embolization through alterations in blood coagulability. This may result in vascular occlusion and femoral head ischemia. Several investigators have reported an increase in serum cortisol levels in patients with excess alcohol intake and osteonecrosis.[130,147] This further gives credence to the proposed common mechanism with that of corticosteroid induced osteonecrosis.

Gout and Hyperuricemia

A review of several series of "idiopathic osteonecrosis" reveals a number of patients with hyperuricemia or clinical gout. Although commonly perceived to be an associated factor, the link between gout and osteonecrosis is not clearly established. Many of the patients in these studies presented with multiple risk factors such as alcoholism or steroid ingestion, making it difficult to ascertain the true etiologic relationship.[84]

Idiopathic Osteonecrosis

Up to 25% of all patients presenting with osteonecrosis of the femoral head present without an associated etiology.[59,80,107,121] Idiopathic osteonecrosis is a diagnosis of exclusion and a diligent search for underlying risk factors is warranted because decision making in the treatment process may vary. Many mechanisms of disease have been proposed, however none have been proven. Once bone cell death occurs, the pathophysiology follows a course similar to other forms of nontraumatic osteonecrosis.

Pathophysiology

Although the exact inciting event or initiating factor has not been discovered, it is well recognized that the initial insult to the femoral head is a disruption of the blood supply. This disruption can

take several different forms. In traumatic osteonecrosis it has been shown that the major arterial supply to the femoral head is disrupted in a somewhat acute fashion.[6,24,34,61] Even in this seemingly well understood mechanism, there has been some disagreement in the literature regarding the actual vascular disruption. Arnoldi and Linderholm[6] found that venous drainage was impaired more frequently than arterial supply following femoral neck fracture.

In nontraumatic osteonecrosis the mechanisms of vascular disturbance are even less well understood. Most recently, fat embolism, venous stasis, increased interosseous pressure, and alterations in fat metabolism have been popular theories of the mechanisms of disease.[39,60,69,86,172] A review of the literature reveals that there is no one mechanism that can explain the onset of all types of osteonecrosis. Glimcher and Kenzora[70] have formulated the theory of accumulative cell stress in order to explain a multifactorial cause of nontraumatic osteonecrosis. Most cases are in all likelihood caused by many factors and rarely by an instantaneous or sudden solitary phenomenon that results in bone ischemia. As these factors interplay in the development of the condition, the cells become progressively compromised until they reach an irreversible state and are no longer able to maintain their cellular equilibrium. The final stress that may overwhelm the system could indeed be in the form of persistent intraosseous hypertension, direct cellular toxic effect, or increased stores of marrow fat. Once this final insult is delivered, the tissue decompensates to a state of cell necrosis.

As with ischemia and infarction in other tissues, this state of demise can be brought about either by interruption of the arterial supply or by occlusion of venous drainage that results in stasis and gradual oxygen starvation.[86] In experimentally induced osteonecrosis, the first histologic changes occur not in the bone itself, but in the marrow elements.[68] At 2 to 4 days following ischemia there is loss of cellular detail with resultant edema and increased intraosseous pressure. As the pressure increases, it further compromises venous return, increases venous stasis and further raises intraosseous pressure. The lacunae are still occupied by osteocytes at this time and indeed necrotic osteocytes may appear normal by light microscopy for weeks. The presence of empty lacunae, a histologic hallmark of osteonecrosis, therefore, is a later feature of bone death (Fig. 21–2).[125]

The resultant necrotic trabeculae are not a source of pain nor are they biomechanically unsound.[22] Thus, it is not the dead bone, per se, that causes

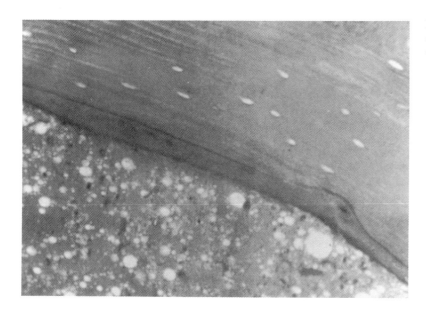

Fig. 21–2. Histologic section of trabecular bone demonstrating empty lacunae, a trait of osteonecrosis.

clinical symptoms. The relentless progression to subchondral fracture and femoral head collapse cannot be explained on the basis of bone ischemia and bone cell death alone. Rather, it is the inevitable, yet often futile attempt at biologic repair and revascularization that persistently leads to head collapse and destruction of the joint surfaces.[28,68,143] If these biologic processes were allowed to progress, in an uninterrupted fashion, one might expect the femoral head to revascularize and repair itself without subsequent collapse.[124]

In order to understand the mechanisms leading to subchondral fracture and femoral head collapse, as well as the staging systems used in osteonecrosis, it is necessary to review the histopathology of the reparative process of bone. Of paramount importance is an understanding of the differences between the revascularization and repair processes of cancellous bone and cortical bone. In the reparative process of cancellous bone, new cells and capillaries invade the marrow vascular spaces between the dead trabeculae. These new cells form osteoblasts that line the dead trabeculae and are responsible for appositional new bone formation. Thus, in cancellous bone, new bone formation occurs *prior* to osteoclastic resorption of the necrotic trabeculae. Cancellous bone does not heal by "creeping substitution." Unlike cancellous bone, however, cortical bone (compact bone) undergoes osteoclastic resorption prior to new bone formation. This area of resorbed compact bone may then act as a stress riser for the development of small fractures produced by continued force application in that area.

In the case of the femoral head, both of these reparative processes are taking place simultaneously.[27,69] In the cancellous portion, appositional new bone formation occurs along the dead trabeculae (Fig. 21–3). As this process continues, the thickened trabeculae give an appearance of increased bone volume or sclerosis when viewed roentgenographically (Fig. 21–4). This process, however, rarely proceeds for more than 4 to 5 mm.[7,70,143] This front of appositional new bone is seen roentgenographically as the classic sclerotic segmental line of demarcation in osteonecrosis. At the peripheral margins, in the area of the subchondral plate, the reparative process follows the process appropriate for cortical or compact bone. The

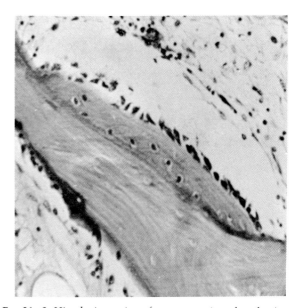

Fig. 21–3. Histologic section of osteonecrotic trabeculae (empty lacunae) with subsequent appositional new bone formation. (From Sevitt, S.: Avascular necrosis and revascularization of the femoral head after intracapsular fractures. J Bone Joint Surg, 46B:286, 1964.)

Fɪɢ. 21–4. Section of femoral head demonstrating restricted area of appositional new bone formation. Seen roentgenographically as a sclerotic rim surrounding the osteonecrotic lesion.

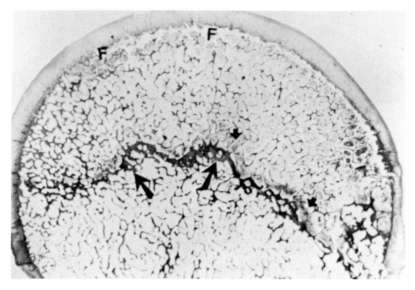

peripheral lateral margin seems to be the area where subchondral osteoclastic resorption first occurs (Fig. 21–5).[69] This extensive resorption occurs in three dimensions at a junction between the advancing front of new bone apposition and the subchondral plate itself. This subchondral stress riser, under the enormous shear stresses placed on the femoral head, gives rise to small fractures, that propagate along the subchondral region, paralleling the articular cartilage and advancing through the region of dead cancellous bone. The difference in elastic modulae between the compact subchondral bone and the cancellous bone of the central portion of the femoral head gives rise to a biomechanical pathway through which the fracture propagates (Fig. 21–6). Roentgenographically this subchondral fracture gives rise to the crescent sign, which is nearly pathognomonic for osteonecrosis (Fig. 21–7). Once the subchondral fracture occurs, support is

lost for the overlying articular cartilage and femoral head flattening occurs.[27,28,59,69,107,115,160] As the process continues, extensive collapse of the subchondral bone and severe deformity of the head become evident. Osteocartilaginous flaps develop leading to further joint incongruity and joint destruction.

Clinical Presentation and Natural History

Osteonecrosis of the femoral head most commonly presents with insidious onset; it is usually characterized by intermittent episodes of pain in the groin, knee, buttock or trochanteric region, with or without associated limp. At times, the onset of symptoms may be sudden and severe, as in

Fɪɢ. 21–5. Osteoclastic resorption recurring in an area of compact bone, similar to that which occurs in the subchondral plate.

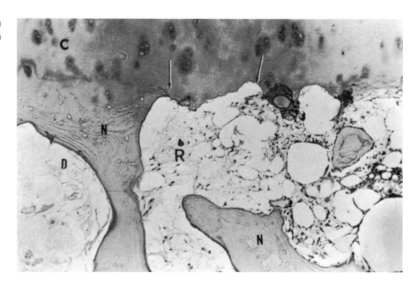

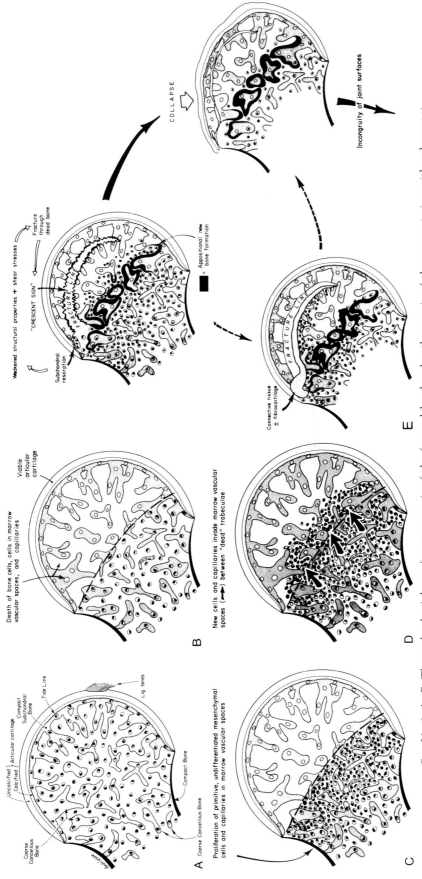

Fig. 21–6. A–E. The pathophysiology of osteonecrosis of the femoral head and pathogenesis of the crescent sign with subsequent development of degenerative arthritis of the hip. (From Kenzora IE, Glimcher MJ: Pathogenesis of idiopathic osteonecrosis: the crescent sign. Ortho Clin North Am, 16:692–693, 1985.

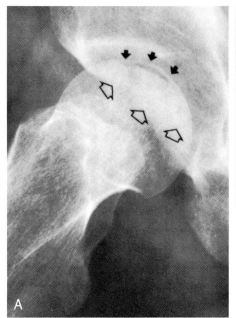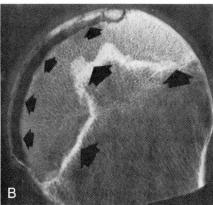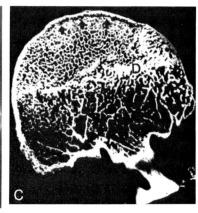

Fɪɢ. 21–7. **A.** Lateral roentgenogram demonstrating a classic crescent sign (small arrows). This finding heralds the onset of Stage 3 disease. Often the sign is more subtle and seen only on CT or MRI images. **B.** Roentgenogram of a 1-cm thick slab specimen again demonstrating the subchondral fracture (small arrows). Also evident is the restricted extent of appositional new bone formation on the necrotic cancellous bone (large arrows). **C.** Microradiograph detailing the subchondral fracture (arrows) and the radiodense band corresponding to the roentgenograms in A and B. (From Kenzora JE, Glimcher MJ: Pathogenesis of idiopathic osteonecrosis: the crescent sign. Orthop Clin North Am 16:685, 1985.)

those cases associated with renal transplantation or sickle cell disease. Although it is seen in both sexes between the third and sixth decades of life, nontraumatic osteonecrosis most typically occurs in males during the fifth decade of life. Radiographs taken during the early stage of disease may be entirely normal or may reveal diffuse or spotty increases in radiodensity within the femoral head representing appositional new bone formation.[59,107,157] As symptoms proceed to more consistent and more intense disabling pain, radiographs proceed through the stages of increasing sclerosis, subchondral fracture, femoral head flattening and joint space destruction. Unfortunately, many patients at the time of presentation have radiographic evidence of subchondral fracture or femoral head collapse.

Even in those cases of late presentation it is of great importance to evaluate and follow the contralateral hip.[38,100,107,112,173] The incidence of bilaterality varies in the literature from 35 to 80%.[57,77,112] In general, it appears that the bilaterality approaches 50% in those cases not associated with corticosteroids and in 70 to 80% of those cases associated with corticosteroids. Despite this high incidence of involvement of both hips, the usual presentation is that of unilateral disease with subsequent progression to the contralateral hip.[38,107,112] It is this "silent hip" that can be diagnosed in the earliest stages of osteonecrosis. Pre-

vention of progression and subsequent joint destruction is most successful in these early stages.[1,10,59,85,136,153,173] If left untreated, an early lesion usually progresses to subchondral fracture and femoral head collapse. Steinberg[157] followed the progression in hips treated nonoperatively. Forty-four of 48 hips showed definite progression and required either femoral head replacement or total hip arthroplasty. Lee[100] followed 11 "silent hips" of idiopathic osteonecrosis and found relentless progression of the disease in all hips. Coste[38] followed the demise of hip function in 38 of 45 patients treated nonoperatively. Nineteen of 24 patients with sufficient followup after nonoperative treatment were rated as poor or very poor by Patterson, et al.[121] Symptomatic treatment with or without nonweight-bearing does not appear to affect the relentless progression to subsequent collapse and deformity of the femoral head. If we are to be successful in preventing destruction and disability in this disorder, early intervention is necessary.

Diagnosis

In many cases of osteonecrosis of the femoral head the diagnosis is readily made. In the symptomatic patient the history and physical examination are often coupled with the classic roentgenographic picture of the segmental wedge-shaped sclerotic line in the superior lateral portion of the femoral head, with or without subchondral fracture and femoral head collapse. Further discussion of the roentgenographic findings in this latter part of the disease process can be found in the section on staging.

The diagnosis of osteonecrosis becomes more difficult when the patient presents early in the course of the disease, prior to any changes on plain roentgenograms.[159] Laboratory investigation is of little help except in confirming the presence of an associated disorder such as sickle cell disease. In an attempt to diagnose this disorder in the "preradiographic" stages it is necessary to resort to other forms of radiographic investigation or to the "functional evaluation of bone."[58,85]

Tomograms are helpful in further defining suspected areas of abnormality on plain roentgenograms. However, prior to substantial appositional new bone formation on the necrotic trabeculae, tomograms will also be normal.

Bone scanning through the use of radionucleotides usually shows increased uptake in the femoral head once the stage of appositional new bone has begun (Fig. 21–8). Early in the investigation of the "silent hip" or in the occasional patient who presents during the early stages of bone ischemia, the bone scan may be either normal or on occasion demonstrate decreased uptake because of decreased blood flow in the region of the femoral head.[25] Although increased uptake will raise the suspicion of a pathologic process and may eventually aid in the diagnosis of osteonecrosis, it is not specifically diagnostic.

More recently, computerized tomography (CT) scanning has been used in the diagnosis of osteone-

crosis. Because of its high resolution, it is able to delineate minor changes in bony architecture (i.e., new bone apposition) that may otherwise be undetected on plain roentgenograms in the early stages of the disease. Very early manifestations of osteonecrosis, including marrow edema and changes in vascularity however, are not depicted. CT scanning has been useful, however, in delineating subchondral fractures that may or may not be apparent on plain roentgenograms.[156] The addition of this information may directly affect the staging and therefore the treatment of the disease.

Magnetic resonance imaging (MRI) has gained acceptance as the imaging modality of choice in the early stages of osteonecrosis of the femoral head.[15,65,78] (Fig. 21–9) Preliminary results indicate that the technique is sensitive to early changes that occur within the marrow elements themselves, as well as the later changes that involve the trabecular bone. The correlation of MR images to histopathology in clinical findings is evolving rapidly.[142] In addition to early diagnosis of the lesion, additional information about the extent of involvement of the femoral head is often gained from the MR image. Observations of the hematopoietic intertrochanteric marrow and its early conversion to fatty marrow in many patients with osteonecrosis may allow the identification of patients at increased risk for osteonecrosis prior to the development of a femoral head lesion.[118]

Although CT scanning still provides better resolution and identification of subchondral fractures, the variation of MR signal intensity in the central region of the lesion shows good correlation with the presence or absence of fracture. Low intensity central regions of T1 weighted images demonstrated an 88% correlation with fractures depicted on CT scanning. In contrast, only one of 13 lesions without fractures (8%) had a low intensity at central region.[118] Much work is currently being done with MR images to depict the morphologic features of osteonecrosis and attempt to classify and stage the lesion based on MR images alone.[19,118,133] In addition, its noninvasiveness and lack of ionizing radiation coupled with its capability of producing images of equal resolution in all planes makes MRI the current state of the art tool for investigation and evaluation of osteonecrosis.

The functional evaluation of bone (FEB) as advocated by Ficat, Arlet, and Hungerford may be another means of diagnosing osteonecrosis in its earliest stages. Taken together, the measurement of intramedullary pressure, intramedullary venography, and core biopsy have demonstrated a high correlation between increased pressure, venous stasis, and osteonecrosis.[58,85] The advent of magnetic res-

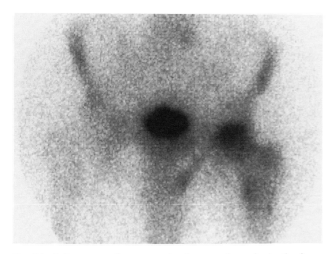

FIG. 21–8. Bone scan demonstrating increased uptake in the femoral head in a patient with osteonecrosis.

FIG. 21–9. MRI scan of the hips. **A.** Coronal image of a patient with severe symptoms of the right hip (Stage 4) and normal x-rays and bone scan in the asymptomatic left hip. **B.** Transverse image of the same Stage 1 lesion of the left hip.

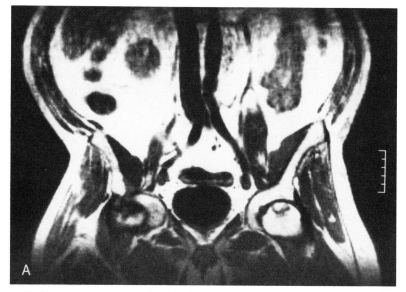

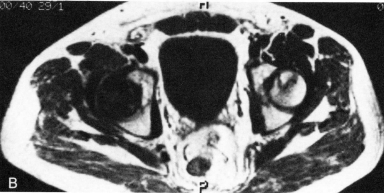

onance imaging obviates the need for this invasive diagnostic technique.

Classification and Staging

The principal importance in staging a disease process is to correlate pathophysiology with appropriately timed therapeutic intervention. The staging system must be concise, easily understood and represent key events in the progression of the disease process (Table 21–3). Elaborate, cumbersome staging systems are less effective in guiding decision making for the practicing orthopedist. In addition, a change in the stage of the disease should indicate either a significant change in the ability to diagnose and effectively treat the disorder (Fig. 21-10).

Marcus, et al., in 1973 offered a 6-part staging sequence for idiopathic osteonecrosis in an attempt to guide diagnosis and treatment.[107] Their attempts at clinical and roentgenographic correlation have subsequently been shown to be inaccurate. The first

two stages demonstrated roentgenographic abnormalities in the femoral head, however, the clinical stage remained asymptomatic. In addition to the realization that some patients present with pain even in the early roentgenographic stages of osteonecrosis, it has now been shown that patients may be symptomatic even prior to the ability to diagnose the disorder on plain roentgenograms. With advances in radiographic technique, it is now possible to diagnose the disorder before the Marcus and Enneking Stage 1 lesion. In this classification, Stages 4 through 6 represent steps in the evolution of degenerative changes including femoral head collapse, joint space narrowing, and acetabular involvement.

In 1980, Ficat and Arlet offered a 5-stage radiologic classification of osteonecrosis in which the clinical manifestations of the Marcus and Enneking system were dropped.[59] In their initial stage at that time, Stage 1, an abnormal uptake on radionucleotide scanning was present in the face of normal anteroposterior and lateral roentgenograms. In Stage 2, AP and lateral roentgenograms became positive with evidence of sclerosis and or cyst formation in the femoral head. Between Stages 2 and

TABLE 21–3. *Various Staging Systems of Osteonecrosis of the Femoral Head*

Stage	MARCUS, ET AL.* (1973)	FICAT AND ARLET (1980–1985)	STEINBERG (1984)	VERNACE (1990)
0		0. Normal x-ray, bone scan abnormal. FEB.[1]	0. Normal x-ray, bone scan	
I	Asymptomatic spotty areas of increased density on x-rays.	I. Normal x-ray Abnormal bone scan	I. Normal x-ray Abnormal bone scan	I. x-ray negative MRI positive
II	Asymptomatic demarcation of infarct zone on x-ray	II. Diffuse porosis sclerosis or cysts	II. Sclerosis and/or cysts A. Mild B. Moderate C. Severe	II. Sclerosis demarcation of infarct bone
		Transition phase -subchondral fracture -head flattening		
III	Onset of pain Subchondral collapse (Crescent sign)	III. Femoral head collapse without secondary joint destruction	III. Crescent sign—no femoral head flattening A. Mild B. Moderate C. Severe	III. Subchondral fracture with normal joint spine Less than 50% More than 50%
IV	Pain with activity Early femoral head collapse (lateral margin only)	IV. Femoral head collapse with secondary joint destruction	IV. Flattening of femoral head without joint narrowing A. Mild B. Moderate C. Severe	IV. Joint narrowing with or without acetabular involvement
V	Pain with activity Further femoral head collapse		V. Flattening with joint narrowing A. Mild B. Moderate C. Severe	
VI	Pain at rest 2° degenerative joint disease		VI. Advanced degenerative changes	

[1]Functional Evaluation of Bone

3, a transitional stage was noted, which represented subchondral fracture in the presence of the crescent sign.[57] Stage 3 was characterized by disruption in the continuity of the epiphysis with partial collapse or flattening of the femoral head. Progressive secondary deterioration of the cartilage as represented by late joint space narrowing and establishment of the typical osteoarthritic changes are characteristic of Stage 4. With the increased use of the functional evaluation of bone, it became possible to diagnose osteonecrosis by core biopsy prior even to the abnormal uptake on the radionucleotide scans. Thus, it became necessary to add Stage 0, which represented normal routine roentgenograms, normal bone scan, and abnormal functional evaluation of bone.[57]

In an attempt to further modify the classification system, Steinberg,[156] in 1984, expanded to a 7-stage system. His stages are similar to those of Marcus and Enneking with the exception of the addition of Stage 0 and the subdivisions of Stages 2, 3, 4, and 5 into subcategories of mild, moderate, and severe in-

volvement of the femoral head at each particular stage. This system is comprehensive and useful in researching various treatment options.

In an attempt to return to simplicity, yet accurately reflect the significant physiologic events and appropriately guide treatment for each stage, the following new classification system is offered.

Stage One. This stage is characterized by an abnormal magnetic resonance imaging scan reflecting changes in the marrow elements and early changes in the trabecular bone that are consistent with the diagnosis of osteonecrosis (Fig. 21–11). This represents the initial pathophysiologic stage of bone ischemia and early repair beginning in the cellular structure of the marrow to osteocyte death and to the very early phase of appositional new bone formation. Plain films and tomograms are normal but radionucleotide scans may be positive.

This stage is a combination of Ficat and Arlet's Stage 0 and Stage 1. With the current wide-spread use of MRI and its reliability in diagnosing osteonecrosis in its earliest stages, the functional evalua-

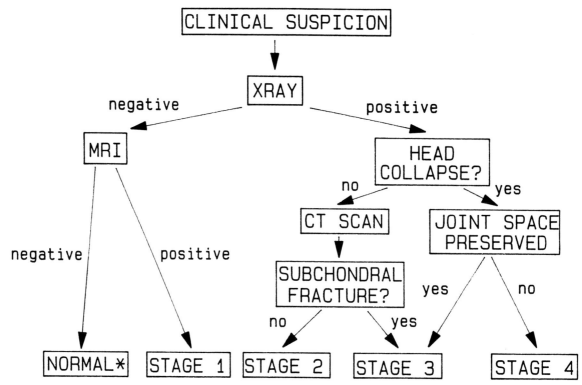

FIG. 21-10. Diagnostic and staging algorithm.

tion of bone via venography and core biopsy is no longer necessary. In addition, because prior treatment recommendations have been similar for Stage 0 and Stage 1 disease, combining these stages does not affect the pathophysiologic interpretation or treatment of early osteonecrosis.

Stage Two. This stage represents the presence of abnormal findings on routine AP and lateral roentgenograms (Fig. 21–12). Patchy sclerosis and cyst formation or evidence of a sclerotic sequestered area may be found. This corresponds to the pathophysiologic stage of appositional new bone formation on necrotic trabeculae. The simultaneous osteoclastic resorption of the ischemic trabeculae in the area of the subchondral plate is also occurring; however, subchondral fracture has not yet occurred.

Stage Three. The hallmark of this stage is the presence of a subchondral fracture, which is represented roentgenographically by the crescent sign (Fig. 21-13). There may be mild flattening of the femoral head but no collapse of the necrotic segment or joint space narrowing is yet present. This stage is further subdivided into Stage 3A (representing less than 50% of the femoral head involved) and Stage 3B (representing greater than 50% of the femoral head involved). The subdivision here is necessary in order to allow continued evaluation and research into the areas of rotational osteotomy, fresh

autogenous grafts, and osteochondral allografts in the treatment of femoral head osteonecrosis.[165] Although not currently useful in an everyday setting, their use in special centers may hinge on the extent of involvement of the femoral head.

Stage Four. In this stage, joint space narrowing, collapse of the femoral head and subsequent progression to the end stage event of degenerative disease occurs (Fig. 21–14).

A review of the treatment options available and their results from the time of femoral head collapse and joint narrowing to complete joint destruction would seem to indicate that no further subdivision of these latter aspects of the disease process is warranted. Further discussion in this regard will be presented in the following section.

Treatment

Even with a concise staging system and a better understanding of the natural history, the treatment techniques employed for osteonecrosis of the femoral head remain controversial. The ability to diagnose osteonecrosis in its "physiologic" (i.e., nonstructural phase) is possible with FEB and MRI scanning. MRI scanning gives us an easier, noninvasive way to diagnose a potentially catastrophic

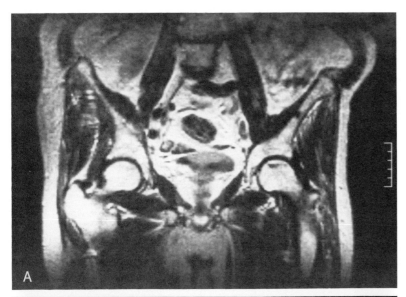

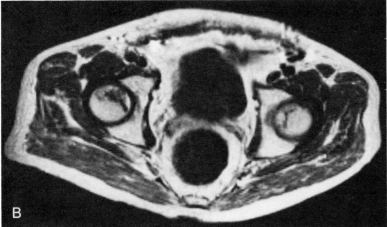

FIG. 21–11. Stage 1. **A.** Coronal images of a patient with right groin pain and an asymptomatic left hip. **B.** Transverse image of the same patient. Roentgenograms and bone scan of the left hip were negative. The images reveal bilateral decreased signal intensity of the femoral heads (Stage 1).

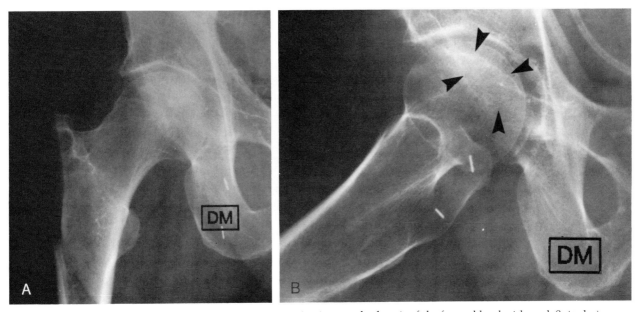

FIG. 21–12. Stage 2. **A.** Anteroposterior roentgenogram suggesting increased sclerosis of the femoral head with no definite lesion seen. **B.** Classic Stage 2 lesion with sclerotic border and no evidence of subchondral fracture (crescent sign).

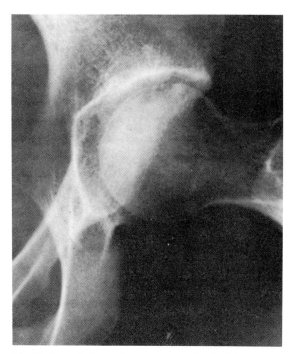

Fig. 21–13. Stage 3. Lateral roentgenograph of classic crescent sign representing subchondral fracture and progression from stage 2 to Stage 3. This is often more subtle and can be seen only on CT or MRI images.

bony disorder prior to actual changes in the bony architecture itself.[36,78,118,133]

An extensive review of the literature is offered on all current treatment modalities available in various stages of osteonecrosis (Table 21-4). A treatment plan is offered based on the relevant pathophysiologic stage of the disease and the review of the results of these various surgical techniques.

Prophylactic Treatment

In several of the conditions associated with osteonecrosis such as renal transplantation, sickle cell disease, and dysbarism, advances have moved us closer to the goal of preventing the disease process.

If modern day standards for decompression from deep-sea diving are followed, including slow resurfacing with staged decompression, virtual elimination of dysbaric osteonecrosis may be possible.

A dramatic decrease in the incidence of osteonecrosis following organ transplantation has been achieved through decreased postoperative corticosteroid doses and alterations in pretransplant renal dialysis protocols.[97,175] These changes in addition to administration of vitamins or phosphate binders where indicated have led to the reduction of osteonecrosis from 17 to 1% in one large series.

TABLE 21–4. *Treatment Options in Osteonecrosis of the Femoral Head*

Nonoperative Management
  Prophylactic Measures
  Symptomatic Treatment
    NSAID, Analgesia
    Limited Weight-Bearing
  Pulsed Electromagnetic Fields
Operative Management
  Femoral Head Preservation
    Core Decompression
    Grafting
      cancellous bone
      cortical bone
      muscle-pedicle bone graft
      free vascularized bone graft
      fresh autogenous graft
      osteochondral allograft
    Electrical Stimulation
    Osteotomy
      angulation
      rotation
  Femoral Head Resurfacing/Replacement
    Cup Arthroplasty
      -standard
      -"adjusted"
    Hemi-Arthroplasty
      unipolar
      bipolar
      hemi-TARA
    Surface Replacement Arthroplasty
    Total Articular Replacement Arthroplasty (TARA)
      -cemented
      -uncemented
    Total Hip Arthroplasty
      -cemented
      -uncemented
      -hybrid
    Hip fusion

Although statistical documentation is lacking, Kenzora feels that the number of patients with SS or SC disease who develop clinically significant osteonecrosis has decreased dramatically over the past 10 years.[97] This decrease is attributed to earlier intervention during a crisis with improved treatment modalities such as exchange transfusion and hyperbaric oxygen.

Control of alcoholism could dramatically decrease the incidence of osteonecrosis. Unfortunately, alcoholism is a widespread social disorder that is clinically beyond our control at this time.

Nonoperative Treatment

Symptomatic Treatment

Osteonecrosis of the femoral head is a progressive disorder.[38,70,100,107,157] Once the diagnosis of osteonecrosis has been made and a lesion larger

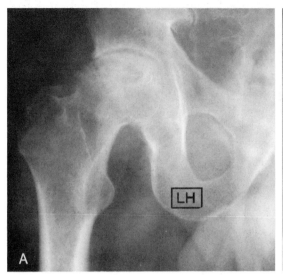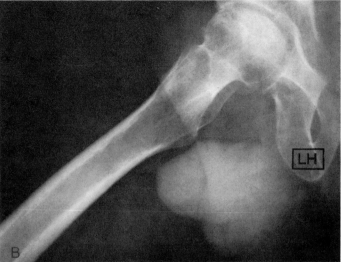

Fig. 21–14. Stage 4. Anteroposterior and lateral roentgenographs demonstrating joint space narrowing following femoral head collapse and signifying progression from Stage 3 to Stage 4 disease.

than 1.5 to 2.0 cm has been localized, early surgical intervention in an attempt to arrest the disease process is warranted in most patients.[97]

Symptomatic treatment, therefore, has a limited role in the treatment of osteonecrosis of the femoral head. This course may be undertaken in those cases that are diagnosed extremely early in Stage 1. These cases would include those diagnosed by magnetic resonance imaging where only pathologic changes in the bone marrow elements are noted. Once bony trabecular changes have occurred and the size of the lesion can be delineated, surgical treatment is warranted. Nonweight-bearing has not been shown to be beneficial in any stage of the pathologic process.

In addition to these rare instances of very early Stage 1 lesions, symptomatic treatment is warranted in high risk medical patients who are not candidates for surgical intervention. Similarly, patients who have reached Stage 3, are not candidates for joint preserving procedures, and those whose symptoms do not yet warrant joint arthroplasty may be treated symptomatically in the interim.

Electrical Stimulation

Several studies have recently reported the use of electrical stimulation in the treatment of osteonecrosis of the femoral head.[1,55,154] Most recently Aaron, et al.,[1] have reported on the use of noninvasive pulsing electromagnetic fields (PEMF) in a comparison study with core decompression. The study included only Ficat Stage 2 and Stage 3 le-

sions and evaluated both clinical and roentgenographic outcome. Stage 2 lesions demonstrated a clinical success rate of 87% with PEMF versus 62% with core decompression (p < 0.025). In Ficat Stage 3 lesions clinical success was noted in 55% of the PEMF group versus 25% of the core decompression group (p < 0.05). As expected, roentgenographic success was reduced in both groups and in both stages, but still showed statistical significance between the PEMF and core decompression groups in Stage 2 lesions (74% versus 38%). There was no statistical difference in roentgenographic success between Stage 3 lesions in the two groups.

The PEMF group was treated by using a single pulse configuration coil placed over the greater trochanter in specially fabricated shorts. The coil was worn for 8 hours per day and the treatment period ranged from 12 to 18 months. Five of 46 patients were noncompliant with treatment, however, there were no complications in the PEMF group. There were two major complications of subtrochanteric fracture in the 44 patient core decompression group.

Although more studies are needed with longer followup, the use of PEMF in the treatment of osteonecrosis is certainly encouraging at this time, especially in hips with documented femoral head collapse (Stage 3). The use of PEMF is also to be considered in patients who are otherwise nonsurgical candidates. If the findings of Aaron, et al.[1] are substantiated in future reports with longer followup, the use of noninvasive PEMF may be indicated in the initial treatment of Stage 1, 2, and 3 lesions.

Operative Treatment

Core Decompression

Core decompression has been advocated as a safe, reliable surgical intervention for the arrest of progression of osteonecrosis of the femoral head when performed in its early stages.[56,57,59,85,86] Prior to the advent of MRI, Ficat and Arlet recommended functional evaluation of bone during Stage 1 of the disease. Included in the examination is a core biopsy in order to histologically prove the presence of osteonecrosis. In the series from the Mayo Clinic, of those patients with a positive diagnosis of osteonecrosis, half required no further treatment at all subsequent to the core biopsy. The remaining patients eventually required surgery because of femoral head collapse and intensification of symptoms. Hungerford, Zizic, and Ficat have reported much higher success rates with core biopsy and decompression.[57,86,175] They have reported 90 to 100% good results on the asymptomatic side of patients with clinically symptomatic disease in the opposite hip. If surgical intervention is undertaken in Stage 1 or Stage 2 of the disease, these authors claim that disease rarely progresses to Stage 3.

Core decompression attempts to reverse the normal pathophysiology of osteonecrosis. The advocates of core decompression also advance the theory that increased marrow pressure is the main factor leading to the ultimate demise of the femoral head.[59,86] Once the initial insult giving rise to bone ischemia occurs, edema and fat cell hypertrophy subsequently develop. Continuation of the cycle occurs and a "compartment syndrome" of the femoral head develops. The increased medullary pressure contributes to an arrest of the reparative process leading to subsequent femoral head necrosis and collapse. The mechanism of action of core decompression is to open the closed bony space and relieve interosseous hypertension. As might be expected, intramedullary pressure tracing at the time of cortex penetration reveals a dramatic drop from the predecompression measurements. Extending the decompression channel into the femoral neck and femoral head further decreases the marrow pressure.[59,85]

In addition to relieving the "compartment syndrome," a well directed core channel also evacuates chronic debris and crosses the sclerotic margins of the reparative zone. (Fig. 21–15) Once the decompression has been achieved, regional revascularization of the femoral head occurs.

This regional revascularization most likely results from an overall increase in blood flow to the femoral head following decompression. Core decompression performed in steroid-induced osteonecrosis of the femoral head in rabbits demonstrated a return to normal or slightly elevated levels of marrow pressure 4 weeks following decompression.[172] The decreased marrow pressure caused by decompression decreases peripheral resistance in the thin walled sinusoids contributing to an increased rate of blood flow. The results of this study support the concept that core decompression is useful in the treatment of the early stages of osteonecrosis.

In addition to its reported ability to halt the progression of the disease, Ficat and Arlet[59] reported that the decompression procedure relieved some

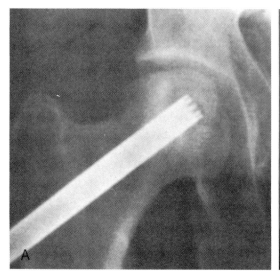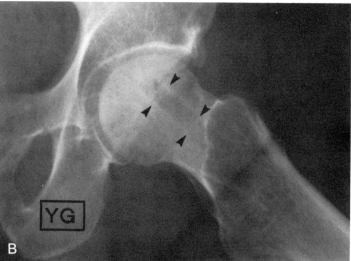

FIG. 21–15. Core decompression. **A.** Trephine in situ during core decompression of an osteonecrotic lesion. **B.** Core tract following decompression procedure.

symptoms. In over half of their cases ". . .the decrease in pain was immediate, having more or less completely disappeared by the evening of surgery." In addition, during injection of saline or contrast media during the functional evaluation of bone, many patients report an onset of pain corresponding to symptomatic complaints. These observations may demonstrate a role for increased medullary pressure itself contributing to the symptoms in some patients. Ficat[57] has divided his long-term results of core decompression into clinical and radiologic results. In a study of 133 hips, with 5-year followup, very good and good results in Stage 1 and Stage 2 were 94 and 98% respectively.

The radiologic progression was worse than the clinical result if one considers either progression to a subsequent stage or evidence of joint space narrowing at followup. Radiographically, Stage 1 hips showed 87% very good or good results and Stage 2 hips showed 67% very good and good results. Most patients who demonstrated joint space narrowing without progression to subsequent stages remained asymptomatic. Hungerford has reported similar results for Stage 1 and Stage 2 osteonecrosis.[85] It is quite evident that the earlier the core decompression is carried out, the better the results. Ficat has noted a decrease in results within Stage 2 in those cases that show a significant sclerotic zone.[57] These cases have had less satisfactory results than those diagnosed earlier in Stage 2, probably because of the author's inability to recognize subchondral fracture without the use of CT scanning or magnetic resonance imaging.

Although many authors have had good results with the use of core decompression in Stage 1 lesions, few have had as good a result as Ficat and Arlet[57] in more advanced lesions.[1,26,136,153,166,173] Camp[26] reported disastrous results with the use of core decompression. This was, however, a multicenter, multisurgeon retrospective analysis of this treatment modality. In other reviews, Warner et al.,[173] reported good to excellent results in 83% of Stage 1 lesions, but only 42% of Stage 2 lesions. Decompression was completely ineffective in any patient once subchondral fracture or collapse had occurred. The results may have been negatively skewed, however, due to a predominantly steroid-associated etiology. Of their patients, 80% had steroid-associated disease and the authors themselves admit to a possible susceptibility bias.

In another study of core decompression and nontraumatic femoral head osteonecrosis, Tooke et al.,[166] had 100% good results in Stage 1 lesions. In Stage 2 lesions 15 of 26 (58%) showed no progression, and 11 of 26 (42%) progressed to Stage 3 lesions. Again, however, there was a significant incidence of steroid associated disease. There was a 50% progression when steroids were continued compared with 22% progression when steroids were discontinued in these patients. The authors concluded core decompression is warranted in Stage 1 and 2 disease, however, patients with steroid-associated conditions should be advised of the high risk of progression. Again, it should be noted that in these studies CT scanning to evaluate an early subchondral fracture line and subsequent reclassification to Stage 3 was not routinely performed.

In summary, although results have been variable and studies have been inconsistent in patient populations and statistical evaluations, core decompression has had good to excellent results in approximately 85 to 100% of Stage 1 lesions. The great variability of results seems to come in Stage 2 lesions where reports of its efficacy are widely divergent. There have been no recent reports to advocate the use of core decompression in Stage 3 or Stage 4 lesions. The nonroutine use of further diagnostic tests (i.e., CT scan) in these studies to confirm Stage 2 versus Stage 3 lesions may account for some of the variability in results. Further studies in this regard as well as closer reporting of associated causes is needed to more precisely define an appropriate group of Stage 2 lesions to treat with core decompression (Fig. 21–16).

Bone Grafting

Not all clinicians agree with the theories and surgical treatment set forth by the advocates of increased marrow pressure. Some investigators believe that the insertion of a bone graft into the necrotic area of the femoral head is both reasonable and necessary to increase the success rate of the procedure.[50,116,126,151]

The removal of a large core of bone from the lateral femoral cortex to the necrotic area of the femoral head leaves a large open channel that is subsequently revascularized along its margins in a distal to proximal direction (Fig. 21–17). It is hypothesized that a race between formation of biologic bony support and collapse of the femoral head takes place with a decompression procedure. In those patients whose treatment is deemed successful, this new bone formation takes place early enough to resist the shear stresses in the femoral head that lead to subchondral fracture. Those patients who fail to

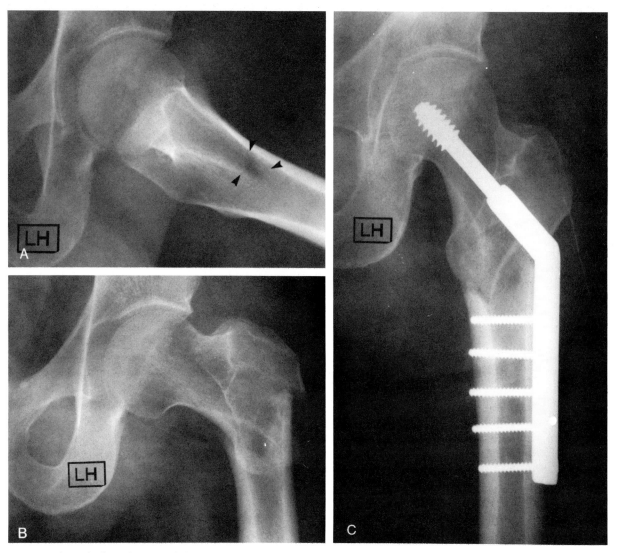

FIG. 21–16. Hole in the lateral cortex of the proximal femur following core decompression procedure. **B.** Subtrochanteric fracture sustained after a fall 2.5 weeks following core decompression. **C.** Subsequent open reduction internal fixation.

develop this bony strut, or who develop it too late in the disease process, progress to subchondral fracture and Stage 3 osteonecrosis. This may explain Ficat's diminishing results with core decompression in late Stage 2 lesions.

If indeed the addition of a cortical strut functions as outlined above and provides additional support to the femoral head, improved results over pure core decompression should be expected. In 1949, Phemister[126] described the use of a cortical bone strut in the technique of treatment of avascular necrosis for nonunion of femoral neck fractures. Two of three patients obtained good results, however, one patient had only 17 months followup. Bonfiglio and Voke[19] reported 75 to 85% good results in traumatic osteonecrosis and 70% good results in cases of idiopathic osteonecrosis. Boettcher and Bonfiglio[18] in 1970 reported on 38 patients with non-

traumatic osteonecrosis of the femoral head and noted only 16 (42%) good results. They noted at that time that those hips in the early stages of osteonecrosis fared much better than those with femoral head collapse. In 1973, Markus, et al.,[107] reported 63% satisfactory results when using Phemister-type bone grafts in the treatment of asymptomatic osteonecrosis.

It would seem then that the use of Phemister-type bone grafts yields 60 to 80% good results when done early in the course of the disease. Penix, et al.,[122] demonstrated that a properly placed cortical graft is effective in reducing the stresses on the femoral head after decompression. An improperly placed graft, however, will not only fail in this regard, but may actually create stress concentrating effects that increase the probability of femoral head collapse. The constraints for graft placement as de-

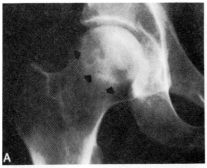
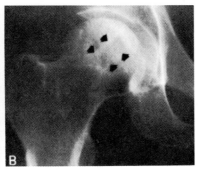
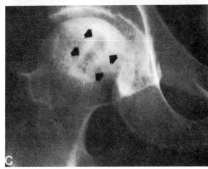

FIG. 21–17. A cylinder of appositional new bone formation seen in the margins of a core decompression tract six months following surgery. This new bone formation may prevent subchondral fracture by resisting shear forces on the femoral head during revascularization of the necrotic fragment. (From Kenzora JE: Idiopathic Osteonecrosis and Treatment Rationale. Orthop Clin North Am, 16:721, 1985.)

fined in this finite elemental analysis study may in part explain the inconsistent results seen in the past with this procedure.

Cortical strut grafting, although currently unpopular, may play a role in the treatment of late Stage 2 disease in which core decompression alone has less predictable results. If cortical grafting is to be undertaken, the graft should extend from the lateral cortex to the subchondral plate and transfix the entire length of the necrotic segment. Improper placement may lead to increased stress and subsequent femoral head collapse.[112]

In an attempt to improve the results of bone grafting for the treatment of osteonecrosis, the concept of muscle pedicle grafting became popular with several investigators. Meyers[114,115] and Baksi[10] have both reported 100% good and excellent results in Stage 1 and Stage 2 lesions. More advanced lesions, however, continue to show much poorer results. Although not as promising, Lee[100] reported 70% good results with quadratus muscle pedicle bone grafting and cancellous bone grafting in Stage 1 and Stage 2. Ficat and Arlet used a rectus femoris muscle pedicle graft and obtained satisfactory results in 11 of 18.[59] Although these results are better than those obtained with Phemister-type grafting, patient populations were relatively small. Further breakdown of early versus late Stage 2 was not available. In addition this vascularized graft is mostly weak cancellous bone and may lose some of the biomechanical advantages demonstrated in the study of Penex, et al.[122]

Still other investigators are using electrical stim-

ulation alone or in combination with core biopsy and bone grafting.[55,153,154] The results from these earliest clinical trials have been encouraging in some respects, yet in others have shown no significant differences with the adjunct of electrical stimulation.

Free vascularized grafts have been used with results similar to those presented above.[63,66,131] Fresh autogenous grafts and osteochondral allografts for the treatment of segmental collapse have been employed by Meyers.[113,115] Early results demonstrate 71% satisfactory results in the overall group and 85% successful results in the nonsteroid group. These advanced surgical techniques are experimental at this time and cannot be advocated for general clinical use.

Osteotomy

As the disease process continues and the osteonecrotic area shows evidence of subchondral fracture and subsequent femoral head flattening and collapse, decompression of the necrotic area with or without bone grafting has proven to be ineffective in halting the progression of the disease. Various osteotomies have been advocated in an attempt to preserve the femoral head in this young patient population.[110,112,117,160,170] Although unpopular in the United States, varus and valgus intertrochanteric osteotomies continue to be performed in Europe. Kerboul[98,112] presented a large series of patients who underwent varus or oblique derotation osteotomies for the treatment of osteonecrosis with mild to severe collapse. After one year, 89% had relief of pain and 60% preserved their functional capacity, these results deteriorated to 47% pain relief and 32% preserved functional capacity at 6-year followup. A major drawback of the procedure seems to be the inability to relieve weight bearing stresses in the osteonecrotic area, even in the modified oblique osteotomy.[9]

In a recent review of the indications and results of intertrochanteric osteotomy, Gottschaok[73] reported on 17 patients below 40 years of age who underwent valgus flexion osteotomy and subsequent fixation with a 95° blade plate. Less than 50% (8 out of 17) had satisfactory results at a mean of 3 years. Five patients required subsequent conversion to total hip arthroplasty within 4 years. Of these cases, 1 required an osteotomy so that the implant could be satisfactorily seated. Patients with metabolic bone abnormalities or those on corticosteroids had an overall worse prognosis. Despite acknowledging a steady deterioration of satisfactory results over time, Maistrelli, et al.,[104] believed the improvements noted lasted a significant period of time to warrant the procedure in a select group of young patients. They found that subsequent total hip arthroplasty was not affected by the osteotomy in most cases.

In an attempt to correct this deficiency, Sugioka[160,161] developed the transtrochanteric anterior rotational osteotomy (Fig. 21–18). In the precollapse phase, 100% of his 13 hips achieved pain relief and showed no evidence of progression or reduction in the range of motion of the hip. In 5 hips that demonstrated mild flattening of the femoral head 80% good results were obtained. Hips that demonstrated more severe collapse did not fare as

well. However, on closer evaluation those heads with less than two-thirds involvement continue to have 100% good results; those with greater than two-thirds of the head involved had good results in only 12 of 18 or 67%. In addition, the overall success rate in steroid-induced necrosis has been less than that in the idiopathic group. With cessation of steroids postoperatively 78% showed good results. With continued administration of steroid after osteotomy only 55% showed good results.

Although these results of postcollapse idiopathic osteonecrosis are certainly encouraging, they have seldom been duplicated by other investigators. Inexperience with this technically demanding procedure has certainly contributed to this deficiency.

Cup Arthroplasty

Cup arthroplasty as popularized by Smith-Peterson has had poor results in the treatment of osteonecrosis of the femoral head. Total capsulectomy, which is performed as a routine part of the procedure, further compromises the vasculature of the femoral head. In addition, because of the loose fitting nature of the cup, the weight-bearing stresses are transmitted through the superior lateral portion of the cup to the superior-lateral osteonecrotic portion of the head leading to further demise and collapse of the femoral head and ultimate implant failure.

A modification of this arthroplasty and its subsequent results were reviewed by Kerboul.[98] This "adjusted cup" arthroplasty was performed with a snugly fitting cup in order to transfer the weight-bearing stresses to the intact portion of the femoral head. Although relatively successful in those cases

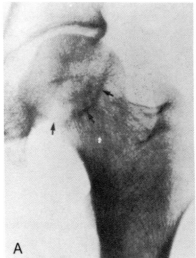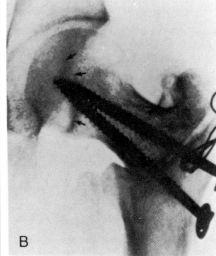

Fig. 21–18. Sugioka spin osteotomy. **A.** Preoperative antero-posterior roentgenogram of a left hip demonstrating sclerotic rim surrounding osteonecrotic lesion (arrows). **B.** Postoperative antero-posterior roentgenogram after 80° anterior rotation. Note the change in position of the sclerotic rim. (From Sugioka Y, et al.: Transtrochanteric rotational osteotomy of the femoral head for the treatment of osteonecrosis: followup statistics. Clin Orthop, 169:115, 1982.)

with a small percentage of femoral head involvement the overall success rate at 1- to 6-year followup was only 66%.

In a further attempt to modify the procedure, Luck described the spherocylindric cup (SCC). A recent review by Sedel, et al.,[141] describes the use of this spherocylindric cup arthroplasty for osteonecrosis of the femoral head in 38 hips with a mean followup of 6 years eleven months. A 79% overall successful outcome was noted in these hips. Five of 7 failures occurred within the first 3 years of the procedure.

Surface Replacement Arthroplasty

Initially viewed as an excellent alternative to the treatment of hip pathology in the younger population, surface replacement arthroplasty has nevertheless had disappointing results.[3,14,119] Dutton, et al.,[52] reviewed 42 hips treated with Tharies surface replacement for osteonecrosis of the femoral head. With a 2-year minimum followup there was an overall 20% failure rate in this population. In addition to the early high failure rate the theoretical advantage of preservation of overall bone stock has not been achieved (Fig. 21–19). Oversized acetabular components and structural allografts often are necessary to reconstruct a Tharies failure.[164] These poor results and technical difficulties with revision do not warrant the use of a surface replacement arthroplasty in the treatment of osteonecrosis of the femoral head. Uncemented surface replacement arthroplasty is currently under investigation, however, long-term followup is not yet available.[4,45]

Hemiarthroplasty

Hemiarthroplasty, and in particular bipolar endoprostheses, have gained wide popularity in the treatment of the latter stages of osteonecrosis.[79] Because of their "conservative" approach to the acetabulum and "preservation" of the articular cartilage, many surgeons view them as an excellent alternative to total hip arthroplasty. Although these implants are useful in the treatment of displaced femoral neck fractures in elderly patients, a review of the literature demonstrates a less satisfactory result when used in the treatment of osteonecrosis.

Cruess, et al.,[41] denounced the theory of articular cartilage preservation with the use of hemiarthroplasty. In a histologic study of canine acetabular cartilage following implantation of cemented hemiarthroplasties, repeated examinations demonstrated

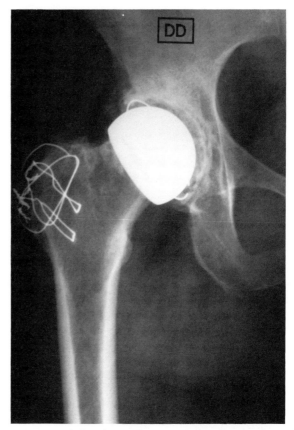

Fig. 21–19. Failed surface replacement arthroplasty with acetabular loosening. Note the loss of bone stock and subsequent need for bone grafting or a large acetabular component during revision surgery.

rapid demise of the articular cartilage with no normal cartilage demonstrable at 6 weeks following implantation. In addition to histologic changes, actual acetabular erosion has been noted by many investigators to occur in 25 to 30% of patients at 3 or more years following hemiarthroplasty (Fig. 21–20). Soreide, et al.,[150] showed accrued frequency of acetabular protrusio of 26%. In addition, older patients or patients with previous hip surgery had a much higher incidence of protrusio.

In an attempt to improve upon the 25 to 50% failure rate experienced with the use of Austin-Moore prostheses at three or more years followup, the low friction bipolar endoprosthesis was introduced.[4,59,121,13] Although it performed better than the Austin-Moore or Thompson prosthesis, the bipolar endoprosthesis has certainly performed below the expectations of the early investigators in this field. Steinberg[158] reported a 50% failure rate with the use of hemiarthroplasty in osteonecrosis of the femoral head. Cabanela and VanDemark[23] reported a failure rate of 23% at an average followup of 2 years. In another group of patients with uncemented femoral stems these investigators reported

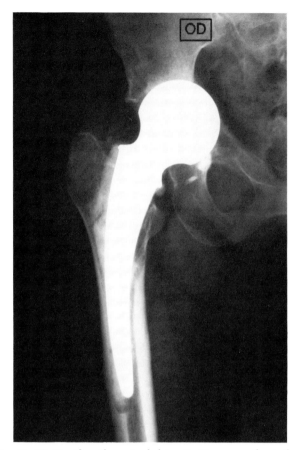

Fig. 21–20. Significantly protruded Austin Moore prosthesis that required a large central bone graft at the time of reconstruction. Acetabular erosion is a common problem with hemiarthroplasty especially in younger individuals or those with previous hip surgery.

a 15% revision rate with an average followup of 28 months.

In another recent report on the use of the bipolar endoprosthesis in osteonecrosis of the femoral head, Desman and Lachiewicz[45] report a 48% satisfactory clinical result at a mean followup period of 4.6 years. In their series, 26 hips were pressfit femoral components; 5 hips had a cemented femoral component. At followup only 9 of 31 hips (29%) required no medication for the treatment of pain. Six hips required occasional use of salicylates; 9 hips required frequent medication; and 7 hips had severe pain in the hips with severe recurrent disability. Three patients who had contralateral total hip arthroplasties had superior pain relief without the need for medication. In addition, acetabular cartilage narrowing or migration was seen in 47% of the hips.

In addition to the high failure rates, several other problems can be identified with the use of hemiarthroplasty. With all hemiarthroplasties, whether cemented or uncemented, violation of the femoral canal seems to result in less than optimal fixation when conversion to total hip replacement is necessary.[51,82,138,152] Conversion to total hip arthroplasty without removal of the femoral stem is an attractive alternative, however, the surgeon's ability to obtain proper soft tissue tension is at times difficult. In addition, each subsequent surgical intervention carries additional morbidity, mortality, and the risk of infection. Dislocations that occur following implantation of bipolar prostheses are more frequently met with the need for open reduction, thus increasing the above risks.

The osteonecrotic patient is in general younger and more active than the osteoarthritic patient.[132,168,169] Dorr et al.,[47] have demonstrated a significant decrease in functional results in younger patients with femoral neck fractures treated with bipolar hemiarthroplasty versus total hip arthroplasty. In this study, pressfit bipolar replacement was highly unacceptable, whereas cemented bipolar replacement yielded similar short-term pain scores, but significantly decreased functional scores in comparison to total hips. With time the functional results continued to deteriorate in the bipolar group while they continued to improve in the total hip group.

In summary, the unacceptably high failure rates coupled with several problems that may be encountered during conversion arthroplasty make hemiarthroplasty an unattractive alternative to the treatment of osteonecrosis following femoral head collapse. Although they felt their results were reasonable, Cabanela and VanDemark[23] stated that "... it is obvious, looking at the clinical results, that their overall quality (bipolar hemiarthroplasty) is inferior to that of a similar group of total hip arthroplasty patients. Indeed, the majority of the patients with good results complained of occasional pain, very often located in the groin, that we think arises in the acetabulum."

Total Hip Arthroplasty

Total hip arthroplasty has revolutionized the orthopaedic surgeon's approach to hip pathology. Although extremely successful in the treatment of hip arthritis in the elderly patient population, the enthusiasm for using total hip arthroplasty in the young patient with osteonecrosis has been tempered by several factors.[31,71,75,105,140] First and foremost is the fear of long-term complications of total hip arthroplasty in young patients. Chandler, et al.,[31] reports a 57% incidence of loosening at 5 years in total hip arthroplasty performed in patients less than 30 years old. Although this is certainly an alarming rate and cause for concern in performing this procedure in young patients a careful review of this paper reveals that a well done total hip arthroplasty in a well educated young patient carries a significantly higher rate of success. Chandler's paper is a retrospective study of total hip arthroplasty performed between 1970 and 1972 by 10 different orthopaedic surgeons with no patient- or disease-matched control group. In addition the surgical technique was deemed inadequate in the vast majority of those cases that failed (Fig. 21–21). So many variables were present in this review, the authors concluded that ". . . this study was considered to be too small to yield data for calculations of statistical significance." In a similar report of total hip arthroplasties in patients less than 45 years old, Dorr, et al.,[48] reported an overall 72% satisfactory result after 5 years. When patients with satisfactory surgical technique were reviewed, the authors report a 93% satisfactory clinical result. Ranawat, et al.,[128] reported a 90% good or excellent result in patients with degenerative joint disease between the

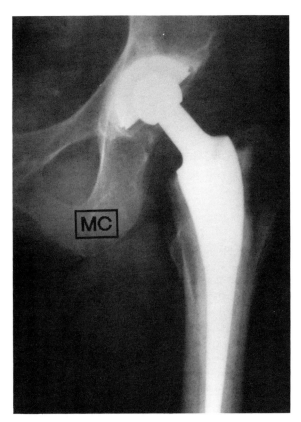

Fɪɢ. 21–21. Cemented total hip arthroplasty demonstrating good surgical technique with acetabular coverage, cement pressurization on both sides of the joint, good femoral component positioning and adequate cement mantle distal to the tip of the femoral prosthesis.

ages of 40 and 60. Although great concern is still warranted in performing total hip arthroplasty in young patients, the grave results often quoted from the papers of Chandler and Dorr should not dissuade the surgeon because much better results were noted when proper technique was used.

The second major area of concern aside from age is the common concern that patients with osteonecrosis obtain a less consistent result than patients with osteoarthritis.[37,128,137] Although many patients who were in need of revision surgery or who showed early signs of loosening in Chandler's series carried the diagnosis of avascular necrosis, it is also true that everyone of these patients had previous surgery on the affected hip. In addition, poor surgical technique contributed to 16 of 18 failures in this group. Dorr reported on 28 hips with osteonecrosis and found an 82% satisfactory result at 5 years. In comparison, 34 hips with osteoarthritis had a 79% satisfactory result. Although osteonecrosis comprised only 11% of the patient population in the paper by Ranawat, et al., these patients accounted for 50% of the revisions performed in that group. It should be noted, however, that 4 of 5 revision operations were done for fractured stems, which is less of a problem with modern alloys and larger femoral components. Although many orthopaedists use the literature cited above as evidence for the restrictive use of total hip arthroplasty in patients with osteonecrosis and the subsequent support of modalities such as hemiarthroplasty, a closer inspection reveals a different set of justifiable claims.

Engh, et al.,[54] reported on 35 cementless total hip arthroplasties performed for the treatment of osteonecrosis of the femoral head. Early symptomatic complaints, such as start-up pain and nonspecific thigh discomfort, spontaneously resolved to give 100% satisfactory results at 2.4 years followup. Although further clinical trials are needed and longer followup necessary, the use of cementless fixation in younger patients is promising (Fig. 21–22).

In a direct comparison of osteonecrosis and osteoarthritis patients following total hip arthroplasty, Ritter and Meding[132] found that although the osteonecrosis group was statistically significantly younger than the osteoarthritis group, there was no significant difference in long-term complications with their total hip arthroplasties. At followup ranging from 3 to 10 years, the revision rate in the osteonecrotic group was only 1.5%, whereas that in the osteoarthritic group was 3.5%. When considering socket demarcation, DeLee and Charnley[43] found no statistical difference between the osteonecrotic and osteoarthritic groups. Similarly,

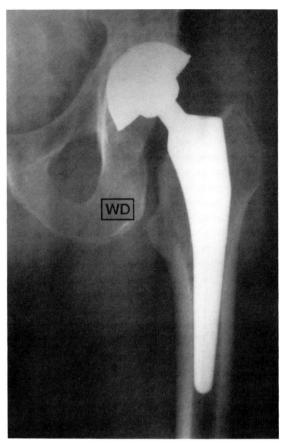

FIG. 21–22. Uncemented, porous ingrowth total hip replacement in a young individual with osteonecrosis of the femoral head. Note the good acetabular component coverage and appropriately sized femoral component.

Lord, et al.,[102] found that the results of uncemented hip arthroplasties in osteonecrotic and osteoarthritic patients were similar in regard to long-term successful pain scores.

A prospective controlled study was conducted at the Rothman Institute to evaluate the results of 84 total hip arthroplasties performed in patients with osteonecrosis versus 438 total hip arthroplasties performed in patients with osteoarthritis. All operations were performed at Pennsylvania Hospital by the same group of surgeons using a supine position, trochanteric osteotomy, and placement of cemented Charnley components. Preoperative demographic data was similar in both groups with the exception of mean age at the time of surgery and the number of conversion arthroplasties in each group. The osteonecrotic population was statistically younger (55.8 years versus 64.3 years, p < .05). In addition a statistical significance (p < .01) existed in the greater number of conversion arthroplasties performed in the osteonecrotic group.

Postoperatively, as was the case preoperatively, Charnley class and Charnley hip grading scores were similar in both groups. There was no statisti-

cal difference in overall revision rates. At a mean followup of 7.2 years (range 2.5 to 14.4 years) the revision rate in the osteonecrotic group was 9.5%. Comparatively with a mean followup of 8.4 years (range 2.2 to 16.6 years) the revision rate in the osteoarthritic group was 8.7%. Statistical significance was found in regard to the weight of the patient in that those weighing greater than 185 pounds at the time of surgery and followup demonstrated a threefold increase in the revision rate in both groups. Although an increase in the revision rate in the osteonecrotic group may be expected based on the younger age[31,37,48] and the greater number of conversion arthroplasties[88,138,152] this was not the case.

Hip Fusion

Because of the exceedingly high incidence of bilateral disease and osteonecrosis of the femoral head, hip fusion is seldom indicated as a treatment alternative. Consideration should be given to this treatment option in the very young patient with unilateral post-traumatic osteonecrosis that has progressed to Stage 4 disease and is symptomatically uncontrollable with nonoperative means. Fusion is contraindicated with any evidence of involvement of the opposite hip. In addition, the failure rate has been high because of the collapse and avascularity of the femoral head.

Practical Treatment Guidelines Based on Staging

In review of the treatment options available, it becomes clear that few are available to the community-based orthopedist that are both technically reproducible and that give consistently good results. Major research centers should continue their investigation into the use of implantable electrical stimulation, osteotomies, vascularized bone grafts, and osteochondral allografts. However, these procedures cannot be generally recommended for the treatment of osteonecrosis of the femoral head. A practical treatment algorithm is offered in Figure 21–23. Appropriate treatment can only be started after an osteonecrotic lesion has been appropriately staged.

Normal

Patients with clinical symptoms of hip or groin pain who have been evaluated with appropriate ra-

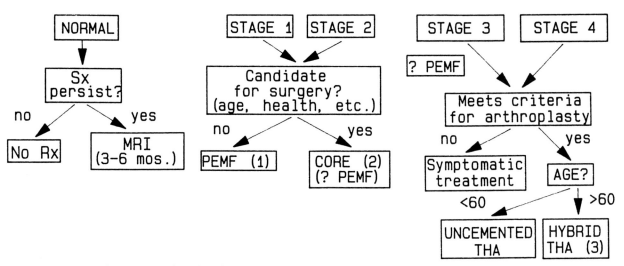

FIG. 21–23. Practical treatment algorithm for osteonecrosis of the femoral head.

diologic studies, all of which are normal, should be followed for persistence of their symptoms. If their symptoms resolve with symptomatic treatment, no further intervention is needed unless their symptoms reappear at a later date. In this instance, or in the instance of persistent symptoms despite symptomatic treatment with rest and nonsteroidal anti-inflammatory drugs, an MRI scan should be repeated 3 to 6 months after the initial evaluation because a lesion may become apparent in those few patients with initial false negative scans.

Stages 1 and 2

Treatment is recommended in all patients in this precollapse phase of osteonecrosis because the vast majority will progress in time. It must be stressed that nonsymptomatic "silent hips" should be treated similarly to those patients who present with a symptomatic Stage 1 or Stage 2 lesion.

In those patients who are candidates for surgical intervention based on age, health, and overall acceptable medical profile, core decompression is recommended. As previously stated, treatment with noninvasive pulsed electromagnetic fields, once further studied, may replace core decompression as the treatment of choice in this precollapse phase. The practitioner is asked to stay current in this regard to the further development of this treatment option and subsequent recommendations to its widespread use.

Stages 3 and 4

In general, once collapse has occurred the only surgical treatment option that gives consistent results is total hip arthroplasty. Once again, the use

of noninvasive PEMF may gain a wider acceptance in the treatment of Stage 3 lesions. In those patients who have progressed to Stage 3 or Stage 4 roentgenographically and do not yet meet the accepted criteria for arthroplasty (i.e., pain, function, disability) symptomatic treatment is indicated. In

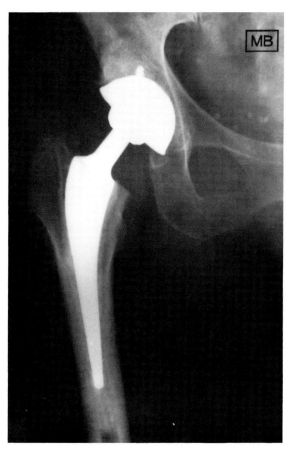

FIG. 21–24. "Hybrid" total hip replacement. Notable is the uncemented porous ingrowth screw-held acetabular component in a well placed cemented femoral component with good cement technique.

those patients failing nonoperative treatment, total hip arthroplasty is the procedure of choice. In those patients less than 60 years of age an uncemented, biologic ingrowth prosthesis is recommended on both the acetabular and femoral sides. In those patients greater than 65 years of age a hybrid total hip arthroplasty with a screw-held porous ingrowth acetabular component and a cemented femoral component is recommended (Fig 21–24). These are general guidelines in relation to age and other factors, such as those considered in performing primary total hip arthroplasty for osteoarthritis, should be considered.

References

1. AARON RK, LENNOX D, BUNCE GE, EBERT T: The conservative treatment of osteonecrosis of the femoral head: a comparison of core decompression and pulsing electromagnetic fields. Clin Orthop, 249:209–18, 1989.
2. AMSTUTZ HC, CAREY EJ: Skeletal manifestation and treatment of Gaucher's disease. J Bone Joint Surg, 48A:670, 1966.
3. AMSTUTZ HC, DOREY F, O'CARROLL PF: Tharies resurfacing arthroplasty. Evolution and long-term results. Clin Orthop, 213:92–114, 1986.
4. AMSTUTZ HC, et al.: Porous surface replacement of the hip with chamfer cylinder design. Clin Orthop, 222:140–160, 1987.
4. ANDERSON LD, HAMSA WR, WARING TL: Femoral-head prostheses. J Bone Joint Surg, 46A:1049, 1964.
5. ARKIN AM, SCHEIN AJ: Aseptic necrosis in Gaucher's disease. J Bone Joint Surg, 30A:631, 1948.
6. ARNOLDI CC, LINDERHOLM H: Fractures of the femoral neck. I. Vascular disturbances in different types of fractures, assessed by measurements of intraosseous pressure. Clin Orthop, 84:116, 1972.
7. ARLOT ME, BONJEAN M, CHAVASSIEUX PM, MEUNIER PJ: Bone histology in adults with aseptic necrosis. J Bone Joint Surg, 65A:9, 1983.
8. AXHAUSEN G: Histologische Untersuchungen uber Knochentransplantation am Menschen. Dtsch Z f Chir, 91:388, 1907.
9. BAKER KJ, BROWN TD, BRAND RA: A finite-element analysis of the effects of intertrochanteric osteotomy on stresses in femoral head osteonecrosis. Clin Orthop, 249:183, 1989.
10. BAKSI DP: Treatment of post-traumatic avascular necrosis of the femoral head by multiple drilling and muscle-pedicle bone grafting Preliminary report. J Bone Joint Surg (Br), 65:268–273, 1983.
11. BANKS HH: Factors influencing the result in fractures of the femoral neck. J Bone Joint Surg, 44A:931, 1962.
12. BARNES R: Fracture of the neck of the femur. J Bone Joint Surg, 40B:607, 1967.
13. BECKENBAUGH RD, ILSTRUP DM: Total hip arthroplasty: a review of thirty-three cases with long followup. J Bone Joint Surg, 60A:306, 1978.
14. BELL RS, SCHATZKER J, FORNASIER VL, GOODMAN SB: A study of implant failure in the Wagner resurfacing arthroplasty. J Bone Joint Surg, 67:1165–1175, 1985.
15. BELTRAN J, et al.: Femoral head avascular necrosis: MR imaging with clinical-pathologic and radionuclide correlation. Radiology, 166:215–220, 1988.
16. BISHOP AR, ROBERSON JR, ECKMAN JR, FLEMING LL: Total hip arthroplasty in patients who have sickle-cell hemoglobinopathy. J Bone Joint Surg, 70:853–855, 1988.
17. BOETTCHER WG, et al.: Nontraumatic necrosis of the femoral head. I. Relation of altered hemeostasis to etiology. J Bone Joint Surg, 52A:312, 1970.
18. BOETTCHER WG, BONFIGLIO M, SMITH K: Nontraumatic necrosis of the femoral head. II. Experiences in treatment. J Bone Joint Surg, 52A:322, 1970.
19. BONFIGLIO M, VOKE EM: Aseptic necrosis of the femoral head and nonunion of the femoral neck. J Bone Joint Surg, 50A:48, 1968.
20. BOYD HB, GEORGE IL: Complications of fractures of the neck of the femur. J Bone Joint Surg, 29:13, 1947.
21. BROWN JT, ABRAMI G: Transcervical femoral fracture. J Bone Joint Surg, 46B:648, 1964.
22. BROWN TD, WAY ME, FERGUSON AB: Mechanical characteristics of bone in femoral capital aseptic necrosis. Clin Orthop, 156:240, 1986.
23. CABENELA M, VERDENMARK RD JR.: Bipolar endoprosthesis. Proceedings of the hip society, 12:68, 1984.
24. CALANDRUCCIO RA, ANDERSON WE: Post-fracture avascular necrosis of the femoral head. Clin Orthop, 152:49, 1980.
25. CAMERON RB: Strontium-85 scintimetry in nontraumatic necrosis of the femoral head. Clin Orthop, 65:243, 1969.
26. CAMP JF, COLWELL CW JR.: Core decompression of the femoral head for osteonecrosis. J Bone Joint Surg, 68:1313–1319, 1986.
27. CATTO M: A histological study of avascular necrosis of the femoral head after transcervical fracture. J Bone Joint Surg, 47B:749, 1965.
28. CATTO M: The histological appearances of late segmental collapse of the femoral head after transcervical fracture. J Bone Joint Surg, 47B:777, 1965.
29. CHANDLER F: Aseptic necrosis of the head of the femur. Wis Med J, 35:609, 1936.
30. CHANDLER FA: Coronary disease of the hip. J Intern Coll Surg, 11:34, 1948.
31. CHANDLER HP, REINECK FT, WIXSON RL: A five year review of total hip replacements in patients under the age of 30—with emphasis on loosening. Orthop Trans, 3:303, 1979.
32. CHRYSSANTHOU CP: Dysbaric osteonecrosis: etiological and pathogenetic concepts. Clin Orthop, 130:94, 1978.
33. CHUNG SMK, ALAVI A, RUSSELL MO: Management of osteonecrosis in sickle-cell anemia and its genetic variants. Clin Orthop, 130:158, 1978.
34. CLAFFEY TJ: Avascular necrosis of the femoral head. J Bone Joint Surg, 42B:802, 1960.
35. COCKSHOTT WP: Hemoglobin SC disease. J Fac Radiol, 9:211, 1958.
36. COLEMAN BG, et al.: Radiographically negative avascular necrosis detection with MR imaging. Radiology, 168(2):525–528, 1988.
37. CORNELL CN, SALVATI EA, PELLICCI PN: Long-term of total hip replacement in patients with osteonecrosis. Orthop Clin North Am, 16:757–769, 1985.
38. COSTE F, et al: Evolution de l'osteonecrose primitive de la tete femorale (O.N.P.) et perspectives therapeutiques. Presse Medicale, 73: 263, 1965.
39. CRUESS RL: Experience with steroid-induced avascular necrosis of the shoulder and etiologic considerations regarding osteonecrosis of the hip. Clin Orthop, 130:86, 1978.

40. Cruess RL, et al.: Aseptic necrosis following renal transplantaion. J Bone Joint Surg, 50:1577, 1968.

41. Cruess RL, et al.: The response of articular cartilage to weight-bearing against metal. J Bone Joint Surg, 66:592, 1984.

42. Cushing EH, Stout AP: Gaucher's disease with report of a case showing bone disintegration and joint involvement. Am Surg, 12:539, 1926.

43. DeLee JG, Charnley J: Radiological demarcation of cemented sockets in total hip replacement. Clin Orthop, 121:20, 1976.

44. Deleeuw HW, Pottenger LA: Osteonecrosis of the acetabulum following radiation therapy: a report of two cases. J Bone Joint Surg, 70:293–299, 1988.

45. de-Meulemeester FF, Rozing PM: Uncemented surface replacement for osteonecrosis of the femoral head. Acta Orthop Scand, 4:425–429, 1989.

46. Desman SM, Lachiewica PF: The bipolar endoprosthesis in avascular necrosis of the femoral head. J Arthroplasty, 3: 131, 1988.

47. Door LD, et al.: Treatment of femoral neck fractures with total hip replacement versus cemented and noncemented hemiarthroplasty. J Arthroplasty, 1:21, 1986.

48. Door LD, Takei GK, Conaty JP: Total hip arthroplasties in patients less than forty-five years old. J Bone Joint Surg, 65A:464, 1983.

49. Dubois EL, Cozen L: Avascular (aseptic) bone necrosis associated with systemic lupus erythematosus. JAMA, 174:108, 1960.

50. Dunn AW, Grow T: Aseptic necrosis of the femoral head. Clin Orthop, 122:249, 1977.

51. Dupont JA, Charnley J: Low-friction arthroplasty of the hip for the failures of previous operations. J Bone Joint Surg, 54:77, 1972.

52. Dutton RO, Amstutz HC, Thomas BJ, Hedley AK: Tharies surface replacement for osteonecrosis of the femoral head. J Bone Joint Surg, 65:1225–1237, 1982.

53. Engel IA, et al.: Osteonecrosis in patients with malignant lymphoma. Cancer, 48(5):1245, 1981.

54. Engh CA, Gloss FE, Bobyn JD: Biologic fixation arthroplasty in the treatment of osteonecrosis. Orthop Clin North Am, 16:771–787, 1985.

55. Efetkhar SA, et al.: Osteonecrosis of the femoral head treated by pulsed electromagnetic fields (PEMFs): a preliminary report. *In*: Hungerford DS(ed): The Hip. St. Louis, Mosby, pp. 306–330, 1983.

56. Ficat RP: Treatment of avascular necrosis of the femoral head. Hip, 1983, pp. 279–95.

57. Ficat RP: Idiopathic bone necrosis of the femoral head (review article). J Bone Joint Surg, 67B:3, 1985.

58. Ficat RP, Arlet J: Diagnostic de l'osteonecrose femoro-capitales primative au stade I (stade pre-radiologique). Rev Chir Orthop, 54:637, 1968.

59. Ficat RP, Arlet J: Ischemia and Necrosis of Bone (edited by Hungerford DS), Baltimore, Williams & Wilkins, 1980.

60. Fisher DE: The role of fat embolism in the etiology of corticosteroid-induced avascular necrosis: clinical and experimental results. Clin Orthop, 130:68, 1978.

61. Frangakis EK: Intracapsular fractures of the neck of the femur. J Bone Joint Surg, 48B:17, 1966.

62. Freund E: Bilateral aseptic necrosis of the femoral head. Ann Surg, 104:100, 1936.

63. Fujimaki A, Yamauchi Y: Vascularized fibular grafting for treatment of aseptic necrosis of the femoral head: Preliminary results in four cases. Microsurgery 4(1):17–22, 1983.

64. Garden RS: Low angle fixation in fractures of the femoral neck. J Bone Joint Surg, 43B:647, 1961.

65. Genez BM, et al.: Early osteonecrosis of the femoral head: detection in high-risk patients with MR imaging. Radiology, 168(2):521–524, 1988.

66. Gilbert A, Judet H, Judet J, Agatti A: Microvascular transfer of the fibula for necrosis of the femoral head. Orthop, 9:885, 1986.

67. Glimcher MJ, Kenzora JE: The biology of osteonecrosis of the human femoral head and its clinical implications. I. Tissue biology. Clin Orthop, 138:284, 1979.

68. Glimcher MJ, Kenzora JE: The biology of osteonecrosis of the human femoral head and its clinical implications. II. The pathological changes in the femoral head as an organ and in the hip joint. Clin Orthop, 139:283, 1979.

69. Glimcher MJ, Kenzora JE: The biology of osteonecrosis of the human femoral head and its clinical implications. III. Discussion of the etiology and genesis of the pathological sequelae; comments on treatment. Clin Orthop, 140:273, 1979.

70. Glimcher MJ, Kenzora, JE: Osteonecrosis: The Pathobiology, Clinical Manifestations, Therapeutic Dilemmas. Instructional Course 103, American Academy of Orthopaedic Surgeons, Annual Meeting, Atlanta, 1980.

71. Goldblatt J, Sacks S, Dall D, Beighton P: Total hip arthroplasty in Gaucher's disease. long-term prognosis. Clin Orthop, 228:94–98, 1988.

72. Goodsir J: The mode of reproduction after death of the shaft of a long bone. *In* Turner W (ed): The Anatomical Memoirs of John Goodsir, Edinburgh, Adam and Charles Black, p. 465, 1968.

73. Gottschalk, F: Indications and results of intertrochanteric osteotomy in osteonecrosis of the femoral head. Clin Orthop, 249:219, 1989.

74. Graham S, Blacklock JWS: Gaucher's disease; a clinical and pathological study. Arch Dis Child, 2:267, 1927.

75. Hanker GJ, Amstutz HC: Osteonecrosis of the hip in the sickle-cell diseases. Treatment and complications. J Bone Joint Surg, 70(4):499–506, 1988.

76. Harrington KD, et al: Avascular necrosis of bone after renal transplantation. J Bone Joint Surg, 53A:203, 1971.

77. Hauzeur JP, Pasteels JL, Orloff S: Bilateral nontraumatic aseptic osteonecrosis in the femoral head: an experimental study of incidence. J Bone Joint Surg, 69:1221–1225, 1987.

78. Hauzeur JP, et al: The diagnostic value of magnetic resonance imaging in non-traumatic osteonecrosis of the femoral head. J Bone Joint Surg, 71(5):641–649, 1989.

79. Hedley AK, Kim W: Prosthetic replacement in osteonecrosis of the hip. Inst Course Lect, 32:265–271, 1983.

80. Herndon JH, Aufranc OE: Avascular necrosis of the femoral head in the adult. Clin Orthop, 86:43, 1972.

81. Hippocrates: The Theory and Practice of Medicine. New York Philosophical Library, p. 177, 1964.

82. Hoagland T, Razzano CD, Marks KE, Wilde AM: Revision of Mueller total hip replacement. Clin Orthop, 161:180, 1981.

83. Hopson CN, Sivehaus SW: Ischemic necrosis of the femoral head: treatment by core decompression. J Bone Joint Surg, 70A:1048, 1988.

84. Hunder GG, Worthington JW, Bickel WH: Avascular necrosis of the femoral head in a patient with gout. JAMA, 203:101, 1968.

85. Hungerford DS: Bone marrow pressure, venography, and core decompression in ischemic necrosis of the femoral head. *In* The Hip: Proceedings of the Seventh Open Scientific Meeting of the Hip Society. St. Louis, Mosby, pp. 218–237, 1979.

86. HUNGERFORD DS, LENNOX DW: The importance of increased intraosseous pressure in the development of osteonecrosis of the femoral head: implications for treatment. Orthop Clin North Am, 16:635–645, 1985.

87. HUNGERFORD DS, ZIZIC TM: Alcoholism associated ischemic necrosis of the femoral head: early diagnosis and treatment. Clin Orthop, 130:144, 1978.

88. HUNTER GA, WELSH RP, CAMERON HU, BAILEY WH: The result of revision of total hip replacement. Clin Orthop, 161:180, 1981.

89. ISOMO SS, WOOLSON ST, SCHURMAN DJ: Total joint arthroplasty for steroid-induced osteonecrosis in cardial transplant patients. Clin Orthop, 217:201–208, 1987.

90. JACOBS B: Epidemiology of traumatic and nontraumatic osteonecrosis. Clin. Orthop, 130:51, 1978.

91. JAFFE HL, POMERANZ MM: Changes in the bones of extremities amputated because of arteriovascular disease. Arch Surg, 29:566, 1934.

92. JONES JP JR, BEHNKE AR JR.: Prevention of dysbaric osteonecrosis in compressed-air workers. Clin Orthop, 130:118, 1978.

93. JONES JP JR, ENGLEMAN EP: Osseous avascular necrosis associated with systemic abnormalities. Arthritis Rheum, 9:728, 1936.

94. KAHLSTROM SC, BURTON CC, PHEMISTER DB: Aseptic necrosis of bone. Surg Gynecol Obstet, 68:129, 1939.

95. KATZ JF: Recurrent avascular necrosis of the proximal femoral epiphysis in the same hip in Gaucher's disease. J Bone Joint Surg, 49A:514, 1967.

96. KAWASHIMA M, TORISU T, HAYASHI K, KITANO M: Pathological review of osteonecrosis in divers. Clin Orthop, 130:107, 1978.

97. KENZORA JE: Treatment of idiopathic osteonecrosis: the current philosophy and rationale. Orthop Clin North Am, 16:717, 1985.

98. KERBOUL M, THOMINE J, POSTEL M, MERLE D'AUBIGNE R: The conservative surgical treatment of idiopathic aseptic necrosis of the femoral head. J Bone Joint Surg, 56B:291, 1974.

99. KIMMELSTIEL P: Vascular occlusion and ischemic infarction in sickle cell disease. Am J Med Sci, 216:11, 1948.

100. LEE CK, HANSEN HT, WEISS AB: The "silent hip" of idiopathic ischemic necrosis of the femoral head in adults. J Bone Joint Surg, 62A:795, 1980.

101. LOONEY WB: Late effects of early medical and industrial use of radioactive materials: part II and III. J Bone Joint Surg, 38A:175, 1956.

102. LORD GA, HARDY JR, KUMMER FJ: Uncemented total hip replacement. Clin Orthop, 141:2, 1979.

103. LUCK JV: Bone and Joint Diseases. Springfield, Charles C. Thomas, 1950.

104. MAISTRELLI G, FUSCO U, AVAI A, BOMBELLI R: Osteonecrosis of the hip treated by intertrochanteric osteotomy. A four to 15 year follow-up. J Bone Joint Surg, (Br), 70(5):761–766, 1988.

105. MALLORY TH, BALLAS S , VANATTA G: Total articular replacement arthroplasty. A clinical review. Clin Orthop, 185:131–136, 1984.

106. MANKIN HJ, BROWER TD: Bilateral idiopathic aseptic necrosis of the femur in adults: "Chandler's disease." J Hosp Joint Dis, 23:42, 1962.

107. MARCUS ND, ENNEKING WF, MASSAM RA: The silent hip in idiopathic aseptic necrosis-treatment by bone grafting. J Bone Joint Surg, 55A:1351, 1975.

108. MARKHAM TN: Ann Arbor case reports: aseptic necrosis in a high-altitude flier. J Occup Med, 9:123, 1967.

109. MATSUO K, et al.: Influence of alcohol intake, cigarette smoking and occupational status on idiopathic osteonecrosis of the femoral head. Clin Orthop, 234:115, 1988.

110. MASUDA T, et al.: Results of transtrochanteric rotational osteotomy for nontraumatic osteonecrosis of the femoral head. Clin Orthop, 288:69–74, 1988.

111. MCCARTHY E: Aseptic necrosis of bone. Clin Orthop, 168:216, 1982.

112. MERLE D'AUBIGNE R, et al.: Idiopathic necrosis of the femoral head in adults. J Bone Joint Surg, 47B:612, 1965.

113. MEYERS MH, JONES RE, BUCHOLZ RW, WENGER DR: Fresh autogenous grafts and osteochondral allografts for the treatment of segmental collapse in osteonecrosis of the hip. Clin Orthop, 174:107–112, 1983.

114. MEYERS MH: Surgical treatment of osteonecrosis of the femoral head. Instr Course Lect, 32:260–265, 1983.

115. MEYERS MH: The treatment of osteonecrosis of the hip with fresh osteochondral allografts and with the muscle pedicle graft technique. Clin Orthop, 130:202, 1978.

116. MEYERS MH, HARVEY JP JR, MOORE TM: Treatment of displaced subcapital and transcervical fractures of the femoral neck by muscle-pedicle-bone graft and internal fixation. J Bone Joint Surg, 55A:257, 1973.

117. MILLIS MM: Biplane intertrochanteric osteotomy for osteonecrosis. Presented at the Symposium on Osteotomy of the Hip and Knee, Boston, 1986.

118. MITCHELL DG, et al.: Magnetic resonance imaging of the ischemic hip: alterations within the osteonecrotic, viable and reactive zones. Clin Orthop, 244:60, 1989.

119. MURRAY WR, VAN-METER JW: Surface replacement hip arthroplasty: results of the first seventy-four consecutive cases at the University of California, San Francisco. Hip, pp. 156–166, 1982.

120. MUSSO ES, MITCHELL SN, SHINK-ASCANI M, BASSETT CA: Results of conservative management of osteonecrosis of the femoral head: a retrospective review. Clin Orthop, 207:209–215, 1986.

121. PATTERSON RJ, BICKEL WJ, KAHLIN DC: Idiopathic avascular necrosis of the head of the femur. J Bone Joint Surg, 46A:267, 1964.

122. PENIX AR, et al.: Femoral head stresses following cortical bone grafting for aseptic necrosis: a finite-element study. Clin Orthop, 173:159, 1983.

123. PHEMISTER DB: Changes in bones and joints resulting from interruption of circulation. I. General consideration and changes resulting from injury. Arch Surg, 41:436, 1940.

124. PHEMISTER DB: Fractures of neck of femur, dislocations of hip, and obscure vascular disturbances producing aseptic necrosis of head of femur. Surg Gynecol Obstet, 59:415, 1934.

125. PHEMISTER DB: The recognition of dead bone based on pathological and X-ray studies. Ann Surg, 72:466, 1920.

126. PHEMISTER DB: Treatment of the necrotic head of the femur in adults. J Bone Joint Surg, 31A:55, 1949.

127. PROSNITZ LR, et al.: Avascular necrosis of bone in Hodgkin's disease patients treated with combined modality therapy. Cancer, 47:2793, 1981.

128. RANAWAT CS, ATKINSON RE, SALVATI EA, WILSON PD JR.: Conventional total hip arthroplasty for degenerative joint disease in patients between the age of forty and sixty years. J Bone Joint Surg, 66A:745, 1984.

129. REICH RS, ROSENBERG NJ: Aseptic necrosis of bone in caucasians with chronic hemolytic anaemia due to combined sickling and thalassemia traits. J Bone Joint Surg, 35A:894, 1953.

130. Rico H, et al.: Increased blood cortisol in alcoholic patients with aseptic necrosis of the femoral head. Calcif Tissue Int, 37:585, 1985.

131. Rindell K, Solonen KA, Lindholm TS: Results of treatment of aseptic necrosis of the femoral head with vascularized bone graft. Ital J Orthop Traumatol, 15(2):145–153, 1989.

132. Ritter MA, Meding JB: A comparison of osteonecrosis and osteoarthritis patients following total hip arthroplasty. A long-term follow-up study. Clin Orthop, 206:139–146, 1986.

133. Robinson HJ Jr, Hartleben PD, Lund G, Schreiman J: Evaluation of magnetic resonance imaging in the diagnosis of osteonecrosis of the femoral head: accuracy compared with radiographs, core biopsy, and intraosseous pressure measurements. J Bone Joint Surg, 71(5):650–663, 1989.

134. Russell J: An essay on necrosis. Section I. General remarks and description of appearances. Clin Orthop, 130:135, 1978.

135. Russell J: Practical Essay on a Certain Disease of the Bones Termed Necrosis. Edinburgh, Neill and Co, 1794.

136. Saito S, Ohzono K, Ono K: Joint preserving operations for idiopathic avascular necrosis of the femoral head. Results of core decompression, grafting and osteotomy. J Bone Joint Surg, (Br), 70(1):78–84, 1988.

137. Saito S, et al.: Long-term results of total hip arthroplasty for osteonecrosis of the hip. Clin Orthop, 244:198–207, 1989.

138. Sarmiento, A, Gerard FM: Total hip arthroplasty for failed endoprostheses. Clin Orthop, 137:112, 1978.

139. Schein AJ, Arkin AM: Hip involvement in Gaucher's disease. J Bone Joint Surg, 24:396, 1942.

140. Scott RD, Urse JS, Schmidt R, Bierbaum BE: Use of TARA hemiarthroplasty in advanced osteonecrosis. J Arthroplasty, 2:225–232, 1987.

141. Sedel L, Travers V, Witvoet J: Spherocylindric (Luck) cup arthroplasty for osteonecrosis of the hip. Clin Orthop, 219:127–135, 1987.

142. Seiler JG, Christie MJ, Homra L: Correlation of the findings of magnetic resonance imaging with those of bone biopsy in patients who have stage I or stage II ischemic necrosis of the femoral head. J Bone Joint Surg, 91(1):28–32, 1989.

143. Sevitt S: Avascular necrosis and revascularization of the femoral head after intracapsular fractures. J Bone Joint Surg, 46B:270, 1964.

144. Sherman M: Pathogenesis of disintegration of the hip in sickle cell anemia. Southern Med J, 52:632, 1959.

145. Sherman MS, Phemister DB: The pathology of ununited fractures of the neck of the femur. J Bone Joint Surg, 29A:19, 1947.

146. Siegling JA: In discussion of "Necrosis of Femoral Head and Sickle-Cell Anemia." Presented at the Annual Meeting of the American Orthopaedic Association, Colorado Springs, 1966.

147. Smals A, Kloppenborg P: Alcohol-induced pseudo-Cushing's syndrome. Lancet, 1:1369, 1977.

148. Smith EW, Conley CL: Clinical features of the genetic variants of sickle cell disease. Bull Johns Hopkins Hosp, 94:289, 1954.

149. Solomon L: Mechanisms of idiopathic osteonecrosis. Orthop Clin North Am, 16(4):655, 1985.

150. Soreide O, Skjaerven R, Alho A: The risk of acetabular protrusion following replacement of the femoral head. Acta Orthop Scan, 53:791, 1982.

151. Springfield DS, Enneking WJ: Surgery for aseptic necrosis of the femoral head. Clin Orthop, 130:175, 1978.

152. Stambough JL, et al.: Conversion total hip replacement: Review of 140 hips with greater than 6 year follow-up study. J Arthroplasty, 1(4):261, 1986.

153. Steinberg ME, et al.: Osteonecrosis of the femoral head: results of core decompression and grafting with and without electrical stimulation. Clin Orthop, (249):199–208, 1989.

154. Steinberg ME, et al.: Electrical stimulation in the treatment of osteonecrosis of the femoral head, a one year follow-up. Orthop Clin North Am, 16:747–756, 1985.

155. Steinberg ME, et al.: Treatment of avascular necrosis of the femoral head by a combination of bone grafting, decompression, and electrical stimulation. Clin Orthop, 186:137, 1984.

156. Steinberg ME, Hayken GD, Steinberg DR: A new method for evaluation and staging of avascular necrosis of the femoral head. *In:* Arlet J, Ficat RP, Hungerford DS: (eds.) Bone Circulation. Baltimore, Williams & Wilkins, pp. 398–403, 1984.

157. Steinberg ME, Hayken GD, Steinberg DR: The "conservative" management of avascular necrosis of the femoral head. In: Arlet J, Ficat RP, Hungerford DS (eds.) Bone Circulation. Baltimore, Williams & Wilkins, pp. 334–337, 1984.

158. Steinberg ME, Unger AS: Femoral endoprosthetic replacement in younger patients. Presented to the American Academy of Orthopaedic Surgeons, 52nd Annual Meeting, Las Vegas, Nevada, 1985.

159. Stulberg BN, et al.: A diagnostic algorithm for osteonecrosis of the femoral head. Clin Orthop, 249:176–82, 1989.

160. Sugioka Y: Transtrochanteric anterior rotational osteotomy of the femoral head in the treatment of osteonecrosis affecting the hip: a new osteotomy operation. Clin Orthop 130:191, 1978.

161. Sugioka Y, Katsuki I, Hotokebuchi T: Transtrochanteric rotational osteotomy of the femoral head for the treatment of osteonecrosis. Clin Orthop, 169:115, 1982.

162. Tanaka KR, Clifford GO, Axelrod AR: Sickle-Cell anemia (Homozygous S) with aseptic necrosis of the femoral head. Blood, 11:998. 1956.

163. Thibodeau AA, Ames DL: Idiopathic avascular necrosis of the femoral head in adults. J Bone Joint Surg, 50A:836, 1968.

164. Tooke SM, Amstutz HC, Delaunay C: Hemiresurfacing for femoral head osteonecrosis. J Arthroplasty, 2:125–133, 1987.

165. Tooke SM, Amstutz HC, Hedley AK: Results of transtrochanteric rotational osteotomy for femoral head osteonecrosis. Clin Orthop, 224:150–157, 1987.

166. Tooke SM, et al.: Results of core decompression for femoral head osteonecrosis. Clin Orthop, 288:99–104, 1988.

167. Trueta J, Harrison MHM: The normal vascular anatomy of the femoral head in adult man. J Bone Joint Surg, 35B:442, 1953.

168. Vernace JV, Balderston RA, Booth RE Jr, Rothman RH: The results of Charnley total hip arthroplasty in osteonecrosis versus osteoarthritis. Presented 57th annual meeting American Academy Orthopaedic Surgeons, New Orleans, February 8–13, 1990.

169. Vernace JV, Balderston RA, Booth RE Jr, Rothman RH: The results of Charnley total hip arthroplasty in osteonecrosis versus osteoarthritis. Submitted for publication, April, 1990.

170. Wagner H, Bauer W: Five year follow-up of intertrochanteric osteotomy for ischemic necrosis of the femoral head. Presented at the Symposium on Osteotomy of the Hip and Knee, Boston, 1986.

171. WANG G, SWEET DE, REGER RI, THOMSON RC: Fat cell changes as a mechanism of avascular necrosis of the femoral head in cortisone-treated rabbits. J Bone Joint Surg, 59A:729, 1977.

172. WANG GJ, DUGHMAN SS, REGER SI, STAMP WG: The effect of core decompression on femoral head blood flow in steroid-induced avascular necrosis of the femoral head. J Bone Joint Surg Surgery, 67A:121, 1985.

173. WARNER JJ, PHILIP JH, BRODSKY GL, THORNHILL TS: Studies of nontraumatic osteonecrosis. The role of core decompression in the treatment of nontraumatic osteonecrosis of the femoral head. Clin Orthop, 225:104–127, 1987.

174. WOODHOUSE CF: Dynamic influences of vascular occlusion affecting the development of avascular necrosis of the femoral head. Clin Orthop, 32:119, 1964.

175. ZIZIC TM, HUNGERFORD DS: Osteonecrosis of bone. *In* Kelley WN, Harris ED, Ruddy S, Sledge CB (eds): Textbook of Rheumatology, 2nd Ed. Philadelphia, Saunders, 1985.

Total Hip

Operative Technique for Primary Total Hip Arthroplasty Using the Hardinge Approach

GEORGE R. PAYNE

Primary total hip arthroplasty is a demanding, yet predictably rewarding, surgical procedure. It should be approached with this attitude. Meticulous surgical technique and strict attention to detail is required for a satisfactory long-term result. A well performed total hip arthroplasty should resemble a symphony of motion. Each step is carefully performed and in combination results in a well orchestrated total hip replacement.

Anesthesia

Primary total hip arthroplasty has been performed routinely under spinal or epidural anesthesia at the Pennsylvania Hospital. This has proven to ensure adequate anesthesia for an appropriate length of time and has the advantages of reducing blood loss and thromboembolic complications, and preserving the mental acuity of the elderly patient. Hypotensive anesthesia also has been used and can significantly reduce blood loss. A program of autologous blood donation has been instituted, which minimizes the need for banked blood. This essentially eliminates the problem of transfusion reactions and transmission of diseases such as hepatitis and AIDS. The more complex reconstructions and revision procedures require greater flexibility in terms of operating time and in these situations continuous spinal or epidural anesthesia or general anesthesia should be considered.

Clean Operating Room and Prophylactic Antibiotics

Numerous studies support the use of a laminar air flow system to reduce wound contamination and lower infection rates. The vertical laminar air flow system in conjunction with operating suits and body exhaust systems have been shown to significantly reduce infection rates. After spinal anesthesia has been administered, the patient is brought into the laminar air flow enclosure where the patient is positioned and the limb prepared for surgery.

Prophylactic antibiotics are administered prior to surgery and many authors have substantiated their effectiveness in reducing infection rates. An antistaphylococcal antibiotic such as a first generation cephalosporin (Cephazolin Sodium 1 gram) is administered within one-half hour prior to surgery. At closure a second gram is given intravenously and continued for 48 hours.

Surgical Procedure Using the Modified Hardinge Approach to the Hip

A modification of the lateral muscle splitting approach to the hip described by Kevin Hardinge has been found by the authors to be a useful and effective alternative to trochanteric osteotomy.[1] The authors have used the trochanteric osteotomy as described by Sir John Charnley. This has been a dependable approach, with superlative exposure, and the opportunity to develop a meticulous technique of cementation. The only disadvantage of trochanteric osteotomy has been a 1% rate of nonunion. Despite this excellent rate of success and a high overall level of surgical satisfaction with trochanteric osteotomy, in certain patients an alternative approach that does not elevate the trochanter is useful.

Patient Selection

Those patients most ideally suited for the modified Hardinge approach are patients with osteopenic bone, slender elderly females, and patients who had prior surgical compromise of the greater trochanter but whose hip joint is not significantly distorted. Those individuals who have severe osteoporosis, particularly those with rheumatoid arthritis, tend to have bone of such diminished strength that fixation of a detached trochanter is technically unsatisfactory and despite special precautions the trochanter frequently separates. Special wiring techniques, trochanteric caps, and gentleness may be to no avail in preventing separation. Certainly, in these individuals it is a significant advantage to preserve the integrity of the trochanter.

The slender elderly female patient has a low risk of trochanteric loosening with cemented total hip replacements and therefore any compromise in the quality of this cement technique is less critical. Although the exposure gained with the modified Hardinge approach is less dramatic than with trochanteric osteotomy, the slender supple female usually provides ample exposure for a technically satisfactory total hip replacement using this exposure.

Patients who have had prior surgical compromise of the greater trochanter but whose hip joint is not significantly distorted also are candidates for the modified Hardinge approach. Certain patients such as those with prior intertrochanteric fractures or prior Thompson prostheses will have had compromise of the greater trochanter that would result in compromised healing potential. Nonetheless, their hip joint is not so distorted that one needs to resort to a trochanteric osteotomy.

Certain patients require greater exposure of the hip joint for a satisfactory total hip replacement. These patients are best suited for trochanteric osteotomy and thus represent a relative contraindication to the modified Hardinge approach. The young muscular male patient requires the most precise and meticulous implantation of the prosthesis and therefore is best served by elevation of the trochanter with its maximum exposure. In our experience these young patients with good bone stock have an extremely low rate of trochanteric detachment.

The obese patient also is a candidate for trochanteric osteotomy. For the most part obese patients are by definition contraindicated as candidates for total hip replacement. Nonetheless, the obese patient occasionally requires surgery and in these individuals there is again a demand for perfect fixation whether it is cemented or uncemented. This optimum fixation is best achieved by the greater exposure provided by trochanteric osteotomy.

Positioning the Patient

The modified Hardinge approach is performed at Pennsylvania Hospital in the supine position. The supine position allows for exact determination of the pelvic position in both the sagittal and coronal planes. This position also allows for direct measurement of leg length equality. The operating table is placed in a perfectly flat position. This prevents distortion of the body and thus miscalculation of component positioning. The patient is centered on the operating table so the sacrum is over the kidney rest or midportion of the table. The patient should be brought to the edge of the table so that the operative hip slightly overhangs the edge of the table. A sacral pad constructed of folded sheets is placed directly beneath the patient's sacrum. The dimensions of this pad are approximately 2 in. in thickness, 12 in. in length, and 6 in. in width. This modest elevation of the sacrum allows the fat and soft tissues about the trochanter to fall posteriorly away from the incision, thereby minimizing the amount of tissue that must be dissected in the lateral approach. A footrest is fixed to the operating table so that the surgical hip is flexed 40°. Both arms are placed on armboards and secured at a position of 90° of abduction to provide adequate room for the surgeon and the first assistant. The operating table is then placed in 5° of Trendelenberg in order to keep the pelvic veins and the veins of the contralateral leg empty during the procedure. The table is also inclined 5 to 10° away from the operative surgeon to improve visualization of the acetabulum during the procedure.

Preparation of the Operative Hip

Plastic adhesive drapes are used to isolate the operative field from the perineum and adjacent skin. The skin is defatted with Freon or ether. A large U-drape is placed isolating the perineum and abdomen from the hip. A second drape is then placed transversely above the level of the iliac crest completing the isolation of the wound area from the abdomen and thorax. Knee high supportive stockings are placed on the patient. Finally, the operative extremity is draped 1 in. above the level of the patella. A flexible adhesive electrocautery pad is taped to the opposite thigh. The foot is then placed in the leg holder. Prior to the surgeon leaving the operating room, the operating lights are adjusted. The function of laminar air flow and body exhaust systems are checked. A final discussion with the operating nurse is held to be certain that any special equipment needed for this case is available and in good working order. Administration of prophylactic antibiotics is confirmed with the anesthesiologist.

The operative field is then scrubbed for 10 minutes with Betadine soap. This is followed by a 10 minute preparation with Betadine solution, which is followed by alcohol, and then the area is dried. The limb is then removed from the leg holder by the circulating nurse and the surgeon grasps the foot with a double thickness stockinette. An impermeable drape is placed across the bottom of the operating table and brought up to the level of the patient's buttocks. This drape protects the surgeon from contamination by the operating table. The stockinette is unrolled to the level of the midthigh. A 1-in. sterile gauze strip is then wrapped around the leg to secure the stockinette in position and allow palpation of the anatomic landmarks, particularly the medial malleolus. This allows accurate assessment of the leg lengths during the surgical procedure.

The limb is then draped sterilely using two full size sheets, which are brought beneath the leg and buttock and held above the level of the iliac crest with towel clips. A double sheet is then placed transversely across the abdomen above the level of the iliac crest. Finally, an impermeable U-drape is brought beneath the leg and buttock and held again with two towel clips. The clean air room is then "sealed" at the head of the operating table with two sterile adhesive drapes.

Using a sterile pen, anatomic landmarks and the incision are outlined on the skin. The greater trochanter is outlined and the iliac crest and femoral shaft are palpated. The skin incision is then superimposed. Large crosshatchings are then drawn to indicate the position of retention sutures and act as guides to skin closure. Finally, iodine-impregnated plastic drapes are applied over the entire area of the skin.

Skin Incision

The hip is flexed 40°, steadied on the footrest, and slightly adducted. The skin incision is then outlined as previously mentioned with a marking pen. The incision is approximately 10 in. in length, extending 3 in. proximal to the trochanter and 7 in. distal to the trochanter. The incision is centered on a point 1 cm anterior to the apex of the vastus lateralis ridge. It extends distally by a gentle curve, ending at the juncture of the middle and proximal thirds of the thigh, which is at the center of the femoral shaft. The proximal limb of the incision is inclined posteriorly 45° and ends 3 in. proximal to the greater trochanter. The length of the incision depends on the size of the patient and the degree of obesity. Crosshatching is also marked on the skin for accurate skin closure (Fig. 22–1).

The skin incision is performed and carried sharply through the subcutaneous tissues down to the fascia lata. The fat is not reflected away from the fascia lata because this would create undesirable dead space. The anterior subcutaneous flap is retracted using a sponge and a Hibbs retractor. The posterior flap is held by the first assistant and compressed with a large sponge. The surgeon achieves

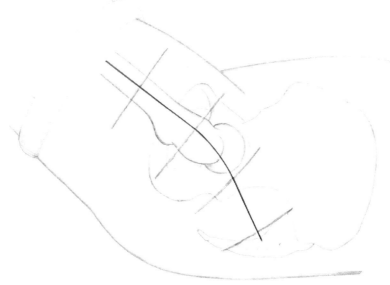

Fɪɢ. 22–1. Skin incision and landmarks.

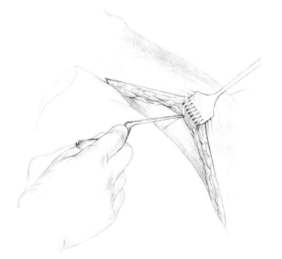

FIG. 22–2. Skin retraction and careful superficial hemostasis.

homeostasis using the electrocautery and bayonet forceps (Fig. 22–2).

Incision of the Fascia Lata

The incision through the fascia lata follows the line of the skin incision. The scalpel is used to penetrate the fascia lata distal to the greater trochanter where there is a natural plane between the fascia lata and the vastus lateralis. This allows safe entrance into the compartments (Fig. 22–3). The incision in the fascia lata is then extended distally using heavy Noble-Mayo scissors. The incision is not carried distal to the skin incision nor undermined. The leg is then slightly abducted and the incision in the fascia lata carried proximally in the line of the skin incision. During this proximal dissection,

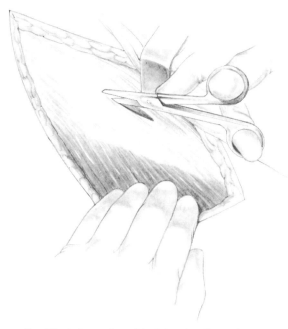

FIG. 22–4. Extension of incision distally with scissors.

the surgeon must be careful not to allow the deep arm of the scissors to enter and transect the fibers of the gluteus maximus. The fascial incision also must be 2 to 3 mm posterior to the tensor fascia femoris muscle to prevent excessive bleeding (Fig. 22–4).

The posterior fascial structures are gently retracted posteriorly and using the heavy scissors, the trochanteric bursa is incised in the plane between the vastus lateralis muscle and the trochanteric bursa.

At this juncture, the fibers of the gluteus maximus are split proximally using firm thumb dissection (Fig. 22–5). For the right hip, the surgeon's left hand and left thumb perform this muscle splitting maneuver. For the left hip, the surgeon's right hand

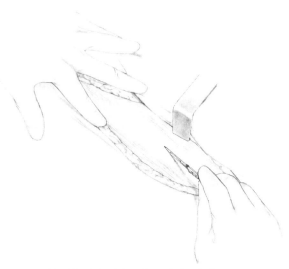

FIG. 22–3. Incision through fascia lata.

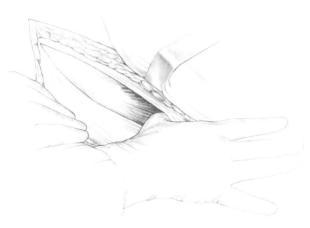

FIG. 22–5. Splitting of the gluteus maximus muscle.

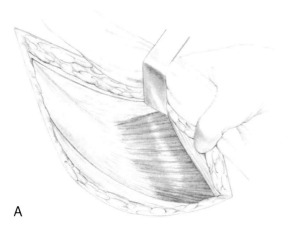

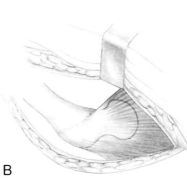

FIG. 22–6. A. Retraction of anterior fascia and identification of anterior posterior borders of gluteus medius muscle. **B.** The location of the femoral neck and head is shown.

A   B

and right thumb perform this maneuver. The posterior soft tissue flap can then be easily mobilized and a large sponge packed proximally to achieve homeostasis. The anterior flap of the fascia lata is retracted with the Hibbs retractor (Fig. 22–6A) and the fascia is dissected anteriorly and proximally off the gluteus medius. At this point, the gluteus medius muscle and greater trochanter are well exposed (Fig. 22–6B). It is not necessary to dissect the interval between the gluteus medius muscle and the anterior capsule.

Splitting the Gluteus Medius and Minimus

The basic premise of the modified Hardinge approach is to develop an anterior flap composed of the anterior portion of the vastus lateralis, the anterior capsule of the hip, and the anterior third of the gluteus medius and minimus muscles to allow exposure of the hip joint. The location of the muscle split is determined by the relative angle of the femoral neck. In those individuals with a varus neck shaft angle, the split is made relatively anteriorly and only a small portion of the gluteus medius is reflected anteriorly, i.e., approximately 25%. In individuals with a valgus neck shaft angle, the split is made more posteriorly carrying 35 to 40% of the gluteus medius fibers anteriorly with almost a horizontal split in the gluteus medius muscle. All else being equal, it is better to have a small segment of the gluteus medius muscle anteriorly because this muscle tissue is at risk of being denervated during the procedure and stability is compromised as one makes the split more posteriorly into the gluteus medius musculature.

The muscle split in the gluteus medius is made using a sharp Cobb elevator beginning just proxi-

mal to the gluteus medius tendon and dissecting through the muscle belly in line with the fibers (Fig. 22–7). This split is carried proximally to a point 3 to 4 cm from the tendinous tissue. The surgeon should be cautious about extending this incision too far proximally because damage to the superior gluteal nerve and vessels can occur with subsequent denervation of the anterior muscle fibers. It should be recalled that the neurovascular structures course beneath the gluteus medius from a posterior to an anterior direction and can be easily traumatized. The split is carried distally with the Cobb elevator until tendinous tissue is encountered. The authors find it convenient to develop this split using the index finger of one hand and the Cobb elevator in the other hand. Once the gluteus medius is penetrated, the surgeon will confront a fatty layer beneath which is found the gluteus minimus muscle. The surgeon may then elect to either bypass this muscle belly by retracting it anteriorly, or split the gluteus minimus as well. The surgeon

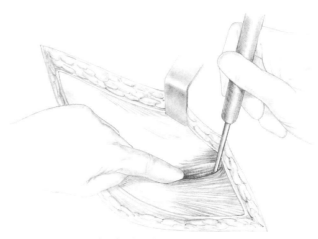

FIG. 22–7. Longitudinal split of the anterior one-third of the gluteus medius muscle using a Cobb nail.

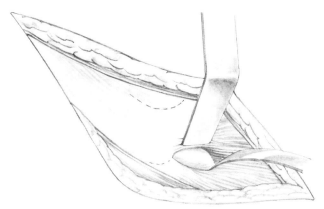

Fig. 22–8. Retraction of the split anterior and posteriorly with retractors.

is then down to the level of the hip capsule, which is cleaned with a Cobb elevator.

A Hibbs retractor or blunt-tipped Homan retractor are placed anteriorly, retracting the interior fibers of the gluteus medius and minimus. The second blunt-tipped Homan retractor is placed posteriorly around the femoral neck retracting the bulk of the gluteus medius muscle posteriorly (Fig. 22–8). The gluteus medius tendon is then split using the electrocautery. The tendon is split down to the bone of the greater trochanter. The capsule will then be well visualized in the depths of the wound. The capsule is then inspected and cleared once again. The capsule itself is incised parallel to the superior aspect of the femoral neck. This is extended to the bony rim of the acetabulum. This horizontal capsular incision is made slightly more posteriorly than the muscle split itself. This horizontal incision will allow easy dislocation of the hip and good visualization of the acetabulum (Fig. 22–9).

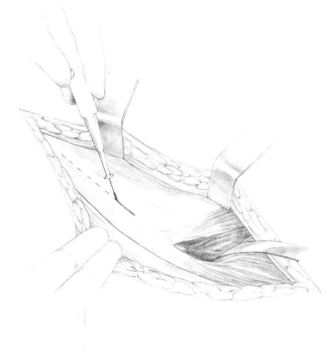

Fig. 22–10. Longitudinal split of the vastus lateralis muscle with Bovie coagulator.

Vastus Lateralis Incision

The anterior one-third of the vastus lateralis is now incised longitudinally using the electrocautery beginning at the trochanteric ridge and extending distally 7 to 8 cm (Fig. 22–10). This muscle is split down to the lateral aspect of the femur. The vastus lateralis flap is dissected subperiosteally in an anterior direction. A Bennet retractor is then placed around the femur medially to reflect the vastus lateralis flap anteriorly (Fig. 22–11).

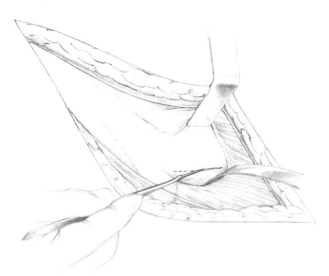

Fig. 22–9. Superior capsular incision.

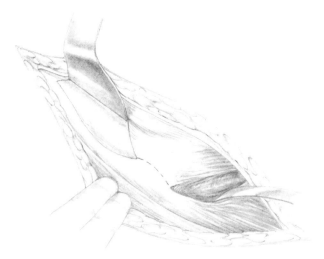

Fig. 22–11. Identification of the gluteus medius/vastus lateralis conjoined tendon.

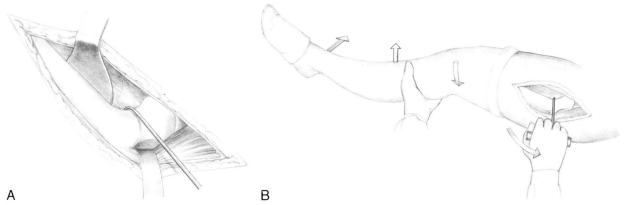

Fig. 22–12. A. Completion of anterior exposure prior to dislocation. **B.** Dislocation of the hip involving a direct lateral pull with the hook and an adduction/external rotation force on the leg.

Transection of the Bridging Gluteus Medius and Anterior Capsule

There now remains an anterior bridge of soft tissue along the greater trochanter between the incision in the vastus lateralis and the incision in the gluteus medius and superior capsule. This bridge consists of the anterior fibers of the gluteus medius. This bridge of soft tissue is incised through the tendon in a gentle arc along the anterior aspect of the greater trochanter connecting the incisions between the vastus lateralis and the gluteus medius split (Fig. 22–11). Ideally, good soft tissues are present on both sides of this arc to allow effective repair during closure. Using the cutting current and tooth forceps, this bridge of soft tissue is dissected from the anterior part of the greater trochanter developing a flap in continuity consisting of the anterior portion of the gluteus medius, the anterior hip capsule, and the anterior portion of the vastus lateralis. This is now carried medially with the second assistant retracting the flap with the Hibbs retractor and the surgeon gradually externally rotating the leg and continuing this dissection with the cutting current. The capsule is elevated off the anterior femoral neck and the dissection carried medially until the medial aspect of the neck of the femur is exposed and one is able to palpate the lesser trochanter. At this point there is generally sufficient exposure and relaxation to allow for a gentle dislocation of the hip.

Dislocation of the Hip

A bone hook is placed around the neck of the femur anteriorly and the leg externally rotated to allow for dislocation of the hip (Fig. 22–12). Forced torque on the femur is contraindicated because of the risk of fracture. If dislocation is difficult, addi-

tional capsule must be released or overhanging osteophytes removed.

Once dislocation has been achieved, the leg is placed in a position of adduction across the operating table with slight external rotation.

Amputation of the Femoral Head and Neck

A femoral rasp, the size of which is determined from the previous use of templates on the x-rays, is now placed on the anterior aspect of the femur and the planned femoral neck cut marked using the coagulation current. After this mark is inscribed, two blunt-tipped Homan retractors are placed about the femoral neck to protect the soft tissues. The head and neck are amputated using a power saw (Fig. 22–13). Often, the surgeon inadvertently anteverts this cut. Careful orientation of the flexed knee perpendicular to the floor prevents this error. Ideally the cut is made in neutral to 10° of anteversion. The femoral head should be stabilized with a towel

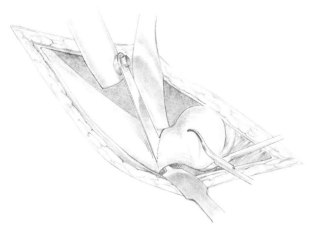

Fig. 22–13. Osteotomy of the femoral neck.

clip by the first assistant while the femoral neck cut is being made. The head is removed and inspected. The disease is carefully noted. The head should be saved for bone graft and this should be emphasized to the scrub nurse so that it will not be inadvertently passed off the table.

Acetabular Exposure

The first retractor placed is the anterior acetabular retractor. For easier exposure, the limb is maintained in slight adduction. A small plane is created between the anterior wall of the acetabulum and the anterior capsule using the Cobb elevator. A blunt-tipped Homan retractor is then placed in the twelve o'clock position anterior to the acetabulum and beneath the capsule. The second assistant can then easily retract the anterior soft tissues.

A second spiked Müller acetabular retractor is then placed in the superior aspect of the acetabulum retracting the superior capsule in a cranial direction. This would be placed at nine o'clock for a right hip and three o'clock for a left hip. The exact placement of the retractor is outside of the labrum and inside of the capsule. Using an impactor and mallet, the surgeon then drives this retractor into the ilium in a slightly cranial direction. If the tip is driven directly perpendicular to the axis of the body, the tip may perforate the dome of the acetabulum. This could become exposed during the reaming process. The handle of this retractor is stabilized by the first assistant.

In order to allow mobilization of the proximal femur and good exposure of the acetabulum, a relaxing incision is routinely made in the anterior capsular flap. A Kelly hemostat is inserted between the iliopsoas muscle and the capsule anteriorly in line with the pubofemoral ligament. The capsule is then incised from medial to lateral. At this point, increased mobilization of the femur in a posterior direction is possible.

A third acetabular retractor is now placed inferiorly. Two varieties of Müller retractors are available for this purpose both exhibiting a double curvature. A large retractor is available for large male patients and conversely a smaller inferior acetabular retractor is available for small female patients. This retractor is placed into the ischium inferiorly rather than directly beneath the inferior acetabular osteophytes. If osteophytes are used for anchorage, they frequently fracture and create a difficult problem in exposure. The blade of the retractor should rest on the neck of the femur rather than on the cut surface, thus allowing a second assistant to retract

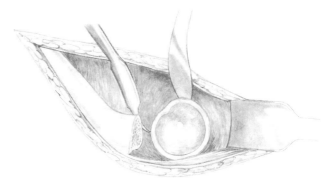

Fɪɢ. 22–14. Placement of the acetabular retractors.

the proximal femur easily in a posterior and inferior position (Fig. 22–14).

If further exposure is needed, a final and fourth retractor may be placed in the posterior position using a small spiked Mueller retractor outside of the labrum but inside the capsule. Care must be exercised not to injure the sciatic nerve. At this juncture, the leg should be placed in slight adduction and crossed gently over the opposite extremity at the level of the ankle. Excellent acetabular exposure is now generously achieved.

Preparation of the Acetabulum for Reaming

Defining the bony margins of the acetabulum is necessary for accurate acetabular component positioning. For these limits to be evident, the glenoid labrum must be excised. This excision is performed by making a transverse incision in the labrum at the six o'clock position. The labrum is then grasped with Kocher forceps and a scalpel is used to sweep the interior bony margin of the acetabulum thus excising the labrum completely (Fig. 22–15). Only the superficial portion of the transverse ligament of the fovea is excised. The contents of the fovea are sharply excised with a Kocher knife or with a cutting current. A small bleeder is frequently encountered in the depths of the fovea which can be controlled using an Adson hemostat and the electrocautery. It is not necessary to excise or uncover "a buried fovea" that is completely covered by osteophytes, since the medial reaming will accomplish this goal.

If osteophyte formation has occurred, creating a sphere of the acetabulum of greater than 180°, the osteophytes are removed with a rongeur until a hemisphere of 180° is created. The soft tissue must first be dissected from the outer portions of the osteophytes. Excessive bone should not be removed inferiorly because the inferior retractor may lose its purchase.

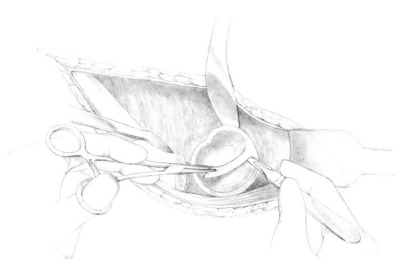

Fig. 22–15. Excision of the glenoid labrum.

Reaming of the Acetabulum

The acetabulum is now reamed using power graters. Reaming begins with the 44 or 48 mm reamers depending on the size of the acetabulum. These smaller reamers are used for initial medialization of the acetabulum. Prior to reaming, the tilt of the pelvis is noted by determining the plane between the two anterior superior iliac spines. The reamer is then held in the position that is desirable for the final seating of the acetabular component (Fig. 22–16). The desired position of the acetabular component is neutral to 5° of anteversion and 35 to 40° of inclination from the horizontal axis of the pelvis. Because of an approximate 20 to 30° anterior tilt to the pelvis on the operating table, the acetabular reamer must be held in this degree of antiversion. Acetabular reaming is continued in two mm increments using the power graters. Proper orientation is maintained throughout the reaming process. Preoperative templating and direct observation of the

size of the acetabulum will determine the final size of the acetabular reamer. During the reaming process, the surgeon must constantly check the acetabulum to be certain that he has not reamed centrally beyond the floor of the fovea. The mouth of the acetabulum should also be reamed slightly larger with the final reamer to prevent any overhang of the acetabular rim. Repeated early trial insertions of the acetabular components prevent excessive reaming. Reaming is complete when the dimensions of the bony acetabulum appear to cover completely the appropriate acetabular component. The final grater is removed from the power reamer and inserted in the acetabulum in the position of the final acetabular component. Appropriate bony coverage of the grater is noted. It is also tested for concentric reaming by noting the stability of the grater and testing for adequate seating by placing an Adson hemostat through several of the grater holes to make certain it is up against the acetabular floor (Fig. 22–17). If complete bony coverage is not evi-

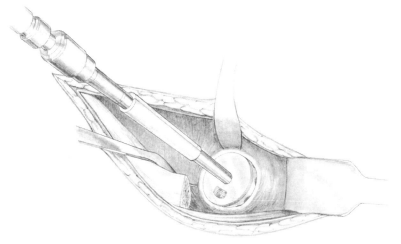

Fig. 22–16. Reaming of the acetabulum.

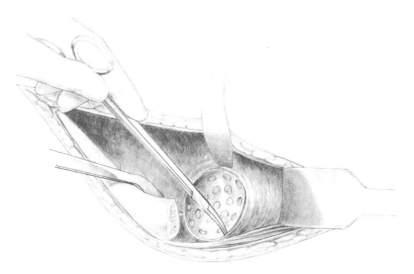

FIG. 22–17. The last reamer is used as a trial. The intimacy of contact of the reamer with the underlying bone is checked with a curved hemostat.

dent or the reaming is not concentric, then further centralization with the reamer is necessary. If the floor of the fovea has been reached with the reamer and bony coverage is still inadequate, bone grafting of the roof of the acetabulum may be necessary.

Curettage and Final Cleansing of the Acetabulum

The residual articular cartilage and fibrous tissue must be completely removed from the inner aspect of the acetabulum. This is accomplished with varying sizes of Mueller curettes and angled curettes. If acetabular cysts are encountered, they first must be emptied of their contents prior to bone grafting (Fig. 22–18).

Pulsatile Lavage and Final Preparation of the Acetabulum

Copious irrigation of the acetabulum and surrounding soft tissues are then performed with antibiotic irrigation. A Bacitracin mixture is currently

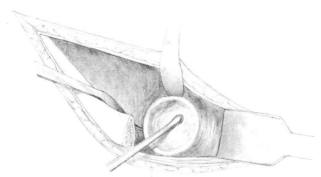

FIG. 22–18. Curettage of the acetabulum.

used. The acetabulum is dried and a slurry of bone graft obtained from reamings of the femoral head is placed in the fovea and in any acetabular cysts.

Introduction of the Acetabular Component

The acetabular component is inserted in a position identical to the position of reaming. The surgeon palpates the pelvic landmarks at this juncture to confirm the tilt to the pelvis in the transverse axis of the anterior superior iliac spines (Fig. 22–19). The acetabular component is inserted on the socket holder (Fig. 22–20). and held in 35 to 40° of inclination from the horizontal axis of the pelvis and neutral to 5° of true antiversion (Fig 22–21). Medialization of the acetabular component is accomplished first by placing an impactor on the lateral aspect of the socket holder and seating the component medially with a mallet (Fig. 22–22). Once medialization has been accomplished, final seating of the metal cup is accomplished by impacting the socket holder with a mallet. Care is taken to make certain the component remains in the appropriate position during seating. The acetabulum is then irrigated and the component is checked for proper seating by placing the curved Adson hemostat through the central hole in the metal cup to make certain it is sitting on the floor of the acetabulum. If this has not been accomplished, further impacting is necessary. Care should be taken not to fracture the acetabulum. Once proper seating has been accomplished, the component is checked for stability. Further stability is then achieved by placing three to four large self-tapping screws through the central holes in the

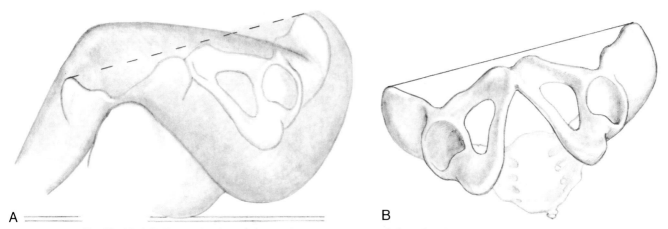

Fig. 22–19. A,B. Determination of the precise transverse axis of the pelvis by palpation of the iliac crest.

metal cup and one to two small self-tapping screws in the peripheral holes of the metal cup (Fig 22–23). This is done in a routine fashion using the appropriate size drill and checking screw size with a depth gauge. The large central screws should be preferably placed in a position of 180° arc superiorly. This will avoid placing the screws in a position near the sciatic nerve or anterior neurovascular structures. Once the peripheral screws are tightened, the central screws are once again tightened. The outer margins of the acetabulum are then palpated to make certain no screws are protruding through the rim of the acetabulum. The acetabulum is once again irrigated and a slurry of bone graft is placed in the remaining large central holes. The most central hole in the peripheral recesses in the metal cup are then cleaned of debris to allow proper seating of the polyethylene liner. The polyethylene liner with the 28 mm inner diameter is seated in the metal cup. A definite "clunk" is noted when the liner is appropriately seated. The liner also has a 10° marginal extension that should be placed posteriorly or poste-

rolaterally depending on the degree of antiversion of the metal cup. The stability of the polyethylene liner should be tested by placing the curved Adson hemostat beneath the rim of the liner. It should not dislodge easily (Fig. 22–24).

Insertion of the acetabular component is now complete. The lower retractor is removed and a decision is made regarding whether further removal of inferior osteophytes will be necessary. Three to four millimeters of inferior osteophyte can be retained without fear of impingement. Excessive re-

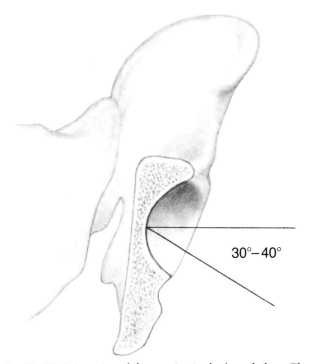

Fig. 22–21. Orientation of the reaming in the frontal plane. The horizontal direction is used to medialize the location of the cup in order to obtain proper coverage. The oblique orientation (30 to 45° depending on the anatomy of the acetabulum) is used to position the cup correctly.

Fig. 22–20. Careful placement of the final acetabular component into the prepared bed.

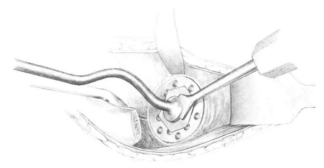

FIG. 22–22. Firm impaction of the acetabular component. The second impactor is used to properly medialize the component prior to final impaction.

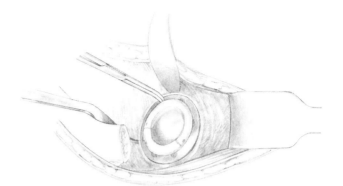

FIG. 22–24. Insertion of the polyethylene liner.

moval of inferior acetabular bone may detach the origin of the medial capsule and render the hip unstable. Each acetabular retractor is then removed individually and the socket is once again irrigated and inspected.

Elevation of the Leg

Prior to beginning work on the femoral side, the limb is elevated, the foot is dorsiflexed and the calf massaged to aid venous circulation and decrease venous stasis.

Exposure of the Proximal Femur

Unlike the trochanteric osteotomy approaches, the femur is placed in a position of modest external rotation, i.e., 45° and crossed over the opposite thigh. A large laparotomy sponge is used to isolate the proximal femur and the femur is elevated using the Mueller inferior acetabular retractor placed into the lesser trochanter. In obese patients, a second retractor, such as the Bennet retractor, is placed beneath the greater trochanter to retract the posterior flap. A generous exposure of the proximal femur is

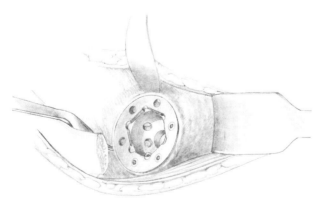

FIG. 22–23. Supplemental cancellous screw fixation for the cup.

now available for broaching and reaming (Fig. 22–25). Forced rotation in adduction of the femur should not be performed since avulsion of the greater trochanter can occur particularly in the osteoporotic elderly individual.

Opening the Femoral Canal

Excess soft tissue is excised from the tip of the greater trochanter. This allows reaming and broaching of the medial margin of the greater trochanter and avoids a varus positioning of the component. A small straight curette is introduced into the femoral canal in a neutral orientation (Fig. 22–26). The second assistant should use his or her hand to create a target at the distal femur and an imaginary plane is envisioned in both the anterior posterior and lateral positions to guide the curette. The fluted reamer is then introduced into the femoral canal to a level appropriate to the size component templated on the preoperative x-rays. The reamer is pushed into varus and valgus positions upon withdrawal to open up the canal and remove cancellous bone in the proximal femur, but in proportions smaller than those for the implant (Fig. 22–27).

Broaching the Femur

The femoral broach is introduced in a neutral position (varus-valgus) and in neutral version (Fig. 22–28). Rotation is judged in relation to position of the flexed leg. Broaching is begun with the 7.5 mm broach. This is progressively enlarged in 2.5 mm increments. Preoperative templating of the x-rays is used as a guide to the final size of the femoral component. The broach is introduced each time to its full depth. If significant resistance is met, broaching should continue with a series of small inward and then outward taps. This is continued until full cortical seating has been accomplished. This can be

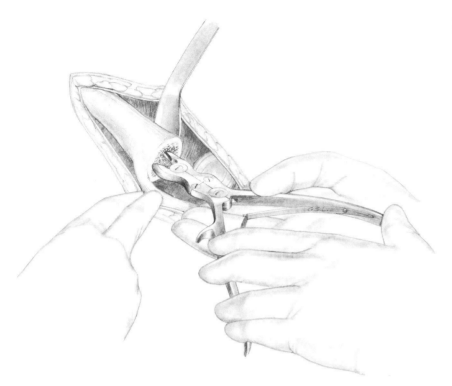

determined by an upward change in pitch as the broach is being seated. As the surgeon gains experience with this maneuver, full seating can be readily determined. The final seating and sizing is determined by the pitch and degree of resistance. This is ultimately more accurate than templating or x-ray.

Trial Reduction

The hip is reduced and stability and leg length are assessed (Fig. 22–29). The first step in this evaluation is to place longitudinal traction on the leg while the hip is in a neutral position. In a typical male, less than 1 mm of distraction between the femoral head and socket is possible. In a more supple female 1 to 2 mm of distraction is typical. Excess distraction indicates laxity of soft tissues and a lack of restoration of leg length. There may be several causes. The cup may be placed in too high a position or the femoral component was placed in too low a position with excessive resection of the femoral neck or the components are too small.

If at this juncture the soft tissues about the hip appear excessively tight with incomplete extension of the hip, the cause is usually an excessively low position of the cup or retention of excessive femoral neck or inappropriately large components. These errors can be accomodated only by changing the femoral neck length or converting to a lateral offset femoral component.

The position of mating of the femoral component and socket is noted. Symmetric mating should be seen when the hip is in the neutral position.

The hip is checked for stability in both flexion and extension. The hip is flexed to 90° and adducted with both internal and external rotation. If dislocation occurs, impingement is present or the components are maloriented or inadequate soft tissue tension is present. With the hip in extension

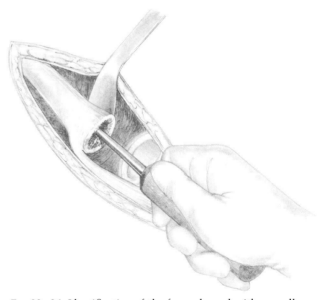

Fɪɢ. **22–26.** Identification of the femoral canal with a small curette.

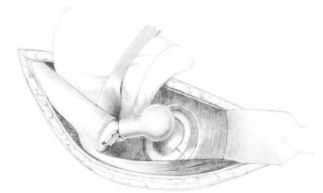

FIG. 22–29. Trial reduction using the broaches and trial head neck sizes.

achieved by increasing the neck length. This is desirable if the limb remains shortened. If, however, leg lengths are equal, a lateral offset trial component should be used to achieve stability in an attempt to maintain equal leg lengths. Stability, however, is more important than equal leg lengths. Therefore, unequal leg lengths should be sacrificed if this is the only way to gain stability. Achieving hip stability on the operating table has made postoperative dislocation in primarily total hip arthroplasty a rare complication.

Insertion of the Femoral Prosthesis

The hip is dislocated and exposure of the proximal femur is once again obtained in the previously described manner. The broach is removed with the extractor and the femoral canal is copiously irrigated. The surgeon's gloves are then changed and the appropriate size femoral component is placed into the femoral canal using the impactor. Appropriate version is maintained during insertion of the prosthesis. The femoral component is then seated into position with a mallet to the position previously obtained by the broach (Fig. 22–30). The femoral component should be well seated at this juncture. A 28 mm trial femoral head is placed on the femoral component using the same neck length. The hip is once again reduced and then tested for stability as previously described. If the hip is unstable at this point, a change in neck length may be necessary. This should be done in lieu of leg length equalization. The hip is then dislocated and exposure of the proximal femur once again obtained. A trial femoral head is removed and the Morris taper is cleaned. The appropriate 28 mm femoral head is then placed on the Morris taper and seated in position with the impactor (Fig. 22–31). The retractors are removed and the hip is once again reduced after the socket has been irrigated and inspected to be

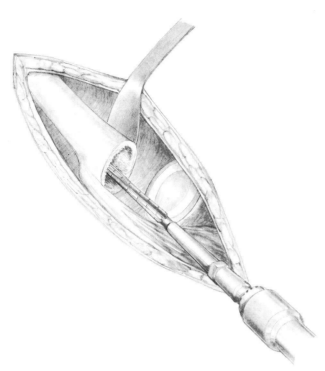

FIG. 22–27. Gentle insertion of the power reamer.

stability is evaluated by external rotation and adduction.

The last step is evaluation of leg length. With both limbs in the neutral position, the medial malleoli are approximated and the leg length is estimated. This is a precise and easy system to determine the leg lengths.

If the hip is unstable due to inadequate soft tissue tension, then increased stability can be

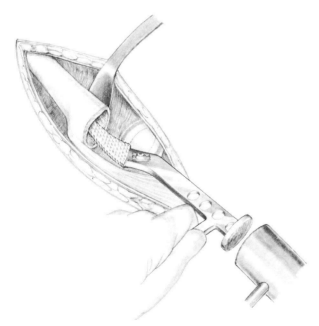

FIG. 22–28. Broaching the femur.

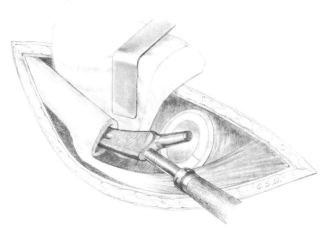

FIG. 22–30. Inserting the femoral prosthesis.

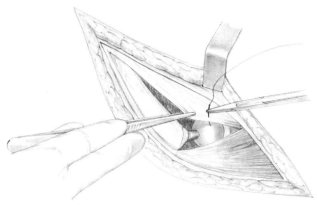

FIG. 22–32. Closure of the anterior gluteus medius/vastus lateralis flap using interrupted suture.

certain there is no debris in the wound. Direct visualization of the reduction must occur so the capsule and other soft tissue is not trapped between the femoral head and the socket. Stability and leg lengths are rechecked. The wound and components are thoroughly irrigated. The wound is now ready for closure.

Wound Closure

Prior to closure of the wound, the area is again inspected for debris and for bleeding. Two suction drains are then inserted. They are placed within the hip joint and brought through the skin anteriorly approximately 3 in. forward of the wound margin. Care must be taken during subsequent closure not to suture in the drains.

Capsular Closure

A careful capsular closure should be performed along the lines of the superior capsular incision.

This is achieved with interrupted figure-of-eight No. 1 vicryl sutures. The surgeon should not confuse gluteus minimus fibers with the capsular tissue. The tendinous insertion of the gluteus minimus and medius muscle are reapproximated to the remaining tendon on the anterior trochanter using interrupted figure-of-eight No. 1 vicryl sutures (Figs. 22–32, 22–33). The split in the gluteus medius muscle fibers can be closed with a running suture of No. 1 vicryl. Likewise, the fascia of the vastus lateralis can be repaired with a running suture of No. 1 vicryl (Fig. 22–34). The wound is again irrigated and the fascia lata is reapproximated with interrupted sutures of No. 1 vicryl in a figure-of-eight fashion. The subcutaneous layers are then co-

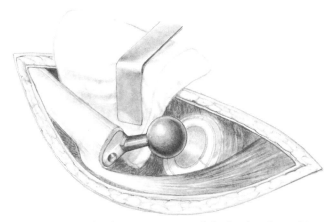

FIG. 22–31. Final reduction using a modular head neck combination.

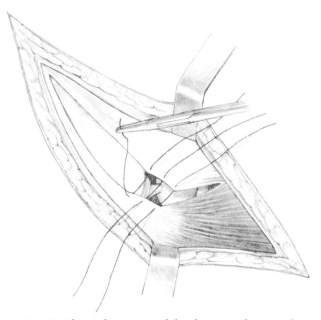

FIG. 22–33. The tendinous area of the gluteus medius muscle is attached with special care.

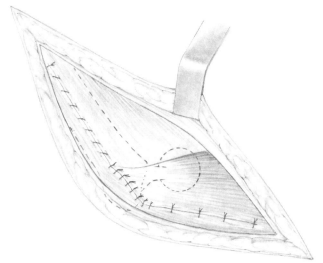

F ɪɢ. 22–34. Closure of the gluteus medius/vastus lateralis flap is completed.

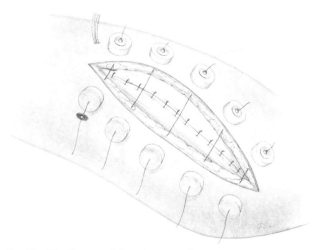

F ɪɢ. 22–35. Closure of deep fascia with interrupted suture. Closure of subcutaneous tissue with retention sutures. Subsequently the skin is closed in a routine fashion.

piously irrigated. The adhesive drape is then removed from the margins of the wound. Large retention sutures to obliterate the dead space are then inserted as described by Charnley and this is followed by closure of the subcutaneous tissues with interrupted 3-0 vicryl suture (Fig. 22–35). The skin edges are approximated with staples. The staples are placed at 4 mm intervals.

Final Dressing of the Wound

The wound is carefully wiped with a sponge wetted with antibiotic solution to remove any residual blood. The wound surface is then dried and finally wiped with Betadine solution. A nonadherent dressing is then applied and held in place with tape.

Abduction Splint

A padded abduction splint is applied on the operating table before the patient leaves the operating theater. The sacral pad should also be removed. This can result in a sacral decubitus if inadvertently left beneath the patient.

After Care

Patients are generally mobilized the day after surgery beginning ambulation with the use of a walker or crutches. For cemented hips, full weight-bearing is allowed immediately and with uncemented hip replacement incremental weight-bearing over a period of 3 months is advised.

The dressings and drains are removed at 48 hours and the wound is left exposed to the air. Betadine solution is applied twice daily until the wound is completely healed. Retention sutures are removed at 1 week and the skin staples at 2 weeks. Patients generally are discharged at 10 to 14 days.

Careful postoperative education is mandatory pertinent to the type of hip implant utilized and the stability of the hip noted at surgery. Infectious precautions are carefully reviewed in writing with the patient prior to discharge.

Reference

1. Hardinge K: The direct lateral approach to the hip. J Bone Joint Surg (Br), 64:17–19, 1982.

CHAPTER TWENTY-THREE

Uncemented Total Hip Arthroplasty

RICHARD H. ROTHMAN
TIMOTHY H. IZANT

Introduction

In the two decades since total hip replacement has been introduced into the United States, there has been a dramatic improvement in the quality of life that can be offered to the older individual afflicted with arthritis of the hip. There has been a steady improvement in the technology associated with this procedure leading frequently to better operative results as measured in terms of safety, efficacy, and durability.

The early techniques of cement fixation produced unacceptable radiographic loosening and clinical failure rates in young, overweight, and male patients. Improvements in cement fixation techniques, such as bone preparation, cement porosity reduction, and pressurization have significantly improved loosening rates and clinical outcome. The gold standard for an elderly female undergoing hip arthroplasty is cemented fixation. However, uncemented fixation has gained broad acceptance in the orthopaedic community based on the favorable results of a few clinical series with short-term followup data.

The two major considerations today in clinical research regarding hip arthroplasty are: first, should one abandon cemented fixation for cementless fixation, and second, if one does abandon cement, what portion of our patient population is most appropriate for cementless fixation. Additional subsidiary issues may be addressed in order to resolve these two questions.

Definitions of clinical failure rate vary among reporting research centers, making comparisons difficult. Several criteria for failure can be considered, including radiographic observations (demarcation, migration, cement fracture), clinical failure (pain, function, limited motion), and revision rates. Wejkner[138] has pointed out that: "If the reoperation rate of 4% (between 5 and 10 years) in the present study had been used as indicator of the results, a true picture would not have been obtained because

the actual rate of clinical failure during that period was 8%." This discrepancy between clinical failure and revision rate has been pointed out by others. It should be remembered that radiologic failure generally occurs first, followed by clinical failure with progressive pain, loss of function, and, at last, revision surgery. The lowest rate of failure generally is the reoperation rate because of the patient's skepticism about the dependability and durability of secondary surgery, advanced age, or greater medical and surgical risks.

Many authors have analyzed in detail the radiographic findings in postoperative hip arthroplasty patients attempting to correlate the radiographic findings with pain, function, and durability. Previous data[72] indicated that certain stigmata such as high grade femoral demarcation at the bone cement interface correlated strongly with unsatisfactory followup clinical scores. This is in contrast to the benign impact of socket demarcation. We have further noted that certain aspects of femoral cementing technique are strong predictors of later aseptic loosening. It is generally presumed that radiographic loosening will correlate with, and predict, clinical failure. It is important to isolate those radiographic aspects that have a particularly ominous connotation such as granuloma formation at the tip of the cemented femoral stem.[67]

Several radiographic criteria have been proposed for evaluating both cemented and uncemented fixation. The most widely used criteria were those defined by Harris[61] for cemented fixation, and by the PCA group[69] and Engh[40] for uncemented fixation. In fact, the necessary data are yet to be developed to correlate the radiographic stigmata with actual pathologic inspection of the hip either during revision surgery or in postmortem studies. Carlsson[18] demonstrated a poor correlation between radiographic data and the actual findings during revision surgery. He noted that 35% of sockets with radiographic signs of migration were in fact found to be stable. Similarly, in uncemented hips, Cook[27] concluded that "radiographic and clinical findings were unreliable in predicting the presence or extent of bony ingrowth in either femoral or acetabular components." More precise methods of radiographic evaluation will be necessary before we can extrapolate radiographic findings to anatomic fixation. Newer techniques such as roentgen stereophotogrammetric analysis (RSA) using tantalum bone markers may improve the precision of our radiographic definition of fixation.[95] An excellent review of the issue of radiographic definition of loosening was presented by Brand and coauthors.[12]

It has been suggested, first by the Mayo Clinic group,[126] that there is an exponential rate of acetabular loosening relative to the linear rate of femoral loosening. The implication emerges that the cemented socket is a vulnerable area for long term successful results. This has led certain surgeons to recommend abandonment of cement for socket fixation and the use of the so-called "hybrid hip."[56] In examination of our own cemented Charnley hip fixations with a 10-year survivorship analysis, Hozack[65] demonstrated the probability of socket survival at 10 years to be 99% using early cement techniques (Fig. 23–1).[66] Similar data, showing excellent cemented socket survival have been presented by others.[19,92,139] McCoy and coauthors[91] in reviewing a 15 year followup study of Charnley low friction arthroplasties, have demonstrated a 98% socket survivorship. Carlsson,[18] from Sweden, demonstrated a 100% socket survival at 10 years. Thus, it is certainly questionable whether the cemented socket should be abandoned and it may be difficult to develop data to support this hypothesis.

General Characteristics of Clinical Series

As an individual surgeon reviews the various series of hip arthroplasty, one must carefully construct the characteristics of the institution or institutions reporting before extrapolating this data to one's own situation. One would expect the data from a joint reconstruction center to be better than that of conglomerates representing regional or countrywide experience. In a similar vein, surgery performed by a senior hip surgeon would be expected to be better than that performed by individuals with various levels of surgical experience. Other factors should be considered, such as the selection process for surgical candidates and the nature of the disease being treated. Obviously, primary and secondary surgery should be segregated.

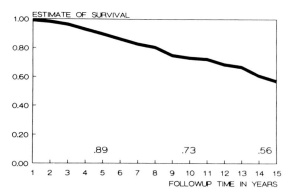

Fig. 23–1. Kaplan-Meier survivorship curve for acetabular revision (From Hozack WJ, Rothman RH: Long-term survival of the Charnley low-friction total hip arthroplasty. Semin Arthroplasty, 1:5, 1990.)

Ideally, comparative or controlled series should be developed wherein one surgical group uses a variety of implants or techniques, thereby generating fewer variables and allowing for stronger conclusions. Unfortunately, few surgical series exist with this type of comparative data.[2,20,111,125,130]

It is generally understood today that patient selection is a strong predictor of durability of hip implants. Factors such as weight, age, sex, and activity level will affect long-term durability.[65,72,111,133] Thus, when comparing the outcomes of various series in terms of wear, breakage, or aseptic loosening, one must keep in mind these factors. The dramatic negative effect of youth was first pointed out by Chandler and others in 1981.[22,26,29,31,108] These considerations help to identify the youthful, active male as a potentially good candidate for uncemented fixation even in the absence of long-term data.

As one attempts to weigh the virtues of cemented versus uncemented fixation, there must be a constant awareness of the dramatic improvement achieved with contemporary cement technique. In 1982, Harris[57] demonstrated a significant reduction in femoral loosening with contemporary cement fixation with a definite radiographic loosening rate of only 1.1% at 3 years. Later data, further emphasizing the contrast between the primitive techniques of cement fixation and modern usage have been presented by a wide diversity of investigators.[28,58,60,61,107,111]

It is obvious, as one contemplates the decision to use cemented or cementless fixation that one must not confuse poor outcomes resulting from errors in implant design with poor outcomes resulting from the method of fixation. With cemented implants, it is generally conceded that certain design considerations such as a broad medial wall and a straight stem will have a beneficial effect.[60] Metal backing of a polyethylene socket was introduced to distribute the joint forces evenly throughout the acetabulum, thereby lessening acetabular wear. Metal backing has gained general acceptance,[57] however improvement in acetabular survival remains to be proven. Our own group, as well as Ritter, has demonstrated the negative effect of a large diameter femoral head[7,110] on acetabular survival. The Muller curved stem has been implicated in a variety of series studying cemented fixation.[104,109,111,133]

Controversy remains regarding the best surface for a cemented femoral component. Ling[86] has presented persuasive evidence on the virtues of a polished femoral stem in contrast to the general trend in the United States to accept precoated or roughened stems that allow a stronger mechanical interlock between metal and methylmethacrylate. Charnley[25] also felt that subsidence could lead to a final stable position.

Similar problems exist with the uncemented components. A substantial incidence of thigh pain has been noted by a variety of authors using femoral designs with a large intramedullary rod.[39,64,69] By contrast the use of a flat wedge-shaped femoral implant has resulted in a considerably lower incidence of thigh pain in our own experience and in others.[63,145] Thus it will be critical to assess diligently whether it is the design of the implant rather than the mode of fixation that affects pain and loosening.

Uncemented Prosthetic Components—Materials

A wide array of materials have been utilized to create components for uncemented hip replacement. Four major groups of materials compromise the field: metals, ceramics, polymers, and composites. The two most common groups of metals used are the titanium alloys and the cobalt chrome alloys. Both of these groups have high strength and good corrosion resistance, although the rate of corrosion of the titanium base alloys is roughly one half that of the cobalt chrome group. For a given component cross section, the modulus of elasticity of titanium is also roughly one half that of the corresponding cobalt chrome alloy. The theoretical advantage of a lower modulus of elasticity, closer to that of bone, is a more physiologic transfer of load from the component to the cortical bone. One disadvantage of titanium alloys is notch sensitivity, especially of concern with the application of porous ingrowth surfaces. Stainless steel components have

less applicability for uncemented use because of material properties. Stainless steel is weaker in fatigue strength and has a greater corrosion potential when used as a porous ingrowth surface.

Ceramic total hip replacements of aluminum oxide have been used in Europe for well over 10 years. The modulus of elasticity of ceramic aluminum oxide is significantly higher than cobalt chrome, but its wear and corrosion characteristics are excellent. Polymers have been used both as components themselves and as coatings for femoral prostheses that have a metallic core. Two such examples are polyacetyl polymer, which is used in the isoelastic hip prosthesis, and the polytetrafluroethylene (proplast) polymer that has been used to coat a more conventional Aufranc-Turner prosthesis.

Macrolock and Microlock Designs

The first major group of noncemented implants use the common mechanical principle of a press fit macrolock type of design. Austin Moore and Thompson prostheses are examples of the press fit macrolock concept. Freeman and Ring have used acetabular components fixed by a polyethylene peg. Another example of the macrolock concept on the acetabular side is the screw-in cup with outer threads for fixation. On the femoral side Mittelmeier has advocated a ribbed prosthesis while Lord has advocated a Madreporique design using 1-mm diameter balls that are sintered onto a femoral stem.

The second major group of prostheses are the porous ingrowth or micropore prostheses. This group uses the concept of bony ingrowth into small pores that provide microlock fixation in tension, compression, and shear. The three major types of porous ingrowth surfaces include: fiber mesh sintered composites, sintered porous beads, and plasma flame sprayed. Fiber mesh composites are composed primarily of titanium and titanium alloys. The porous wire mesh is bonded to the metal substrate with a sintering process leaving a porosity of roughly 50%, with a mean pore size of 200 to 300 microns. Metal powder or macro beads also can be sintered to a solid substrate and yield porosities of 30 to 50% with pore diameters from 100 to 400 microns. The AML and the PCA prostheses are examples of this type of bony ingrowth component. It must be remembered that to form either the fiber mesh composite or the sintered bead composite, significant heating of the metal substrate must take place to achieve bonding. These significant temperature elevations produce weakening of either the cobalt-chrome or the titanium substrate.

Plasma flame sprayed technology involves the use of a heated powder that is propelled onto a substrate. The advantage of this technology is that the core metal of the prosthesis does not have to be significantly heated, thus the substrate in not weakened. However, the disadvantages of plasma spray surface are irregular pore size and poorer interpore connection space. Retrieval studies have found bony ingrowth into all the porous surfaces, but mostly at sites of fixation pegs or screws.

The steps required for establishment of a successful bone prosthesis interface are similar to those described for fracture healing. The basic science of this process has been best studied in the fiber mesh ingrowth and sintered bead ingrowth systems. As in the case of fracture healing, the steps most commonly described are the inflammatory, reparative, and remodeling phases.

The inflammatory phase begins at the time of surgery when the prosthesis is introduced into the intramedullary canal of the femur or into the acetabulum of the pelvis. Blood and marrow elements are mixed with a typical inflammatory exudate at the surgical site. As the inflammatory phase subsides, the hematoma is replaced by osteoprogenitor mesenchyme. The primitive tissue may form either fibrous tissue or healing bone depending upon numerous local factors.

The reparative phase of porous ingrowth is heralded by the formation of woven bone. There is usually little or no cartilaginous component of this reparative response. Galante has shown that at 1 week the first trabeculae of this bony response may be seen within the void spaces of the porous implant. At this stage it can be shown that the initial trabeculae of woven bone appear simultaneously at all depths of the porous structures, thus indicating that bony ingrowth does not necessarily begin peripherally and proceed toward the core of the prosthesis. With maturation of these woven bony trabeculae there is formation of an interlocking grid with the metal fibers.

Perhaps as early as 2 weeks after implantation, osteoblasts may be seen outlining the original bony trabeculae. These osteoblasts signify the initiation of appositional bone formation on the initial primary membranous bone. Galante has shown demarcation between woven and lamellar bone 4 to 6 weeks after porous component implantation.

Many agents have been studied in an effort to enhance the biologic response for bony ingrowth and to shorten the interval between the subsequent stages of the reparative and remodeling phases. Most of these agents have demonstrated little, if any, transitional benefit, and none have demonstrated a long-term enhancement of bony ingrowth fixation.

Trancik[132] reported that indomethacin, aspirin, and ibuprofen had an inhibitory effect upon porous ingrowth in an animal model. This suggests that anti-inflammatory medicines may be contraindicated in the perioperative time period.

Synthetic calcium phosphates in the form of mineral hydroxyapatite and tricalcium phosphate have been used as bone grafting agents. These synthetic materials have a function as grouting agents and promote earlier stability of the femoral stem in dogs. The ultimate interface strength and quantity of bone ingrowth have not been shown to be greater with these agents. However, greater amounts of bone proliferation have been observed histologically at earlier time periods. The use of such agents may allow for full weight-bearing at earlier time periods, however more research is needed.

Electrical stimulation has been examined using pulsed electromagnetic fields and the common results of these animal studies have shown no long-term effect on bony ingrowth. There is conflicting data regarding whether electrical stimulation accelerates the ingrowth process or gives higher shear strength interfaces early in the healing process.

In the operating room, surgeons frequently use bone autografts or allografts as grouting agents to augment fixation of cementless total joint prostheses. As yet, no study has demonstrated an enhanced biologic effect of this surgical strategy. Indeed, there may be initial resorption of this implant material that might possibly contribute to prolonged inflammatory and early reparative phases of the bony ingrowth process. The basic science of autograft and allograft function especially in the role of revision surgery with cementless components needs further animal study.

Two animal studies have demonstrated the detrimental effect of diphosphonates on biologic fixation. A 76% reduction in the strength of fixation was found after 8 weeks in EHDP treated animals. This same study also indicated that gamma radiation and indomethacin have significant inhibitory effects 4 weeks after surgery in rabbits. Methotrexate and systemic steroids may also cause retardation of the bony ingrowth response.

The influence of aging on bony ingrowth is not well defined at this time. A recent study has shown a decrease in bone formation with age in dogs and indeed these findings may coincide with the often prolonged healing time for fractures in elderly patients. Also, the effect of active osteoporosis on the bony ingrowth process is unknown at this time.

Design Considerations For Cementless Components

The design factors that are applicable to all uncemented systems are initial stability of the prosthesis, proximity of the prosthesis to opposing bone, modulus of elasticity, proximal stress transfer, low friction and wear characteristics, modularity, biocompatibility, implant retrieval technology, and pore size.

Initial Stability

In order for a stable bone-component interface to arise, gross motion must not be present between the prosthesis and bone. For the porous ingrowth subset of prostheses, studies in animals demonstrated that 6 weeks is necessary for early remodeling and maturation of the cortical interface to form a stable interlock. For humans this stable time period may take up to 12 weeks. Clinically, if gross motion is present at the time of implantation, it is unlikely that a stable interface will be achieved. We must suppose that some degree of micromotion is present because of the dynamic loading of the prosthesis with its greater modulus of elasticity compared to bone. But if the micromotion is less than the pore size, the implant will be able to be stabilized by the maturing, woven bone that coalesces at the interface. Animal studies have shown that if gross motion is present between the prosthesis and its bony bed, fibrous tissue will proliferate and not form a stable interface.

On the femoral side a number of general categories of prostheses can be identified. One large subset is the group that require intramedullary reaming for an essentially intramedullary device that also has proximal support at the femoral neck. Examples of this type of prosthesis are the AML and the Harris-Galante (Fig. 23–2) femoral components. A variation of this design incorporates intramedullary fixation with a curved stem, such as the PCA (Fig. 23–3).

Another large group of femoral components are those that utilize a wedge fit; intramedullary reaming is not required. These prostheses have a broad proximal area that fills the metaphyseal portion of

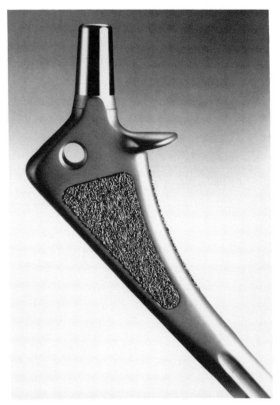

Fɪɢ. 23–2. Harris-Galante total hip prosthesis.

the femur and a narrower distal portion that allows for a three-point fixation to the diaphysis of the femur. Examples of this type of prosthesis include the Taperloc (Fig. 23–4) and Gemini femoral designs. In a cadaver study at our institution using Taperloc and cemented components, Sharkey[122] evaluated micromotion under axial and rotational loading. The results showed that the amount of micromotion occurring in the cementless Taperloc stem was comparable to that of a cemented component. Furthermore, stability for the two types of components was similar.

A third group of femoral designs matches the bone both proximally and distally with modular subcomponents. These designs attempt to improve proximal stress transfer and center the component distally. Examples of this design are the S-ROM and Omniflex systems.

Engh and others have shown that early clinical failure of uncemented femoral components has been caused by undersizing within the femoral canal. The fourth group of femoral designs addresses this issue with custom-made components. The rationale of custom-made components has been to achieve a greater degree of fill of the femoral canal and to improve initial stability. This technique is accomplished either with the use of preoperative

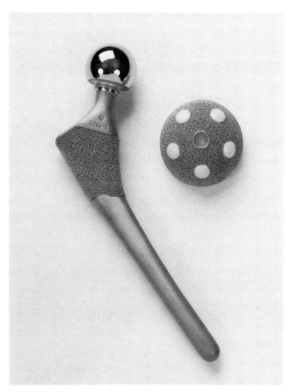

Fig. 23–3. PCA total hip prosthesis.

computer-assisted design and computer-assisted manufacturing (CAD/CAM), or with intraoperative laser measurements and manufacturing.[99] Amstrutz, Bargar, and Stulberg have reported on their early results using custom implants in patients with significant anatomic deformity. Their results[4,8,128] are not inferior to contemporary uncemented total hip arthroplasty (THA). However, the off-the-shelf designs (OFS) are recommended for routine THA. The disadvantages of custom components include high costs (custom components and CT scan), inaccuracy of final fit, inadequacy of in-

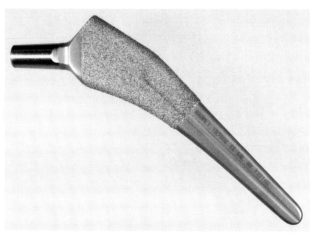

Fig. 23–4. Taperloc system.

struments for insertion, and inability to perform mechanical testing on the component. Capello[17] also points out that maximizing the fill of the femoral canal may further increase proximal stress shielding, despite adequate fit.

In addition to initial stability to axial and bending forces, femoral designs must provide stability to rotational stresses. Greater rotational micromotion has been observed in some femoral designs with uncemented fixation compared to cemented fixation.[100,120] The "out of plane" rotational forces are considerable with stair climbing and upon rising from a chair. Early failures and thigh pain in uncemented femoral fixation may be caused by failure of rotational fixation.

On the acetabular side, many different designs have been studied, including hemispherical, truncated cone, and cylindrical shapes. The nonhemispherical shapes are reamed to provide immediate stability. The bony ingrowth hemispherical components are anchored by screws that compress the prosthesis into the subchondral bone. Some designs have pegs, spikes, or pins to provide additional fixation.

The use of supplemental acetabular screws has been associated with intrapelvic vascular penetration. Anatomic studies by Keating and Wasielewski [81,137] have identified the anterior-superior quadrant of the acetabulum as a high risk for vascular complication when using screw fixation.

The prostheses themselves may be threaded and numerous screw-in types of mechanisms have been attempted, but short term results have been disappointing. The specifics of each design will be discussed under the section on clinical data.

Proximity of the Uncemented Component to Bone

This principle may appear obvious at first, however, it is extremely important that the bone-component interface be as great a surface area as possible. Inadvertent reaming or utilization of a broach that is too large will decrease the surface area available for stabilization of the uncemented component. This factor is especially critical in prostheses that require bony ingrowth. Bone has been shown to transcend small gaps of up to 1.5 mm, although the bony ingrowth will occur at a slower rate. In one experimental acetabular model, a 0.5-mm gap was associated with a paucity of bony ingrowth in that area. Obviously, the greater the surface area of intimate contact, the greater the early stability of the implant with respect to its bony host.

Modulus of Elasticity

For a given component size, the modulus of elasticity between the various metals, polymers, composites, and ceramics varies greatly. Given our initial principles of immediate stability and maximization of bony contact, the sizes of the prostheses are largely dictated by the bony anatomy, especially on the femoral side. For a large male patient, these prostheses can be quite massive and a large cobalt-chrome prosthesis may be extremely stiff. This principle led to the development of the so-called isoelastic prosthesis as developed by Mathis and Morscher. As the modulus of elasticity of the uncemented femoral component more closely approximates that of cortical bone, we should expect to see less in the way of long-term bony changes associated with stress shielding. These considerations have been studied more closely on the femoral than on the acetabular side.

Proximal Stress Transfer

This principle applies to the femoral component and its relationship to the metaphyseal and diaphyseal regions of the proximal femur. With large, stiff, metal femoral components that have tight, distal apposition, and thus significant load transfer capability, the entire proximal femur may be shielded from the dynamic loading stress that is necessary for healthy bone maintenance. Current femoral designs emphasize the ability of a given prosthesis to stress the metaphyseal cortex of the femur. Femoral shaft designs that are tapered distally theoretically allow for a gradual transfer of forces to the cortical bone. This is in contrast to the femoral designs that have a broad distal end, which causes a sharp transfer of forces to the diaphysis.

The addition of a collar to the femoral design has been used to increase proximal stress transfer. Clinically, other factors such as high modulus of elasticity or large component size have outweighed any benefit from a collar. Theoretically, a collar may block subsidence, thereby preventing stable fixation over time.

For bony ingrowth prostheses, the roughened surface is usually limited to the metaphyseal region of the component and is absent from the diaphyseal portion. With intimate bony contact and maturation of a stable bony ingrowth interface, efficient stress transfer to the metaphyseal cortex is indeed possible.

With femoral component designs that incorporate a significantly lower modulus of elasticity with dynamic loading, the prosthesis itself bends enough to provide proximal femoral stress transfer. The theoretical answer to this problem is the design of Morscher that has an isoelastic modulus with respect to the proximal femur. For a given size the titanium alloy prostheses have half the stiffness of the cobalt chrome prostheses; thus proximal stress transfer is more critical in the larger cobalt chrome femoral components.

Low Friction and Wear Characteristics

These principles have largely been discussed in a previous chapter on the basic science of total hip arthroplasty. Thirty-two millimeter femoral heads have been associated with greater volumetric wear[87] and significantly higher acetabular revision rate.[96] In general, the smaller head sizes of 22 and 28 mm impart less torque to the acetabular component and result in less acetabular loosening. The ceramic prostheses especially have excellent wear and friction coefficients.

Modularity of Components

As has been stated before, the femoral designs of uncemented prostheses require initial stability with maximization of contact to bone. At the same time it must be remembered that the principles of capsular tension and leg length equality must be considered at the time of surgery. With cemented prostheses it may be possible to use the cement mantle to achieve the equalization of leg lengths and normalization of capsular tension that provide stability for the femoral acetabular articulation. For most uncemented hip systems there is one position of that particular femoral component in a given femoral canal that is most stable. Given that constraint, it is extremely advantageous to have regular and lateral offset femoral necks as well as modularity of neck lengths available to the surgeon. An example of this capability is demonstrated by the Taperlock system, (Fig. 23–5) which for any given femoral component size using a 28-mm head, there are 14 possible combinations of offset and neck length that assist the surgeon in achieving maximization of capsular tension and leg length equality.

One disadvantage of modular components is their potential for disassembly within the patient associated with a dislocation.[13,46,83,141] Disassembly can occur at the liner-cup interface, at the femoral head and mortise-taper junction, or with displacement of the femoral acetabular component in a bipolar prosthesis.

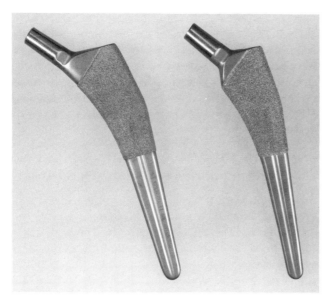

FIG. 23–5. Lateralized (left) and standard offset Taperloc stems.

Biocompatibility

Orthopaedic implants have a broad range of interrelationships with their human hosts. These interactions include both local and systemic effects involving primarily the elements that are incorporated into the uncemented prosthesis. The metallic ions may induce inflammatory, immunologic, metabolic, and carcinogenic activity.

The first critical interaction of the various materials is at the level of the femoral and acetabular bone. As we have seen before, the various metals, polymers, ceramics, and composites are inert with respect to their abilities to form a stable bony interface. Although methylmethacrylate may form such a boundary, unfortunately, it is not uncommon for methylmethacrylate to induce a biologic lytic response of the local bone. This response is indeed what the surgeon is trying to avoid by switching to an uncemented hip system. However, it must be remembered that the surface area for release of elements into the systemic circulation with these metal porous ingrowth systems may be five to ten times the surface area of cemented implants. It must also be remembered that loosening and wear increase this release rate greatly.

Aseptic loosening has been reported with titanium alloy femoral heads secondary to osteolysis induced from metallic debris.[88,93] Furthermore, this metalosis has been observed with titanium alloy beads, without concurrent acetabular or femoral loosening.[11] Newer techniques of implanting nitrogen ions onto the femoral head may improve resistance to wear and corrosion as well as fatigue properties.

The systemic effect of biomaterials is of greater concern with uncemented hip arthroplasty. For the cobalt-chrome prostheses, the critical elements are chromium, cobalt, and nickel. For the titanium alloys the critical elements include titanium and vanadium. Galante studied baboons in which titanium, aluminum, and vanadium composites were implanted from 3 weeks to 10 years. At the time of sacrifice, titanium concentrations in the lungs, spleen, and regional lymph nodes were elevated. Woodman has studied the effect of porous coated implants of cobalt, chromium, and nickel in the New Zealand white rabbit. No overt clinical disease was noted. However, increases in chromium, cobalt, and nickel concentrations were found in the urine, feces, and serum of all experimental animals. The long-term metabolic effect of these elements on human biologic systems remains incompletely studied.

Of greater concern is the incidence of carcinogenesis associated with these implants. Carcinogenesis in animals has been shown for chromium and nickel; cobalt is greatly suspected of having a carcinogenic role.[9] Implant site tumors are an infrequent occurrence, however, there have been three case reports of tumors associated with total hip replacement. Two malignant fibrous histiocytomas have been associated with the implantation of a Charnley-Mueller and a McKee-Ferrer prosthesis. Also, an osteosarcoma has been associated with an uncemented Ring prosthesis. These neoplasms developed between 2 and 5 years after implantation of the total hip replacement. There has been no study examining the incidence of remote site tumors with respect to patients who have metal implants.

Implant Removal

The technology must be present for each of the given systems so that the surgeon may remove a given prosthesis without undue destruction of the bony substrate. Theoretically the larger fixation devices require more exposure and possibly more bony destruction to effect a successful implant removal. Of great concern are the bony ingrowth prostheses that form a bond to diaphyseal bone and thus require violation of diaphyseal bone to remove the prosthesis.

Femoral components that have a broadening of the tip are especially difficult to extract without causing significant bone loss, diaphyseal fractures, or large cortical windows. On the acetabular side as well, thought must be given to possible salvage procedures when evaluating the various acetabular component designs. Ideally, only a minimal amount of bone should have to be removed in order to extricate a given prosthesis. The macrolock nonporous ingrowth prostheses have an advantage in that a smooth interface may be preserved when removing the implant.

Pore Size for Porous Ingrowth Prostheses

Many authors have studied the effect of pore size on the ability to form a strong interface both with respect to shear and tension forces. The summation of animal data suggests that the optimum pore size is between 100 and 400 microns. Bobyn and Pilliar examined a bead sintered system with various pore sizes. Their groups included pore sizes of 20 to 50, 50 to 200, 200 to 400, and 400 to 800 micron range. Their data clearly showed an increase in shear strength of the 50 to 200 and 200 to 400 pore size groups. Groups below 50 and above 400 showed significantly less shear strength.

Clinical Series

The era of metallic implants for hip endoprostheses began over 40 years ago with the Austin Moore prosthesis, and long-term clinical studies are available demonstrating its efficacy. Twenty years ago both Ring and Savash began with metal on metal, nonporous, uncemented replacement of both the acetabulum and femur. By the middle and late 1970s several European centers were begining clinical trials on a wide variety of uncemented designs. Every major survivorship analysis of cemented fixation demonstrates a progressive loss of fixation with time.[3,65,92,94,104,111,144] Although limited data are available in the United States, Engh[36] has implied that once stable fixation has occurred, the outcome does not deteriorate with time.

A further advantage proposed for uncemented fixation is that bone loss will not occur even in the face of loosening, in contrast to the dramatic granulomatous destruction of bone that occurs with loose, cemented implants. Although this would appear to be so, European investigators have greater long-term experience with uncemented fixation. Zweymuller[143] holds a dissenting point of view that loose uncemented implants can indeed lead to loss of bone. "Cementless disease" may become a clinical entity with uncemented component loosening as we gain more long term followup data.

A third potential advantage of cementless total

hip replacement was demonstrated by Kim[82] with an unusually low incidence of thromboembolism. That this observation can be validated in other ethnic groups and in controlled studies remains to be proven. Factors such as reduced operative time, younger patient population and healthier patients, may produce lower overall complication rates.

Uncemented Data—Primary Total Hip Replacement

Little interest remains in the press fit designs such as the smooth Moore stem because of their relatively poor performance.[105] In Europe, the major emphasis has been on a macrointerlock system, whereas in the United States, microinterlock has been stressed. First, the European experience will be reviewed, although reliable conclusions are difficult because many of the major series are reported by the designer of the implant.

An excellent review of the European experience using uncemented prostheses has been presented by Morsher.[97,98] He concludes his review by emphasizing that the best indication for cementless endoprostheses is in revision arthroplasty. This is because of the potential to replace lost bone stock. He emphasizes the short-term followup of most European series with the exception of the Ring and Mittelmeier implants.

One of the earliest and largest series was reported by Ring. Over 3000 uncemented hip prostheses were implanted over two decades at first using a metal-on-metal configuration, and then using metal-on-plastic. His 5-year followup clinical results on 471 prostheses were reported in 1983. The design of the femoral component is an intramedullary macrolock stem with a lateral fin to control rotation. The prosthesis is not modular. On the acetabular side there is a polyethylene cup secured by an osseous peg of the Freeman design. The femoral component comes in three sizes. Of 1797 uncemented metal-on-metal implants, 85% had an excellent rating at 1-year followup; at 5 years 81% were rated excellent. The loosening rate for the metal-on-metal prostheses was 0.5% per year. For the metal-on-plastic prosthesis, 94% demonstrated an excellent result at 1- to 3-year followup.

In the contemporary series of the metal-on-plastic prosthesis, 164 patients were evaluated at 1 to 3 years. There was no evidence of migration or loosening of the acetabular component. The femoral component demonstrated demarcation in 10 patients, however, these changes were not associated with a poor clinical result. In 1985, Mittelmeier[94] reported on his first decade of experience with his Autophor system. He noted 67% excellent or good results at 7 years. The femoral loosening rate was 3.2% at 9 years and the acetabular loosening rate was 0.8%. In contrast to these results, which he considered satisfactory, Mallory and coauthors[101] reported a 3-year average followup with 69 Mittelmeier arthroplasties: 27% were revised. With this short-term followup, radiographic analysis showed 82% of the patients to have acetabular radiolucencies and 47% to have femoral radiolucencies. Groher[51] also reviewed the Mittelmeier implant in 257 patients with satisfactory results in 79%, with a mean 2-year followup. Only 5 of the remaining 22 hips were painless.

Lord[89] reviewed his experience with the Madreporique implant. This hip system has a femoral design of large beads sintered onto the metallic femoral stem. The beads employed were not designed for porous ingrowth, but rather to serve as a large interface macrolock within the femoral canal. Lord's acetabular prosthesis is a threaded ring in the shape of a truncated ellipsoid forming the outer metallic shell. Within the outer shell lies a polyethylene liner for articulation with the femoral head. Lord's latest prosthesis is modular.

In 1982, Lord reported on a series of 1509 patients. At 5 years of followup the clinical results of 235 prostheses demonstrated a 83% good or excellent rating. The best results were obtained in younger patients, "about or younger than 50 years." Midthigh pain was commonly present for 12 to 18 months and disappeared in most cases.

In general, good stability was noted without sinkage, cortical atrophy or scalloping. Positive images of bony ingrowth were reported in 23% of the patients. If radiolucent lines were present, they were evident at 1 year and it was suggested that these radiolucent lines could disappear with some resolution of the thigh pain.

Dislocation occurred in 4.5% of Lord's series indicating an abnormally high rate of instability. There is no mention made of the alignment of the acetabular components, but difficulty might have been encountered with initial placements of the threaded, truncated cone acetabular design. Twenty-three femoral shaft fractures were encountered at the time of insertion of the femoral component. The reason for this difficulty with revision is in part related to the roughened surface along the entire length of the intramedullary femoral stem. It is of interest that he concluded that "cement is useless in most arthroplasties." He further states that "in the revision of a previously cemented total

hip . . ., new cement appears to be particularly harmful."

In an attempt to minimize stress shielding of the proximal femur caused by excessive rigidity of metallic femoral components, Morscher has developed the isoelastic hip. This design utilizes a femoral component with a central core of titanium, and is surrounded by a polyacetyl resin that has a similar modulus of elasticity compared to cortical bone. The femoral component, in addition, has a metallic femoral head that is not modular. The femoral prosthesis itself is self-locking with a proximal fixation screw. The acetabular component utilizes polyethylene pegs and is self-locking.

The clinical results reported by Morscher and Dick in 1983 were excellent.[97,98] Of 240 patients with a followup of 6 to 48 months, 221 rated their hip as excellent or good, 9 as satisfactory, and only 10 were not satisfied with their pain relief. A change in femoral design was initiated in 1977. With a maximum followup of 5.5 years, the polyethylene cups were described as having good acceptance with none demonstrating either loosening or migration. The authors described increased sclerosis of the pelvis in the weight-bearing portion of the acetabulum and these changes were noted to stabilize at 1 year.

Most of the cementless acetabular components were inserted opposite cemented Mueller prostheses. As yet, there have been no revisions required for primary acetabular loosening. There was an infection rate of 2.0% requiring reoperation. An interesting and wide divergence of quality of result has been noted by others with this implant. Bombelli and coauthors[5] followed a group of 400 patients with a minimum review time of 2 years. Ninety-two percent were considered good with a 0.8% revision rate. Of note, 23% sustained intraoperative femoral fractures. Other reviews of this implant are in marked contrast and less satisfactory. Rosso[113] presented a 5-year review of the RM isoelastic total hip noting very good or good results in only 59% of patients. Only 36% of his patients were symptomfree. Jakim[73] in a review of 34 RM isoelastic hips, noted a 32% revision rate with less than a 4-year followup. Nine percent had good results.

Other isoelastic prostheses such as the Butel[14] showed evidence of a better outcome. Forty-two of 47 patients followed for a minimum of 5 years resulted in good or excellent results. Seven of 51 were rated failures. Tullos[133] reported on a dismal experience with a low modulus porous-coated femoral component of Proplast, a material similar to Teflon. He found a 36% clinical failure rate at 3 years, with 5 revisions in 47 hips. Examination of the 5 retrieved implants noted failure of the coating within its substrate. He concluded that "the coating had insufficient strength to withstand normal weight bearing loads."

The series reported by Zweymuller[143–145] are of particular interest. He has designed a cementless press fit prosthesis using titanium. The femoral component is a flat wedge-shaped design.[134] He demonstrated that, with a 3- to 4-year mean followup, 97% of his patients achieved good relief of pain.

This group of patients and series of reviews was of particular interest to the authors of this review because they have also noted a relative freedom from thigh pain using a flat wedge-shaped design. This same phenomenon had been noted earlier by Evarts[63] using a generally similar femoral design. It is possible that the wedge-shaped design allows subsidence to a point of stability and thereby improves rotational stability. It has been pointed out recently by Whiteside[140] that torsional stability may be the critical element in the fixation of the uncemented stem. If this is so, it is possible that the flat wedge-shaped implant will prove superior to the current rod-like components that have gained favor. Certainly, in order to achieve this rotational stability, subsidence must be possible. A collared implant would thus seem disadvantageous. Zweymuller emphasizes the extreme biocompatibility of titanium, which allows for bone to directly oppose the metal surface without fibrous interposition. This concept of "osseointcgration" of titanium implants has been described in a series of articles by Carlsson and Albrektsson.[1,21]

The studies by Zweymuller based on his clinical experience are of interest. They first suggest that late signs and symptoms of loosening can occur with uncemented implants and that bone lysis also can occur with loosening of the prostheses. Not surprisingly, he concludes that cement should be avoided whenever possible, particularly in revisional surgery, in the face of osteoporosis.

In the United States, the greatest in-depth experience has been gained by Engh and is reported in a series of presentations.[34–37,41,42] In a review of his 343 porous surface femoral prostheses studied with a mean 5-year followup, he noted a 3.5% revision rate and "end of stem pain" in 7.8% of patients. He estimated 78% radiographic bony ingrowth, or osteointegration, at 2 years. The certainty of estimating bony ingrowth by x-ray and the challenges to its validity have been previously noted.[27] It should be appreciated that the quality of this result, in terms of both pain and revision rate, appears inferior to that of the contemporary series of cemented

stems. Engh[36] also addressed the issue of femoral bone resorption and noted that "bone resorption is neither severe nor progressive beyond the first or second postoperative year." Proximal stress shielding occurred only in bone ingrowth stems. The stem diameter is critical. Stems equal to or greater than 13.5 mm showed five times the resorption of those 12 mm or less. Stems that were fully coated and two-thirds coated also showed greater resorption than those that were only proximally coated.

Femoral fractures have been observed in many uncemented designs, especially early in the surgeon's learning curve. In Engh's series, 3% of the patients sustained intraoperative femoral fracture, of which only one-half were recognized at the time of surgery. Incomplete and complete fracture patterns have been observed in the proximal femur and about the tip of the component. In a study on insertional fractures using a Taperloc prosthesis in a cadaver model, Sharkey[123] tested axial and rotational stability with loads simulating single-leg stance and stair-climbing both before and after fracture and with the addition of A-O cerclage wire fixation after fracture. Ninety percent of the components demonstrated decreased axial and rotational stability following fracture. The long-term clinical sequelae of intraoperative fracture have yet to be determined. However, loss of initial rigid stability can be expected following a fracture, possibly leading to fibrous ingrowth and a higher incidence of early pain. A group of 10 patients who sustained intraoperative femoral fractures during uncemented total hip arthroplasty were matched for age, sex, weight, diagnosis and length of followup to a control population by Sharkey.[124] The mean length of followup was 2.3 years. No significant difference in either clinical or radiographic results was found between the two groups.

The AML implant was studied using survivorship techniques by Krevolin[84] who demonstrated a survival rate at 4 years of 99% for those 55 or older and 97% for those under age 55. He concludes, in comparing his data with the Cornell and Ranawat series, that there was no significant difference between these two studies.

The HGP implant (Fig. 23–6) was reviewed in a series of 163 primary hip replacements from Rush-Presbyterian and St. Luke's Medical Center and Massachusetts General Hospital with a minimum 2-year followup.[85] Ninety-one percent had good or excellent hip scores but 9% had significant pain and 8% continued to limp. Femoral revisions were undertaken in 3% for aseptic loosening. No socket had been revised for loosening.

The PCA femoral stem has been used extensively

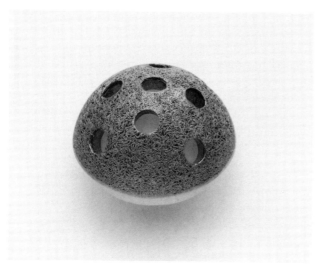

Fig. 23–6. HGP II acetabular prosthesis.

in the United States. Hungerford[69] in a review of 579 PCA hips with a 1- to 5-year followup noted a revision rate of 1.2% with undersizing as the common factor causing failure. Herberts[64] in a Scandinavian multicenter study of the PCA stem reviewed 420 arthroplasties. At 1-year followup 14% of the patients had thigh pain that diminished at 2 years to 3%. No revisions were noted. He states that "cementless porous coated prostheses are not as effective in relieving pain during the first 1 to 2 years as cemented devices are."

The PCA implant was also studied prospectively by Callaghan.[16] Thigh pain was noted in 18% at 1 year and 16% at 2 years. Twenty-eight percent had a moderate or severe limp at 2 years. Progressive loosening of beads was observed from the femoral component in 24% and from the acetabular component in 18%. The authors were concerned by pro-

gressive radiolucent lines, bead loosening, and persistent, albeit minor, thigh pain.

A review of PCA implants in the elderly by Hungerford[68] indicated that most would obtain good or excellent clinical results and therefore there should not be an arbitrary age limit for cementless total hip patients.

Few comparative series are available in which the same group of surgeons compare their results with cemented and noncemented hips. Roraback[114] compared his results of 65 PCA hips with 65 HD2 cemented hips in a short-term review of 6 to 12 months. They concluded that the cementless scores, although initially inferior, approximated the cemented scores after 1 year.

In a prospective comparative series on 87 cemented Pennsylvania and 117 cementless Taperloc hips with a minimum 2-year followup at our institution, Rothman[115] concluded that clinical and radiographic results were equivalent despite a significantly larger number of younger, heavier male patients in the cementless group. (Fig. 23–7). Examples of Taperloc components in place are shown in Figures 23–8 and 23–9.

Enhancement of biologic fixation by hydroxyapatite coating is an attractive concept that has been studied by Geesink.[49,50] His studies indicated that hydroxyapatite (HAP) coatings "permit an implant fixation far superior to current methods using either cemented or cementless techniques." Jasty[74] also demonstrated significant enhancement of bony ingrowth with HAP coating. Animal studies[102,131] of HAP implants demonstrated increased bone deposits at earlier time periods, without evidence of deterioration of HAP coating, or delamination of the coating from the implant.

Fig. **23–7.** Preoperative and postoperative Charnley scores for Taperloc uncemented hip.

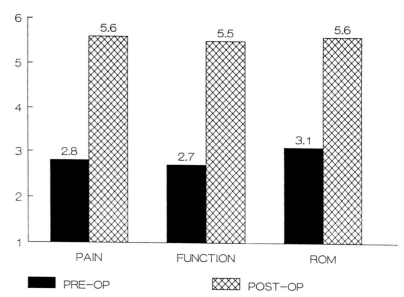

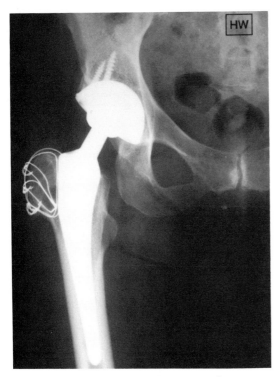

Fig. 23–8. Standard offset Taperloc stem with osteotomy.

Uncemented Revision Total Hip Replacement

The use of cementless revision for failed cemented hip arthroplasty is gaining general acceptance. Although intermediate and long-term data are, as yet, not available, acceptance is based on the dismal results of cemented revisions because of the poor interlock available between cement and bone. Second, the use of uncemented revisions presents the opportunity for restoration of lost bone stock with grafting. Whether these premises will, in fact, result in long-term success remains to be proven.

Engh[36,37] has presented his experience with cementless revision with 160 hips followed for an average of four years. He has tabulated his data and compared these with the other major revision series. On the femoral side, possible and definite instability was noted in 4% of patients, 1% of whom received the AML stem. On the acetabular side, possible and definite instability was noted in 22% of his overall series. Of these, 41% of his Mecron ring series and 9% of his porous cups were unstable. Hungerford[70] recently reviewed the rationale for cementless revision, also identifying the poor microinterlock as a reason to abandon polymethylmethacrylate in revision surgery. His own experience, with a PCA cementless revision, consists of 75 cementless hip revisions with 2 years or more of followup. All patients had grafting, including either

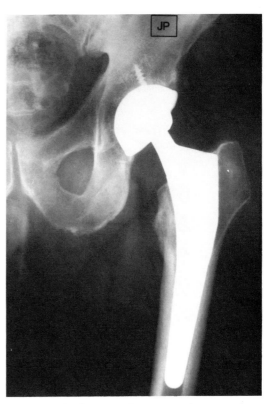

Fig. 23–9. Lateral offset Taperloc stem with universal acetabulum.

autografts or allografts. Ninety percent of patients measured 80 points or better on the Harris hip scale. Two patients required revision. Most encouraging was the dramatic reconstruction of bone stock.

Hedley[62] also reviewed his revision experience with the PCA cementless implant. Sixty-one hips were followed for greater than 1 year, with a mean followup of 21 months. Two required revision, with 90% achieving a good or excellent clinical evaluation. They note no graft resorption with this short-term followup.

Gustilo[52–54] has reported on his experience with cementless revision using the Bias stem (Fig. 23–10). An example of a revision using a Bias femoral component can be seen in Figure 23–11. Gustilo has analyzed 31 hips with a 3- to 6-year followup. An average postoperative hip score of 81 was achieved and appeared to improve with time. Two patients required revision.

Harris[61] has reported results of cementless revisions. Twenty-three patients were available for a minimum 2-year followup. Seventy-three percent of these had good or excellent results. No revisions were noted. Galante[48] reported his cementless revision series using the Harris-Galante implant in 38 patients and the Bias implant in 62. The followup period averaged 30 months with a 2- to 4-year

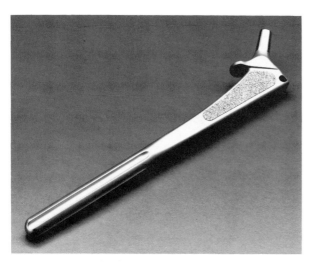

FIG. 23–10. Bias total hip prosthesis.

range. Good or excellent results were obtained in 64% with a revision rate of 8%.

Representing the European experience, Lord[90] presented a review of 284 revisions using his own implant for cementless fixation. At 5 years, excellent or good results were obtained in 73% of patients.

Thus it appears that the overall data relevant to cementless revision surgery is short-term and marginal in quality. Hopefully, the quality of results noted will improve with time and will exceed that obtained with cemented revision.

The ultimate justifications for uncemented hip arthroplasty will rest with the absence of late deterioration as measured by clinical performance and lower revision rates relative to the 10 and 15 year data available with contemporary cemented arthroplasty.

References

1. ALBREKTSSON T, ALBREKTSSON B: Osseointegration of bone implants: a review of an alternative mode of fixation. Acta Orthop Scand, 58:567, 1987.
2. ALHO A, SOREID EO, BJERSAND AJ: Mechanical factors in loosening of Cristiansen and Charnely arthroplasties. Acta Orthop Scand, 55:261, 1984.
3. AMSTUTZ HC, YAO J, DOREY FJ, NUGENT JP: Survival analysis of T-28 hip arthroplasty with clinical implications. Orthop Clin North Am, 19:491, 1988.
4. AMSTUTZ HC, NASSER S, KABO JM: Preliminary results of an off-the-shelf-press system. Clin Orthop, 249:60, 1989.
5. ANDREW TA, FLANAGAN JP, GERUNDI NIM, BOMBELLI R: The isoelastic non-cemented total hip arthroplasty: Preliminary experience with 400 cases. Clin Orthop, 206:127, 1986.
6. AUGUST AC, ALDAM CH, PYNSENT PB: The McKee-Farrar hip arthroplasty: a long term study. J Bone Joint Surg, 68B:520, 1986.
7. BALDERSTON RA, FRANKEL A, BOOTH RE, ROTHMAN RH: Radiographic demarcation of the acetabular bone cement interface: the effect of femoral head size. Proceedings of the 56th Annual Meeting of the AAOS, Las Vegas, p. 79, 1989.
8. BARGAR WL: Shape the implant to the patient: a rationale

FIG. 23–11. Revision of cemented total hip using Bias femoral stem. **A.** Preoperative. **B.** Posteroperative.

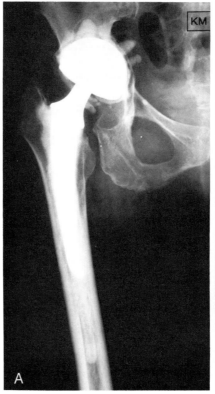
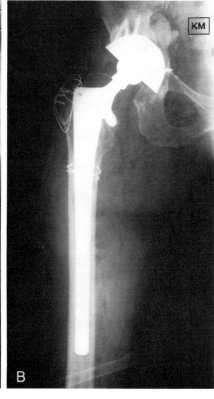

for the use of custom-fit cementless total hip implants. Clin Orthop, 249:73, 1989.

9. BLACK J: Metallic ion release and its relationship to onco-genesis. *In* The Hip: Proceeding of the 13th Hip Society. p. 199, 1985.

10. BLACK J: Editorial: does corrosion matter? J Bone Joint Surg, 70B:517, 1988.

11. BLACK J, et al: Metallosis associated with a stable titanium-alloy femoral component in total hip replacement: a case report. J Bone Joint Surg, 72A:126, 1990.

12. BRAND RA, PEDERSEN D, YODER SA: How definition of "loosening" affects the incidence of loose total hip reconstructions. Clin Orthop, 10:185, 1986.

13. BUECHE MJ, HERZENBER JE, STUBBS BT: Dissociation of a metal-backed polyethylene acetabular component: a case report. J Arthroplasty, 4(1):39, 1989.

14. BUTEL J, ROBB JE: The isoelastic hip prosthesis followed for five years. Arch Orthop Scand, 59:258, 1988.

15. BUTLER CA, JONES LC, HUNGERFORD DS: Initial implant stability of porous coated total hip femoral components: a mechanical study. Proceeding of the Orthopaedic Research Society, p. 423, 1988.

16. CALLAGHAN JJ, DYSART SH, SAVORY CG: The uncemented porous-coated anatomic total hip prosthesis: two-year results of a prospective consecutive series. J Bone Joint Surg, 70A:337, 1988.

17. CAPELLO WN: Fit the patient to the prosthesis: an argument against the routine use of custom hip implants. Clin Orthop, 249:56, 1989.

18. CARLSSON AS, GENTZ C: Radiographic vs. clinical loosening of the acetabular component in non-infected total hip arthroplasty. Clin Orthop, 185:145, 1984.

19. CARLSSON AS, GENTZ C, SANZEN L: Socket loosening after arthroplasty: radiographic observations in 241 cases up to 15 years. Acta Orthop Scand, 57:97, 1986.

20. CARLSSON AS, LINDBERG HO, SANZEN L: Loosening of the socket in a 35 millimeter snap fit prosthesis and the Charnley hip prosthesis: a roentgenographic evaluation of 321 cases operated upon because of osteoarthritis. Clin Orthop, 228:63, 1988.

21. CARLSSON L, ROSTLUND T, ALBREKTSSON T, BRANEMARK P: Osseointegration of titanium implants. Acta Orthop Scand, 57:285, 1986.

22. CHANDLER HP, REINICK FT, WIXSON RL, MCCARTHY JC: Total hip replacement in patients younger than 30 years old: a five year follow-up study. J Bone Joint Surg, 63A:1426, 1981.

23. CHARNLEY J, CUBIC Z: The 9 and 10 year results of the low friction arthroplasty of the hip. Clin Orthop, 95:9, 1973.

24. CHARNLEY J: Low Friction Arthroplasty of the Hip: Theory and Practice. New York, Springer-Velag, 1979.

25. CHARNLEY J: Long term results of low friction arthroplasty. *In* The Hip. Proceedings of the 10th Hip Society. p. 42, 1982.

26. COLLIS DK: Cemented total hip replacement in patients who are less than 50 years old. J Bone Joint Surg, 66A:353, 1984.

27. COOK SD: Studies of retrieved human porous coated implants. Presented at Cement vs. Cementless THR—Is the Wrong Question. Boston, Sept. 28, 1988.

28. CORNELL CN, RANAWAT CS: The impact of modern cement techniques on acetabular fixation in cemented total hip replacement. J Arthroplasty, 1:197, 1986.

29. CORNELL CN, RANAWAT CS: Survivorship analysis of total hip replacements: results in a series of patients who were less than 55 years old. J Bone Joint Surg, 68A:1430, 1986.

30. DOHMAEY Y, et al.: Reduction in cement-bone interface shear strength between primary and revision arthroplasty. Clin Orthop, 236:214, 1988.

31. DORR LD, TAKEI GK, CONATY JP: Total hip arthroplasties in patients less than 45 years old. J Bone Joint Surg, 65A:474, 1983.

32. DUNN AW, HAMILTON LR: Muller curved stem total hip arthroplasty: long term follow-up of 185 consecutive cases. South Med J 79:698, 1986.

33. EFTEKHAR NS: Long term results of cemented total hip arthroplasty. Clin Orthop, 225:207, 1987.

34. ENGH CA: Principles, techniques, results, and complications with a porous-coated sintered metal system. Instr Course Lect, 35:169, 1986.

35. ENGH CA, BOBYN JG, GLASSMAN AH: Porous coated hip replacement: the factors governing bone ingrowth, stress shielding and clinical results. J Bone Joint Surg, 69B:45, 1987.

36. ENGH CA: Results of cementless revision for failed cemented total hip arthroplasty. Presented at Cement vs. Cementless THR—Is the Wrong Question. Boston, Sept. 28, 1988.

37. ENGH CA, GLASSMAN AH, GRIFFIN WL, MAYER JG: Results of cementless revision for failed cemented total hip arthroplasty. Clin Orthop, 235:91, 1988.

38. ENGH CA, BOBBYN JG: The influence of stem size and extent of porous coating on femoral bone resorption after primary cementless hip prosthesis. Clin Orthop, 231:7, 1988.

39. ENGH CA, MASSIN P: Primary total hip replacement using the AML stem. Presented at Cement vs. Cementless THR—Is the Wrong Question. Boston, Sept. 28, 1988.

40. ENGH CA, BOBYN JD: Biological Fixation in Total Hip Arthroplasty. Slack, Thorofare, NJ, 1985.

41. ENGH CA, GRIFFIN WL, MARX CL: Cementless acetabular components. J Bone Joint Surg, 72B:53, 1990.

42. ENGH CA, MASSIN P: Cementless total hip arthroplasty using the anatomic medullary locking stem: results using a survivorship analysis. Clin Orthop, 249:141, 1989.

43. ESKOLA A, et al: Cementless revision of aggressive granulomatous lesions in hip replacements. J Bone Joint Surg, 72B:212, 1990.

43A. FITZGERALD RH JR: The infected prosthetic joint: approaches to therapy and results. Presented at Cement vs. Cementless THR—Is the Wrong Question. Boston, Sept. 28, 1988.

44. FITZGERALD RH JR, BRINDLEY GW, KAVANAGH BF: The uncemented total hip arthroplasty: intraoperative femoral fractures. Clin Orthop, 235:61, 1988.

45. FOWLER JL, GIE GA, LEE AJC, LING RSM: Experience with the exeter total hip replacement since 1970. Orthop Clin North Am, 19:477, 1988.

46. FRIEDMAN RJ: Displacement of an uncemented femoral component after dislocation of a total hip replacement: a case report. J Bone Joint Surg, 71A:1406, 1989.

47. FUCHS MD et al.: Results of acetabular revisions with newer cement techniques. Orthop Clin North Am, 19:649, 1988.

48. GALANTE JO: Results of cementless revision total hip arthroplasty with titanium fiber metal components: two to four year follow-up. Presented at Cement vs. Cementless THR—Is The Wrong Question. Boston, Sept. 28, 1988.

49. GEESINK RGT, DE GROOT K, KLEIN CPAT: Chemical implant fixation using hydroxyl-apatite coatings: the development of a human total hip prosthesis for chemical fixation to bone using hydroxyl-apatite coatings on titanium substrates. Clin Orthop, 225:147, 1987.

50. GEESINK RGT, DE GROOT K, KLEIN CPAT: Bonding of bone to apatite coated implants. J Bone Joint Surg, 70B:17, 1988.

51. GROHER W: Uncemented total hip replacement. Can J Surg 26:534, 1983.
52. GUSTILO RB, BECHTOLD JE, GIACCHIETIO J, KYLE RF: Rationale, experience and results of long-stem femoral prosthesis. Clin Orthop, 249:159, 1989.
53. GUSTILO RB: Revision of femoral component loosening with titanium ingrowth prosthesis and bone grafting. Instr Course Lect 35:161, 1986.
54. GUSTILO RB, KYLE RF: Revision total hip replacement with titanium ingrowth prosthesis and bone grafting—for failed cemented femoral component loosening. Presented at Cement Vs. Cementless THR—is the Wrong Question. Boston, Sept. 28, 1988.
55. HADDAD RJ, COOK SD, BRINKER MR: A comparison of three varieties of noncemented porous-coated hip replacement. J Bone Joint Surg, 72B:2, 1990.
55A. HALLEY DK, CHARNLEY J: Results of low friction arthroplasty in patients 30 years of age or younger. Clin Orthop, 112:180, 1975.
56. HARRIS WH, MALONEY WJ: Hybrid total hip arthroplasty. Clin Orthop, 249:21, 1989.
57. HARRIS WH, MCCARTHY JC, O'NEILL DA: Femoral component loosening using contemporary techniques of femoral cement fixation. J Bone Joint Surg, 64A:1063, 1982.
58. HARRIS WH, MCGANN WA: Loosening of the femoral component after use of the medullary plug cementing technique: follow-up note with a minimum 5 year follow-up. J Bone Joint Surg, 68A:1064, 1986.
59. HARRIS WH, PENENBERG BL: Further follow-up on socket fixation using a metal-backed acetabular component for total hip replacement: a minimum 10 year follow-up study. J Bone Joint Surg, 69A:1140, 1987.
60. HARRIS WH, DAVIES JP: Modern use of modern cement for total hip replacement. Orthop Clin North Am, 19:581, 1988.
61. HARRIS WH, KRUSHELL RH, GALANTE JO: Results of cementless revision of total hip arthroplasties using the Harris-Galante prosthesis. Clin Orthop, 235:120, 1988.
62. HEDLEY AK, GRUEN TA, RUOFF DP: Revision of failed total hip arthroplasties with uncemented porous-coated anatomic components. Clin Orthop, 235:75, 1988.
63. HEINER JP, EVARTS C: Total hip arthroplasty: biological fixation: a preliminary report. Proceedings of the 54th Annual Meeting of the AAOS. p. 138, 1987.
64. HERBERTS P, MALCHAU H, ROMANUS B: Uncemented total hip replacements in young adults—a Scandinavian multicenter PCA study. Presented at Scandinavian Orthopaedic Association. Arhus, Denmark, June 8–11, 1988.
65. HOZACK WJ, et al.: Survivorship analysis of 1041 Charnley total hip arthroplasties. Proceedings of the 55th Annual Meeting of the AAOS. Atlanta, p. 116, 1988.
66. HOZACK WJ, ROTHMAN RH: Long-term survival of the Charnley low-friction total hip arthroplasty. Sem Arthroplasty, 1:3, 1990.
67. HUDDLESTON HD: Femoral lysis after cemented hip arthroplasty. J Arthroplasty, 3:285, 1988.
68. HUNGERFORD DS: Cementless prosthesis in the elderly. Presented at Cement vs. Cementless—THR is the Wrong Question. Boston, Sept. 28, 1988.
69. HUNGERFORD DS: The PCA femoral stem. Presented at Cement vs. Cementless—THR is the Wrong Question. Boston, Sept. 28, 1988.
70. HUNGERFORD DS, KRACKOW KA, JACOBS MA, LENOX DW: Cementless revision of failed THR using the PCA total hip system. Presented at Cement vs. Cementless—THR Is the Wrong Question. Boston, Sept. 28, 1988.
71. HUNGERFORD DS, JONES LC: The rationale of cementless revision of cemented arthroplasty failures. Clin Orthop, 235:12, 1988.
72. IANNOTTI JP, et al.: Aseptic loosening after total hip arthroplasty. J Arthroplasty, 1:99, 1986.
73. JAKIM I, BARLIN C, SWEET MBE: RM isoelastic total hip arthroplasty: a review of 34 cases. J Arthroplasty, 3:191, 1988.
74. JASTY MJ, et al.: Localized osteolysis in stable, nonseptic total hip arthroplasty. J Bone Joint Surg, 68A, 912, 1986.
75. JASTY M, et al.: Stimulation of bone ingrowth into porous surfaced total joint prosthesis by applying a thin coating of tricalcium phosphate-hydroxyapatite. Presented at Cement vs. Cementless—THR is the Wrong Question. Boston, Sept. 28, 1988.
76. JASTY M, HARRIS WH: Salvage total hip reconstruction in patients with major acetabular bone deficiency using structural femoral head allografts. Presented at Cement vs. Cementless—THR is the Wrong Question. Boston, Sept. 28, 1988.
77. JOHNSTON RC, CROWNINSHIELD RD: Roentgenologic results of total hip arthroplasty: a ten-year follow-up study. Clin Orthop, 181:92, 1983.
78. JONES LC HUNGERFORD DS: Cement disease. Clin Orthop, 225:192, 1987.
79. KAVANAGH BF, ILSTRUP DM, FITZGERALD RH: Revision total hip arthroplasty. J Bone Joint Surg, 67A:517, 1985.
80. KAVANAGH BF, FITZGERALD RH: Multiple revisions for failed total hip arthroplasty not associated with infection. J Bone Joint Surg, 69A:1144, 1987.
81. KEATING EM, RITTER MA, FARIS PM: Structures at risk from medially placed acetabular screws. J Bone Joint Surg, 72A:509, 1990.
82. KIM Y, SUH J: Low incidence of deep vein thrombosis after cementless total hip replacement. J Bone Joint Surg, 70A:878–882, 1988.
83. KITZIGER KJ, DELEE JC, EVANS JA: Disassembly of modular acetabular component of a total hip replacement arthroplasty: a case report. J Bone Joint Surg, 72A:621, 1990.
84. KREVOLIN JL, POLANDO GH, SAAS HA, GREENWALD AS: Survivorship analysis of cemented and porous coated hip implant series. Proceedings of the Orthopaedic Research Society, p. 463, 1988.
85. KRUSHELL R: Primary THR using the HGP hip replacement: minimum 2 year follow-up. Presented at Cement vs. Cementless—THR is the Wrong Question. Boston, Sept. 28, 1988.
86. LING PA: Cemented total hip replacement—Long Term results 11-16 years. Presented at Cement vs. Cementless—THR is the Wrong Question. Boston, Sept. 28, 1988.
87. LIVERMORE J, ILSTRUP D, MORREY B: Effect of femoral head size on wear of the polyethylene acetabular component. J Bone Joint Surg, 72A:518, 1990.
88. LOMBARDI AV, MALLORY TH, VAUGHN BK, DROUILLARD P: Aseptic loosening in total hip arthroplasty secondary to osteolysis induced by wear debris from titanium-alloy modular femoral heads. J Bone Joint Surg, 71A:1337, 1989.
89. LORD GA: Madreporique stemmed total hip replacement: five years clinical experience. J Royal Soc Med, 75:166, 1982.
90. LORD G, MAROTTE J, GULLIAMON J, BLANCHARD J: Cementless revisions of failed aseptic cemented and cementless total hip arthroplasties. Clin Orthop, 235:67, 1988.
91. MCCOY TH, SALVATI EA, RANAWAT CS, WILSON PD: A 15 year follow-up study of 100 Charnley low friction arthroplasties. Orthop Clin North Am, 19:467, 1988.

92. McGann WA, Welch RB, Picetti GD: Acetabular preparation in cementless revision total hip arthroplasty. Clin Orthop, 235:35, 1988.

93. McKellop HA, Sarmiento A, Schwinn C, Ebramzadeh E: In vivo wear of titanium-alloy hip prostheses. J Bone Joint Surg, 72A:512, 1990.

94. Mittelmeier: Report on the first decennium of clinical experience with a cementless ceramic total hip replacement. Acta Orthop Belg, 51:367, 1985.

95. Mjoberg B, et al.: Mechanical loosening of total hip prostheses: a radiographic and roentgen stereophotogrammetric study. J Bone Joint Surg, 68B:770, 1986.

96. Morry BF, Ilstrup D: Size of the femoral head and acetabular revision in total hip replacement arthroplasty. J Bone Joint Surg, 71A: 50, 1989.

97. Morscher EW: European experience with cementless total hip replacements. *In* The Hip. Proceedings of the 11th Hip Society, p. 190, 1983.

98. Morscher EW: Cementless total hip arthroplasty. Clin Orthop, 181:76, 1983.

99. Mulier JC, et al.: A new system to produce intraoperatively custom femoral prosthesis from measurements taken during the surgical procedure. Clin Orthop, 249:97, 1989.

100. Nunn D, Freeman MAR, Tanner KE, Bonfield W: Torsional stability of the femoral component of hip arthroplasty: response to an anteriorly applied load. J Bone Joint Surg, 71B:452, 1989.

101. O'Leary JFM, et al.: Mittelmeier ceramic total hip arthroplasty. J Arthroplasty,

102. Oonishi H, et al.: The effect of hydroxyapatite coating on bone growth into porous titanium alloy implants. J Bone Joint Surg, 71B:213, 1989.

103. Pavlov PW: A 15 year follow-up study of 512 consecutive Charnley-Muller total hip replacements. J Arthroplasty, 2:151, 1987.

104. Pellicci PM, et al.: Long term results of revision total hip replacement: a follow-up report. J Bone Joint Surg, 67A:513, 1985.

105. Phillips TW, Messieh SS: Cementless hip replacement for arthritis: problems with smooth surface Moore stem. J Bone Joint Surg, 70B:750, 1988.

106. Poss R, et al.: The effects of modern cementing techniques on the longevity of total hip arthroplasty. Clin Orthop North Am, 19:591, 1988.

107. Ranawat CS, Atkinson RE, Salvati EA, Wilson PD: Conventional total hip arthroplasty for degenerative joint disease in patients between the ages of 40 and 60 years. J Bone Joint Surg, 66A:745, 1984.

108. Reikeras O: A ten year follow-up of Muller hip replacements. Acta Orthop Scand, 53:919, 1982.

109. Ring PA: Uncemented total hip replacement. J Royal Soc Med, 74:19, 1981.

110. Ritter MA, Campbell ED: Long term comparison of the Charnley, Muller, trapezoidal-28 total hip prostheses: a survival analysis. J Arthroplasty, 2:299, 1987.

111. Roberts DW, Poss R, Kelley K: Radiographic comparison of cementing techniques in total hip arthroplasty. J Arthroplasty, 1:241, 1986.

112. Roberts JA, Finlayson DF, Freeman PA: The long term results of the Howse total hip arthroplasty: with particular reference to those requiring revision. J Bone Joint Surg, 69B:545, 1987.

113. Rosso R: Five year review of the isoelastic RM total hip endoprosthesis. Arch Orthop Trauma Surg, 107:86, 1988.

114. Rorabeck CH, Bourne RB, Nott L: Cemented vs. non-cemented total hips: a preliminary report. J. Bone Joint Surg, 69B:508, 1987.

115. Rothman RH, Hozack WJ, Booth RE, Balderston RA: A prospective comparative study of cement vs. cementless total hip arthroplasty. (unpublished)

116. Rubash HE, Harris WH: Revision THA of cemented femoral components using modern cement techniques—six year average follow-up. J Bone Joint Surg, 69B:509, 1987.

117. Russotti GM, Coventry MB, Stauffer RN: Cemented THA using contemporary techniques—a minimum five year follow-up study. Presented at Cement vs. Cementless—Is THR the Wrong Question. Boston, Sept. 28, 1988.

118. Salvati EA, et al.: A ten year follow-up study of our first 100 consecutive Charnley total hip replacements. J Bone Surg, 63A:753, 1981.

119. Sarmiento A, Natarajan V, Gruen TA, McMahon, M: Radiographic performance of two different total hip cemented arthroplasties. Orthop Clin North Am, 19:505, 1988.

120. Schneider E, et al.: A comparative study of the initial stability of cementless hip prostheses. Clin Orthop, 248:200, 1989.

121. Schwartz JT, Mayer JG, Engh CA: Femoral fracture during non-cemented total hip arthroplasty. J Bone Joint Surg, 71A:1135, 1989.

122. Sharkey PF, Albert TJ, Hume EL, Rothman RH: Initial stability of a collarless wedge-shaped prosthesis in the femoral canal. Sem Arthroplasty, 1:87, 1990.

123. Sharkey PF, Wolf LW, Hume EL, Rothman RH: Insertional femoral fracture: a biomechanical study of femoral component stability. Sem Arthroplasty, 1:91, 1990.

124. Sharkey PF, Hozack WJ, Rothman RH, Booth RE: The clinical significance of intraoperative femoral fractures in cementless total hip arthroplasty. (unpublished)

125. Snorason F, et al.: The Mittelmeier hip prosthesis—a clinical, radiographic and scintimetric evaluation. Acta Orthop Scand, 59–84, 1988.

126. Stauffer RN: Ten year follow-up study of total hip replacement with particular reference to roentgenographic loosening of the components. J Bone Joint Surg, 64A:983, 1982.

127. Stromberg CN, Herberts P, Ahnfelt L: Revision total hip arthroplasty in patients younger than 55 years old: clinical and radiologic results after 4 years. J Arthroplasty, 3:47, 1988.

128. Stulberg SD, Stulberg BN, Wixson RL: The rationale, design characteristics, and preliminary results of a primary custom total hip prosthesis. Clin Orthop, 249:79, 1989.

129. Sudman NE, Havelin LI, Lunde OD, Rait M: The Charnley vs. the Christiansen total hip arthroplasty: comparative clinical study. Acta Orthop Scand, 54:545, 1983.

130. Sutherland CJ, Wilde AH, Borden LS, Marks KE: A ten year follow-up of 100 consecutive Muller curved stem total hip replacement arthroplasties. J Bone Joint Surg, 64A:970, 1982.

131. Thomas KA, et al.: Biologic response to hydroxyapatite-coated titanium hips: a preliminary study in dogs. J Arthroplasty, 4(1):43, 1989.

132. Trancik T, Mills W, Vinson N: The effect of indomethacin, aspirin, and ibuprofen on bone ingrowth into a porous-coated implant. Clin Orthop, 249:113, 1989.

133. Tullos HS, McCaskill BL, Dickey R, Davidson J: Total hip arthroplasty with a low modulus porous coated femoral component: a progress report. J Bone Joint Surg, 66:888, 1984.

134. Turner TM, et al.: A comparative study of porous coatings in a weight bearing total hip arthroplasty model. J Bone Joint Surg, 68A:1396, 1986.

135. Turner RH, Mattingly DA, Scheller A: Femoral revision total hip arthroplasty using a long stem femoral component: clinical and radiographic analysis. J Arthroplasty, 2:247, 1987.

136. Van der Schaaf DB, Deutman R, Mulder TJ: Stanmore total hip replacement: a 9-10 year follow-up. J Bone Joint Surg, 70B:45, 1988.

137. Wasielewski RC, Cooperstein LA, Kruger MP, Rubash HE: Acetabular anatomy and the transacetabular fixation of screws in total hip arthroplasty. J Bone Joint Surg, 72A:501, 1990.

138. Wejkner B, Stenport J: Charnley total hip arthroplasty—10 to 14 year follow-up study. Clin Orthop, 231:113, 1988.

139. Welch RB, McGann WA, Picetti GD: Charnley low friction arthroplasty: a 15 to 17 year follow-up study. Orthop Clin North Am, 19:551, 1988.

140. Whiteside LA: Stability of cementless femoral component in total hip replacement. Presented at Cement vs. Cementless—THR is the Wrong Question. Boston, Sept. 28, 1988.

141. Woolson ST, Pottorff GT: Disassembly of a modular femoral prosthesis after dislocation of the femoral component: a case report. J Bone Joint Surg, 73A:624, 1990.

142. Wroblewski BM: 15 to 21 year results of the Charnley low friction arthroplasty. Clin Orthop, 211:30, 1986.

143. Zweymuller K, Semlitsch M: Concept and material properties of a cementless hip prosthesis system with a1 to 03 ceramic ball heads and wrought ti-6AL-4V stems. Arch Orthop Trauma Surg, 100:229, 1982.

144. Zweymuller K: A cementless titanium hip endoprosthesis system based on press fit fixation: basic research and clinical results. Instr Course Lect 35:203, 1986.

145. Zweymuller KA, Lintner FK, Semlitsch MF: Biologic fixation of a press fit titanium hip joint endoprosthesis. Clin Orthop, 235:195, 1988.

CHAPTER TWENTY FOUR

The Rheumatoid Hip

ANTHONY S. UNGER
CHITRANJAN S. RANAWAT
RANDALL J. LEWIS

Hip joint disease is infrequent early in the clinical course of rheumatoid arthritis. In patients with established disease, however, the incidence of radiographic hip joint disease approaches 50% Once hip disease manifests itself clinically, the symptoms tend to progress rapidly, and require evaluation by an orthopaedic surgeon. Initial therapy should consist of appropriate conservative care delivered in conjunction with the patient's rheumatologist. However, if pain and disability are significant and do not respond to conservative management, surgical intervention must be considered.

This chapter discusses the unique characteristics of hip surgery in patients with rheumatoid arthritis. The preoperative evaluation, clinical manifestations, and surgical options in the treatment of these patients is discussed. As in all orthopaedic patients, the first formal therapy should consist of conservative care. This chapter, however, does not provide an extensive description of these modalities.

General Considerations

Because of the diffuse and chronic nature of rheumatoid disease a thorough preoperative multisystem evaluation should be performed before surgical therapy is contemplated. The patient should be evaluated from both the medical and orthopaedic standpoint. Evaluation by an occupational therapist, physical therapist, and, if appropriate, a social worker, is recommended. Because of the systemic nature of the disease, rheumatoid arthritis must be treated by a multidisciplinary approach.

Patients with rheumatoid arthritis frequently are steroid-dependent. Because of the chronic nature of the steroid administration these patients are susceptible to intraoperative and postoperative complications. If a patient is identified as being steroid-dependent he should be prophylactically administered intravenous steroid preparations. The steroid preparations should be continued for a minimum of 5 days postoperatively. The oral medications can be started immediately. In the period during which the steroid is administered intravenously, we recommend that the patient be treated with a histamine H-2 receptor antagonist.

A thorough search for occult infection should be performed prior to surgery. The oral cavity should be examined. Any sign of gingival infection or tooth abscess is a contraindication for surgery. The patient also should be evaluated for urinary tract infection. Frequently, rheumatoid arthritis patients who are steroid-dependent are not symptomatic for urinary tract infections, therefore, a urine culture should be sent for analysis prior to surgery. In addition, examination of the lower extremities, particularly the feet, should be performed in search of hidden sources of infection in the toes or nails. Any open wound, chronic infection, osteomyelitis, or chronically infected joint replacement are contraindications for total joint replacement. However, the patient who previously had a septic joint that has been adequately treated and reimplanted may be considered for joint replacement.

Preoperative evaluation of a patient with rheumatoid arthritis should always include evaluation of the cervical spine. Because of the possibility of cervical cord impingement during intubation, lateral views in flexion and extension should be performed prior to surgery. If cervical instability is severe and neurologic involvement is suggested, elective arthroplasty may be deferred until surgical stabilization has been obtained. In addition, any patient with cervical instability should be brought to the operating room with the appropriate cervical orthosis in place. This avoids inadvertent damage to the cervical cord during anesthesia. A patient with lower extremity weakness or signs of myelopathy should undergo detailed neurologic evaluation prior to surgery.

Patients with rheumatoid arthritis frequently have involvement of the temporomandibular joint, making oral intubation difficult, and, at times, impossible. The use of nasal intubation, fiber optic assistance, and regional anesthesia should be considered. Preoperative evaluation by an anesthesiologist will help avoid unnecessary delays.

The rehabilitation potential of the patient with rheumatoid arthritis should be accurately assessed prior to surgery. The goals set by the surgeon should be realistic for the patient's medical, social, and economic needs. An evaluation by the social worker, occupational therapist, and physical therapist often provides valuable information about rehabilitation potential and the reasonableness of the surgical plans. Arrangements should be made prior to surgery for out-patient physical therapy, post-hospital placement, and extended rehabilitation programs.

A decade ago, patients with rheumatoid arthritis who required extensive reconstruction always underwent the lower extremity surgery first, generally beginning with the hips. The rationale was that walking with crutches following hip or knee surgery would damage reconstructed upper extremity implants, and that patients should be off crutches prior to addressing upper extremity problems. Lower extremity procedures were felt to be more predictable, and hip replacement more reliable than knee replacement.[12,13,26]

Ten years of experience has changed some of our priorities. We still believe that lower extremity procedure should be performed first. Because hip and knee reconstructions are now regarded as being equally reliable and durable, the patient is offered reconstruction of the more painful or disabling joint first. When the hands and arms are so severely affected that they cannot functionally grasp assistance devices to help support the patient during ambulation, shoulder, elbow, and hand reconstruction occasionally may be performed as the first step, followed later by hip and knee surgery.

When hip surgery is contemplated, the knee, ankle, and foot should be carefully evaluated. The foot should be examined for painful plantar callosities and subluxations of the metatarsalphalangeal joints. If the foot is painful, forefoot reconstruction may be recommended before hip surgery. The ankle and subtalar joints should be similarly evaluated. The degree of flexion contracture and arthritis in the knee must be ascertained. The coexistence of a significant flexion contracture or deformity in the

knee may prevent satisfactory reconstruction of the hip. In particular, if the knee is ankylosed or has a flexion contracture of more than 30° with varus or valgus alignment of 30° or more, knee surgery may need to be performed prior to the hip surgery. Ipsilateral single-stage hip and knee operations ordinarily are not recommended. Hip surgery should be performed first followed by knee surgery 2 weeks later. However, in the extenuating circumstances, the knee can be reconstructed first, followed by the hip surgery.[10,25,31,36]

Bilateral hip surgery is frequently required in rheumatoid arthritis. The major indication for bilateral procedures is severe debilitating disease that would prevent ambulation after a single procedure. The overall health of the patient must be ascertained before contemplating a single-stage bilateral procedure. Single-stage bilateral procedures should not be performed on patients with significant cardiovascular and pulmonary disease or on elderly patients. Although the incidence of thrombophlebitis is not greater in a single stage bilateral procedure, the medical complications are significantly increased with a single-stage bilateral procedure.[28,32,33,35,48] Salvati, et al.[49] has reported the blood loss to be approximately 30% higher with single-stage bilateral hip arthroplasty when compared to separate procedures. In addition, the duration of surgery was almost doubled and the only death in the series occurred in a single-stage bilateral procedure because of massive fat embolism. Bilateral surgery should only be contemplated in healthy patients who have severe bilateral disease that would significantly impair their ability to ambulate after a single procedure. If any question exists about the overall health of the patient, a single hip procedure should be performed, separated by a 1- to 2-week interval from the next procedure. In the interim, between the first and second operations, the patient should be kept at bed rest if ambulation is impossible.

Clinical Manifestations of the Rheumatoid Hip

Synovitis

Destruction of the hip in rheumatoid arthritis results from inflammatory synovitis. Early in the disease, patients may present with nonspecific hip pain and x-rays may show no evidence of joint space narrowing. Over the long term, this synovitis will lead to destruction of the hip joint. In the early phases of the disease, without radiographic evidence of cartilage destruction, the patient should be followed and treated by a rheumatologist with antiarthritic drugs. Intra-articular steroid injections are not recommended. Sterile preparation of the skin around the hip is difficult in the office setting and we are fearful of contamination of the joint, which may compromise reconstruction at a later date. Injections may lead to a temporary increase in intra-articular pressure and possibly compromise femoral head vascularity. Synovitis alone usually can be controlled by medical management.

Joint Contractures

Joint contractures about the hip occur because of the chronic synovitis in the joint. The most frequent deformity around the hip joint is a flexion and adduction contracture. The flexion contracture results from anterior scarring and shortening of the iliofemoral ligament. Over time, the scar becomes thick, contracture becomes fixed, and the patient begins to compensate for the loss of hip extension by accentuating the lumbar lordosis. This may lead to both lumbar spine and knee complaints. Hip flexion contracture should be carefully evaluated because it may impair reconstruction of the hip joint. At the time of surgery, an attempt should be made to eliminate all of the flexion contracture. In most patients with rheumatoid arthritis, however, a 10 to 15° flexion contracture will stretch out after total hip replacement. For the patient with a severe flexion contracture, particularly of both hips, bilateral single-stage hip replacements may be necessary. In such cases a generous capsulotomy and release of the anterior structures is necessary to ensure adequate exposure of the hip joint and prevent improper orientation of the components.

Adduction contractures occur in the rheumatoid patients with long-standing disease. Aside from the difficulties with gait and perineal hygiene, adductor contracture may compromise postoperative care of the hip. If the patient is unable to abduct the hip to 0°, an adductor tenotomy may be necessary prior to hip reconstruction. If the adductors are not released and the extremity cannot be placed in a safe abducted position, the patient will be susceptible to postoperative dislocation.

Protrusio Acetabuli

Protrusio acetabuli (Fig. 24–1) is common in patients with advanced rheumatoid arthritis. Once recognized protrusio is progressive. As the protrusio progresses the joint reactive forces are concentrated on the medial wall of the acetabulum, increasing the rate of medial migration of the femoral head. Once the head of the femur reaches Koehler's line, serious consideration should be given to hip reconstruction. Surgery is recommended in rheumatoid arthritis because of the progressive nature of the protrusio and the difficulties with reconstruction once the migration has become severe. The degree of protrusio can be measured by the method described by Ranawat (Fig. 24–2).[46,47] Because optimal hip reconstruction requires normalization of the center of rotation, an aggressive approach to patients with significant protrusio is recommended.

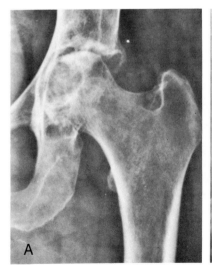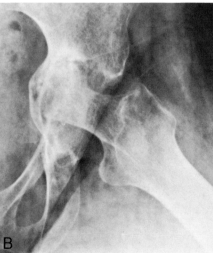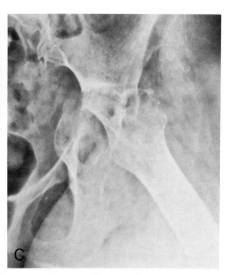

FIG. 24–1. Progression of protrusio acetabuli. **A.** Initial roentgenogram. **B.** Four years later. **C.** Six years later.

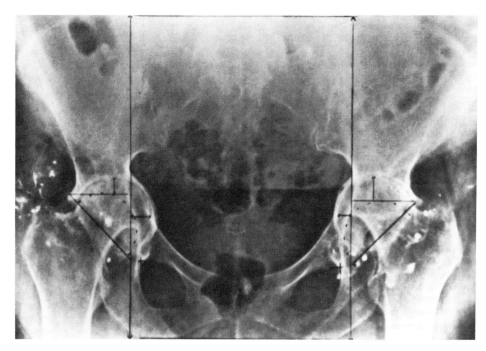

Fɪɢ. 24–2. One-fifth of the height of the pelvis approximates the height of the acetabulum. A point is located 5.0 mm lateral to the intersection of Kohler's line and Shenton's line. A vertical line is drawn from this point superiorly to a second point; the distance equals one-fifth the height of the pelvis. A perpendicular line is then drawn laterally from this second point to a third point that is drawn at one-fifth the height of the pelvis. The vertical and horizontal lines mark the medial and superior boundaries of the normal acetabulum. The amount of medial and superior protrusion can be measured relative to these lines. (From Ranawat CS, Zahn MG: Role of bone grafting in correction of protrusio acetabuli by total hip arthroplasty. J Arthroplasty, 1:131, 1986.)

Ankylosis

End stage rheumatoid arthritis occasionally results in ankylosis of the hip joint. In patients who do not have rheumatoid disease, ankylosis in good position frequently results in a stable situation. Unfortunately, the patient with rheumatoid arthritis is often severely compromised by an ankylosed hip. The ankylosis of the hip frequently results in increased stresses on other diseased joints of the lower extremity, compromising these joints and leading to rapid deterioration. If ankylosis occurs in an adducted, fixed position, disability from the ipsilateral knee and perineal hygiene occurs. Therefore, in those patients who have end stage rheumatoid arthritis with an ankylosed hip, "takedown" of the ankylosis may be recommended. Although the procedure is formidable, the results in general lead to an excellent outcome. Frequently, patients with ankylosed hips are non-ambulatory and by reconstructing the hip joints they regain their ambulatory status and can sit comfortably in chairs. At the very least, perineal care is facilitated by restoring mobility to the hip joint. If the patient has no potential for ambulation because of severe knee or upper extremity involvement, an osteotomy to facilitate perineal care can be performed rather than arthroplasty.

Acetabular Bone Loss

The term protrusio acetabuli delineates loss of the medial wall of the acetabulum. Other forms of acetabular bone loss occur in rheumatoid arthritis as well. Patients with protrusio acetabuli frequently have coexisting superior bone loss, which presents formidable reconstructive problems to the surgeon. Anterior and posterior wall bone loss occurs frequently as well. When severe acetabular bone loss is identified, we recommend aggressive surgical reconstruction consisting of prosthetic replacement with supplemental bone graft. When the column is deficient it may be necessary to use acetabular reinforcing devices.

Avascular Necrosis

Coexisting avascular necrosis is a common occurrence in patients with rheumatoid arthritis. In the majority of cases the avascular necrosis is secondary to long term steroid administration. When avascular necrosis does occur it is symptomatic and progressive in patients with rheumatoid arthritis. The treatment of this condition usually consists initially of conservative therapy followed by total joint replacement when the patient becomes severely symptomatic. We do not feel that core decompression, osteotomy, or hemiarthroplasty is appropriate for patients with rheumatoid arthritis. Because the level of activity of the patients with rheumatoid arthritis is very low, a total joint replacement should be recommended over the hemiarthroplasty.

Other Coexisting Conditions

Patients with rheumatoid arthritis may have other coexisting conditions, such as acetabular dysplasia. In the early stages of the disease, before significant degenerative changes have occurred, acetabular dysplasia may be treated by pelvic or femoral osteotomies. In the later stages of the disease, when there is joint destruction, total joint replacement using standard reconstructive techniques for acetabular dysplasia is recommended. Acetabular autogenous bone grafts or allografts should be used to restore the deficient anatomy. Customized or miniature components may be necessary.

Surgical Options

Synovectomy

There are few reports of the results of synovectomy for hip disease in patients with rheumatoid arthritis. We have little experience with this procedure and in general do not recommend it. Cruese[16] felt that the procedure was indicated early in the disease and that results on short followup were satisfactory. Wilkinson[63] reported very poor results after synovectomy of the hip. Eyring, et al.[21] felt that synovectomy of the hip could best be performed through an anterior approach without dislocation of the hip, hopefully preventing damage to the posterior retinacular vessels. This approach, however, affords only a limited view of the hip joint and a complete synovectomy cannot be performed. The posterior approach with dislocation of the hip can jeopardize the blood supply to the femoral head by interfering with the intrasynovial vessels. Synovectomy has a limited role in the treatment of hip disease in patients with rheumatoid arthritis.

Total Joint Replacement

Cemented Total Hip Replacement

Cemented hip replacement is the mainstay in the treatment of hip disease in patients with rheuma-

toid arthritis. Studies of total hip replacement in patients with osteoarthritis have revealed excellent durability and functional outcomes on long-term followup.[4,7,9,14,17,18,27,34,50,54,57] Although few long-term studies pertain strictly to patients with rheumatoid arthritis, the reported results have been excellent.[2,3,5,11,24,29,45,62] A study at The Hospital for Special Surgery revealed excellent results on long-term followup in patients with rheumatoid arthritis who underwent total hip replacement (Fig. 24–3).[59] At an average of 12 years followup (10 to 17 years), 81% of the patients had satisfactory results. The revision rate including infection was 16.7%. The revision rate for mechanical loosening was 13.3%. Survivorship analysis of this same group demonstrated that 93% of the hips survived to the 9 year interval.

Poss, et al.,[43,45] have shown that patients with rheumatoid arthritis who underwent total hip replacement were functioning extremely well at an average followup of 7 years. Although the radiographic results suggested that long-term failure might occur because of acetabular loosening, the results were comparable to those obtained in the osteoarthritis population. Welch and Charnley[62] reported 95% excellent results in 307 hips, with an average of 32.3 months followup. Colville, et al.,[11] reviewed 378 Charnley low friction arthroplasties with followup from 1 to 6 years; 95% had excellent pain relief on followup and 98.5% felt that the additional mobility makes the hip replacement a recommendable procedure.

Long-term followup studies of total hip replacement in rheumatoids have revealed a propensity toward acetabular failures. At the Hospital for Special Surgery there were 4 times the number of acetabular revisions compared to femoral revisions at 12

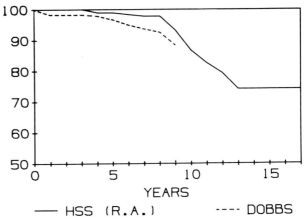

Fig. 24–3. Survival curves of the Hospital for Special Surgery study compared with Dobbs study.

years average followup.[59] Radiographically, loose acetabular components were 5 times more prevelant. Stauffer[54] has also demonstrated that the rheumatoid total hip replacement fails more often on the acetabular side. In the osteoarthritis group, 28.5% of the femoral components were loose by radiographic analysis compared to 7.0% of the acetabular components. However, the rheumatoid population had the reverse situation. Twelve percent of the femoral components were loose, compared with 35% of the acetabular components.

The preponderance of acetabular failures on long-term followup probably has several causes. First, the quantity of bone stock available for reconstruction in the rheumatoid hip is usually reduced. Second, the quality of the bone is unsatisfactory; it is often osteoporotic and fatty, and its mechanical strength is diminished. Third, it is difficult for the surgeon to achieve an optimal interface with the raw bleeding surfaces of this poor quality bone.

Because of the limited demands in mobility of the patient with rheumatoid arthritis, there is less reservation about recommending cemented total hip replacements to patients under 50 years of age than other groups of patients. Several studies have indicated very poor results in the osteoarthritis and avascular necrosis population for the chronologically young.[6] However, in polyarticular disease, a chronological age of under 50 is not a contraindication for a cemented total hip replacement. In those patients who are under 50 years of age, with monoarticular disease, and excellent bone stock uncemented total joint replacement may be considered.

Uncemented Total Hip Replacement

Uncemented total hip replacement may have a role in the treatment of patients with rheumatoid arthritis. Engh has not reported a significant difference in the survivorship of uncemented total hip replacement for the osteoarthritis patient population vs. the rheumatoid population. He did, however, note less bone ingrowth fixation in patients with rheumatoid arthritis. Cementless reconstruction of acetabular defects seems to us to have advantages over cemented total hip replacement. Initial reports of these techniques are encouraging and we believe they offer long-term advantages over the cemented cup.

Over the last 3 years we have gained considerable experience in the use of hydroxylapatite coated implants in patients with rheumatoid arthritis. Uncemented total hip replacement reconstructions have been performed in 10 patients with severe rheumatoid disease. All of these patients were steroid-dependent. At an average followup of 2 years, all of the hips are performing extremely satisfactorily. There are no radiographic signs of loosening and all of the bony defects had been reconstructed. We believe that the hydroxylapatite coated implant may offer significant advantages over porous coated implants. Because patients with rheumatoid arthritis are in a catabolic state and the presence of systemic steroids may interfere with bony ingrowth, we feel that the use of a hydroxylapatite coated implant on either a macro or micro-structured substrate has significant advantages over the porous coated implants.

In spite of our excellent success, using the hydroxylapatite coated implant in patients with rheumatoid arthritis, we still feel that more information needs to be gathered on the long-term results of uncemented hip replacements before it becomes a standard treatment. Since the results obtained with cemented implants in the low-demand population are both predictable and durable, we still continue to recommend cemented arthroplasty for the majority of our patients with severe rheumatoid disease.

Surface Replacement Arthroplasty

Surface replacement arthroplasty evoked substantial interest in the late 1970s, but after relatively short followup the procedure had an unacceptably high failure rate. Several reasons for the frequent failures were postulated: the thin polyethylene acetabular component was flexible and did not provide a stable interface over time; the large diameter arthroplasty produced increased friction, which creates high torque stresses at bone cement interface; avascular necrosis of the femoral head and neck underneath the femoral component and stress-shielding led to femoral loosening and femoral neck fractures. Although the failure rate of this procedure was no higher in patients with rheumatoid arthritis when compared to other populations we feel that the failure rate of 20% to 30% at less than 5 years followup is not acceptable and we do not recommend this procedure.[1,23,55,60]

Hemiarthroplasty

In his initial report of 1957, Moore[39] discussed the results of 6 patients with rheumatoid disease who underwent endoprosthetic replacement. On followup, 2 of the 6 were rated as good; 4 were rated as poor. Salvati, et al.,[50] also reported disappointing results with the use of the Moore prosthesis with 6 of 11 rheumatoid patients rated as fair or poor at 8 years followup. Sarmiento,[51] in contrast, stated that 81.3% of the rheumatoids were satisfactory at a mean followup of 4 years.

Recent reports have generated enthusiasm for bipolar endoprosthesis in the treatment of subcapital hip fractures and aseptic necrosis.[19] There are, however, several reasons *not* to recommend this procedure to the rheumatoid patient. The bipolar prosthesis, despite the inner bearing, is still a metal on cartilage arthroplasty, a situation that invariably leads to cartilage degeneration. Certainly, in the rheumatoid, because the cartilage is diseased, this procedure is inappropriate. Even in the fracture patient, the presence of abnormal acetabular cartilage is generally a contraindication to hemiarthroplasty. Long-term followup of at least one bipolar device has revealed protrusio to be a long-term problem.[52] In the rheumatoid hip, the incidence and severity might well be expected to be worse.

Patients with symptomatic rheumatoid disease who sustain intracapsular hip fractures are generally best treated by total hip replacement. The impacted subcapital hip fracture (Garden I or II) can be effectively treated with percutaneous Knowles pins, unless significant joint destruction has occured. If any question exists, we prefer primary total hip arthroplasty for hip fractures in rheumatoid patients, as well as other patients with pre-existing arthritis of the hip.

Arthrodesis

Hip arthrodesis has little role in the treatment of patients with rheumatoid hip disease. This procedure, although ideal for a young patient with osteoarthritis, is contraindicated in most patients with rheumatoid arthritis. The loss of hip motion causes transfer of abnormal stresses to the other joints of the lower extremity and the lumbosacral spine. The increased stresses are poorly tolerated by other joints already compromised by the rheumatoid process, and the end result can be a deterioration of the patient's ambulatory ability. The only role for hip arthrodesis in the rheumatoid patient is in a young, active patient with monoarticular disease.

Osteotomy

Osteotomy also has a limited role in the treatment of the rheumatoid hip. As discussed previously, it may be recommended for a patient with congenital hip dysplasia if the joint can be congruently reduced. This occurs occasionally only in the juvenile rheumatoid arthritis patient. Most adult rheumatoids are best treated with a total hip replacement. In the nonambulatory patient with a nonpainful, ankylosed hip, osteotomy occasionally is recommended to improve perineal care.

Surgical Techniques

Approaches

Surgical approaches to the rheumatoid hip are no different from those ordinarily used by the surgeon for other entities. Any approach that provides adequate exposure for optimal positioning of the component can be used. Despite a reported higher rate of dislocation, we prefer the posterior approach for most primary procedures. Trochanteric osteotomy, although it facilitates exposure, should be used judiciously because of the osteoporotic rheumatoid bone that may compromise trochanteric attachment and healing. It is recommended for revision surgery and special situations when wider exposure is needed.[41,58,61]

Acetabular Preparation

Meticulous acetabular preparation is important when the surgeon elects to use cemented total hip replacement in the patient with rheumatoid arthritis. Acetabular component fixation may be compromised by the relatively soft bone stock of the rheumatoid arthritic patient and the difficulty in achieving optimal cement fixation in the soft vascular rheumatoid bone. Care should be taken during the reaming process so that the structurally supportive subchondral bone is not lost. Removal of this subchondral end plate of bone exposes the bleeding cancellous surface beneath, and makes support of the component and cement fixation difficult. A useful technique to prevent this technical mishap involves using hand curettage to remove the panus and debris from the acetabulum and using the reamer only to remove adherent cartilage. Cement fixation is then achieved by making multiple anchoring holes in the subchondral bone.

Because many patients with rheumatoid arthritis regularly take aspirin or nonsteroidal anti-inflammatory agents that interfere with platelet function, good cement technique may be difficult to achieve. Bleeding from exposed bone surfaces compromises the ability of the surgeon to pressurize cement into the interstices of the bone. We, therefore, have relied heavily on the use of hypotensive general anesthesia to minimize the bleeding from these exposed bony surfaces, and use both the pulsating lavage and topical hemostatic agents.

Component Selection

Most available total hip systems can be used for the reconstruction of the patient with rheumatoid hip disease. There is no clear scientific evidence demonstrating the superiority of either chrome-cobalt or titanium alloys or of one modern stem design over another. The system chosen by the surgeon should, therefore, be one with which he is most familiar, provided that a few factors are kept in mind. First, the surgeon should try to optimize acetabular component survival by reducing abnormal stresses at the bone-cement interface. This can be achieved by using an acetabular component with the thickest polyethylene mantle that is possible. Metal backing also may promote uniform stress distribution. Femoral component selection should achieve 80% filling of the medullary canal with metal, and 20% with polymethylmethacrylate so that optimal material structure is obtained. In addition, frictional forces and transmitted torque stresses at the bone-cement interface can be reduced by the selection of a small diameter femoral head such as a 28 mm or a 26 mm.

Protrusio and Acetabular Defect Reconstruction

Surgical reconstruction of protrusio acetabuli and other acetabular defects should be directed toward correcting the bone deficiencies and restoring the center of rotation to its normal position.[30,37,38,53] Previously, Ranawat, et al.,[46] found a high incidence of acetabular radiographic bone cement radiolucency in hips in which the component was positioned 1.0 cm medially or superiorly beyond the anatomic center of rotation. Crowinshield[15] has demonstrated by in vitro studies that forces on the medial wall can be reduced by lateralizing the cup to its true anatomic center of rotation. Management of protrusio acetabuli to normalize the center of rotation is best treated as follows:[47]

1. If the protrusio is less than 5.0 mm and the medial wall appears strong, a bone graft is not necessary.
2. If the protrusio is greater than 5.0 mm an autogenous bone graft should be used. (We prefer bone graft over a protrusio ring or shell.) A bone graft can be procured from the autogenous femoral head (Fig. 24–4). It should be sliced into the appropriate size and thickness with an oscillating saw and then mortared into place with a small amount of polymethylmethacrylate. After the cement has hardened a second batch of cement should be used to seat the acetabular compo-

FIG. 24–4. **A.** Preoperative x-ray depicting medial wall bone loss of 7.0 mm. Superior bone loss measures 3.0 mm. **B.** Postoperative reconstruction by autogenous medial bone graft to restore center of rotation.

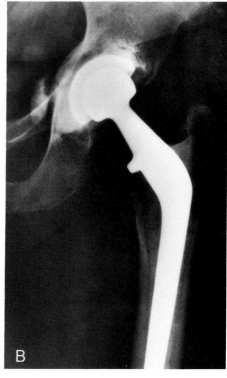

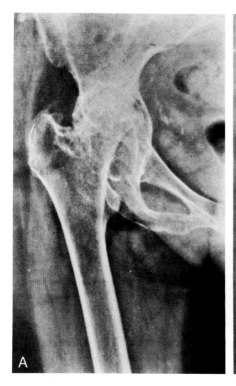 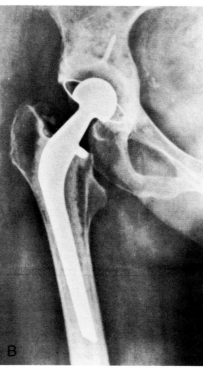

FIG. 24–5. **A.** Preoperative x-ray with superior and medial protrusion. **B.** Postoperative x-ray after medial and superior bone grafting. (From Ranawat CS, Zahn MG: Role of bone grafting in correction of protrusio acetabuli by total hip arthroplasty. J Arthroplasty, 1:131, 1986.)

nent. An alternative method of managing a moderate protrusio is the use of an oversized uncemented cup. The oversized uncemented cup transfers the stress to the mouth of the acetabulum. Morselized autogenous bone graft is placed behind the socket to reconstitute the medial wall.

3. If the medial wall defect is deficient it should be reconstructed with a substantial bone graft. A protrusio ring, uncemented oversized cup, or specialized cup may be used in addition. The relative merits of these devices are unknown, and longer followup is needed to determine the advantages of one device over another.

Specific Recommendations for the Management of Acetabular Defects

Contained acetabular defects, such as a large bone cyst, should be packed with morselized autogenous bone graft. Structural acetabular deficiencies, particularly in the weight-bearing dome, are best treated with corticocancellus autogenous bone grafts or allografts (Figs. 24–5, 24–6). These grafts can be fixed to the pelvis, using cancellous bone screws or titanium mesh, as necessary. Anterior or posterior column defects are best treated with large cortical cancellous bone grafts supplemented with reinforcing rings or similar devices.

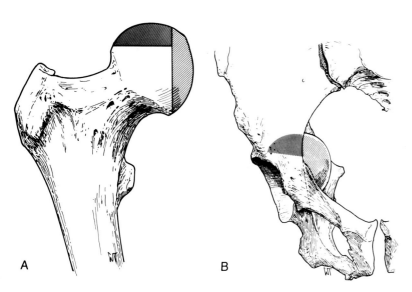

FIG. 24–6. **A.** Resection lines after dislocation for superior and medial bone grafts. **B.** Bone grafts in position; cement and acetabular component placed over graft. (From Ranawat CS, Zahn MG: Role of bone grafting in correction of protrusio acetabuli by total hip arthroplasty. J Arthroplasty, 1:131, 1986.)

A   B

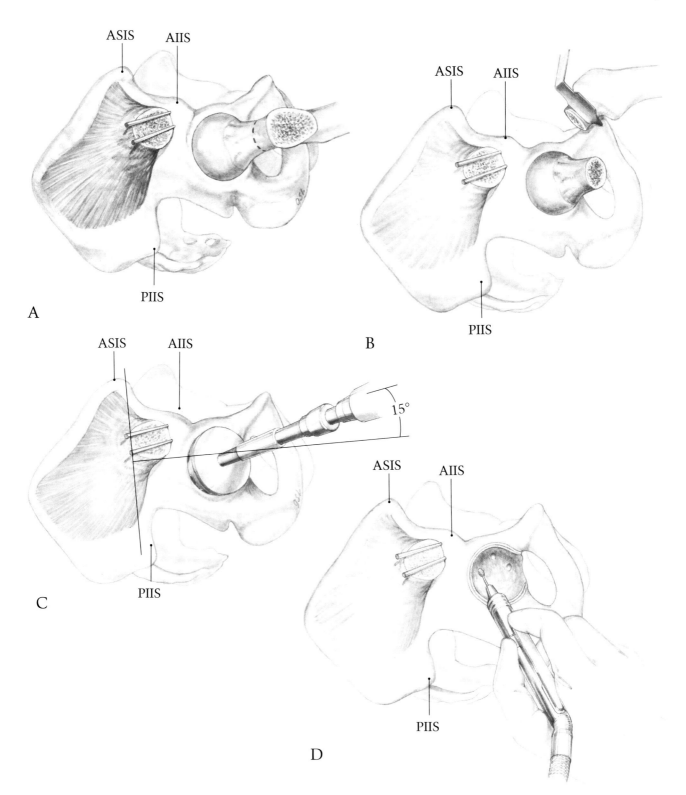

Fig. 24–7A. Operative view of an ankylosed hip. A trochanteric osteotomy has been made. The trochanteric fragment is retracted proximally and held with two Steinman pins. The resection line on the femoral neck is indicated B. The femoral neck osteotomy has been performed. The femur can either be retracted anteriorly, as depicted in the drawing, by a bent Homan retractor, or posteriorly. **C.** The protruding fragment of femoral neck and head is removed using either a bone saw or a rongeur. The true acetabulum is then best found by reaming through the ankylosed heads starting with a small 46.0 mm reamer. In this way the subchondral plate can be identified. D. The subchondral plate of the remaining femoral head is chipped away using a high speed burr. When the remaining femoral head is removed, the true confines of the acetabulum are identified. Acetabular preparation then can be undertaken in a usual manner. ASIS = Anterior superior iliac spine. AIIS = Anterior inferior iliac spine. PIIS = Posterior superior iliac spine.

Ankylosis Takedown (Fig. 24–7)

The reconstruction of a previously ankylosed rheumatoid hip is one of the most challenging procedures that the orthopaedic surgeon encounters. The procedure can be facilitated by the incorporation of the following techniques: A trochanteric osteotomy should be routinely performed. The femoral neck should be osteotomized with the femoral head in situ. The true acetabular component position is best found by reaming through the ankylosed femoral head starting with a very small reamer. In this way the subchondral plate can be identified. Once the subchondral plate of the femoral head is identified it can be chipped out using a small curette or high speed burr. The femoral head once removed, defines the bony confines of the true acetabulum.

Postoperative Complications

Thromboembolic Disease

The incidence of thromboembolic disease in patients with rheumatoid arthritis undergoing total hip replacement is similar to that in osteoarthritic patients. Poss, et al,[44] reported the incidence of deep vein thrombosis as 1.5% and that of pulmonary embolism as 1.0%. Coville, et al,[11] found a 1.3% incidence of deep venous thrombosis in 278 patients with rheumatoid arthritis. Arden, et al.,[2] detected deep vein thrombosis in 4.75% of patients with rheumatoid arthritis undergoing total hip replacement compared with 7.7% of osteoarthritis patients. This difference, however, reflected the difference in the average age of the two groups. We feel that all patients should receive antithrombotic prophylaxis.

Infection

Patients with rheumatoid arthritis are at increased risk for infection following total hip arthroplasty. Poss, et al.,[44] reported that patients with rheumatoid arthritis have 2.6 times greater risk of infection than osteoarthritics. Charnley[8] stated that the rheumatoid arthritis patient has an incidence of infection that is 1.5 times greater than the average. Arden, et al.,[2] showed that rheumatoid patients have a threefold increase in infection after total hip replacement. In our long-term followup study at The Hospital for Special Surgery,[59] 3.4% of the revisions were for late infection. This represented 20% of the overall revision rate. With time, late infection may be a significant cause of failure in patients who have undergone total hip replacement for rheumatoid arthritis.

Dislocations

Postoperative dislocation occurs in rheumatoids at a rate that is similar to that in patients with osteoarthritis.[22] Coville, et al.,[11] found a dislocation rate of 0.7%. Poss, et al.,[44] stated that the dislocation rate following total hip replacement, at his institution, was 2.3%. The dislocation rate in patients with rheumatoid arthritis was 1.5%. We have not found that the dislocation rate in patients with rheumatoid arthritis is different from that obtained in those with osteoarthritis.

Summary

Rheumatoid hip disease frequently results in destruction of the joint and causes considerable disability. The evaluation of rheumatoid patients must be comprehensive, with input from the rheumatologist, occupational therapist, social worker and physical therapist. When surgical reconstruction is recommended, it is most often a cemented total joint replacement. Recent studies have demonstrated that total hip arthroplasty is both satisfactory and durable in the patient with rheumatoid arthritis. Attention should be directed to restoration of the center of rotation, reconstruction of bone defects, meticulous cement technique, optimal position and selection of components, and the utilization of absolute aseptic techniques. The role of uncemented total hip arthroplasty should be limited until longer followup is available. Other procedures such as surface replacement arthroplasty, fusion, osteotomy, endoprosthetic replacement, and synovectomy are of limited value, even in the young rheumatoid patient.

Note: The authors wish to thank Margaret McDonald for technical assistance.

References

1. Amstutz HC, Graff-Radford A, Gruen TA, Clarke IC: Tharies surface replacements: a review of the first 100 cases. Clin Orthop, 134:87, 1978.

2. ARDEN GP, ANSELL BM, HUNTER MJ: Total hip replacement in juvenile chronic polyarthritis and ankylosing spondylitis. Clin Orthop, 84:130, 1972.

3. ARDEN GP, TAYLOR AR, ANSELL BM: Total hip replacement using the McKee-Farrar prosthesis in rheumatoid arthritis. Still's disease and ankylosing spondylitis. Ann Rheum Dis, 29:104, 1970.

4. BECKENBAUGH RD, ILSTRUP DM: Total hip arthroplasty: a review of three hundred and thirty-three cases with long term follow-up. J Bone Joint Surg, 60A:306–313, 1978.

5. BRYAN RS, SCOTT WT, BICKEL WH: Results of surgical management of the hip in patients with rheumatoid arthritis or rheumatid spondylitis. *In* Cruess RL, Mitchell NW (eds): Surgery of Rheumatoid Arthritis. Philadelphia, Lippincott, p. 63. 1971.

6. CHANDLER HP, REINECK FT, WIXSON RL, MCCARTHY JC: Total hip replacement in patients younger than thirty years old. J Bone Joint Surg, 63A:1426, 1981.

7. CHARNLEY J: Low Friction Arthroplasty of the Hip: Theory and Practice. New York, Springer, 1977.

8. CHARNLEY J: Post-operative infection after total hip replacement with special reference to air contamination in the operating room. Clin Orthop, 87:167, 1972.

9. CHARNLEY J, CUPIC Z: The nine and ten year results of the low-friction arthroplasty of the hip. Clin Orthop, 95:9–25, 1973.

10. CLAYTON ML: Surgery of the lower extremity in rheumatoid arthritis. J Bone Joint Surg, 45A:1517, 1963.

11. COLVILLE J, RAUNIO P: Total hip replacement in juvenile rheumatoid arthritis. Acta Orthop Scand, 50:197, 1979.

12. CONARY JP, NICKEL VL: Functional incapacitation in rheumatoid arthritis: a rehabilitation challenge. J Bone Joint Surg, 53A:624, 1971.

13. CONARY JP: Surgery of the hip and knee in patients with rheumatoid arthritis. J Bone Joint Surg, 55A:301, 1973.

14. COVENTRY M.: Ten year results of total hip arthroplasty. Orthop Trans, 5439:350, 1981.

15. CROWNINSHIELD RD: A stress analysis of acetabular reconstruction in protrusio acetabuli. J Bone Joint Surg, 65A:495, 1983.

16. CRUESS RL: Synovectomy of the hip in rheumatoid arthritis. *In* Cruess RL, Mitchell NS (eds): Surgery of Rheumatoid Arthritis. Philadelphia, Lippincott, p 59, 1971.

17. DELEE JG, CHARNLEY J: Radiological demarcation of cemented sockets in total hip replacement. Clin Orthop, 121:20–32, 1976.

18. DOBBS HS: Survivorship of total hip replacements. J Bone Joint Surg, 62B:168, 1980.

19. DRINKER H, MURRAY WR: The universal proximal femoral endoprosthesis. J Bone Joint Surg, 61A:1167, 1979.

20. ENGH CA, BOBYN JD, GLASSMAN AH: A study of factors governing bone ingrowth, stress shielding, and clinical results with porous coated hip replacement. J Bone Joint Surg, 698:45, 1987.

21. EYRING EJ, LONGERT A, BASS JC: Synovectomy in juvenile arthritis. J Bone Joint Surg, 53A:638, 1971

22. FACKLER CD, POSS, R: Dislocation in total hip arthroplasties. Clin Orthop, 151:169, 1980.

23. FREEMAN MAR (ed.): Total surface replacement hip arthroplasty. Clin Orthop, 134:2, 1978.

24. FREEMAN PA, LEE P, BRYSON TW: Total hip joint replacement in osteoarthrosis and polyarthritis: a statistical study of the results. Clin Orthop, 95:224–230, 1973.

25. FREEMAN PA, STURROCK RD: Surgery of the weight bearing joints in rheumatoid arthritis. *In* Buchanan WW, Dick WC (eds.): Recent Advances in Rheumatology. Edinburgh, Churchill Livingstone, p. 138, 1976.

26. GRANT GH: The philosophy of surgery in rheumatoid arthritis. J Bone Jont Surg, 46A:904, 1964.

27. GRIFFITH MJ, SEIDENSTEIN MK, WILLIAMS D, CHARNLEY J: Eight year results of Charnley arthroplasties of the hip with special reference to the behavior of cement. Clin Orthop, 137:24–36, 1978.

28. HARDAKER WT, OGDEN WS, MUSGRAVE MD, GOLDNER JD: Simultaneous and staged bilateral total knee arthroplasty. J Bone Joint Surg, 60A:247, 1978.

29. HARRIS J, LIGHTOWLER CDR, TODD RC: Total hip replacement in inflammatory hip disease using the Charnley prosthesis. Br Med J, 2:750–752, 1972.

30. HASTINGS DC, PARKER SM: Protrusio acetabuli in rheumatoid arthritis. Clin Orthop, 108:76, 1975.

31. HEAD WD, PARADIES LH: Ipsilateral hip and knee replacements as a single surgical procedure. J Bone Joint Surg, 59A:352, 1977.

32. JAFFE WL, CHARNLEY J: Bilateral Charnley low-friction arthroplasty as a single operative procedure: a report of fifty cases. Bull Hosp Joint Dis, 32:198–214, 1971.

33. JOHNSON KA: Arthroplasty of both hips and both knees in rheumatoid arthritis. J Bone Joint Surg, 57A:901, 1975.

34. LAZANSKY MG: Ten-year results of Charnley total hip replacement. Orthop Trans, 5:350, 1981.

35. LIPSCOMB PR: Reconstructive surgery for bilateral hip disease in the adult, J Bone Joint Surg, 47A:1, 1965.

36. LIPSCOMB PR: Surgery for rheumatoid arthritis-timing and techniques: summary. J Bone Joint Surg, 50A:614, 1968.

37. MCCOLLUM DE, NUNLEY JA: Bone grafting in acetabular protrusion: a biologic buttress in the hip. *In* The Hip: Proceedings of the Sixth Open Scientific Meeting of the Hip Society. Mosby, St. Louis, p. 124, 1978.

38. MCCOLLUM DE, NUNLEY JA, HARRELSON JM: Bone grafting in total hip replacement for acetabular protrusion. J Bone Joint Surg, 62A:1065, 1980.

39. MOORE AT: The self locking metal hip prosthesis. J Bone Joint Surg, 39A:811, 1957.

40. OH I, HARRIS WH: Protrusio acetabuli and total hip replacement: bone grafting and use of protrusio shell. Orthop Trans, 3:276, 1979.

41. PARKER HG, et al.: Comparison of pre-operative, intraoperative, and early post-operative total hip replacements with and without trochanteric osteotomy. Clin Orthop, 121:44 1976.

42. PETERSON LFA: Surgery for rheumatoid arthritis-timing and techniques: the lower extremity. J Bone Joint Surg, 50A:587, 1968.

43. POSS R: Total hip replacement. Orthop Clin North Am, 6:801, 1975.

44. POSS R, EWALD FC, THOMAS WH, SLEDGE CB: Complications of total hip replacement arthroplasty in patients with rheumatoid arthritis. J Bone Joint Surg, 58A:1130, 1976.

45. POSS R, et al.: Six to eleven year results of total hip arthroplasty in rheumatoid arthritis. Clin Orthop, 182:109, 1984.

46. RANAWAT CS, DORR LD, INGLIS AE: Total hip arthroplasty in protrusio acetabuli of rheumatoid arthritis. J Bone Joint Surg, 62A:1059, 1980.

47. RANAWAT CS, ZAHN MG: Role of bone grafting in correction of protrusio acetabuli by total hip arthroplasty. J Arthroplasty, 1:131, 1986.

48. RITTER MA, RANDOLPH JC: Bilateral total hip arthroplasty: a simultaneous procedure. Acta Orthop Scand, 47:203–208, 1976.

49. SALVATI EA, HUGHES P, LACHIEWICZ P: Bilateral total hip replacement arthroplasty in one stage. J Bone Joint Surg, 60A:640, 1978.

50. Salvati EA, Wilson PD: Long term results of femoral head replacement. J Bone Joint Surgery, 55A:516, 1973.
50A. Salvati EA, et al.: A ten-year follow-up study of our first one hundred consecutive Charnley total hip replacements. J Bone Joint Surg, 63A:753, 1981.
51. Sarmiento A: Austin Moore prosthesis in the arthritic hip. Clin Orthop, 82:16, 1972.
52. Soreide O, Molster A, Raugstad TS: Replacement with the Christiansen endoprosthesis in acute femoral neck fractures, a five year followup study. Acta Orthop Scan, 51:137, 1980.
53. Sotelo-Garza A, Charnley J: The results of Charnley arthroplasty of the hip performed for protrusio acetabuli. Clin Orthop, 132:12, 1978.
54. Stauffer RN: Ten-year follow-up study of total hip replacement: with particular reference to roentgenographic loosening of the components. J Bone and Joint Surg, 64A:983, 1982.
55. Steinberg ME (ed.): Surface replacement arthroplasty of the hip. Orthop Clin North Am, 13:661, 1982.
56. Stinchfield FE, et al.: Late hematogenous infection of total joint replacement. J Bone Joint Surg, 62A:1345, 1980.
57. Sutherland CJ, Wile AH, Borden LS, Marks KE: A ten-year follow-up of one hundred consecutive Muller curved-stem total hip replacement arthroplasties. J Bone Joint Surg, 64A:970, 1982.
58. Thompson RC, Culver JE: The role of trochanteric osteotomy in total hip replacement. Clin Orthop, 106:102, 1975.
59. Unger AS, Inglis AE, Ranawat CS, Johansen N: Total hip arthroplasty in rheumatoid arthritis: a long term follow-up study. J Arthroplasty 2:191, 1987.
60. Wagner H: Surface replacement arthroplasty of the hip. Clin Orthop, 134:102, 1978.
61. Weisman HS, et al.: Total hip replacement with and without osteotomy of the greater trochanter: clinical and biomechanical comparisons in the same patient. J Bone Joint Surg, 60A:203, 1978.
62. Welch RB, Charnley J: Low-friction arthroplasty of the hip in rheumatoid arthritis and ankylosing spondylitis. Clin Orthop, 72:22–32, 1970.
63. Wilkinson MC: Synovectomy for rheumatoid arthritis. Clin Orthop, 100:125, 1974.
64. Barrack RL, Newland CC: Uncemented total hip arthroplasty with superior acetabular deficiency: femoral head autograft techniques and early clinical results. J Arthroplasty 5:159, 1990.
65. Engh CA, Massin P: Cementless total hip arthroplasty using the anatomic medullary locking system. Clin Orthop 249:141, 1989.

CHAPTER TWENTY-FIVE

Proximal Femoral Replacement

RICHARD LACKMAN

Reconstruction of proximal femoral defects has long been a difficult challenge for the hip surgeon. In order to be successful, proximal femoral reconstruction must provide a stable articulation with a functional range of motion and possess the inherent strength necessary to withstand the stresses of repetitive weight-bearing.

Early attempts at prosthetic reconstruction usually entailed the use of a long-stemmed prosthesis, often bolstered with methylmethacrylate. Unfortunately, device failure was common. During the past 10 years, however, advances in metallurgy techniques and prosthetic design have resulted in the availability of "custom" prostheses that are capable of replacing proximal femoral defects and are strong enough to withstand the stresses of their environment for long periods.

Other reconstructive options also exist. Proximal femoral allografts have received little enthusiasm because of the high incidence of stress fracture. Composite reconstructions consisting of a long-stemmed prosthesis combined with a proximal femoral allograft are also possible.[1] The theoretical advantage of this technique over proximal replacement prostheses is that the former hopefully re-establishes bone stock through incorporation of the allograft. Whether or not this goal is actually achieved is not yet known because long-term followup is not available. Use of these composites does incur several problems not encountered with use of the prosthesis alone, namely the high infection and nonunion rates associated with the use of massive allografts.

In order to put this situation in proper perspective it is important to consider the age and prognosis of the patient. Proximal replacement prostheses are a very good option in elderly people and the most common indications here include metastatic proximal femoral destruction and salvage for failed total hip arthroplasty.[2] Younger adults with a limited life expectancy are also excellent candidates. Those younger, active patients who may have a long life expectancy, such as following resection of

a low grade sarcoma, are reasonable candidates to consider for allograft-prosthesis composite reconstruction.

Proximal femoral replacement prostheses (Fig. 25–1) are a valuable addition to the hip surgeon's armamentarium and should, as mentioned, have a long survival when used in appropriate patients. These prostheses can articulate with either a bipolar type hemiarthroplasty or with a conventional total hip cup. This author prefers the former be-

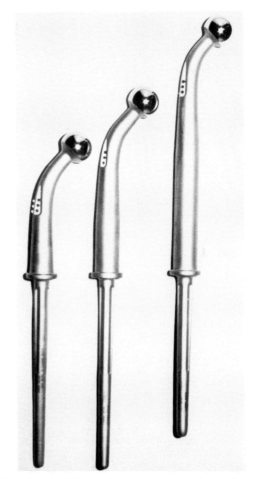

FIG. 25–1. Proximal femoral replacement prostheses showing incremental replacement lengths.

cause the bipolar probably yields a more stable articulation in this situation, though either should provide satisfactory results if well executed.

Two factors are crucial to joint stability following proximal femoral replacement. The first is that the prosthesis must be put in tightly because any toggle whatsoever will predispose to dislocation. Graduated replacement lengths are necessary because it is very difficult to tell preoperatively which replacement length will be needed. A complete set of prostheses involves having replacement lengths varying from 9 cm to 25 cm at 2 cm intervals. It is difficult to go much beyond 25 cm of replacement length without running out of femur length for stem fixation. Replacement lengths shorter than 9 cm can usually be accomplished with calcar replacement prostheses.

Second, accurate anteversion is needed to prevent posterior dislocation. Twenty to twenty-five degrees of femoral anteversion is probably optimal. Retention of the hip capsule and careful capsular repair adds greatly to early hip stability as will firm reattachment of the greater trochanter to the shoulder of the prosthesis. When dealing with primary tumors, however, these options are often not feasible because good resection technique for these lesions usually requires sacrifice of the hip capsule and greater trochanter. In these instances the author prefers to place the patients postoperatively in a walking abduction spica cast incorporating the pelvis and involved thigh only and allowing free motion at the knee. The hip is placed in abduction and slight flexion and maintained in the cast for 6 weeks. The cast is then removed and the patients are permitted unrestricted hip range of motion.

Surgical Technique

Although proximal femoral resection can be performed via any approach that provides extensive exposure, the "Y" incision is probably optimal because it provides good anterior and posterior exposure without sacrificing any major structure (Fig. 25–2). This incision is based with the junction of the "Y" at the greater trochanter. The anterior and posterior limbs are then extended each at 60° from the long axis.

The incision is carried sharply through the skin and subcutaneous tissues. (Fig. 25–3) The deep fascia is then split in line with its fibers beginning distally and working proximally toward the junction of the "Y." The posterior limb is then extended through the deep fascia of the gluteus maximus and

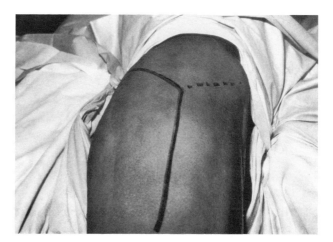

Fɪɢ. 25–2. The posterolateral approach is easily converted to a "Y" approach for extensile exposure of the hip.

this muscle is then split bluntly in line with its fibers as with a typical posterolateral approach. The anterior limb is then carried through the deep fascia and the few remaining fibers of the gluteus maximus.

One can then elevate the proximal flap (Fig. 25–4) by retracting the anterior portion of the gluteus maximus proximally, thus exposing the underlying gluteus medius and minimus. Posterior retraction of the posterior flap will expose the main insertion of the gluteus maximus on the posterior aspect of the proximal femur.

The gluteus maximus insertion (Fig. 25–5) is then divided close to the femur. Great care should be taken to perform this division one layer at a time because several perforating vessels are frequently encountered. In the fatty tissues just deep to this tendon lies the sciatic nerve which can easily be identified in this location and must obviously be protected (Fig. 25–6).

The short external rotators (Fig. 25–7) can then

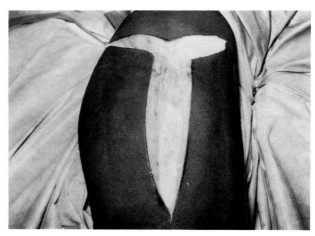

Fɪɢ. 25–3. The skin and subcutaneous tissue are incised.

be incised and retracted as per the usual posterolateral hip approach. If necessary, the sciatic nerve can then be traced all the way proximally to the sciatic notch, which facilitates its protection.

The next step is to place a large clamp under the gluteus medius and minimus to separate these muscles from the underlying hip capsule. If the greater trochanter is to be resected with the specimen, division of the insertion of the gluteus medius and minimus is performed. Retraction of these muscles proximally then exposes the hip capsule. (Fig. 25–8).

If the trochanter is to be osteotomized for later reattachment (as in the case of failed joint salvage or metastatic disease) then the origin of the vastus lateralis is incised (Fig. 25–9) to expose the underlying vastus ridge on the lateral surface of the proximal femur. The origin of the vastus lateralis is then retracted distally (Fig. 25–10) and the greater trochanter is then osteotomized (Fig. 25–11).

The leg is then externally rotated to expose the lesser trochanter (Fig. 25–12) and the iliopsoas insertion on this structure is identified and divided. One can then dissect under the quadriceps femoris to expose the posterior, lateral, and anterior surfaces of the proximal femur (Fig. 25–13).

The femur can then be osteotomized (Fig. 25–14). The proximal femoral fragment is then abducted to allow division of any medial soft tissue attachment (i.e., the abductor insertion). A capsulotomy or capsulectomy is then performed (Fig. 25–15) as required. The proximal femur is then removed from the field, (Fig. 25–16).

The femoral shaft is then reamed appropriately (Fig. 25–17). Once reaming is completed and the prosthesis is inserted in the femoral shaft (Fig. 25–18), a closed reduction can be performed (Fig. 25–19).

The proper length of the femoral replacement can be now determined. It should be noted that the femur should be placed in 20° of anteversion. It should also be placed in as much soft tissue tension as is reasonably possible in order to prevent dislocation. A reduction that requires moderate force and leaves no toggle whatsoever is desirable. Once the prosthesis is cemented in place the hip capsule can be repaired (Fig. 25–20). Good capsular repair adds considerably to the postoperative stability of these prostheses. With the capsule repaired, the trochanter can then be reattached to the shoulder of the prosthesis. This step further increases the postoperative stability (Fig. 25–21). In those patients with primary tumors when it is necessary to excise completely the hip capsule and the greater trochanter,

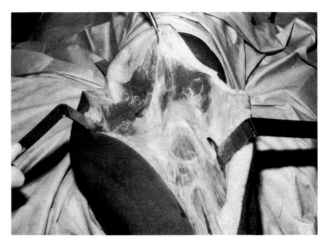

Fɪɢ. 25–4. Anterior, superior, and posterior flaps are created.

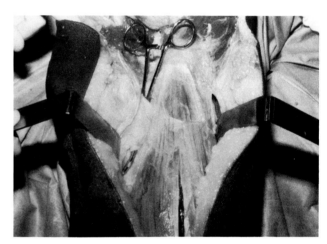

Fɪɢ. 25–5. The gluteus maximus insertion is identified and incised.

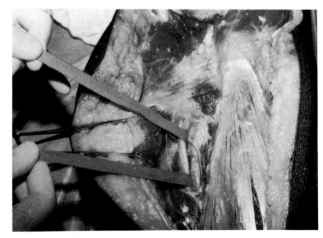

Fɪɢ. 25–6. The sciatic nerve is identified beneath the retracted gluteus maximus insertion.

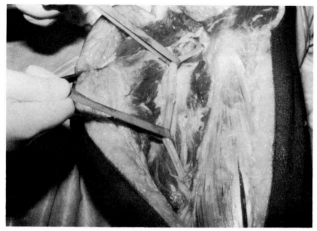

Fig. 25–7. The sciatic nerve can be fully exposed after division of the short external rotator muscles.

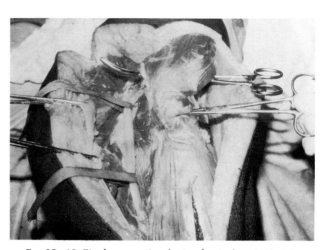

Fig. 25–10. Final preparation for trochanteric osteotomy.

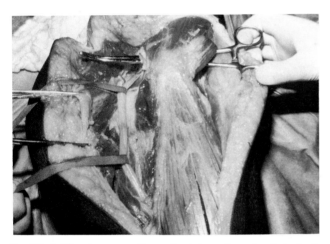

Fig. 25–8. The gluteus medius and minimus insertion is incised.

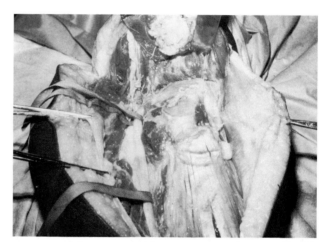

Fig. 25–11. The greater trochanter is retracted proximally following osteotomy.

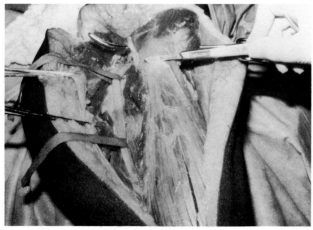

Fig. 25–9. When the greater trochanter can be saved, the vastus lateralis origin is incised prior to trochanteric osteotomy.

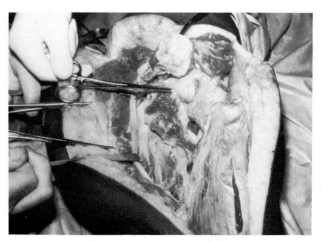

Fig. 25–12. The iliopsoas tendon is identified at its insertion on the lesser trochanter.

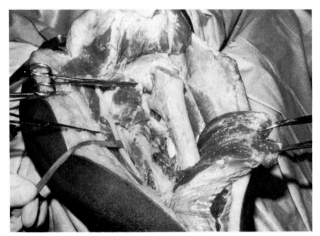

FIG. 25–13. The proximal femoral shaft is exposed.

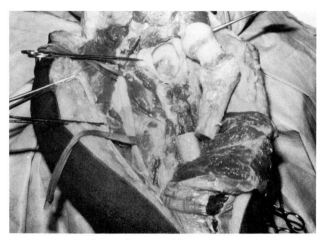

FIG. 25–16. The diseased proximal femur can now be removed.

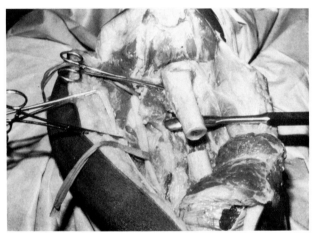

FIG. 25–14. The femur is then osteotomized at the desired location.

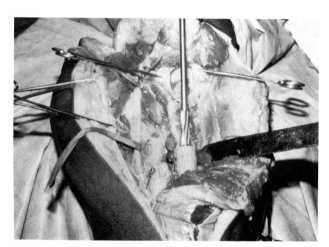

FIG. 25–17. The femoral shaft is reamed to accommodate the stem of the prosthesis.

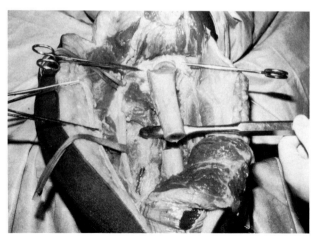

FIG. 25–15. The hip capsule is visualized and incised or resected.

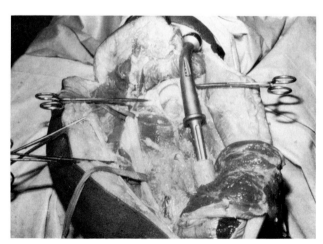

FIG. 25–18. The prosthesis is inserted into the femoral shaft.

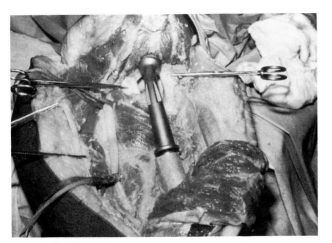

FIG. 25–19. A trial reduction is then performed.

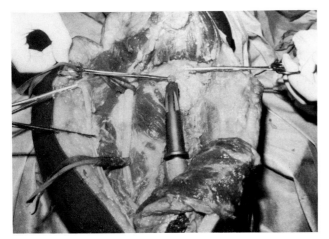

FIG. 25–20. The hip capsule, if still present, is repaired.

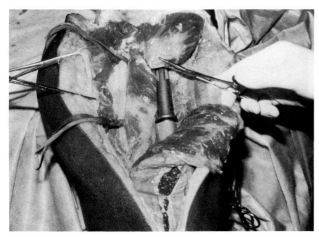

FIG. 25–21. The greater trochanter is reattached to the shoulder of the prosthesis.

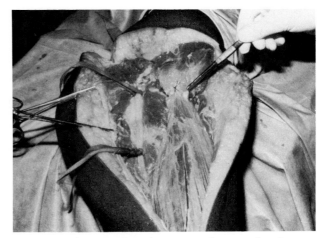

FIG. 25–22. The vastus lateralis is repaired to provide soft tissue coverage over the prosthesis.

the prostheses are much less stable and usually require a walking abduction hip spica cast for the first 6 weeks until healing is complete. With the trochanter reattached, the vastus lateralis is repaired (Fig. 25–22) giving good soft tissue coverage over the prosthesis. The deep fascia is then repaired in the usual fashion with interrupted sutures (Fig. 25–23) followed by the usual closure of the more superficial tissues and the skin.

Figure 25–24 shows a patient with extensive destruction of the proximal femur secondary to metastatic hypernephroma treated by resection and proximal femoral replacement. The trochanteric wires typically break during the first 3 months following surgery, but the trochanter is fixed in scar tissue and usually migrates little.

The patient shown in Figure 25–25 is a 60-year-old female who had previously undergone curettage and internal fixation. This recurred leaving no al-

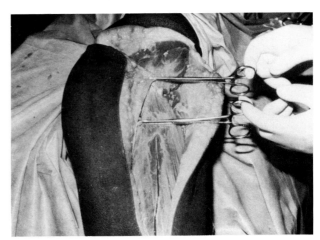

FIG. 25–23. The fascia lata and superficial tissues are closed in the usual fashion.

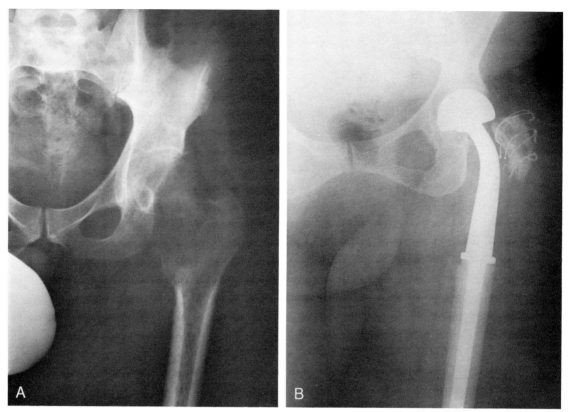

FIG. 25–24A,B. Metastatic hypernephroma treated with a proximal femoral replacement bipolar prosthesis.

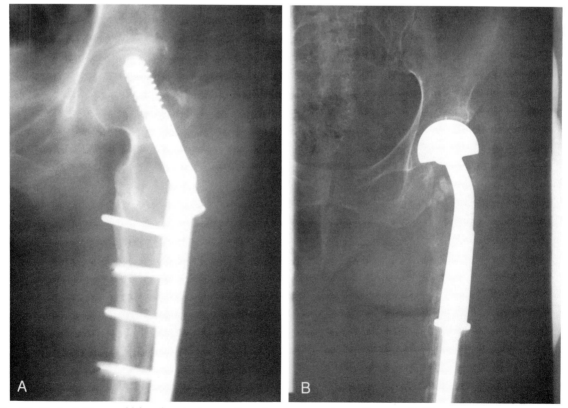

FIG. 25–25. **A.** A 60-year-old female prior to resection of a recurrent giant cell tumor. **B.** The same patient 6 years later.

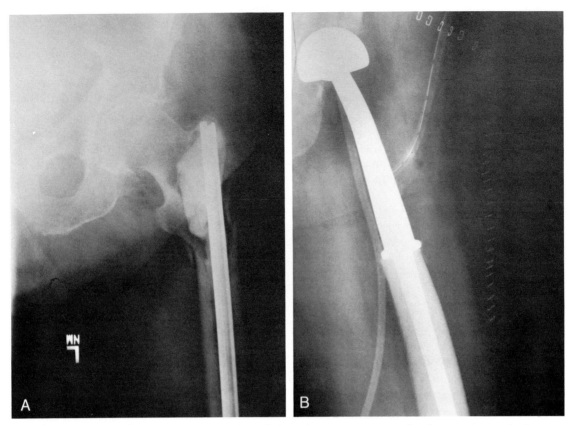

FIG. 25–26A,B. Failed internal fixation of a pathologic fracture reconstructed with a custom prosthesis.

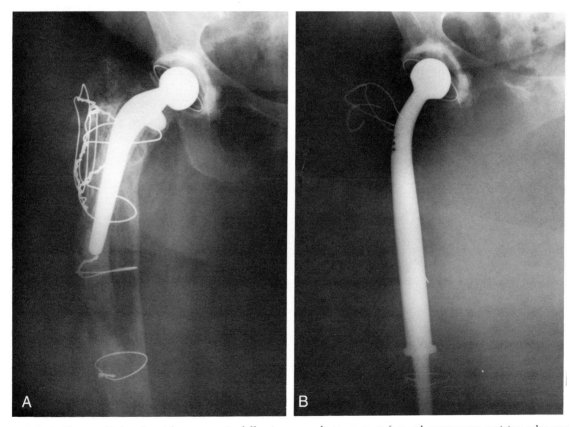

FIG. 25–27A,B. A 70-year-old female with severe pain following several attempts at femoral component revision who was treated successfully with excision and proximal femoral replacement.

ternative but resection and again a proximal femoral replacement bipolar prosthesis was used. This patient remained tumor-free and essentially asymptomatic 6 years following surgery.

Another indication for proximal femoral replacement is shown in Figure 25–26. This 70-year-old male had persistent pain and inability to bear weight several months after an attempt at internal fixation of a pathologic fracture. This patient's hip was reconstructed with a custom prosthesis and he remained ambulatory until his demise 3 years later.

The patient in Figure 25–27 was a 70-year-old female with Paget's disease. She presented with severe right hip pain following several revisions of her femoral total hip component. This was treated by excision of the deficient proximal femur and prosthetic reconstruction. This patient was asymptomatic and ambulatory at last followup 3 years after surgery.

In summary, proximal femoral replacement prostheses are a valuable addition to our surgical skills. Proper execution of this procedure requires a thorough knowledge of the anatomy involved and careful attention to surgical technique. When properly done, however, this operation can preserve nearly normal function in patients otherwise left with few viable alternatives.

References

1. HEAD WC, et al.: Proximal femoral allografts in revision total hip arthroplasty. Clin Orthop, 225:22–36, 1987.
2. SIM FH, et al.: Hip salvage by proximal femoral replacement. J Bone Joint Surg, 63: 1228–39, 1981.

CHAPTER TWENTY-SIX

Revision of Failed Cup Arthroplasty

WILLIAM G. STEWART

A revision of a failed cup arthroplasty is indicated when the overall result of the hip reconstruction is less than the patient and the surgeon anticipated. Revision for infection is covered in a separate chapter. The debridement in an infected cup is less demanding than in a cemented total hip because of the absence of the acrylic material.

Indications

The most common indications for revision of a cup arthroplasty are pain and limitation of motion. Early instability is a more rare but always possible reason for another operation. The hip that dislocates in the immediate postoperative period can usually be stabilized by a closed reduction and immobilization in a hip spica for a period of 6 to 8 weeks. However, the chronically dislocating cup arthroplasty requires an open procedure to regain stability. It can be evaluated radiologically at the extremes of motion with push-pull techniques. Tomograms and CAT scans are helpful in evaluating the area of deficient bone. Examination under general anesthesia with the image intensifier often indicates dynamically where and why the cup dislocates. At revision surgery, bone grafting and tendon transfers usually stabilize the situation. Postoperatively, a short-leg, single hip spica will protect the revision in a good position until scar tissue supplements the stability.

Revision Operations

The most common indication for revision in the young patient who meets the criteria for a cup arthroplasty—young, good bone stock, good musculature, and cooperative—is limited range of motion of the joint. Pain can also be a reason for revision.

There are three basic types of operations for this revision.

Repeat Cup Arthroplasty

A repeat cup arthroplasty can often remove both the cause of the limitation of motion and the pain. Excision of all heterotopic bone and accompanying scar tissue will free up a hip joint that is tethered. It may not be necessary to re-ream the femoral head and the acetabulum depending on the appearance of the fibrocartilage (Fig. 26–1). Removal of bone overgrowth around the femoral neck and the acetabulum can result in restoring a good range of motion of the hip without removing the cup. Reaming the femoral head and acetabulum to bleeding cancellous bone when a sclerotic corn is found and replacing the cup can restore painless hip function.

Bipolar Reconstruction

In this age group, when there has been aseptic necrosis of the femoral head under the cup, yet the acetabulum is covered with good fibrocartilage, a bipolar type hip reconstruction has been carried out with excellent results (Figs. 26–2, 26–3). Minimal protection is necessary because of the mature fibrocartilage over the acetabulum. A press fit or porous coated femoral component is used in this situation. Because of the limited long-term experience available with porous coated prostheses, the press fit component may be preferable.

When there has been failure of maturation of the fibrocartilage on the acetabular side of a failed cup arthroplasty, reconstruction has been accomplished by once again reaming the acetabulum to bleeding cancellous bone and then using a bipolar device as noted above. An alternative to the bipolar prosthesis is the use of a porous coated acetabulum appliance. The long-term followup in these situations is

449

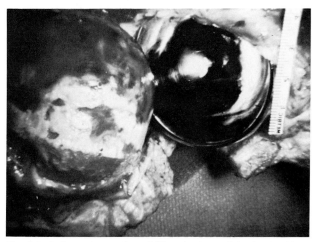

FIG. 26–1. Appearance of good fibrocartilage of the femoral head under a cup. The operation was performed 18 years prior to death.

not yet available. The early results appear to be satisfactory.

Revision of a failed cup arthroplasty in the elderly patient is usually undertaken for the same reasons as in the younger patient. If increasing deformity, decreased range of motion and hip pain can no longer be tolerated, then revision is necessary. Also, in the elderly patient, when the fibrocartilage over the acetabulum is intact, a bipolar ace-

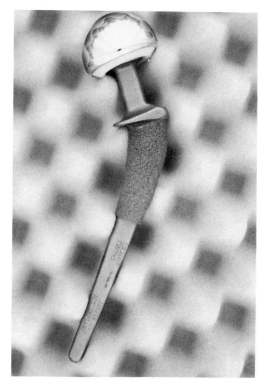

FIG. 26–3. Photo of porous coated bipolar hip replacement.

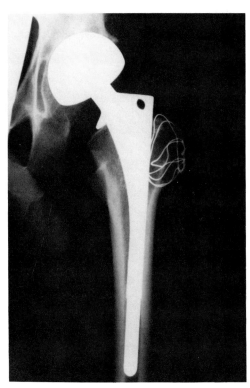

FIG. 26–2. X-ray appearance of a bipolar type reconstruction used in revision of cup arthroplasty.

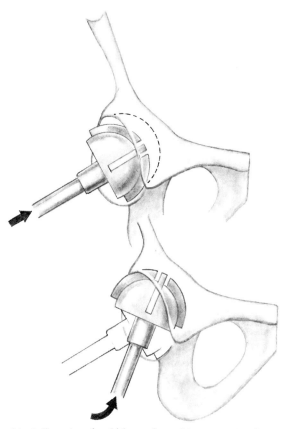

FIG. 26–4. Reaming should be performed in a superior direction rather than toward the medial pelvic wall.

tabular component with a porous coated or cemented femoral component is favored.

Cemented Total Hip

The third revision option is the conversion of a cup arthroplasty to a cemented total hip arthroplasty. Fixation of the femoral component does not present a difficult problem. However, it is failure of the acetabulum in fixation with methyl methacrylate that influences the results of revision after cup arthroplasty. The stability of the socket, particularly with regard to protrusio, must be addressed. Bone graft either of a composite or morselized nature should be used to support the medial pelvic wall. All fibrocartilage should be removed from the acetabulum by changing the shape of the acetabular dome or by vigorous reaming of the weight-bearing surface. Careful attention to the direction of the reamer will prevent violation of the medial pelvic wall (Fig. 26–4).

Summary

The cup arthroplasty represents a "conservative" approach to hip reconstruction. One of its primary advantages is that it does not compromise bone stock on either side of the joint. Avoiding the necessity of removal of acrylic cement in a revision situation is a great advantage. The potential future pitfalls of porous coating are also avoided in a second operation. Overall success in the revision of the failed cup arthroplasty should approach those of a primary hip reconstruction.

CHAPTER TWENTY-SEVEN

Acetabular Revision

WILLIAM J. HOZACK
ROBERT E. BOOTH

Introduction

Acetabular revision in total hip arthroplasty presents a wide scope for discussion. There are numerous scientific principles painstakingly learned over time through basic research and clinical experimentation to which the hip reconstructive surgeon must adhere if consistent and reliable results are to be achieved. This is especially true in acetabular reconstruction for primary degenerative arthritis but it is also true for more complicated problems such as congenital dysplasia of the hip or protrusio acetabuli. However, in acetabular revision surgery, problems are encountered that test these scientific principles to the limit, perhaps even past. In these situations, it is the surgeon's ability not only to adhere to the scientific principles but also to express adaptability and ingenuity that will extricate him from the variety of situations that occur.

The goal of this chapter is to stress the scientific principles that can be applied in acetabular revision surgery. However, as the problems get more complex, it will become apparent that artistic ingenuity and adaptability begin to play a more prominent role. It must be stressed, however, that this improvisation should not come from a vacuum, rather, it should be based on a firm grasp and complete understanding of all the accepted scientific principles. Only then can the surgeon, both as scientist and artist, have consistent and successful results.

Classification of Acetabular Deficiencies

The American Academy of Orthopedic Surgeons (AAOS) Committee on the Hip, classification scheme for acetabular deficiencies,[12] shown below, is simple, useful, and should be adopted (Figs. 27–1 to 27–5).

AAOS Classification of Acetabular Deficiencies

Type 1—Segmental
    A. Peripheral (rim)
    B. Central (medial wall absent)
Type 2—Cavitary
    A. Peripheral
    B. Central (medial wall intact)
Type 3—Combined Cavitary/Segmental
Type 4—Pelvic Discontinuity
Type 5—Arthrodesis

The surgeon must be prepared to deal with any single defect or combination of defects as they occur. The most important tool available in assessing potential deficiencies is the plain radiograph, which must be analyzed critically. Regular computerized tomography or three dimensionally reconstructed computerized tomography can be helpful but are expensive tests that usually not are necessary (Fig. 27–6). There will be times, however, when the deficiency is not apparent until the revision procedure is actually underway. At these times, it is the ability of the surgeon to properly identify defects as they occur and to orient himself to the pathologic anatomy that ultimately determines the quality of the reconstruction.

Preoperative Planning

No facet of the reconstructive procedure should be left to chance. In order to avoid a compromise of surgical technique or prosthetic selection, careful preoperative planning is essential.

An expanded inventory of component types and sizes must be available. At the Rothman Institute both cemented and cementless acetabular components are stocked, ranging in size from an offset-bore 36-mm diameter component to an 80-mm diameter component. Although we also have bipolar components available, we currently are not in favor of using them. With a wide range of component

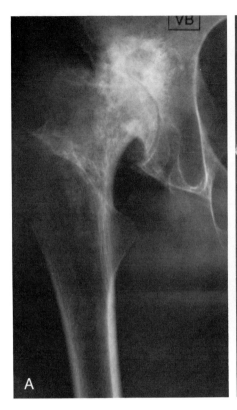
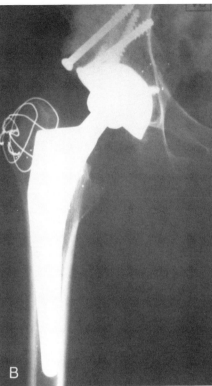

FIG. 27–1. **A.** Preoperative x-ray demonstrating a typical segmental peripheral defect, in this case a superior segmental defect. **B.** Postoperative x-ray demonstrating reconstruction of the acetabulum using an acetabular bone graft (autograft femoral head) fixated with two cancellous screws. An uncemented acetabular component was used in this case. The small metallic markers in the acetabulum and femur are tantalum beads used to measure micromotion of the components.

choices at hand, custom components have not been necessary although some surgeons continue to explore the possibilities of custom component application.

A wide variety of polyethylene insert sizes must be available (22 mm, 26 mm, 28 mm, 32 mm). Occasionally, in an isolated acetabular revision, the size of the insert will be dictated by the femoral

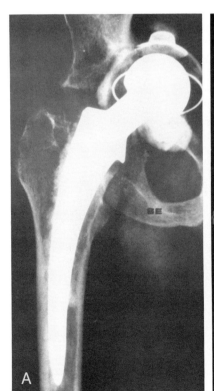
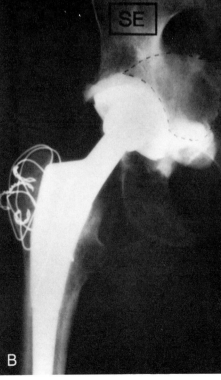

FIG. 27–2. **A.** Preoperative x-ray demonstrating a central segmental defect with a deficient medial acetabular wall. **B.** Postoperative x-ray showing restoration of the anatomic axis of the acetabulum using a large femoral head allograft and a cemented cup.

FIG. 27–3. **A.** Preoperative x-ray demonstrating an extensive cavitary defect, located both medially and in the peripheral superior area. The components are fixed with radiolucent cement. **B.** Postoperative x-ray demonstrating restoration of the acetabular anatomy and filling of the cavitary peripheral defect with bone graft fixated with two screws.

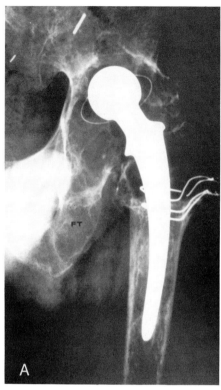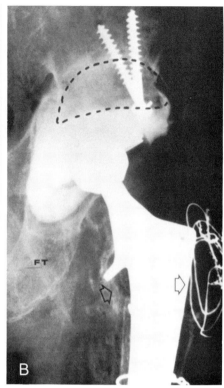

component head size. If the properly matched polyethylene insert is not available, revision of a well fixed, well positioned femoral component may be necessary. A 22 mm insert is useful for the smaller cup sizes in order to allow for sufficient plastic thickness. In general, for those cup sizes below 50 mm, we will choose a 22 mm insert. However, careful forethought must be given to the possibility of instability because the 22 mm head only comes in two lengths. In contrast we stock 28 mm head/

FIG. 27–4. **A.** Preoperative x-ray demonstrating a severe cavitary central defect with the medial wall intact. **B.** Reconstruction of the acetabulum using a large allograft, in this case a distal femoral allograft.

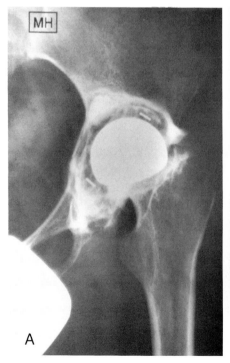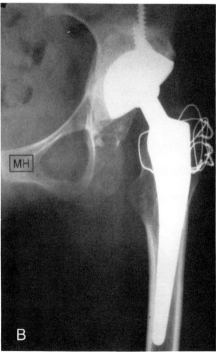

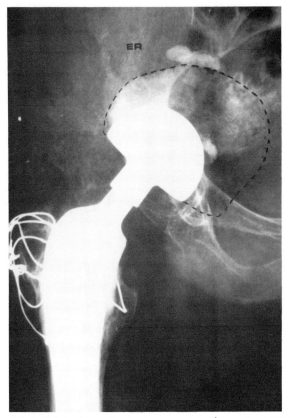

Fɪɢ. 27–5. Pelvic discontinuity is present in this patient. Note that Kohler's line is discontinuous. Failure to reestablish the continuity of the acetabular columns in this patient led to eventual failure of this reconstruction.

neck modular components in −6 mm, −3 mm, 0, +3 mm, +6 mm, +9 mm and +12 mm lengths. The extra-long neck lengths may sometime be necessary to re-establish stability especially if the acetabular construction has been undertaken in a "high" nonanatomic location.

A variety of other equipment can be useful. Cannulated screw sets facilitate bone graft fixation. Pelvic reconstruction plates are sometimes necessary to adequately secure rim grafts. A variety of reamer sizes are useful in properly fashioning the acetabular bed for reconstruction. High speed drills can greatly assist the removal of components and in the preparation of the bone graft.

Crucial to preoperative planning is careful evaluation of the preoperative radiograph.[47] Careful templating of the plain radiographs can prepare the surgeon for the need for bone grafting. In certain instances additional special studies should be obtained. Intrapelvic protrusion of components may warrant a preoperative arteriogram. Furthermore, an additional approach for component removal may be necessary and general surgery consultation may be indicated.[15] If the plain radiographs give a distorted view of the acetabulum, a reconstructed computerized tomography scan can sometimes elucidate the bony deficiencies.[55]

Surgical Approach

The quality of the acetabular reconstruction and its longevity critically depend on the ability of the surgeon to remove the components with a minimum of bone destruction, to evaluate and appreciate the underlying bony deficiencies, and to reconstruct a mechanically sound prosthetic acetabulum.

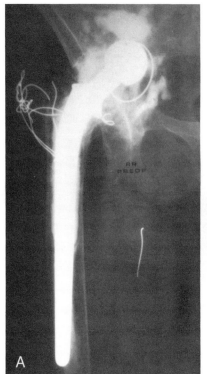

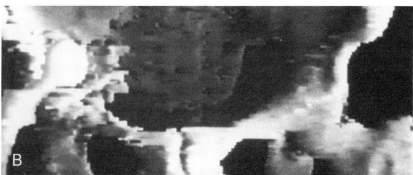

Fɪɢ. 27–6. **A.** Preoperative x-ray demonstrating a severe acetabular deficiency, which is difficult to define on the plain radiograph. **B.** Three dimensional reconstruction using CT scan demonstrates a discontinuity of the anterior pelvic wall.

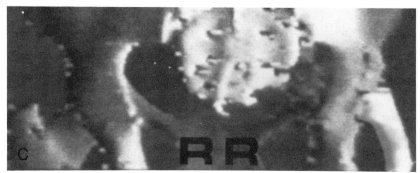

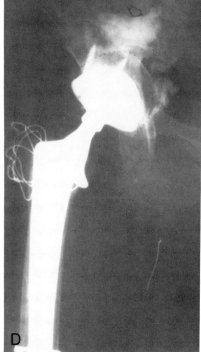

Fɪɢ. 27–6 (*continued*). **C.** The same reconstruction demonstrates that the posterior wall, however, is intact and therefore the reconstruction is facilitated. **D.** Post reconstruction using a whole acetabular graft.

Each of these requirements themselves depend on proper intraoperative exposure. Therefore, the direct lateral approach with trochanteric osteotomy continues to be our preferred approach for acetabular revision surgery.

Specifically, after splitting the fascia lata and gluteus maximus, the anterior and posterior borders of the gluteus medius are carefully identified. The scarred anterior capsule is separated from overlying tissue with a Cobb elevator. A partial anterior capsulectomy is performed. The posterior structures, specifically the small external rotator muscle insertions, are cut from their insertions into the femur and trochanter. Any previous wires around the trochanter are removed. However, it is unwise to excessively traumatize the tissues overlying the trochanter in a vain search for loose wires. The trochanteric bed is outlined with Bovie coagulation. With the anterior and posterior structures reflected, a trochanteric osteotomy is carefully performed with an oscillating saw. A more horizontal saw cut will preserve a cancellous bed for subsequent trochanteric reattachment. An angle of 30° with respect to the transverse plane is best. The trochanter is then retracted proximally. Excessive scarring in the superior capsule can inhibit the proximal reflection of the trochanter. If present, this scar can easily be excised. A superior retractor imbedded into the ilium then retains the trochanter with its attached musculature in the superior position. An anterior blunt Homan retractor is then placed carefully over the anterior pelvic rim and an inferior retractor is placed into the ischium. This inferior retractor displaces the femur posteriorly and inferiorly. In this fashion, superior acetabular exposure is facilitated.

The bony confines of the acetabulum are then defined by careful excision of scar tissue from around the acetabular edges. Manual palpation of the bony edges assists the surgeon during this step. Further exposure of the acetabular anatomy is undertaken after the pre-existing component is removed.

Special approaches may be indicated in special situations. For example, a previous Hardinge approach with inadequate reattachment of the anterior gluteus flap may preclude a proper transtrochanteric approach. Reutilization of the previous approach may be necessary. Intrapelvic protrusion of components may require a separate approach to expose the intrapelvic components or cement.[15]

Component Removal

Several techniques can successfully remove a component. The most useful is to define and enter the interface between the cup and the cement with a specially designed curved osteotome available on the several revision instrumentation sets. Once the cup-cement interface is broken, the component is removed and the underlying cement can be curetted away. Removal of cementless components requires entry into the cup-bone interface. Although more difficult, the curved osteotome is generally successful. With this technique, great care must be taken to preserve the underlying bone.

Cup sectioning with saws, osteotomes, or high speed drills is another popular technique for component removal. After sectioning, the cup will "implode" and removal is facilitated. With the newer high strength metal alloys, this cup sectioning technique can be tedious. A large volume of plastic and metal debris is created during the removal process and must be carefully removed from the wound.

Preparation for Reimplantation

After the component and cement are removed, a fibrous membrane is generally found within the acetabular bed. Gentle curetting of this membrane will expose the underlying bone. If any central segmental defects are present (i.e., any central perforations through the medial acetabular wall) it is wise not to remove too vigorously the overlying fibrous membrane. This membrane can be useful in containing subsequent bone graft and prevent any intrapelvic extrusion. Furthermore, behind this membrane lie venous plexuses that should be left undisturbed.

At this time it is best to re-establish and reidentify the bony rim of the acetabulum. This may require repositioning of retractors. The true anatomic location of the acetabulum must be exposed. Direct palpation of the ischial ramus and superior pubic ramus is of great value in providing the surgeon with the proper orientation. All bony defects must then be analyzed.

Reaming of the acetabular bed should then be undertaken. Reaming has three useful purposes. First, it further cleans the bone. Second, it allows the surgeon to create a fresh surface for the subsequent implantation of a cemented or cementless component. Finally, it allows the surgeon to appreciate the full extent of the bony defects. Reaming should be done carefully. No further protrusion should be created. In addition, the limiting factor for the extent of reaming is generally the anterior-posterior dimension of the acetabulum. Excessive reaming can compromise the already weak anterior and posterior rims and thus compromise the mechanical quality of the subsequent reconstruction.

Acetabular Revision Using Cemented Components

Kavanagh, et al.,[29] reported on 166 cemented revision total hip arthroplasties with a mean followup of 4.5 years (range 2 to 10.5 years). Twenty percent of the cups were radiographically loose at followup: 9% had migrated and 11% had 3 zone demarcation. An additional 8% had evidence of progressive radiolucencies about the cement-bone interface. They found a significantly higher incidence of radiographic loosening of the acetabulum (50%) in those hips in which the acetabulum was initially revised for loosening. They felt that this reflected the inability of the surgeon to attain adequate mechanical interlock between the cement and bone and these revisions. The overall revision rate for this series was 9%.

Callaghan[5] reviewed 139 revision total hip arthroplasties performed at the Hospital for Special Surgery. At a mean of 3.6 years (range 2 to 5 years) 9% of the cups had migrated, and 19% had progressive radiolucent lines. Two other important points are noteworthy. First, on the initial postoperative radiograph (subsequent to the revision) 34% of the acetabular components had a complete three zone radiolucent line, suggestive of failure to achieve initial mechanical fixation. Second, failure to reestablish an adequate anatomic reconstruction of the hip significantly prejudiced the results. Satisfactory clinical and radiographic results were achieved in 81% when the anatomic reconstruction was deemed adequate; only 62% satisfactory results were achieved if the reconstruction was not anatomic. Amstutz[1] reviewed 66 revisions with 1 to 9 years of followup (mean 2.1 years): 10% had circumferential radiolucent lines at the acetabular bone cement interface on initial postoperative x-ray. This increased to 71% at the latest followup.

Marti, et al.,[35] presented a series of 60 revisions with a mean followup of 8.9 years (range 5 to 15 years). They emphasized certain technical aspects of the surgery: a transtrochanteric approach, anatomic cup placement, bone grafting if cup coverage was less than 90%, and meticulous preparation of the acetabular bed with anchoring holes. During their followup, they found only 3 migrated cups, 7 cups with three zone demarcation, and 4 cups with radiolucent lines. They reported a 90% survivorship probability at 9 years in their 60 cemented revisions.

Engelbrecht[17] reported on 134 revision total hip arthroplasties at an average followup of 7.4 years (range 3 to 15.5 years) and found 92% with satisfactory pain relief. An 8.8% failure rate was experienced. Of the 98 cemented cups, one-third had radiographic evidence of loosening. Loosening was significantly correlated with poor acetabular bone stock.

Aside from the Marti series, the clinical and radiographic results of cemented revision for acetabular reconstruction are discouraging (Fig. 27–7). However, some of the blame for these dismal results must lie with the surgeon. As noted by several authors, three zone demarcation of the cup is present on the initial postoperative radiograph in up to one-third of the cases. This failure to achieve an initial mechanical bond of cement to bone directly affects the longevity of the acetabular reconstruction. As Marti, et al., have shown, meticulous attention to surgical technique can give a highly satisfactory long-term clinical and radiographic result in cemented acetabular revisions.

The principles of a cemented acetabulum have been well defined.[10,41] Exposure is key—all the referenced series use the transtrochanteric approach. Prosthesis containment by bone is necessary and failure to achieve adequate coverage for the cup leads to a high failure rate.[47A] However, the critical area of attention lies at the cement-bone interface. Preservation of any remaining subchondral bone is important to maintain normal acetabular stresses and strains.[6] Multiple fixation holes must be cre-

ated as the interface in the revised acetabulum is smooth. These anchoring holes serve as the only means to resist the torsional forces placed on the cup. Pulsatile lavage, meticulous hemostasis, hypotensive anesthesia, and thrombin-impregnated gelfoam packing are important to prevent an interface of blood from forming between the cement and the bone. Proper cement pressurization can also improve the mechanical bond between the cement and bone.[46] Restoration of the anatomic location of the acetabulum during the reconstruction appears to have a beneficial effect on the ultimate result. Bone grafting may be necessary to achieve this goal. Although not usually the source of failure in revision cemented acetabula, the cement-prosthesis interface bond can be enhanced through porous coating or cement precoating of a metal-backed cup. Whether these innovations will improve the longevity of the cemented acetabulum is open to question, as the primary location of failure is the cement bone interface.

Currently, acetabular revision using cemented techniques should be reserved for those cases in which the bone stock is well preserved and in which a mechanically sound interface of cement to bone can be achieved (Fig. 27–8). Poor acetabular bone stock is a contraindication to the use of cement. However, cemented components may be use-

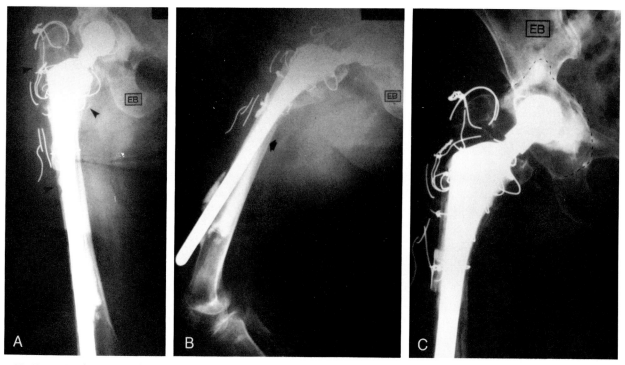

Fig. 27–7. A–C. This patient had undergone three surgical procedures on the right hip. The end result of each is demonstrated in these photos. Cemented revision in this patient is doomed to failure because there is minimal bone stock available for proper mechanical fixation of the cement to the bone.

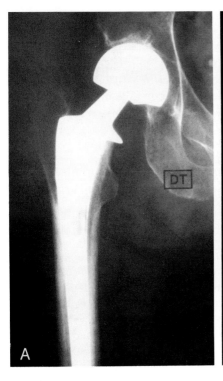
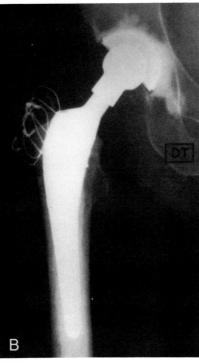

FIG. 27-8. **A.** This patient had been treated for a subcapital hip fracture with an uncemented bipolar component. This patient was experiencing severe pain and had severely reduced function. **B.** Because the bone stock on both the acetabular and femoral sides was well preserved, a mechanically sound interface of cement to bone could be achieved and this patient attained an excellent result with a conversion to a cemented total hip arthroplasty.

ful when large allograft reconstructions are necessary and contact of the prosthesis with host bone is minimal.

Acetabular Revision Using Cementless Components

Very little long-term clinical information is available on the fate of cementless acetabular components with primary or revision total hip arthroplasty.

Engh[18] reviewed 130 smooth threaded cups and 285 porous surfaced hemispherical cups (with additional spike fixation) in 415 primary total hip arthroplasties. At a mean 4.8 years of followup, none of the porous cups demonstrated signs of instability (as measured by migration of over 3 millimeters or a change in inclination of over 8°) and only 2% of these patients had symptoms referable to the cup (e.g., groin or buttock pain). In contrast, at 3.9 years of followup, 21% of the smooth threaded cups were radiographically unstable and 25% of the patients had clinical symptoms. Engh's experience with the threaded acetabular component is contrary to the European experience, however.[34,36A]

Wilson-MacDonald, et al.,[54] reported on 545 cementless uncoated primary polyethylene acetabular components and noted a high rate of loosening over time—70% probability of radiographic loosening

by 9 years. They concluded that direct contact of polyethylene to bone should be avoided because micromotion creates excessive polyethylene debris and subsequent bony erosion. This reflects the experience of Wroblewski, et al.[55A]

Harris and Maloney[24] reported on a series of 126 hybrid primary total hip arthroplasties with an uncemented cup [either acetabular reconstruction component (ARC) or Harris-Galante Prosthesis* (HGP)] and a cemented femoral component. At a mean followup of 42 months (range 24 to 67 months) 96% of the patients had satisfactory clinical scores, 1 acetabular component had migrated 2 mm, and 3 components had a continuous radiolucent line (all less than 2 mm).

In a 2-year followup study of the porous coated anatomic (PCA)* total hip prosthesis, Callaghan, et al.,[4] found that although the satisfactory rating was 94%, progressive loosening of acetabular beads from the porous coat of the cup was identified in 18%. One cup had a change in position but the patient was asymptomatic.

The data on cementless revision of the acetabulum is sparse and is complicated by the need for a variety of bone grafting procedures in these difficult revision situations. Engh, et al.[19] reviewed 160 total hip revisions with a mean followup of 4.4 years (range 2 to 6 years). The review included 107 ace-

*Zimmer, Warsaw, IN.
*Howmedica, Rutherford, NJ.

tabular revisions: 34 porous coated devices (either threaded or hemispherical with spikes) and 73 smooth threaded components. Acetabular instability was defined as migration greater than 2 mm or a change in angle of the cup greater than 5°. Of the smooth threaded cups 32% were unstable at followup and only 3% of the porous coated cups were unstable. Several important points were stressed by the authors. The degree of bone damage to the acetabulum significantly and directly influenced the radiographic results. Stable fixation was achieved in 92% of those acetabula with only minimal bone damage but only in 73% when the acetabular damage was severe. Second, an optimal fit also directly affected the ultimate stability of the cup. If the fit was optimal, only 15% became unstable radiographically but if suboptimal, 34% became unstable.

Hedley[25] reviewed 61 total hip revisions using PCA components with a mean followup of 21 months (range 12 to 15 months). Bone grafting was used in 30 cases to provide adequate coverage and stability for the cups. A porous coated cup was used with two superior pegs available for additional rotational stability. Acetabular migration and loosening was found in 4 cases (6.6%). Hedley did note some settling of sockets especially if large superior or superomedial weight-bearing grafts were used.

McGann[36] reported on 75 acetabular revisions using the Harris-Galante cup (hemispherical with additional screw fixation through holes in the cup) with a mean 14 month followup (range 2 to 36 months). Rigid fixation of the cup was obtained at surgery in all cases. A variety of different defects were grafted. New postoperative lucencies were seen around the cups in 23%—most likely denoting fibrous ingrowth. No cup migration occurred in this short followup.

Emerson, et al.,[16] reported on the use of cementless cups with large allografts during revision arthroplasty. Of 13 threaded cups followed for a mean of 40 months, only 5 were radiologically stable and 4 were clinical failures. Of 46 pressfit porous hemispherical cups (with 4 fins for rim fixation) followed for a mean of 22 months, 7 had migrated and only 1 was a clinical failure.

Because of the relatively short followup periods in the clinical series on cementless acetabular reconstruction, the guidelines for revisional arthroplasty with cementless devices will continue to undergo change in the future. At this time, however, there appear to be several important principles to which the revision surgeon should adhere.

Preparation of the bony bed must be fastidious and careful. If still present, subchondral bone should be preserved. The cortical rims of the acetabulum must be clearly identified and zealously guarded. The acetabular rim is a critical structure to which the cementless cup is anchored. If the rim is discontinuous, it must be reconstructed (usually with graft). For the porous hemispherical cup designs, intimate contact with host bone is required for bony ingrowth. Therefore, careful reaming must be undertaken. Any motion of the reamers in the surgeon's hand will convert a true hemispherical bed into an oblong shape and therefore reduce the area of contact of bone to the cup.

Although a variety of different name brand cementless cups are available, there are only two basic types—threaded and hemispheric pressfit. The threaded cups are designed to gain initial stability through the threaded purchase on bone. Long term stability is through macrointerlock if bone consolidation occurs around the threads and additional microinterlock if a porous coating is added to the cup.[35] A variety of different designs have been available. Overall, however, the clinical results with threaded cups are less than satisfactory. In their testing of in vivo cementless acetabular fixation in dogs, Tooke, et al.,[49] found a higher degree of micromotion and a lower amount of bone contact with the threaded components as compared to a porous coated design. Thus in revisional surgery, when given a choice, it would seem prudent to select a porous coated design and to avoid threaded acetabular components.

The porous coated hemispherical cup designs appear to be the most promising option for revision acetabular surgery. They hold several advantages to the surgeon. Because the acetabulum tends to be somewhat hemispherical (in both primary and revision situations) minimal bone sacrifice is necessary for implantation of the cups (Fig. 27–9). If intimate bone contact can be achieved, bone ingrowth and hopefully permanent fixation can be achieved.[23] On the other hand, fibrous ingrowth can also provide mechanically sound fixation.[49]

Probably the most important requirement for successful cementless acetabular revision is to achieve rigid stability of the cup at the time of implantation. Contact of the cup with an intact acetabular rim is important in achieving this goal. If the rim is deficient, it must be rebuilt. Proper cup sizing at the time of surgery will insure rim contact. Unrestricted reaming of the acetabular bed can destroy the rim and prevent a satisfactory reconstruction. Pressfitting of the cup can give excel-

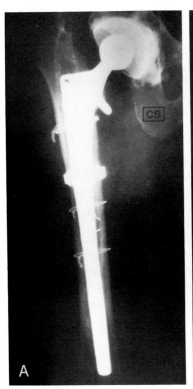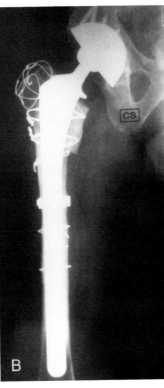

Fig. 27–9. A. Failed total hip arthroplasty with loose cemented acetabular component and loose uncemented femoral component. **B.** Postoperative x-ray demonstrating reconstruction of the acetabulum with uncemented hemispherical cup. The hemispherical shape of this cup allowed the radiographic appearance of this revision acetabulum to mimic that of a primary acetabular component.

lent stability and some surgeons will under-ream the acetabulum and then impact a slightly over-sized cup to insure rim contact. A report by Cheng, et al.,[8] on the effect of sizing mismatch on bone ingrowth into uncemented porous coated acetabular component showed that bone ingrowth at the peripheral one-third of the acetabulum is best achieved by the use of oversized hemispherical components.

However, because the stability of hemispherical cups placed into hemispherical beds is suspect, a secondary means of achieving additional stability of the cup must be provided. This comes in the form of pegs, spikes, pins, or screws. A study by Lachiewiez, et al.,[32] comparing a two-peg design, a three-spike design, and a three-screw design found that the best fixation could be achieved with the hemispherical cup that used three screws through it for additional stability. A clinical study by Haddad, et al.,[22] comparing a three-spike design, a two-peg design, and a three-screw design confirmed the above laboratory findings with the incidence of groin pain being the least (only 2%) in the three-screw design, versus 17% in the three-spike design and 20% in the two-peg design. The other advantage of the hemispherical cup with portals for multiple screws is the ability to transfix acetabular grafts by proper placement of screws to the cup. One potential pitfall with this design is the concern

about the fate of these screws if component migration occurs.

A more practical concern is the anatomical location of the screws used for fixation. Keating, et al.,[30] performed an anatomic study of the structures at risk from medially placed acetabular screws. These structures include the external iliac vein, the obturator artery nerve and vein, and tributaries of the internal iliac vein. They recommended avoiding placing screws in the anterior superior quadrant of the acetabulum. Wasieliewski, et al.,[51] devised an acetabular quadrant system that uses one line drawn from the anterior superior iliac spine through the center of the acetabulum to the posterior fovea. A second line is drawn perpendicularly to the first at the midpoint of the acetabulum. They recommended against screw placement in the anterior superior and anterior inferior quadrants.

Should one choose to perform an acetabular revision with cementless components, several important facts should be kept in mind. The long-term data on the durability of these components are unavailable. Preparation of the bony bed and preservation of the acetabular rims are critical for success. Finally, the initial stability of the cup must be assured through whatever means are necessary or early clinical failure will occur. Most revision acetabular surgery performed at the Rothman Institute is now done using cementless designs. Only longer followup will determine the most appropriate cementless design for revision surgery.

Acetabular Revision Using Bipolar Components

Initial enthusiasm for the application of bipolar sockets to the problem of acetabular revision was stimulated by the reports of Bateman,[2] Scott,[45] and Murray.[37] The concept was to use a well fitted bipolar cup against the acetabular rim as a solution for those cases in which bone stock was inadequate to support a fixed socket. The technical aspects were further emphasized in later followups by Scott[53] and by Murray.[38] The socket must obtain fixation through contact with the intact acetabular rim. Furthermore, the bipolar component must be contained adequately within the acetabular bed to avoid component dislocation. Proper bone grafting techniques must be used. Noncontained peripheral or central segmental defect grafts will not survive against a bipolar prosthesis—inevitable graft dissolution and component migration will ensue.[52] Roberson and Cohen[44] reported on 27 bipolar components used during revision surgery when adequate fixation for a cementless acetabular component could not be achieved. At 2 to 6 years of followup, only 1 case of significant component migration had occurred.

A report by Oschner, et al.[40] of 10 patients who underwent revision total hip arthroplasty using large allografts and bipolar components demonstrated an average of 8 mm of superior migration and 4 mm of medial migration at 2 years of followup. A report by Emerson, et al.,[16] of 37 bipolar revisions demonstrated migration and graft resorption in 50%. In addition, the clinical scores for other bipolar revisions were inferior to those scores for the "fixed-cup" revisions. In their opinion, bipolar devices "should be reserved for low-demand patients in whom a longer and more involved acetabular reconstruction is not indicated." The authors concur with this statement (Fig. 27–10). Furthermore, when the acetabular rim is intact (a prerequisite for the use of a bipolar device) a cementless or cemented fixed cup can invariably be used with a better clinical result.

McGann[36] and Hedley[25] each reported on a specific indication for the bipolar cup in revision arthroplasty. They suggested that a bipolar cup would be useful in those cases in which the abductor musculature was absent or incompetent and in whom recurrent dislocation of the hip was a problem. They each reported on one case in which a revision from a fixed cup to a bipolar cup solved the problem of instability.

Bipolar components should continue to be performed by the revision hip surgeon, but a fixed cup (either cemented or cementless) should be used preferentially.

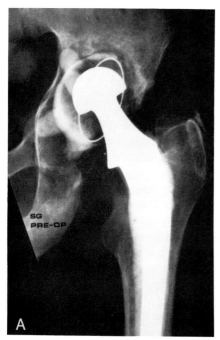 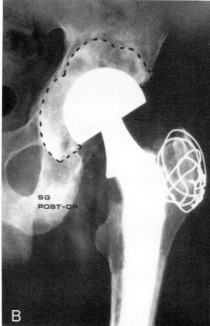 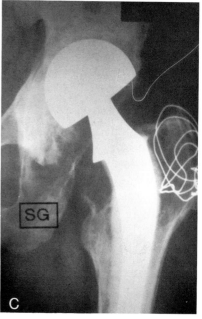

FIG. 27–10. A. Loose cemented acetabular component in a patient with Gaucher's disease. **B.** Reconstruction of the acetabulum with a large allograft femoral head and a bipolar component. **C.** Two years later the Bipolar component had eroded through the bone graft.

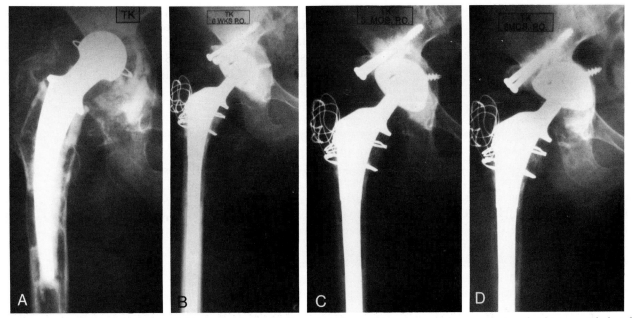

Fɪɢ. 27–11. **A.** Failed cemented total hip arthroplasty. **B.** Reconstruction using uncemented component and a large acetabular allograft. (In this case a distal femur was used.) **C.** Three months postoperatively, there was early resorption of the bone graft. **D.** Six months postoperatively, there was complete resorption of the bone graft medially. With an early loss of the bone graft, the possibility of infection must be considered.

Bone Grafting in Acetabular Revision

The current role of bone grafting for acetabular revision surgery is in flux (Figs. 27–11, 27–12). The pendulum of prejudice has always alternated between biologic and prosthetic answers to operative problems of severe bone deficiency. Currently, popular wisdom would favor the biologic approach with bone grafting being used to restore structural defects, to accelerate and facilitate the healing of bone deficiencies, and to contain methacrylate or to stabilize contemporary cementless components and to restore the normal joint axes critical to the function of contemporary prosthetic designs. The longevity of any artificial implant is necessarily limited, but the replacement of deficient bone stock will prepare the skeleton for a future and hopefully better chance at reconstruction. Further, the clinical results of revision total hip arthroplasty using cement have been poor (see the previous section on acetabular revision using cement).

Most prosthetic implants today enjoy a modular design allowing a small complement of prostheses to accommodate a wide variety of anatomic variations. For some situations, custom designs might be appropriate. However, the uncertainties and vagaries of surgical reconstruction of the acetabulum still demand of the surgeon certain solutions accommodated only by graft. Of the variety of graft materials currently available for reconstructive use,

fresh autograft and frozen or freeze-dried allografts are the most common. Bone graft substitutes may in the future play a larger role. Autograft bone has the best potential for healing to the host bone and for subsequent incorporation and remodeling. Although it takes longer, however, the incorporation of allograft bone is qualitatively the same.[21] Cortical grafts act initially as weight-bearing space fillers, over time becoming a mixture of necrotic and viable bone serving as a scaffold for potential reossification. Cancellous grafts are replaced by creeping substitution and are more rapidly revascularized than cortical grafts. Cancellous grafts may be completely repaired within a several year period.[21]

Allograft carries with it several advantages. There is no limit to the size, shape, or quantity of bone that can be obtained. Femoral heads, femoral condyles, distal femurs, and whole acetabular allografts are most commonly used in revision acetabular surgery. Furthermore, there is no sacrifice of normal structures and there is no donor site morbidity. The potential disadvantages of allograft include the possibility of an adverse immunologic response, the possibility of disease transfer, and the ultimate question of biologic potential.

The experience with structural allografts in revision acetabular surgery has been variable. A canine study of large bone allografts in acetabular reconstruction by Taylor, et al.,[48] found, in well prepared host beds, that both autografts and allografts

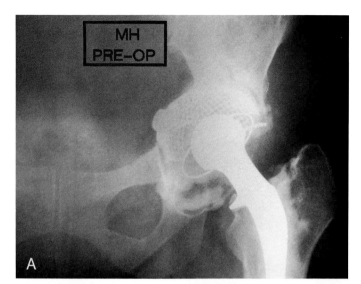

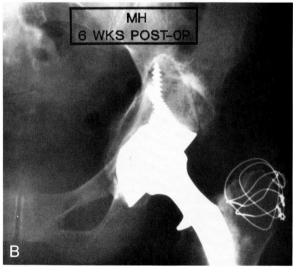
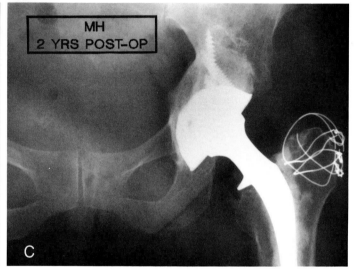

FIG. 27–12. A. Normal preoperative x-ray showing failed cemented total hip arthroplasty. B. Early postoperative X-ray demonstrating large acetabular bone graft. Note that the definition between the bone graft and the patient's own acetabular bone is easy to make. C. Two years postoperatively, the bone graft has completely healed to the patient's pelvis and this patient continues to enjoy excellent function.

showed similar evidence of good healing and incorporation. At 6 months, screws used for fixation continued to provide resistance to motion resulting from rim loads. Finally, bone resorption consistently occurred at the cup graft interface with poor potential for bony ingrowth. Trancik, et al.,[50] reported on 17 acetabular allografts performed during revision total hip arthroplasty with an average followup of 3.5 years (range 2 to 5 years). Six months of postoperative crutch walking was required using the involved limb for balance only. One graft collapsed and was revised, leaving 16 patients with a successful allograft and no evidence of loosening. All 16 grafts appeared to have healed to the host bed. Convery, et al.,[9] reviewed 14 revision total hip arthroplasties using 11 acetabular allografts and 3 iliac crest autografts. With a followup period of 32 months, no autograft failures occurred. Significant migration occurred in 3 of the 14 allograft cases. All grafts united to the host bed.

Jasty and Harris[26] reported on 38 hip reconstructions using allograft femoral heads and cemented cups with a mean followup of 5.9 years (range 4 to 9.1 years). All allografts united but component loosening occurred in 32%. Resorption of the grafts occurred to some degree in 60%. Survivorship analysis predicted a 76% success rate (no acetabular component loosening) at 6 years. The degree to which the graft provided support for the cup had a positive correlation with cup loosening.

Chandler[7] reported on 38 acetabular grafts followed for a mean of 9.5 years (range 6 to 18 years) with 20 autografts and 18 allografts. Of the grafts, 87% were rim or intra-acetabular and subject to weight-bearing forces. Six patients had aseptic loosening of their cemented cup at a mean 8.6 years postoperatively. Five of these 6 had viable graft at subsequent revision and further grafting was not needed. Major graft resorption occurred in 3 cases (1 septic). The authors felt that the results were directly related to technique. It was emphasized that the graft must be positioned beneath a buttress of host bone capable of supporting weight-bearing forces. All screws used for graft fixation should be oriented in the direction of the weight-bearing forces and should be roughly parallel to each other. The threads of the screws should have purchase only on host bone and not in the graft, allowing for impaction.

Emerson, et al.,[16] in reporting their experience with acetabular allografts felt that insufficient mechanical stability of the graft was the primary problem in the difficult revision cases. In particular, they felt that screw fixation alone for rim grafts was insufficient and they recommended the addition of a buttress plate. In their series of 46 cases followed 22 months (range 12 to 32 months) there was only one cup failure. Hedley's experience[25] with 61 revision hip replacements found no graft resorption and he noted consolidation of the medial wall and cancellous hypertrophy in many of the cases in the superior weight-bearing region. Mc-Gann, however, noted that noncontained grafts consistently appeared to resorb.[36]

From this experience, several important issues can be resolved. Foremost, it is essential that several technical considerations are remembered. The quality of the host bed is a critical determinant of the ultimate fate of the graft because from the host is derived the revascularization process. Therefore, decortication to a viable bleeding surface is necessary. This can be accomplished (gently) with circular reamers and high speed burrs. Every attempt must be made to create an absolute conformity of the interface between the graft and the host. Fashioning the host bed and the graft is a three-dimensional problem that can severely test the skills of the surgeon. Most grafts are formed freehand using rongeurs, high speed burrs, or reciprocating saws. An unlimited number and variety of structural shapes can be fashioned and the size and shape of each graft must be carefully studied to provide optimal utilization. A table vise or multiple towel clips serve to stabilize the working model. With experience, the number of passes in and out of the operative field to confirm conformity with the host can be reduced. For those not blessed with three-dimensional psychomotor skills, a cement mold of the defect can be created to serve as a positive template for rough graft fashioning. Judicious use of circular reamers in the acetabular bed can remove a variety of irregular defects and leave a more uniform bed for more facile reconstruction. When incongruities or fissures remain despite the surgeon's best efforts at graft sculpturing, granular graft augmentation is helpful—just as a carpenter would use putty to mask an imperfect joint.

Stabilization of the graft within the host is essential to success. The failure of many grafts may be related to a lack of mechanical stability and inadequate internal fixation. Stability can be achieved in several ways: by exact conformity of the graft in host defects, by the use of turrets or protuberances on the graft to retard rotation, by impaction of the graft into a defect contained by a viable acetabular rim, and subsequently by impaction of a prosthetic cup, or by screw fixation. As recommended by Emerson, et al.,[16] reconstruction plates may be indicated in peripheral grafts not contained by host bone. This is especially important in posterior and posterior-superior grafts, which experience considerable forces during sitting and walking. As emphasized by Chandler,[7] the orientation of the screws is important and the ability to provide compression for the graft is useful.

The design of the cup may play a role in the survival of the underlying grafts. All cemented cups and most hemispherical porous coated cups have no provision for rim fixation of the cup. However, a modification to the hemispherical design to achieve rim contact and rim fixation for the cup may alleviate stresses seen by the underlying bone graft avoiding its collapse and allowing it enough time to remodel. Designs such as the Mallory Head cup* or the Universal cup* may be superior because they provide a means for rim fixation of the cup (Fig. 27–13).

Finally, all grafts must be protected from stress overload until bony incorporation occurs. If all these technical criteria are recalled and accomplished, a successful bone graft becomes likely. At this time, however, it seems prudent to attempt all reconstructions primarily without a structural allograft if possible (Figs. 27–14, 27–15). Using cementless components, gentle reaming should be performed until the anterior-posterior bony rim dimensions limit further expansion. If at this time the cementless component can be inserted with adequate stability and rim support, no structural grafting need be undertaken. However, in many cases of severe acetabular erosion, bone grafting is necessary.

Unsolved Issues

Acetabular Component Position

Restoration of the normal position of the acetabulum is generally considered a prime goal of reconstructive hip surgery. Experience with primary pro-

*Biomet, Warsaw, IN.

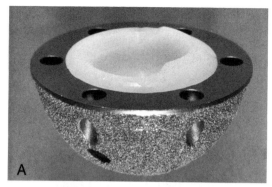

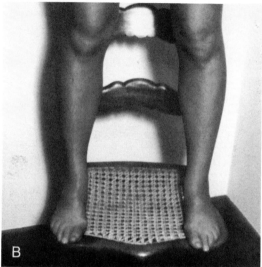

FIG. 27–13. **A.** Photograph of a universal cup (Biomet, Warsaw, IN) demonstrating the peripheral flange that allows fixation of the cup to the rim of the pelvis. **B.** An analogy of this type of fixation can be made to that of a cane chair in which the only stability is obtained from the outer edge of the chair, as demonstrated in this photograph.

trusio acetabuli[3,31,42,43] and congenital dysplasia of the hip[27] has shown that restoration of the normal position gives better clinical and radiographic results. Furthermore, a stress analysis of acetabular reconstruction by Crowninshield[11] found that anatomic position of the cup in protrusio acetabuli was important in reducing the medial bone stresses. Further, a biomechanical analysis of the reconstructed hip by Johnston, et al.[28] found the least hip loading if the cup was placed as medially, anteriorly, and inferiorly as possible. Accordingly, most surgeons prefer to re-establish this anatomic position of the cup at revision surgery even if it means using structural allograft. The counter argument is that resorption of the graft may lead to cup fixation failure. Thus, the idea of acetabular revision with the cup in a "high" position is currently being discussed. The advantages include the ability to avoid grafting and the ability to achieve direct contact of the cementless cup with host bone. The disadvantages include the inferior mechanical properties of the reconstruction and the increased potential for bone impingement and hip instability (Fig. 27–16). A further limitation of this concept of the "high hip center" is that severe thinning of the anterior and posterior acetabular bony columns in the high position may preclude adequate rim contact and proper support of the cementless cup. A recent report by Yoder, et al.[56] suggested that significantly higher rates of femoral loosening and higher (but not significantly so) rates of acetabular loosening are experienced with reconstruction in a high nonanatomic position. The overall weight of the data at this time supports continued efforts to

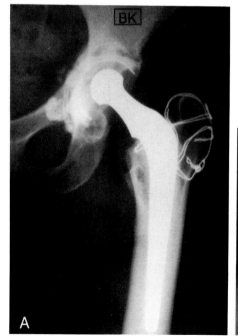

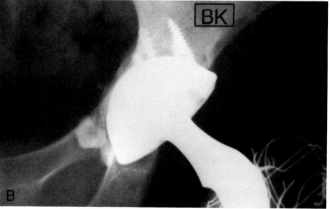

FIG. 25–14. **A.** Preoperative x-ray demonstrating a loose acetabular component with cavitary bone deficiencies. **B.** Postoperative x-ray demonstrating reconstruction of the acetabulum using a large uncemented cup with minimal bone graft.

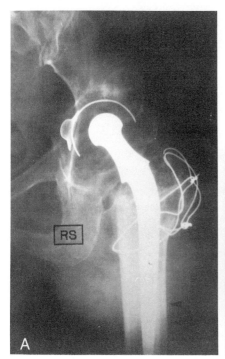

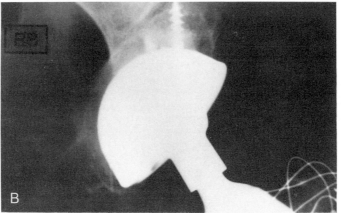

Fɪɢ. 27–15. **A.** Preoperative x-ray showing a bony deficiency very similar to that of Figure 27–14A. **B.** Postoperative x-ray demonstrating a large acetabular cup with an extensive bone graft unlike Figure 27–14B. This patient required a bone graft in order to reconstruct the acetabulum. It is difficult preoperatively to absolutely predict the need for a bone graft.

reconstruct the acetabulum in an anatomic position despite the occasional need for structural allografts.

Cemented Versus Cementless Components Associated With Large Allograft Reconstruction

Bony ingrowth in cementless components is not possible when the component is in contact with structural graft. In fact, Engh suggests that it is unlikely even in areas where particulate graft has been used to fill small defects.[18] Therefore, when a significant portion of the cup is in contact only with graft, many surgeons recommend using a cemented component (Figs. 27–17, 27–18). However, what constitutes a "significant portion of the cup," varies. Chandler[7] will accept 90% graft and 10% host bone. McGann[36] found success by accepting as little as 30% host-bone contact using nonstructural grafts provided that the cup is inherently stable within the pre-existing host bone. He will accept up to 40% of the surface area of the cup being in contact with solid graft (60% host bone). These are approximate guidelines. Only further followup will clarify the answer. Another factor to consider is that bone ingrowth may not be necessary for the cementless cups to survive. If a stable pressfit fibrous ingrowth fixation is achieved, long term clinical success may be possible with cementless cups, regardless of the extent of the underlying graft.

Component Coverage

Failure to provide adequate coverage for the cup has been linked with early component loosening.[33,47A] For this reason, bone grafting procedures became popular for rim deficiencies, especially in reconstructions for congenital dysplasia of the hip. However, long-term followup by Gerber and Harris[20] found a high rate of failure of these lateral grafts at 7 years postoperatively. The question then becomes in revision surgery: how much of the cementless cup can be left uncovered before grafting is needed? In congenital dysplasia of the hip, one solution is to use very small cups. However, the acetabular defect in revision acetabular surgery is generally too large for this solution to be a viable one. On the other hand, reports by Drabu[14] and by Nunn[39] suggest that lack of bone coverage over the lateral surface of the cup did not have adverse effects on the stability and function of the hip. The report by Drabu suggests that proper reaming with some medialization allowed more than 30% of the lateral wall of the cup to remain uncovered without adverse effect. When one considers that nonloaded lateral grafts were likely to resorb, the ability to accept lack of coverage for a cementless cup is attractive. Failure to graft, however, does not solve the problem of bone deficiency should further revisions be necessary. At this time, however, it seems reasonable to accept some degree of lack of coverage for the cup provided that the initial stability of the cup is not compromised. In our experience at the Rothman Institute approximately 25% of the cementless cup

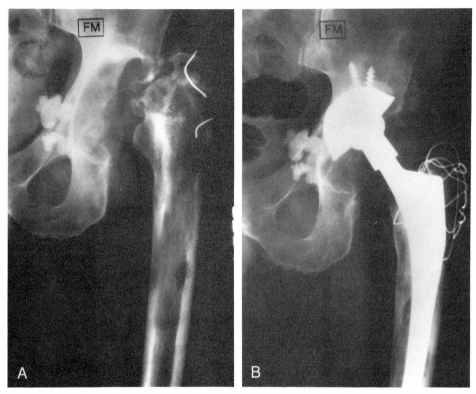

Fɪɢ. 27–16. **A.** Preoperative x-ray showing a resection arthroplasty performed for infection. **B.** Reconstruction of the hip with the acetabular component placed in a high proximal position. Extra stability was obtained in this patient by using a laterally offset femoral component and a long neck. Despite these two additional features, the patient continued to have episodes of hip instability and required postoperative bracing. The potential advantage of avoiding a graft and the ability to achieve direct contact of the cementless cup against host bone in these cases must be weighed against the disadvantages of increased potential for bone impingement and hip instability.

Fɪɢ. 27–17. **A.** Preoperative x-ray demonstrating a failed cemented acetabular component. **B.** Postoperative reconstruction using a large allograft in the acetabulum and the cemented cup against the allograft.

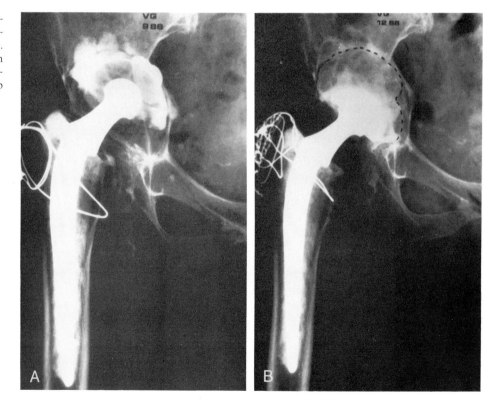

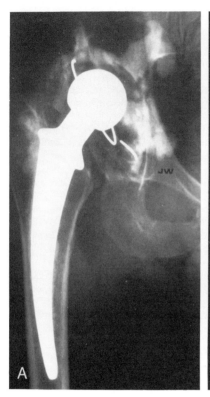 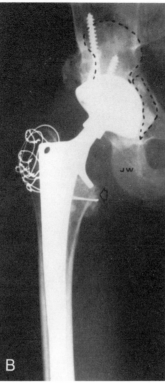

FIG. 27–18. **A.** Preoperative x-ray demonstrating severe loss of bone after loosening of the cemented cup. **B.** Postoperative x-ray demonstrating reconstruction of the acetabulum with large allografts and an uncemented cup. The use of cemented versus cementless components in association with large allograft construction is one of the many unsolved issues in acetabular revision surgery.

can be left uncovered by bone before initial stability is lost.

With these principles in mind the problem of reconstruction can more easily be defined, the solutions can be more satisfactory, and the clinical results can be more enduring.

Conclusions

The problem of acetabular reconstruction in revision hip surgery is complex and the solutions are many and varied. For this reason, it is important that future reports adhere to an accepted classification of acetabular deficiencies. Currently, the AAOS classification advocated by the Hip Society is the best choice.[12] Only then can any meaningful analyses be made of future followup studies and only then can the unresolved issues be answered.

The currently available clinical results in revision acetabular surgery are satisfactory but little long-term data is available. What must be thoroughly understood are the basic principles of acetabular reconstruction which include:

1. Restore the center of rotation.
2. Restore acetabular continuity.
3. Restore acetabular integrity.
4. Prosthesis containment.
5. Graft containment.
6. Rigid graft fixation.

References

1. AMSTUTZ HC, MA SM, JINNAH RH, MAI L: Revision of aseptic loose total hip arthroplasty. Clin Orthop, 170:21–28, 1982.
2. BATEMAN J: Salvage of failed hip arthroplasty using a multiple bearing implant. Orthop Trans, 5:357, 1981.
3. BAYLEY JC, CHRISTIE MJ, EWALD FC, KELLEY K: Long term results of total hip arthroplasty in protrusio acetabuli. J Arthroplasty, 2:275–279, 1987.
4. CALLAGHAN JJ, DYSART SH, SAVORY CG: The uncemented porous-coated anatomic total hip prosthesis. J Bone Joint Surg, 70A:337–346, 1988.
5. CALLAGHAN JJ, et al.: Results of revision for mechanical failure after cemented total hip replacement. J Bone Joint Surg, 67A:1074–1086, 1985.
6. CARTER DR, VASU R, HARRIS WH: Periacetabular stress distributions after joint replacement with subchondral bone retention. Acta Orthop Scand, 54:29–35, 1983.
7. CHANDLER HP, MCCARTHY J, PENNENBERG B, ALLAYNE N: Solid acetabular bone grafts in association with total hip replacement—six year follow-up. Personal Communication.
8. CHENG SL, et al: The effect of sizing mismatch on bone ingrowth into uncemented porous coated acetabular components. Trans Orthop, 36:442, 1990.
9. CONVERY HR, CONVERY M, DEVINE SD, MEYERS MH: Acetabular augmentation in primary and revision total hip arthroplasty with cementless prostheses. Clin Orthop, 252:167–175, 1990.

10. CORNELL CN, RANAWAT CS: The impact of modern cement techniques on acetabular fixation in cemented total hip replacement. J Arthroplasty, 1:197–202, 1986.

11. CROWNINSHIELD RD, BRAND RA, PEDERSEN DR: A stress analysis of acetabular reconstruction for protrusio acetabuli. J Bone Joint Surg, 65A:495–499, 1983.

12. D'ANTONIO JA, et al: Classification and management of acetabular abnormalities in total hip arthroplasty. Clin Orthop, 243:126–137, 1989.

13. DAVIES JP: Fatigue strength of cement-metal interfaces: comparison of porous, precoated, and smooth specimens. Trans Orthop, 34:367, 1988.

14. DRABU KJ, RING PA: Uncemented acetabular cups in dysplastic and protrusio acetabuli. Clin Orthop, 210:173–178, 1986.

15. EFTEKHAR NS, NARCESSIAN O: Intrapelvic migration of total hip prostheses: operative treatment. J Bone Joint Surg, 71A:1480–86, 1989.

16. EMERSON RH, HEAD WC, BERKLACICH FM, MALININ TI.: Noncemented acetabular revision arthroplasty using allograft bone. Clin Orthop, 249:30–43, 1989.

17. ENGELBRECHT DJ, WEBER FA, SWEET MBE, JAKIM I: Long term results of revision total hip arthroplasty. J Bone Joint Surg, 72B:41–45, 1990.

18. ENGH CA, GRIFFIN WL, MARKS CL: Cementless acetabular components. J Bone Joint Surg, 72B:53–59, 1990.

19. ENGH CA, GLASSMAN AH, GRIFFIN WL, MAYER GAG: Results of cementless revision for failed cemented total hip arthroplasty. Clin Orthop, 235:91–110, 1988.

20. GERBER SD, HARRIS WH: Femoral head autografting to augment acetabular deficiency in patients requiring total hip replacement. J Bone Joint Surg, 68A:1241–1248, 1986.

21. GOLDBERG VM, STEVENSON S: Natural history of autografts and allografts. Clin Orthop, 225:7–16, 1987.

22. HADDAD RJ, COOK SD, BRINKER MR: A comparison of three varieties of uncemented porous-coated hip replacement. J Bone Joint Surg, 72B:2–8, 1990.

23. HARRIS WH, et al.: Bony ingrowth fixation of the acetabular component in canine hip joint arthroplasty. Clin Orthop, 176:7–11, 1983.

24. HARRIS WH, MALONEY WJ: Hybrid total hip arthroplasty. Clin Orthop, 249:21–29, 1989.

25. HEDLEY AK, GRUEN TA, RUOFF DP: Revision of failed total hip arthroplasties with uncemented porous coated anatomic components. Clin Orthop, 235:75–90, 1988.

26. JASTY M, HARRIS WH: Salvage total hip reconstruction in patients with major acetabular bone deficiencies using structural femoral head allografts. J Bone Joint Surg, 72B:63–67, 1990.

27. JENSEN JS, RETPEN JB, ARNOLDI CC: Arthroplasty for congenital hip dislocation. Acta Orthop Scand, 60:86–92, 1989.

28. JOHNSTON RC, BRAND RA, CROWNINSHIELD RD: Reconstruction of the hip, a mathematical approach to determine optimum geometric relationships. J Bone Joint Surg, 61A:639, 1979.

29. KAVANAGH BF, ILSTRUP DM, FITZGERALD RH: Revision total hip arthroplasty. J Bone Joint Surg 67A:517–526, 1985.

30. KEATING EM, RITTER MA, FARIS PM: Structures at risk from medially placed acetabular screws. J Bone Joint Surg, 72A:509–511, 1990.

31. LACHIEWICZ PF, et al: Total hip arthroplasty in juvenile rheumatoid arthritis: 2–11 year results. J Bone Joint Surg, 68A:502, 1986.

32. LACHIEWICZ PI, SUH PD, GILBERT JA: In vitro initial fixation of porous-coated acetabular hip components. J Arthroplasty, 4:201–205, 1989.

33. LINDE F, JENSEN J: Socket loosening in arthroplasty for congenital dislocation of the hip. Acta Orthop Scand, 59:254–257, 1988.

34. LORD G, BANCEL P: The madreporic cementless total hip arthroplasty. Clin Orthop, 176:67–76, 1983.

34A. MALLORY TH, et al: Threaded acetabular components: design rationale and preliminary clinical experience. Orthop Rev 17:305–314, 1988.

35. MARTI RK, SCHULLER HM, VESSELAAR PP, HAASNOOT ELV: Results of revision hip arthroplasty with cement. J Bone Joint Surg, 72A:346–354, 1990.

36. MCGANN WA, WELCH RB, PICETTI GD: Acetabular preparation in cementless revision total hip arthroplasty. Clin Orthop, 235:45–46, 1988.

36A. MITTLEMEIER H: Cementless revision of failed total hip replacement with ceramic autophor prosthesis. *In* Welch RB (ed.): The Hip: Proceedings of the 12th Open Scientific Meeting of the Hip Society. St. Louis, Mosby, p. 312–331, 1984.

37. MURRAY WR: Salvage of acetabular insufficiency with bipolar prostheses. In Welch RJ (ed.): Proceedings of the Hip Society. St. Louis, Mosby, pp 296–311, 1984.

38. MURRAY WR: Acetabular salvage in revision total hip arthroplasty using a bipolar prosthesis. Clin Orthop, 251:92–99, 1990.

39. NUNN D: The ring uncemented polyethylene cup in the abnormal acetabulum. J Bone Joint Surg, 69B:756–760, 1987.

40. OCHSNER JL, PENNENBERG BL, DORR LD, CONATY JP: The bipolar endoprosthesis and bone grafting in the management of aseptic acetabular component loosening. Orthopedics, 13:45–49, 1990.

41. OH I: A comprehensive analysis of the factors affecting acetabutar cup fixation and design in total hip replacement arthroplasty. In Welch RB (ed.): Proceedings of the Hip Society. St. Louis, Mosby, p. 110–177, 1983.

42. RANAWAT CS, DORR LD, INGLIS AE: Total hip arthroplasty in protrusio acetabuli of rheumatoid arthritis. J Bone Joint Surg, 62A:1059–1064, 1980.

43. RANAWAT CS, ZANN MG: Role of bone grafting in correction of protrusio acetabuli by total hip arthroplasty. J Arthroplasty, 1:131–137, 1986.

44. ROBERSON JR, COHEN D: Bipolar components for severe periacetabular bone loss around the failed total hip arthroplasty. Clin Orthop, 251:113–118, 1990.

45. SCOTT RD: Use of a bipolar prosthesis with bone grafting in acetabular reconstruction. Contemp Orthop, 9:35–41, 1984.

46. SHELLEY P, WROBLEWSKI BM: Socket design and cement pressurization in the Charnley low-friction arthroplasty. J Bone Joint Surg, 70B:358–363, 1988.

47. SUTHERLAND CJ: Radiographic evaluation of acetabular bone stock in failed total hip arthroplasty. J Arthroplasty, 3:73–79, 1988.

47A. SUTHERLAND CJ, et al: A ten year follow-up of one hundred consecutive curved-stem total hip replacement arthroplasties. J Bone Joint Surg, 64A:970–982, 1982.

48. TAYLOR JK, et al: Large bone grafts in acetabular reconstruction: a canine study. Trans Orthop, 36:230, 1990.

49. TOOKE SM, et al: Comparison of in vivo cementless acetabular fixation. Clin Orthop, 235:253–260, 1988.

50. TRANCIK TN, STULBERG BM, WILDE AH, FIGLIN DH: Allograft reconstruction of the acetabulum during revision total hip arthroplasty. J Bone Joint Surg, 68A:527–533, 1986.

51. WASIELEWSKI RC, COOPERSTEIN LA, KRUGER MP, RUBISH HE: Acetabular anatomy in the trans-acetabular fixation of screws in total hip arthroplasty. J Bone Joint Surg, 72A:501–508, 1990.

52. WILSON MG, et al: The fate of acetabular allografts after bipolar revision arthroplasty of the hip. J Bone Joint Surg, 71A:1469–1479, 1989.

53. WILSON MG, SCOTT RD: Reconstruction of the deficient acetabulum using the bipolar socket. Clin Orthop, 251:126–133, 1990.

54. WILSON-MACDONALD J, MORSHER E, MASAR Z: Cementless uncoated polyethylene acetabular components in total hip replacement. J Bone Joint Surg, 72B:423–430, 1990.

55. WOOLSON ST: Three dimensional bone imaging and preoperative planning of reconstructive surgery. Contemp Orthop, 12:13–22, 1986.

55A. WROBLEWSKI, BM, LYNCH M, ATKINSON JR, DOWSON D, ISAAC GH: External wear of the polyethylene socket in cemented total hip arthroplasty. J Bone Joint Surg, 69B:61–63, 1987.

56. YODER SA, BARAND RA, PEDERSEN DR, O'GORMAN TW: Total hip acetabular component position affects component loosening rates. Clin Orthop, 228:79–87, 1988.

CHAPTER TWENTY-EIGHT

Femoral Revision Arthroplasty

RUSSEL E. WINDSOR
JOHN J. CALLAGHAN
PAUL M. PELLICCI
EDUARDO A. SALVATI

Approximately 90,000 total hip replacements are performed in the United States each year.[57] The operation predictably improves pain resulting from arthritis or failed previous hip operations, such as, open reduction and internal fixation for fracture, proximal femoral osteotomy or arthrodesis. The first report of femoral loosening appeared in 1970.[56] Mechanical failure rates, on the femoral or acetabular side may be as high as 24%.[27] In many instances, however, the failure rates are radiographic rather than clinical and revision arthroplasty for clinically significant mechanical failure is estimated at 1 to 2%.[13,39] However, some reported revision rates are as high as 9%.[36] Radiographic signs of failure may predict future implant failure.

Cementless fixation of total hip replacements has been used to diminish the long-term loosening problem that has developed after cemented total hip arthroplasty. However, there have been no critically controlled studies on this subject and new kinds of failure may develop with this technique. Although there have been improvements in cement and cementless fixation designs, it is reasonable to expect that a small percentage of total joint arthroplasties will still fail. This mostly results because younger active patients are undergoing this procedure.

The surgeon should be aware of the patients' psychological attitude. The patient may become discouraged at the failure of the arthroplasty, which may lead to a breach of confidence in the surgeon. Certainly, the patient will have doubts regarding future success of revision arthroplasty. The hospitalizations and financial burden that are associated with this operation may generate hostile feelings in the patient. Thus, the surgeon should accurately assess the patients' comprehension of the problem and explain it in a way that will enable the patient to participate maximally in the postoperative rehabilitative program.

A distinction should be made between conversion and revision arthroplasty. Conversion total hip arthroplasty is done for unremitting pain caused by failure of a previous orthopaedic operation. These failures may occur after open reduction and internal fixation for proximal femoral fracture when nonunion, malunion, or progressive arthritic change in the joint may occur. Conversion of failed femoral neck osteotomies for congenital dysplasia may present peculiar difficulties because of altered anatomy. Surface replacements have no longer been generally accepted because of the high failure rates, but conversion to a total hip replacement is easier on the femoral side because of the presence of an intact femoral neck. This chapter, however, deals only with revision of the femoral side for failed, aseptic total, and hemiarthroplasty of the hip.

Indications

The femoral side of a hip arthroplasty may fail in a variety of ways. A painful hemiarthroplasty may be inappropriately sized on the acetabular side or become loose. Loosening may be divided into septic and aseptic causes. A cemented total hip femoral component may loosen aseptically over time depending on the patient's age, activity level, and body weight. Cementless implants may fail to adequately bond to the underlying cancellous bone. Incomplete aseptic loosening of the femoral total hip prosthesis may result from good distal but poor proximal fixation, leading ultimately to fatigue failure of the stem itself and fracture (see Chapter 29). Finally, the femoral component may dislocate because of malalignment of the femoral acetabular component. Usually acetabular component malalignment is the cause for dislocation resulting from excessive anteversion or inadvertent retroversion of the cup. However, the femoral component may dislocate because of failure to restore the normal anatomic center of the femoral head, inadequate muscle tensioning, and excessive anteversion or retroversion of the femoral neck. An increased likelihood of excessive femoral component anteversion is found during conversion of a congenitally dislocated hip to total hip arthroplasty because of the inherent femoral neck anteversion present in these dysplastic hips.

Failed Femoral Hemiarthroplasty

The failure rate for femoral endoprosthesis may be as high as 35% after 10 years.[31,48] Failure can result from recurrent subluxation or dislocation, superior migration of the prosthetic femoral head with loss of acetabular cartilage and subchondral bone, painful impingement because of implant contact on normal acetabular bone, and after failed open reduction and internal fixation of a femoral neck fracture.[49] The femoral endoprosthesis may loosen and migrate distally because of femoral neck resorption causing pain and impingement whenever the hip is moved. Bipolar hemiarthroplasties may have an additional problem of disengagement of the head and acetabular component. If the stem is loose or the acetabular cartilage is eroded, revision to a total hip replacement should be performed.

Failed Cemented Total Hip Arthroplasty

A large number of reports describe results, complications, and failure of total hip replacements.[5,10,14,18,26,27,38,43,54] Pain relief and function after primary total hip arthroplasty is predictable. Some failures occur early, whereas others occur late in the postoperative course. Aseptic loosening of cemented femoral components generally occurs earlier than that of cemented acetabular components.[51,53] Femoral stem loosening has been reported to occur in as few as 0.67% and in as many as 20% of the patients undergoing total hip replacements.[11,22,35,47,56] However, these discrepancies may be based on reports of radiographic rather than clinical signs of loosening.

Loosening of the cemented femoral component is classified into four modes according to the region of the femoral shaft where loss of acrylic support occurs.[3] In mode 1 (Piston mode), the entire stem is loose and distal stem migration is observed. In mode 2 (medial midstem pivot mode), there is complete loosening with rocking of the stem in the

proximal-medial and distal-lateral direction. In mode 3 (calcar pivot mode), the distal portion of the femoral stem is loose and the prosthesis rocks with a fixed proximal center of rotation. A "windshield wiper sign" may be observed radiographically that results from the formation of an arc of sclerotic reactive bone caused by the pendulum-like movement of the distal stem. Finally, in mode 4, (cantilever fatigue mode), the distal stem is well fixed but the proximal support is inadequate. This loosening may result in plastic deformation or ultimately femoral stem fracture. Aseptic loosening of the cemented femoral component correlates with varus prosthetic positioning; young, heavy, active males; poor femoral stem design that may include a medial diamond shaped contour; and poor cementing technique.[35,41,50] Femoral component stresses are greatest in the varus position and an incomplete cement mantle ultimately yields poor long-term support and early failure. Surgical attention to the details of cementing, prosthesis selection, and appropriate implant positioning during primary hip arthroplasty results in greater longevity of the initial replacement and a decreased overall femoral revision rate.[4,37]

Component loosening may result from repeated torque caused by the cantilever stresses that are placed across the implant cement-bone interfaces.[74] Metal sensitivity has been implicated as a possible cause for failure.[22] However, the latter observation remains controversial and has only been rarely seen.[29] The rigidity of the metal may result in localized bone resorption at the level of the calcar, which may ultimately cause distal migration and loosening. The loosened femoral stem may result in significant peripheral bone loss caused by the constant pistoning of the implant inside the femoral canal.

Gustilo has classified failure on the femoral side by relating it to bone loss.[25] His type 1A demonstrates minimal endosteal bone loss with an intact circumferential wall. Loosening occurs at the metal-cement interface. There is less than 50% of thinning of the proximal cortices (Fig. 28–1). Type 1B: the same cement-bone interface failure with greater than 50% thinning of the proximal cortices. Canal enlargement is observed but the circumferential wall is intact. Type 2 loosening involves proximal cortical thinning in addition to a lateral wall defect with lateral prosthetic migration. Type 3 demonstrates posteromedial wall deficiency involving the lesser trochanter and significant instability. In Type 4, proximal circumferential bone loss is associated with severe component loosening. This bone loss may result from the histiocytic re-

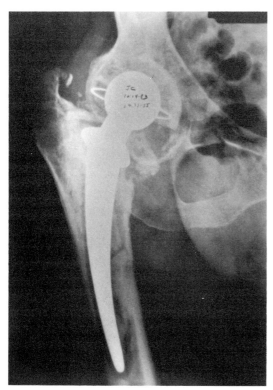

Fɪɢ. 28–1. Anteroposterior radiograph demonstrating Type 1 loosening. Note cortical thinning at distal-lateral cortex.

sponse of fragmented cement after initial prosthetic loosening.

Dislocation of the femoral from the acetabular component following total hip replacement has been reported to have occurred in as few as 0.5% and in as many as 7% of cases.[12,16,44] Malposition of the femoral or acetabular component or both may result in chronic dislocation. The femoral component may dislocate when it impinges on the acetabular component during active hip flexion or extension. Excessive anteversion of the femoral and acetabular components may result in anterior dislocation. Retroversion of the acetabular or femoral component will more commonly result in posterior dislocation. A retroverted acetabular cup with an excessively anteverted femoral component causes impingement and subsequent dislocation. Spinal anesthesia and the use of the posterior approach to the hip without reattachment of the posterior capsule and external rotators have been implicated in more frequent component dislocation.[45]

The incidence of femoral stem fracture varies from 0.23 to 2%.[8,9,13,23] A patient at risk for this failure is the young, heavy, active male with the fracture incidence rising sharply in men over 1.8 m tall and weighing greater than 76 kg. Varus malposition of the femoral prosthesis and metallurgical defects during the manufacturing process also contribute to premature implant failure. Stem designs with a diamond shape cross section, such as the Muller prosthesis and the trapezoidal-28 prosthesis, are particularly prone to failure (see Chapter 29).

Any painful hip replacement should be considered infected until proven otherwise. The diagnosis often is not clear and objective criteria such as an elevated temperature, leukocyte count, or erythrocyte sedimentation rate are undependable and frequently normal despite active joint infection (see Chapter 30).

Last, the patient may sustain a fracture of the femur at or distal to the tip of a well cemented and positioned femoral stem. Traction may not obtain anatomic alignment of the proximal and distal bone fragments and revision of the femoral component to a longer stem design may be required to stabilize the fracture. Most fractures proximal to the implant can be treated well with traction and observation. However, treatment of fractures at the site of the distal tip of the femoral component is controversial. These patients often have osteoporosis and compromised bone stock that inhibits secure fixation of the fracture fragments.

Failed Uncemented Total Hip Replacement

The use of uncemented total hip replacements has risen over the last 5 years. Published results, however, are still short-term compared with those available for cemented total hip replacements.[20] Thus, future modes of femoral component failure may be still undetermined.

Persistent thigh pain at 2 years following uncemented total hip arthroplasty is as high as 17%.[6] This may result from a biologic reaction to the porous coated surface, loosening, or micromotion at the prosthesis-bone interface, where inadequate fixation to trabecular bone is present. Gross loosening of these implants may cause pistoning or distal migration in the canal. The implants may be fixed by fibrous tissue and show no clear radiographic evidence of loosening. Persistent thigh pain may ultimately require revision.

Revision arthroplasty may be necessary for recurrent dislocation. Removal of a well fixed femoral component can be formidable with a high risk of damaging cortical and cancellous bone. Proximal calcar resorption because of stress shielding at the proximal femur has been reported in implants with a high modulus of elasticity, which can result in progressive loosening or fracture of the prosthesis.

Preoperative Evaluation

A careful history and thorough physical examination is mandatory in evaluating patients with failed total hip arthroplasties. Consistently done serial anteroposterior and lateral radiographs should be obtained. Tomography, aspiration, arthrography, and radionuclide scanning may be required depending on the clinical situation. Evaluation of failed total hip arthroplasties by magnetic resonance imaging and computed axial tomography is limited because of metal implant artefacts observed with computed axial tomography and implant voids seen on the magnetic resonance image.

A complete blood cell count with differential leukocyte count should be obtained along with erythrocyte sedimentation rate. If infection is suspected, C-reactive protein levels may also be obtained. Information concerning the patients' initial postoperative course, such as persistent pain, hematoma, drainage, or delayed wound healing, may give insight into the possibility of infection.

At The Hospital for Special Surgery, all patients with a painful total joint arthroplasty are considered infected until proven otherwise. Radiographs may demonstrate cortical erosion but hip aspiration is the definitive diagnostic test. All hips considered for revision arthroplasty undergo an aspiration arthrogram of the hip, done under fluoroscopic control and image intensification. A 20-gauge spinal needle is inserted via an anterolateral approach under strict aseptic technique lateral to the femoral artery and distal to the inguinal ligament. An image intensifier is used to guide the needle toward the prosthetic femoral neck. A short beveled needle will facilitate intracapsular positioning, for successful aspiration. Whether or not fluid is obtained, 1 ml of renografin is injected within the pseudocapsule to assess needle placement. If no fluid can be aspirated and the needle appears well positioned, 3 to 5 mm of injectable sterile saline (without bacteriostatic agent) is injected and withdrawn. This fluid is sent to the microbiology laboratory for culture and sensitivity analysis for aerobic, anaerobic, acid fast bacilli, and fungi. Next, five to 15 ml of contrast liquid is injected depending on the pseudocapsule's capacity and the hip is moved. Anteroposterior, lateral, and oblique radiographs are taken. In some cases of loosening, the contrast medium may fill the radiolucency in the prosthesis-cement or cement-bone interface. If radiopaque cement was used during the first operation, the radiolucent line is opacified by the contrast agent. If radiolucent cement was used, contrast will be clearly seen between the prosthesis and bone. When the arthrogram is difficult to interpret, subtraction arthrography may be performed.[46] The patient's hip must be immobilized because identical superimposable views are required. A preinjection film is then subtracted from a postinjection film, which makes any contrast within the interface more clearly visible. A negative arthrogram does not preclude loosening resulting from filling of the space with fibrous or granulation tissue. In this situation, serial plain radiographs may be more illustrative than the arthrogram.

Standard weight-bearing anteroposterior and lateral radiographs give an accurate indication of the loaded state of the hip. Review of serial standard radiographs may be the most accurate means of diagnosing loosening. Radiolucent lines wider than 2 mm at the bone-cement or prosthesis-cement interface are highly suggestive of loosening. Nonprogressive radiolucencies less than 1 mm are common and may represent no problem.[42] Serial radiographs showing progressive radiolucency or component migration regardless of magnitude represent absolute evidence for loosening.

Distal cement fractures, reported in approximately 1.5% of the cases in the largest reported series[55] may be associated with gross loosening and subsidence of the femoral component. However, 89% of those patients with cement fractures were asymptomatic and only 1 patient was more than mildly asymptomatic. Thus, distal cement fractures do not necessarily signify clinically important femoral component loosening.

Diagnosis of a loose cementless porous coated femoral component may be difficult. Currently, there is inadequate knowledge concerning the amount of ingrowth that is necessary to stabilize a prosthesis in the femoral canal and not cause thigh pain. Radiolucencies may suggest loosening. Arthrography may be helpful but its use has not been documented in the literature. Migration of the implant and a 2-mm radiolucency with complete sclerotic margins around it also signify absolute loosening. Radiographic findings such as calcar resorption, cancellization, cortical condensation and hypertrophy are not yet clinically correlated with cementless implant failure. Calcar resorption raises the possibility of significant stress relief at the proximal femur, which may worsen over time and cause subsequent implant loosening. Long-term followup studies will be needed.

Radionuclide scanning can more subtlety diagnose femoral component loosening. If technetium-99 scanning of the hip shows increased uptake of the tracer 6 or more months following total hip replacement, loosening or infection may be suspected. Differential diagnoses may be made by hip aspiration or gallium-67 (^{67}Ga) citrate scanning. Recently, indium-111 (^{111}In) labelled leukocyte scanning may be more specific in differentiating infection from loosening.

Contraindications

Medical infirmity will contraindicate revision. The patient's cardiovascular, pulmonary, and renal systems should be thoroughly evaluated. Metabolic disorders such as diabetes mellitus and thyroid abnormalities should be controlled before surgery is planned. A relative contraindication to revision arthroplasty is the level of the patient's disability compared to the functional requirement of daily living. If the patient's symptoms do not significantly decrease function then the risks involved with revision arthroplasty may be disproportionate.

Active infection is a relative contraindication to revision arthroplasty. However, infection may not always be clearly demonstrated preoperatively. One positive preoperative aspiration yielding low virulence organisms (e.g., staphylococcus epidermidis) may not always signify a contaminant, if other negative aspirations were obtained. Therefore, preoperative antibiotics should not be administered until fluid and tissue have been obtained during surgery for gram stain and culture tests. The character of the joint fluid and surrounding tissues should be assessed. Tissue should be sent for an immediate frozen section. If a large number of polymorphonuclear leukocytes or organisms are seen, infection should be assumed to be active and revision arthroplasty can be done successfully as a staged procedure (see Chapter 30). Our protocol involves removal of all implants and cement during the first procedure with the limb placed in traction until appropriate cultures and sensitivity tests are obtained. A new total joint arthroplasty is implanted after the patient receives a 6-week course of intravenous antibiotics with minimum serum bacterial titers of 1:8. For certain highly virulent bacteria agents, further delay of reimplantation of at least 6 months, may be required.

Preoperative Planning

Templates should be placed on the preoperative radiographs so that the surgeon can estimate the appropriate stem size, and appropriate offset and neck length of the femoral component (Fig. 28–2).

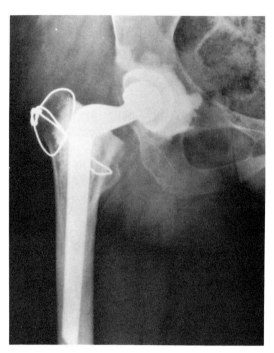

Fig. 28–2. This patient had a dysplastic proximal femur that required a large femoral neck offset.

If the failed component has settled, the center of the femoral head is difficult to assess. In this case, the relationship of the center of the contralateral femoral head with the greater and lesser trochanters can be measured. This analysis can also be done when there is significant bone loss and unclear bony landmarks.

The surgeon should choose the appropriate implant design and type of fixation (i.e., cemented or uncemented). Each revision situation is unique and the method of fixation may depend on the patient's age and the available bone stock. Cementless and cemented forms of fixation should be decided upon preoperatively with cementless fixation chosen for young age and large bone loss whereas cement is used in an older patient with good bone surfaces.

Stems of various lengths should be available at the time of revision, in addition to special cement removing tools.[52] Fiberoptic headlights should be used in all cases to facilitate viewing the intramedullary canal. High speed rotary tools that cut through metal should be available.

Severe proximal bone loss may require a calcar-replacing or custom-designed implant. Patients with congenital hip dysplasia may have an intramedullary canal too small to accept a standard-sized femoral component, so an extra small prosthesis with a decreased femoral neck offset is required.

Autogenous and allogeneic bone graft may be necessary in conjunction with the implant. Large allogeneic bone grafts should be ordered preoperatively. The patient should be appropriately positioned during surgery to obtain sufficient bone graft material. If a massive amount of autogenous bone graft is required the patient should be placed prone initially so that bone can be obtained from the posterior iliac crest. The patient is then placed in the lateral decubitus or supine position according to surgeon preference.

Operative Techniques
Cemented Femoral Components

After the patient has been medically evaluated, and the preoperative planning is complete, revision arthroplasty is performed. Sufficient blood, preferably autologous must be available. Because this operation usually requires more blood than routine total hip arthroplasty, cell-savers may be used. Preoperative antibiotics should be given to all patients. If infection is suspected, antibiotics should be given intraoperatively after tissue is sent for routine culture and sensitivity tests, immediate gram stain, and frozen section. If infection is not present, synthetic penicillinase-resistent antibiotics (e.g., oxacillin, 2 gm) is administered intravenously 1 hour prior to surgery. For minor penicillin allergy, cephazolin is substituted. For major penicillin sensitivity, vancomycin is used. Antibiotics are continued for 4 days until final culture results are available.

The lateral decubitus position is used; bolsters are placed over the pubis, sacrum, and scapula to secure pelvic orientation for accurate positioning of the acetabular cup and sufficient femoral exposure. This position permits bone graft procurement from the posterior iliac crest. We prefer autograft to allograft at The Hospital for Special Surgery. The affected limb is draped free and an intravenous saline bag is placed under the upper thoracic cage to relieve pressure on the brachial plexus.

Previous incisions should be incorporated into the new one wherever possible to avoid making avascular tissue flaps. New incisions should not be made parallel to old ones to avoid potential postoperative skin slough and infection.

Trochanteric osteotomy is used in almost all cases (Fig 28–3). Occasionally, a grossly loose femoral component may come out of the canal easily with an intact cement mantle and trochanteric osteotomy can be avoided. However, removal of the greater trochanter facilitates complete cement removal from the proximal intramedullary cavity. It allows precise adjustment of abductor muscle tension prior to closure, which enhances prosthetic stability and optimize postoperative function.[2]

We utilize laminar flow rooms with hoods and exhaust body systems to minimize potential contamination of the wound. A fiberoptic overhead

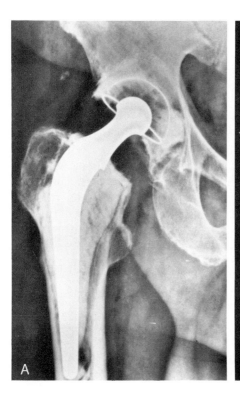
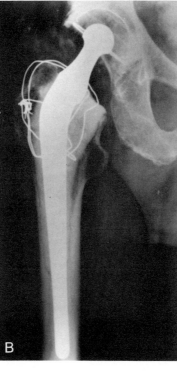

Fɪɢ. **28–3. A.** A loose Charnley total hip prosthesis. **B.** A long-stemmed component was utilized and exposure required greater trochanteric osteotomy.

lamp is used in all cases to facilitate vision of the intramedullary canal.

The incision is extended through the subcutaneous fat, and another longitudinal incision is made across the insertion of the external rotator tendons. A retractor is placed between the obturator externus muscle and gluteus maximus tendon to define the distal border of the capsular incision. The proximal aspect of the gluteus maximus insertion is incised to facilitate exposure.

Trochanteric osteotomy can be done in one of two ways. First, the vastus ridge is exposed and the greater trochanter is osteotomized with a reciprocating saw. Alternatively, the greater trochanter's attachments to the vastus lateralis and abductor muscles may be preserved by a sliding osteotomy that can be reflected superiorly.[24] Previous transtrochanteric wires should be removed, and the trochanteric osteotomy should leave enough bone so that solid reattachment can be accomplished.

The dissection proceeds close to the femur, with care taken to avoid the sciatic nerve. Occasionally, when the posterior aspect of the hip joint is severely scarred, the sciatic nerve should be exposed and protected. By maintaining a subperiosteal femoral exposure the sciatic nerve is safe and a formal exposure is frequently not required.

A complete anterior and posterior capsulotomy is performed to gain full exposure of the hip joint. Both components should be tested for loosening. All visible bone-cement interfaces should be clearly exposed to aid assessment of loosening.

Removal of the femoral component may require flexible osteotomes and high speed rotary burrs to disrupt the cement mantle. A variety of collared extraction devices should be available. The prosthesis is usually removed easily, if there is no porous surface. However, if a porous component is cemented and well fixed, flexible osteotomes and rotary burrs should be used to disrupt the cement prosthesis interface. Some hip systems have their own extraction devices, which should be used. If femoral component removal is not possible with an extraction device, a lateral window can be made on the femur above or just below the distal tip of the prosthesis. A small hole is made so that osteotomes may be used to hammer the prosthesis out of the canal. If a distal window is made, a new long-stemmed device should be inserted with the stem extending beyond the fenestration by a dimension of 3 femoral diameters. Bone stock should be preserved at all times and all fenestrations should be grafted.

A variable amount of cement will come out with the femoral stem and proximal cement removal is easy. However, removal of cement from the distal aspect of the femoral canal is usually difficult and tedious, but all loose cement should be excised. If the cement is well fixed to bone, enough should be removed to provide sufficient space for implantation of a new component. Revision osteotomes can be used with rigid cement reamers to aid in cement removal.[52] Flexible osteotomes are also required to minimize risk of iatrogenic fracture of the femur. Loose cement fragments can be extracted with long pituitary forceps. Frequently, long suction tips are needed to remove bloody debris at the distal aspect of the canal. When a headlight is used, it is helpful to darken the operating room. The surgeon may sit so that the canal is at eye level and parallel to the floor. The surgeon should be patient, because speeding up this stage can result in femoral shaft perforation. If perforation is suspected, the vastus lateralis may be split longitudinally so that the femoral shaft can be directly visualized. Perforation should be noted intraoperatively so that a long-stemmed component may be inserted to bypass the defect, which will need bone graft.

Any exposed trabecular bone should be thoroughly cleaned with pulsatile lavage to allow cement interdigitation. If the patient is not active and over 70 years of age, the entire femoral component can be cemented using a new cement restrictor. Care should be taken to assure proper femoral neck anteversion because the lesser trochanter frequently is not easily seen and trochanteric osteotomy removes an easy reference point. After the new femoral component is inserted, the distance between the center of the femoral head and the lesser trochanter should be the same as the measurement made on the preoperative radiographs, and at the beginning of the operation to preserve leg length equality. Many hip replacement systems have modular femoral heads that can be placed onto a Morris taper, which allows femoral heads with varying widths and neck lengths to be implanted after the prosthesis is cemented into place.

Two transverse and two longitudinal wires are passed through drill holes placed in the proximal femur for later reattachment of the greater trochanter. The transverse wires may be passed through drill holes made in the lesser trochanter or medial aspect of the femoral neck to allow secure wire fixation without risk of contacting the femoral component.

A cement gun containing two packs of acrylic cement is used. Three or four packs are necessary if a long-stemmed component is used. The cement is inserted into the femoral canal under manual pressure using sterile gloves to prevent cement extrusion from perforated areas. Cement removal from these areas should be meticulous so that bone graft can be applied.

The greater trochanter is reattached using wire tighteners and may be tied over wire mesh, if the bone is osteoporotic. The transverse longitudinal wires are passed through drill holes placed in the greater trochanter and the longitudinal wires are passed proximally through the glutei just superior to the trochanter. Square knots are made and the vastus lateralis is reattached to the ridge.

Occasionally, intraoperative fracture may occur because of the compromised nature of the femoral bone stock and circlage wires or a long-stemmed prosthesis can be used to gain adequate control of the fracture fragments. Bone grafting should be done at the fracture site and at any perforation in the femoral cortex.

If there is little trabecular bone available for adequate cement interdigitation, a cementless femoral device may be used. Porous coated implants may be used and should almost completely fill the femoral canal to permit the porous surface to be contiguous with the cortex. Autogenous and allogeneic bone graft fills the space unoccupied by the component. The implant should be press fitted securely to facilitate bone ingrowth. However, in cases of severe bone loss, cementless fixation may be the only viable option, because long-term studies on cemented revision arthroplasties have shown decreased implant longevity when compared with that obtained after primary total hip arthroplasty.[7,33,41] Long-term data on this method is unavailable.

In Type I cement-prosthesis failure with minimal cortical wall bone loss, the prosthesis could be implanted using either cemented or uncemented techniques (Fig. 28–4). If cementless fixation is chosen, bone grafting is usually necessary. In Type II femoral component failure (lateral wall deficiency), a long-stemmed cementless prosthesis can be reinserted with bone graft placed on the lateral aspect to cover the defect. In Type III failure (posteromedial wall deficiency), the cementless porous ingrowth prosthesis should be inserted with bone graft placed at the site of deficient bone. A calcar replacing prosthesis can be used in the elderly patient with limited activity. In Type IV failure (complete proximal femoral shaft deficiency), a porous ingrowth prosthesis can be used with a proximal allograft. Autogenous cancellous bone graft may augment the reconstruction especially in the young patient who will also require protective weight-bearing for 6 to 12 months. In an elderly patient, the proximal allograft can be cemented to the prosthesis as a separate step prior to inserting the distal end into the intramedullary canal.

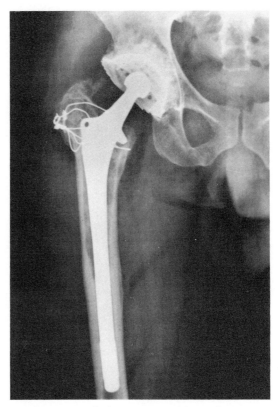

Fig. 28–4. Revision of a loose cemented femoral component using an uncemented prosthetic design.

The treatment of femoral shaft fractures which occur after total hip replacement may vary depending on the location of the fracture and may not always require femoral component revision. Oblique fractures distal to the femoral stem usually heal with traction followed by cast bracing. Serial radiographs should be obtained to assess adequacy of reduction. Unstable fractures at the tip of the femoral stem may be treated by traction and cast bracing if the bone fragments are aligned and contiguous. The patient, however, must be healthy enough to permit long-term bedrest. If the patient's bone stock is adequate, open reduction and internal fixation by plating and grafting of the fracture is possible, but obtaining cortical screw fixation may be difficult. This particular fracture may more predictably heal by converting the femoral component to a long-stemmed prosthesis that extends beyond the fracture a distance 3 times the diameter of the femoral canal. Bone grafting is done at the fracture site (Fig. 28–5). This fixation provides optimum stability and enables the patient to ambulate quickly. If plating is required, carbide or diamond-tipped drills may be necessary to perforate the cement and screws should be placed obliquely to avoid contact with the component's metal surface so that stress risers are eliminated. Comminuted fractures of the

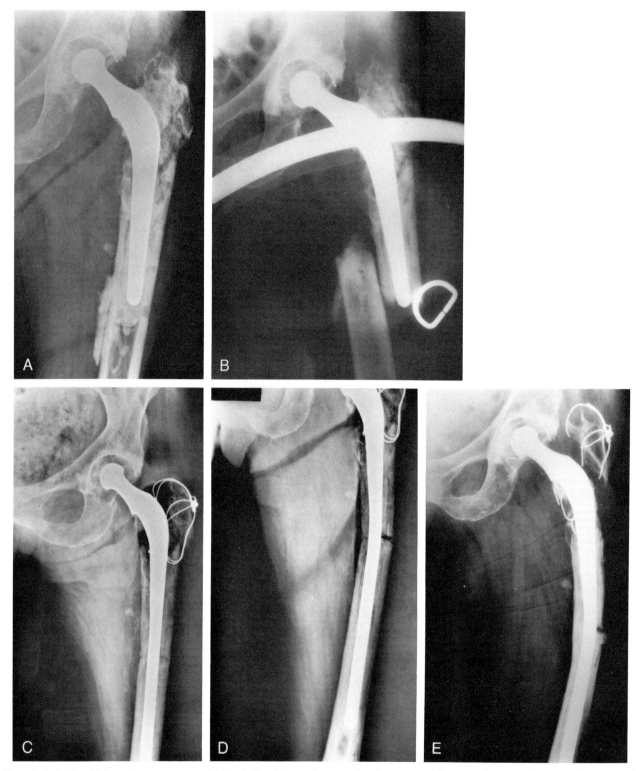

FIG. 28–5. **A.** Total hip replacement was performed after failure of open reduction, internal fixation of intertrochanteric fracture with compression screw, and side plate. Note screwholes. **B.** Fracture occurred at tip of the prosthesis at screw hole site. Traction was inadequate. **C.** Long-stem prosthesis was used to reduce the fracture, but a bone graft was not placed at the fracture site. **D.** Delayed union of fracture with bending of prosthesis at the fracture site. **E.** The fracture healed with bent femoral stem. All fractures should be bone-grafted.

proximal femur should be treated with long-stemmed femoral components, circlage wiring, and bone grafting, provided bone stock is sufficient to allow secure fixation.

Uncemented Femoral Component Revision

The revision of well fixed porous coated or uncemented femoral components may pose the most significant revision challenge. Causes for revision of well fixed cementless implants are: (1) Persistent thigh pain caused by loosening and possible fibrous union of the femoral component to the surrounding trabecular bone. (2) Femoral component malalignment with associated dislocation. (3) Infection. (4) Component breakage because of failure of proximal bone incorporation.

The revision technique involves exposure of the proximal stem, so that flexible osteotomes can disrupt the prosthesis-bone interface. Rigid osteotomes should not be used during this stage to minimize the risk of cortical fracture. Most current prostheses have a porous surface only at the proximal end to facilitate stem removal with standard extraction devices after disruption of the interface. An extraction device alone usually suffices in removing the femoral component if it is united firmly to bone by fibrous tissue. Rarely, a large window is required on the anterior aspect of the femur to allow rotary burrs and flexible osteotomes to further disrupt the prosthesis-bone interface. Where the prosthesis is completely covered with a porous surface, it may be necessary to remove the entire anterior cortex. The anterior cortex is then replaced and fixed by multiple circlage wires after a new implant is inserted. Cementless revision usually involves more blood loss than cemented techniques because of the exposed nature of the underlying bone surfaces. An appropriate amount of blood should be available.

Patients with persistent thigh ache after initial cementless total hip arthroplasty may not wish to receive an uncemented revision prosthesis (Fig. 28–6). A new prosthesis may be cemented into place provided there is good corticocancellous bone stock.

Postoperative Management

Continuous suction drains are used for 24 hours and bed rest is maintained for two days with the operated leg held in abduction by balanced suspension slings. Dangling, standing, and ambulation are usually done on the second postoperative day de-

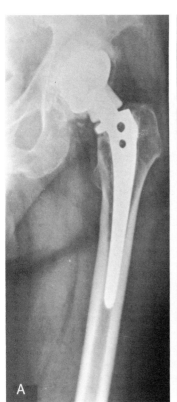
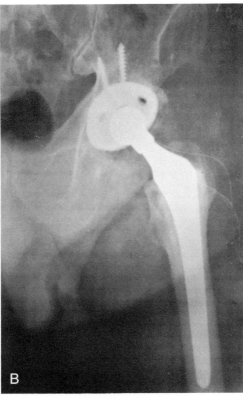

FIG. 28–6. **A.** A loose cementless total hip prosthesis. (Note complete radiolucency around the femoral component.) Also, the acetabular cup is too vertical. **B.** New femoral component was cemented. Acetabular cup was placed more horizontally using a cementless design. This hybrid technique has grown popular recently.

pending on the stability of the reconstruction and the degree of muscle tension on the trochanteric repair. The patient usually stands on the first postoperative day with a tilt table. The patient initially ambulates with a walker and progresses to crutches. One-third to one-half body weight is allowed on the limb for the first two months in order to protect the trochanteric osteotomy. The patient increases weight-bearing over the following 2 months with a cane. The time of protected weight-bearing may be prolonged if bone loss is severe or if the trochanteric reconstruction is tenuous. An abduction splint may be required to protect the repair.

Results

Complications following revision arthroplasty are more frequent than those following primary total hip replacement.[15,17,19] Mortality can be as high as 2% to 3%. Early results of revision arthroplasty may be nearly as good as for primary total hip replacement.[32,57] However, other reports have shown that the failure rate following revision arthroplasty is higher than that following primary total hip replacement. In a study of over 100 patients who underwent revision hip arthroplasty and were followed for an average of 3.4 years, 60% of the hips were rated good or excellent; 23% were fair; 17% were poor.[40] Poor results were caused by deep infection, mechanical failure, and recurrent dislocation. Complications included infection (3.6%), trochanteric problems (13%), mechanical failure (14%), and progressive radiolucencies (26%). It was concluded that the result of revision total hip replacement was comparable to that of original arthroplasty.

The original group of revisions were re-evaluated later and the mechanical rate of failure increased from 14 to 16% and the infection rate rose from 3.6 to 5.5%.[41] With an average followup of 8.1 years, there was a steady increase in mechanical failure to 29%.[41] In the total group of 99 revised hips, 63% had good or excellent results and 7% had a fair result. Eleven hips also were noted to have progressive radiolucency (7 were rated good and 4 fair). Many of these revision total hip replacements were performed before recent advances in materials, technique, and instrumentation. These results deteriorated over time with a mechanical failure rate associated with poor bone quality and inadequate anatomical reconstruction.[7]

In another review of 67 revised total hip replace-

ments followed for an average of 2.5 years, Amstutz, et al., reported an infection rate of 1.5% with a trochanteric complication rate of 7.6%; dislocation or subluxation rate of 21%, and a 7.5% incidence of peroneal nerve palsy. The mechanical failure rate was 9% and progressive radiolucencies were found in 43% of the femoral components and 61% of the acetabular components. The authors felt that the results were poorer than those for index total hip replacement.[1]

Between 1969 and 1978, 206 revision total hip arthroplasties were performed at the Mayo Clinic and the patients were followed for an average of 4 years.[33] The infection rate was 2%, dislocation was found in 12%. The incidence of femoral shaft fracture was 11% (mechanical failure rate was 18%) and a second revision was required in 8% of the patients. Thus, they concluded that the quality of results after an uncomplicated revision arthroplasty was similar to that after primary total hip replacement but serious complications were more frequently encountered, which precluded a successful result.

The initial quality of an uncomplicated revision of a total hip replacement compares favorably with that of a primary total hip replacement. However, the decreased durability of the result has led many surgeons to use cementless systems for revision arthroplasty. Data on revision total hip arthroplasty using cementless techniques are short-term. Lord presented data on 284 revisions of aseptic total hip arthroplasty failures, 213 of which involved cemented implant failures.[34] He obtained a satisfactory result in 70% of the patients reviewed after 5 years. Biologic fixation by bone ingrowth may only be expected under certain conditions such as viable decorticated bone, a tight mechanical fit, and a well designed corrugated implant surface. Bone stock may be preserved but complications appeared no different than in the series of cemented revision arthroplasties, with a 3.3% infection and a 7% dislocation rate. The greater trochanteric fracture rate was 7.5% with a 6.6% rate of femoral shaft fracture. However, it was felt that reconstruction of a failed hip replacement with deficient bone stock could be best achieved by a cementless device and bone graft.[34]

Hedley, et al., reviewed 82 revision arthroplasties performed using noncemented components. Four initial cases used cementless fixation of the femoral component. Frequently custom-designed prostheses were required to assure good intramedullary fit of the prosthesis. Structural bone grafts were used in 30 cases for substantial bone defects. With a 1-year minimum clinical followup, two hips required reoperation for femoral component loosening and excessive leg lengthening. There were 4 dislocations, 1 nerve palsy, and no infections. There was radiographic evidence of symptomatic femoral component toggle; 56 hips were rated clinically excellent or good, 3 hips were fair, and 3 were considered poor, with the cause being symptomatic loosening or femoral component subsidence of up to 5 mm.[30]

Engh, et al., followed 160 revision arthroplasties using cementless fixation of the femoral component for a mean of 4.4 years and felt that success following this procedure depended on the design of the component, surgical technique, and available bone stock.[21] Currently available cementless femoral components have a porous surface only at the proximal end rather than the entire surface to facilitate future device extraction. They examined the radiographic results of the femoral component and only 5 of 127 femoral components (3.9%) met their criteria for fixation failure, which were subsidence and a complete, widening area of radiolucency around the component. Only 1 component with a press fit design failed to achieve stable fixation. If a press fit was not obtained at the time of initial arthroplasty, a 16.7% incidence of radiographic instability was noted. Deep infection occurred in only 1 case. However, nonunion occurred in 10.4% of the trochanteric osteotomies. Patient satisfaction appeared directly related to the stability of the femoral implant. Good initial implant fixation at the isthmus of the femoral canal and evidence of definite migration of the femoral component was only 4% compared with 13% and 36% in other series.[7,14] A good initial press fit correlated with an excellent result with thigh pain being directly related to the success of the femoral component fit.[21]

Gustilo presented a series of 57 hips with an average followup period of 2.8 years. The preoperative Harris hip score improved from 45 to 82 with a 4% dislocation rate, 4% infection, and a 4% revision rate for a loose femoral component. Two years after surgery, 83% of the patients had no pain, 70% had no limp, and 73% used no support. Overall it was felt that the results of total hip arthroplasty with cementless fixation are at least comparable, if not, superior to the use of cemented devices.[25]

Harris reported 71% good and excellent results in 60 patients who were treated with Harris-Galante prostheses for failed, nonseptic, cemented total hip arthroplasties at a minimum followup time of 1 year. Only 1 femoral component that was asymptomatic subsided and 23 hips were followed for more than 2 years.[28]

Long-term results using cementless techniques need to be published and a philosophy of revision using a hybrid cementing technique has evolved (cemented femoral component, noncemented acetabular component). The surgeon may opt for cementless fixation for both femoral and acetabular components in a young patient with adequate bone stock who presents the risk of future mechanical failure because of youth and high activity level. In a population greater than 70 years of age, both components may be cemented if there is excellent bone stock. Long-term clinical results with the hybrid cementing technique are too scant to form specific recommendations. If bone quality is poor, a calcar replacement or cementless prosthetic design with autogenous or allogeneic bone graft may be the only option on the femoral side.

Revision total hip arthroplasty must be considered one of the most challenging operations on the hip joint. The surgeon must plan every operative detail preoperatively and have adequate equipment at his disposal to perform a competent, durable arthroplasty. Clinical results are related to available bone stock, the condition of the surrounding musculature, and the number of previous revision arthroplasties. It is the hope that further advances in technique and design will allow revision arthroplasty to more predictably approach that of primary total hip replacement.

References

1. Amstutz HC, Ma SM, Jinnah RH, Mai L: Revision of aseptic loose total hip arthroplasties. Clin Orthop 170:21, 1982.
2. Amstutz HC, Maki S: Complications of trochanteric osteotomy in total hip replacement. J Bone Joint Surg, 60A:214, 1978.
3. Amstutz HC, et al.: Loosening of total hip components: cause and prevention. *In* The Hip: Proceedings of the Fourth Open Scientific Meeting of the Hip Society. St. Louis, Mosby, 1976.
4. Andriacchi TP, et al.: A stress analysis of the femoral stem in total hip prostheses. J Bone Joint Surg, 58A:618, 1976.
5. Beckenbaugh RD, Ilstrup DM: Total hip arthroplasty. J Bone Joint Surg, 60A:306, 1978.
6. Callaghan JJ, Dysart SH, Savory CG: The uncemented porous-coated anatomic total hip prosthesis. J Bone Joint Surg, 70A:337, 1988.
7. Callaghan JJ, et al.: Results of revision for mechanical failure after cemented total hip replacement. J Bone Joint Surg, 67:1074, 1985.
8. Carlsson AS, Gentz CF, Stenport J: Fracture of the femoral prosthesis in total hip replacement according to Charnley. Acta Orthop Scand, 48:650, 1970.
9. Charnley J: Fracture of femoral prostheses in total hip replacement. Clin Orthop 111:105, 1975.
10. Charnley J: Low Friction Arthroplasty of The Hip. New York, Springer-Verlag, 1979.

11. CHARNLEY J, CUPIC Z: The nine and ten year results of the low friction arthroplasty of the hip. Clin Orthop, 95:9, 1973.

12. CHARNLEY J, CUPIC Z: Etiology and incidence of dislocation in Charnley low friction arthroplasty. Centre for Hip Surgery, Wrightington Hospital, Internal Publication, No. 46, 1974.

13. COLLIS D: Femoral stem failure in total hip replacement. J Bone Joint Surg, 59A:1033, 1977.

14. COLVILLE J, RAUNIO P: Charnley low friction arthroplasties of the hip in rheumatoid arthritis. J Bone Joint Surg, 60B:498, 1978.

15. DUPONT JA, CHARNLEY J: Low friction arthroplasty of the hip for failure of previous operations. J Bone Joint Surg, 54B:77, 1972.

16. EFTEKHAR NS: Dislocation and instability complicating low friction arthroplasty of the hip joint. Clin Orthop, 121:120, 1976.

17. EFTEKHAR NS: Replacement of failed total hip prostheses in the absence of infection: low friction arthroplasty technique. *In* The Hip: Proceedings of the Fourth Open Scientific Meeting of The Hip Society. St. Louis, Mosby, 1976.

18. EFTEKHAR NS: Mechanical failure in low friction arthroplasty. Instr Course Lec, 24:230, 1977.

19. EFTEKHAR NS, et al.: Revision arthroplasty using Charnley low friction arthroplasty technique. Clin Orthop, 95:48, 1973.

20. ENGH CA: Hip arthroplasty with a Moore prosthesis with porous-coating: a five year study. Clin Orthop, 176:52, 1983.

21. ENGH CA, GLASSMAN AH, GRIFFIN WL, MAYER JG: Results of cementless revision for failed cemented total hip arthroplasty. Clin Orthop, 235:91, 1988.

22. EVANS EM, et al.: Metal sensitivity as a cause of bone necrosis and loosening of the prosthesis in total joint replacement. J Bone Joint Surg, 56B:626, 1974.

23. GALANTE JO, ROSTOKER W, DOYLE JM: Failed femoral stems in total hip prostheses. J Bone Joint Surg, 57A:230, 1975.

24. GLASSMAN AH, ENGH CA, BOBYN JD: A technique of extensive exposure for total hip arthroplasty. J Arthroplasty, 2:11, 1987.

25. GUSTILO RB, PASTERNAK HS: Revision total hip arthroplasty with titanium ingrowth prosthesis and bone grafting for failed cemented femoral component loosening. Clin Orthop, 235:111, 1988.

26. GRIFFITH MJ, et al.: Eight year results of Charnley arthroplasties of the hip with special reference to the behaviour of cement. Clin Orthop, 137:24, 1978.

27. HARRIS WH: Loosening in The Hip: Proceedings of the Sixth Open Scientific Meeting of the Hip Society. St. Louis, Mosby, p. 161, 1978.

28. HARRIS WH, URUSHELL RJ, GALANTE JO: Results of cementless revisions of total hip arthroplasties using the Harris-Galante prosthesis. Clin Orthop, 235:120, 1988.

29. HARRIS WH, et al.: Extensive localized bone resorption in the femur following total hip replacement. J Bone Joint Surg, 58A:612, 1976.

30. HEDLEY AK, GRUEN TA, RUOFF DP: Revision of failed total hip arthroplasties with uncemented porous-coated anatomic components. Clin Orthop, 235:75, 1988.

31. HOOTNICK DR, BIERBAUM BE: Total hip replacement for failed femoral endoprostheses. Orthop Rev, 9:97, 1980.

32. JONES JM: Revisional total hip replacement for failed ring arthroplasty. J Bone Joint Surg, 61A:1029, 1979.

33. KAVANAUGH BF, ILSTRUP PM, FITZGERALD RH: Revision total hip arthroplasty. J Bone Joint Surg, 67A:517, 1985.

34. LORD G, MAROTTE HJ, GUILLAMON JL, BLANCHARD JP: Cementless revisions of failed aseptic cemented and cementless total hip arthroplasties: 284 cases. Clin Orthop, 235:67, 1988.

35. MARMOR L: Femoral loosening in total hip replacement. Clin Orthop, 121:116, 1976.

36. MCBEATH AA, FOLTZ RN: Femoral component loosening after total hip replacement. Clin Orthop, 141:66, 1979.

37. MCNIECE GM, AMSTUTZ HC: Stresses in prosthesis stems and supporting acrylic: a finite element study of hip replacement. Transactions of the Twenty-Second Annual Meeting of the Orthopaedic Research Society. 1976.

38. MILLER J, et al.: Pathophysiology of loosening of femoral components in total hip arthroplasty. *In* The Hip: Proceedings of the Sixth Open Scientific Meeting of The Hip Society. St. Louis, Mosby, 1978.

39. PELLICCI PM, SALVATI EA, ROBINSON HJ: Mechanical failures in total hip replacement requiring reoperation. J Bone Joint Surg, 61A:28, 1979.

40. PELLICCI PM, WILSON PD, SLEDGE CB: Results of revision total hip replacement. *In* The Hip. Proceedings of the Ninth Open Scientific Meeting of The Hip Society. St. Louis, Mosby, 1981.

41. PELLICCI PM, et al.: Long term results of revision total hip replacement: a follow-up report. J Bone Joint Surg, 67A:513, 1985.

42. RECKLING FW, ASHER MA, DILLON WL: A longitudinal study of the radiolucent line at the bone cement interface following total joint replacement procedures. J Bone Joint Surg, 59A:355, 1977.

43. RIEDL K, REICHELT A: Repeated operations after total arthroplasty of the hip joint *In* Aschwend N, Debrunner HV (eds.): Total Hip Prosthesis. Baltimore, Williams & Wilkins, 1976.

44. RITTER MA: Dislocation and subluxation of the total hip replacement. Clin Orthop, 121:92, 1976.

45. ROBINSON RP, ROBINSON HJ, SALVATI EA: Comparison of the trans trochanteric and posterior approach for total hip replacement. Clin Orthop, 147:143, 1980.

46. SALVATI EA, et al.: Subtraction technique in arthrography for loosening of total hip replacement fixed with radiopaque cement. Clin Orthop, 101:105, 1974.

47. SALVATI EA, et al.: Radiology of total hip replacements. Clin Orthop, 121:74, 1976.

48. SALVATI EA, WILSON PD: Long-term results of femoral head replacement. J Bone Joint Surg, 55A:516, 1973.

49. SARMIENTO A, GERARD FM: Total hip arthroplasty for failed endoprostheses. Clin Orthop, 137:112, 1978.

50. SIMON SR, et al.: Friction of total hip prostheses and its relationship to loosening. J Bone Joint Surg, 57A:226, 1975.

51. STAUFFER RN: Ten-year follow-up study of total hip replacement. J Bone Joint Surg, 64A:983, 1982.

52. STUHMER G, WEBER BG, MATHYS R: New set of instruments for the removal of implant and bone cement in the replacement of hip prostheses. *In* Gschwend N, Debrunner HV (eds.): Total Hip Prosthesis. Baltimore, Williams & Wilkins, 1976.

53. SUTHERLAND CJ, WILDE AH, BORDEN LS, MARKS LE: A ten-year follow-up of one hundred consecutive Muller curved-stem total hip replacement arthroplastie. J Bone Joint Surg, 64A:970, 1982.

54. VOLZ RG, BROWN FW: The painful migrated united greater trochanter in total hip replacement. J Bone Joint Surg, 59A:109, 1977.

55. WEBER FA, CHARNLEY J: A radiological study of fractures of acrylic cement in relation to the stem of a femoral head prosthesis. J Bone Joint Surg, 57B:297, 1975.

56. WILSON JN, SCALES JT: Loosening of total hip replacements with cement fixation. Clin Orthop, 72:145, 1970.

57. WILSON PD, et al.: Total prosthetic replacement of the hip. J Clin Orthop, 23, 1978.

CHAPTER TWENTY-NINE

Revision of Fractured Femoral Stem Components

RUSSELL E. WINDSOR
JOHN J. CALLAGHAN
PAUL M. PELLICCI
EDUARDO A. SALVATI

Although fracture of the femoral component of a total hip replacement is an uncommon mode of mechanical failure, when it does occur, symptoms may be dramatic. In addition, it presents the surgeon with one of the more challenging problems in surgical revision of total hip arthroplasty in general. This chapter reviews the problem of femoral stem fracture, evaluates the mechanism of stem failure, and provides long-term followup of The Hospital for Special Surgery experience in revision arthroplasty for fractured femoral components. The techniques of revision also will be presented to enable the surgeon to handle this difficult problem.

Historical Review

The literature suggests that the incidence of femoral stem fractures varies according to the material, device used, and the patient population. Charnley[6] estimated an incidence of 0.23% in a review of his first 6,500 total hip arthroplasties. Carlsson reported a 0.67% incidence of stem fracture in Charnley prostheses inserted in Malmo, Sweden.[4] More recently Wroblewski updated the incidence of stem fracture to be 1.15% in the Charnley "flat back" prosthesis performed at Wrightington, England.[18] Martens reported an alarming 11% incidence of stem fracture in the early designs of the Charnley and Mueller prostheses.[13] In the largest series of fractured femoral components reported to date (58 stems), other than the Wrightington experience (120 stems), Chao estimated the fracture incidence in all prostheses performed at the Mayo Clinic to be 0.6%.[5]

Weight appears to be an important variable when considering the population at risk for stem fail-ure.[14] The average patient weight in the series reported by Galante was 90 kilograms.[10] Collis estimated that if only those patients taller than 1.8 m and heavier than 91 kg were considered, the incidence of stem fracture would be 33% in his series.[7] In Charnley's experience a 6% incidence of fracture was calculated for patients weighing more than 88 kg.[6] The patients who present with stem fractures at The Hospital for Special Surgery are heavier and taller on average when compared to the population with femoral component loosening.[3] Clinical factors other than body habitus that have been mentioned as contributing to stem fracture include high activity level, limitation of hip motion, and bilateral hip disease.[8]

Roentgenographic evaluation of cases of femoral component fracture demonstrates loosening, lack of support at the level of the calcar femorale, and varus positioning as the most common findings. Charnley[6] reported the incidence of subsidence before stem fracture to be 40% and Wroblewski[18] in the later followup series estimated a 77% subsidence rate. Chao,[5] however, did not find subsidence to be a problem with stem fracture in the Mayo Clinic study.

Lack of support at the level of the calcar femorale, either by proximal loosening or resorption of bone causing Gruen's cantilever bending mode of failure,[11] has been implicated in most large series. The condition puts the femoral component especially at risk when the distal aspect of the stem is well fixed in the cement mantle. In this way cantilever bending would be the sole cause for fatigue fracture in the proximal and middle third of the component. Chao reported 62% proximal loosening in the femur and 8% proximal bone loss without loosening in the 37 stems that were serially followed before fracture.[5]

Varus positioning has been implicated in the initial Charnley series and in the other smaller series of stem fractures. Andriacchi, et al., demonstrated that a varus positioning combined with loss of proximal cement support and reabsorption of the calcar femorale produced stem stresses of a magnitude that, if applied cyclically over a period of time, could conceivably produce the types of fatigue failure observed clinically.[1] In Wroblewski's[18] series 56% of the stems were initially placed in varus and Chao[5] cited a 42% incidence of varus stem alignment in the Mayo Clinic series.

Although one may be led to believe that the present use of super alloys and bioingrowth prostheses will make stem fracture a problem of the past, some recent reports suggest that this might not be the case. The fracture of the forged vitallium prosthesis has been reported,[4] and Lord[12] reported a 0.27% incidence of stem fracture with his cementless madreporic prosthesis. Revising the retained distal fragment in an ingrowth prosthesis may pose an extreme surgical challenge, which may require extensive femoral fenestrations in these particular cases.

Metallurgic Considerations

Femoral component fracture occurs by the mechanism of fatigue failure. All structures, if repetitively stressed at a sufficiently high level for a certain number of cycles, will ultimately fail by this mechanism. Fatigue failure has three stages: (1) initial fatigue damage leading to crack initiation; (2) crack propagation until the remaining uncracked cross section becomes too weak to sustain the loads that are imposed; and (3) final sudden fracture of the remaining intact cross section. This failure usually begins at the anterolateral corner of the femoral stem in the cross-sectional direction and in the middle third of the stem in the longitudinal direction because the tensile stresses placed on a femoral component are highest and directed longitudinally and posteriorly at these areas (Figs. 29–1, 29–2). When evaluating the fractured stem at the fracture site, tide marks radiate away from the site of crack initiation which is usually located at the anterolateral corner of the femoral stem cross section. These "clamshell-like" or "conchoidal" arrest marks indicate fatigue failure.[8] In some instances, especially with the trapezoidal-28 (T-28) fractured stems retrieved at The Hospital for Special Surgery, medial secondary cracks were present suggesting that tensile stresses are produced and maintained

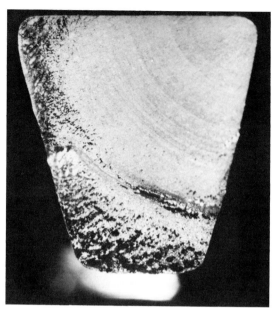

Fig. 29–1. Cross-sectional view of T-28 prosthesis at the site of fracture. Clamshell-like markings extend in a radial configuration from the site of crack initiation (upper right corner of prosthesis) at the anterolateral corner of the prosthesis.

on the medial surface as well. The stresses on this medial surface are thought to be primarily compressive, however, we hypothesize that because of the trapezoidal cross section of this particular prosthesis, the residual tensile stresses may result from compressive yielding of the material in this region. This may be the reason for these medial cracks.[2]

The mechanical properties of the implant materials available in the 1970s and in the early 1980s also must be considered when discussing femoral component failure. All the prostheses retrieved at The Hospital for Special Surgery and all other prostheses retrieved and reported in the literature, except for one forged vitallium stem were made of casts from cobalt or annealed stainless steel. The use of the newer alloys by the orthopedic industry in manufacturing prostheses should significantly decrease but probably not eliminate the problem of femoral component failure of cemented prostheses.[9] (Table 29–1).

Finally, metallurgic defects can contribute to stem fracture. These defects can cause fatigue crack initiation. The most common defect observed with annealed 316 stainless steel is large course crystals in the normally very fine-grained structure. Other defects observed in annealed stainless steel are large inclusion bodies and inclusion stingers. The most common defect reported in cast chromium cobalt alloys has been microporosity. These pores can be generated in castings when the molten metal solidifies, resulting in volume reduction (shrinkage porosity), or when dissolved gas is ex-

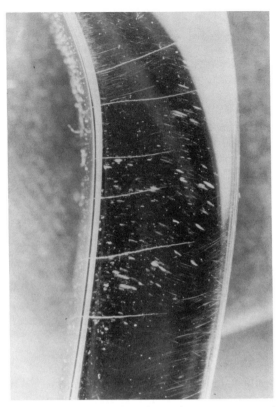

Fɪɢ. **29–2.** Secondary medial cracks on the same T-28 prosthesis as shown in Figure 29–1.

pulsed (gas porosity). Carbide segregation, undissolved master alloy, and nonmetallic inclusions are other defects reported with cast cobalt-chromium alloys.[8]

The Hospital For Special Surgery Experience

The first revision for fracture of a femoral component at The Hospital for Special Surgery was performed in April, 1974, 15 months after the prosthesis had been inserted. Between that time and April,

1984, 71 patients presented with 72 fractured femoral stems at that institution. Long-term clinical and roentgenographic evaluation was performed on 53 fracture stems revised from 1974 to 1982. These years were selected to coincide with two previously reported revision study groups from our institution.[3,16] These two previous reports involved revisions done before 1979, and the second report also studied revisions done between 1979 and 1982. This allowed us to compare the results of revision for fracture of the femoral component to revision surgery for other forms of mechanical failure, mainly, loosening.

Demographic Data

Table 29–2 illustrates the female to male ratio, age at primary and revision arthroplasty, longevity of the stem, height, weight, and condition of the contralateral hip, ipsilateral knee, and low back in the fractured stem patient population. In addition, these figures are separately listed for the three most commonly revised fractured femoral stems: the T-28, Mueller, and Charnley.

There was a large male to female ratio (50:22) when evaluating the data for all patients, and this was also true for the three separately evaluated groups of patients. The Mueller stem population had the highest male to female ratio, 17:4. This finding of male predominance is distinctly different than the ratios seen for mechanical failure for other reasons, that is, loosening. The male to female ratio obtained by combining the Pellicci and Callaghan study was 75:123 (Table 29–3). The average age of fractured stem revision was 62 years. The average age of the T-28 group was younger (57) than those of the fractured Mueller and Charnley groups (66 and 67, respectively). The fractured T-28 prostheses were placed in younger patients, with an average age of 50 compared to the Mueller and Charnley patients, whose average age was 59. The average age

TABLE **29–1.** *Mechanical Properties of Implant Materials*

Type of Alloy	Yield Strength ($\times 10^2$ MPa)	Fatigue Strength ($\times 10^2$ MPa)
Annealed 316 stainless steel[9]	2.07	1.52
Cast Co-Cr-Mo alloy[9]	5.18	2.55
Cold worked 316 stainless steel	6.90	2.90
Forged Co-Cr-Mo alloy	8.98	7.59
Hot isostatic pressed Co-Cr-Mo-alloy	8.40	7.65
Titanium alloy (Ti6A14V)	8.63	5.52
Hot forged MP 35 N alloy	9.65	6.21
Cold worked MP 35N alloy	15.88	8.98

TABLE 29–2. Demographic Data on Patients Revised for Fracture of the Femoral Component

	Number Prostheses	Number HBS Primary	Female and Male	Age at Revision	Age at Primary	Longevity Of Stem In Years	Height (cm)	Weight (kg)	Prosthesis In Patients Less Than 60 kg	Contralateral Hip Prosthesis	Contralateral Hip Disease	Significant Back Pain	Significant Knee Pain
All prostheses	72	55	22:50	62.2 (26–84)	55.5 (22–77)	6.8 (1.2–11)	169 (140–192)	81.5 (48–120)	7	31	13	11	6
T-28	29	22	9:20	57 (26–83)	50.1 (23–77)	6.9 (3–10)	167.5 (140–192)	78.8 (48–116)	5	13	3		
Mueller	21	18	4:17	66 (26–78)	59.4 (22–76)	6.6 (1.2–11)	171.7 (140–812)	84.2 (49–115)	1	7	5		
Charnley	16	13	6:10	67.3 (45–83)	59.8 (40–76)	7.6 (3–10)	170 (150–180)	83.9 (60–120)	0	11	2		

at revision was actually older for the fractured stem patients (62) when compared to other patients with different modes of mechanical failure (59). This is especially apparent for Mueller's and Charnley's populations (average age 66 and 67, respectively).

Patients with fractured stems were taller on average (169 cm) compared to other patients with mechanical failure (165 cm). This was more apparent in the Charnley and Mueller groups in which the average height was 172 and 170 cm respectively. The patients in the fracture stem group also were heavier (average weight 81.5 kg) compared to patients with other forms of failure (average 72.5 kg). However, 7 prostheses fractured in patients weighing less than 60 kg. Five of these fractures involved a T-28 stem, one occurred in a Mueller prosthesis, and one developed in a custom-designed femoral stem. Sixteen patients gained more than 5 kg while their prostheses were in place (5 to 23 kg) and 5 patients lost more than 5 kg (5 to 21 kg).

Thirty-one patients had a contralateral total hip replacement (43%); the percentage was highest with the Charnley prosthesis (69%). The percentage of patients with contralateral arthroplasties in the patients that had component failure for other reasons than femoral stem fracture was 28.5%. Contralateral hip disease was present in another 18% of the patients with femoral stem fracture. Significant back pain was present in 11 patients (15%) and significant ipsilateral knee pain was noted in 6 patients (8.2%).

The right femoral component was fractured in 33 cases, the left in 37 and both in 1 case. The diagnosis at the time of the initial arthroplasty was osteoarthritis in 52 patients, aseptic necrosis in 9, trauma in 4, rheumatoid arthritis in 3, congenital hip dislocation in 3 and slipped capital femoral epiphysis in 1 patient.

Clinical data concerning the acute versus chronic presentation of symptoms was obtained from the patients' charts or by telephone interview. In addition, the longevity of the initial femoral component was calculated and the patients were grouped by the year the component was implanted (Table 29–4) and the year the component was revised (Table 29–5).

Thirteen patients (18%) admitted to grossly abusing their prostheses. The two most common activities were daily running or playing tennis. One patient had even run a marathon. Three patients had fallen and sustained acute trauma that immediately caused pain; two of these patients fell from a ladder. Thirty-nine patients felt an acute onset of pain while walking or rising from a chair. Eleven pa-

TABLE 29–3. *Demographic Data on Patients Revised for Mechanical Failure Other Than Fracture of the Femoral Component*

	Hips	Age (Years)	Height (cm)	Weight (kg)	Bilateral	Sex (female-male)
Pellicci	96	59.6	—	—		59:35
Callaghan	104	59.3	165	72.5	28.5	64:40
Total	200	59.5				123:75

tients presented after having pain over a 2 to 3 day period. Nineteen patients had more gradual symptoms up to several months and, in fact, one of these was diagnosed only because the patient had an abdominal radiograph for an unrelated problem. Several patients required a high index of suspicion by the clinician and the diagnosis was made only after fluoroscopic examination and spot films of the stem were obtained with the thigh in different positions.

The fractured femoral component population consisted of 29 T-28, 21 Mueller, 16 Charnley, 2 Bechtol, 2 Aufranc, and 2 custom-designed prostheses. The longevity of the stems averaged 6.8 years with the shortest period of implantation 15 months and the longest period 11 years. The longevity of the T-28, Mueller, and Charnley prostheses were 6.9, 6.6, and 7.6 years, respectively. Only 1 stem fractured less than 2 years after implantation, 14 between 2 and 5 years, and 57 greater than 5 years after implantation. The year of implantation did not affect longevity; however, the majority of the fractured stems were implanted between the years of 1973 and 1975. These were the three years when most of the T-28 prostheses were used at The Hospital for Special Surgery. It is curious to note that 13 of 29 T-28 stem fractures occurred in patients with a diagnosis other than osteoarthritis. This observation may be accounted for by the younger age

of this group of patients at the time of primary revision arthroplasty who most likely developed arthritis from a condition other than idiopathic primary osteoarthritis.

Roentgenographic Evaluation

Roentgenographic measurements were made on all patients using the same variables used by Chao.[5] These variables were:

1. Cement thickness of less than 2 mm at the proximal medial, midmedial, distal medial, proximal lateral, midlateral, and distal lateral levels of the stem-cement complex.
2. Any cement voids of more than 4 mm.
3. Stem position of more than 3° of varus orientation.
4. Cancellous bone beneath the area of attachment at the calcar femorale more than 2 mm thick that was not removed during insertion of the stem.
5. Buildup of cement more than 2 mm in height at the base of the femoral neck.
6. Limb length discrepancy of more than 2 cm.
7. Trochanteric nonunion.
8. Cancellous bone at the greater trochanter that was not removed and replaced with cement.

TABLE 29–4. *Distribution of Fractured Stems By Year Implanted*

Year Inserted	Number of Fractured Stems Implanted Per Year	Average Longevity of Stems Implanted Per Year (months)
1970	1	95
1971	—	—
1972	8	77
1973	15	80
1974	24	82
1975	12	82
1976	4	79
1977	2	49
1978	5	58
1979	—	—
1980	—	—
1981	—	—
1982	1	25

TABLE 29–5. *Distribution of Fractured Femoral Components By Year of Revision*

Year Revised	Number of Revised Components	Fractured Stem Revisions as a Percentage of All Revisions for Mechanical Failure at the Hospital for Special Surgery
1974	1	25
1975	2	22
1976	2	17
1977	4	19
1978	3	20
1979	4	10
1980	14	30
1981	13	28
1982	9	14
1983	10	11
1984	10	Not Full Year

In addition, the following findings were recorded:

1. Complete radiolucencies around the acetabulum.
2. Acetabular wear greater than 1 mm.
3. Calcar resorption greater than 5 mm.
4. Calcar resorption greater than 1 cm.
5. Distance from the neck-stem junction to the fracture site recorded as a percentage of the entire stem length on the 70 prostheses when the fracture was in the stem (two fractures occurred in the neck).

The evaluation of these 13 variables was performed on 68 stems. Prefracture roentgenographs were not adequate to make these measurements in 4 cases.

The 5 most common roentgenographic findings were varus stem positioning (69%), inadequate calcar cancellous bone removal (62%), cement voids (53%), complete acetabular radiolucencies (44%) and calcar resorption (43%) (Table 29–6). Out of the 21 stems placed in valgus or neutral position only 4 had adequate removal of calcar bone. Stem failure occurred in both the proximal and the middle third of the stem (Table 29–7). The T-28 stems seemed to fail in the proximal aspect of the stem and Mueller stems failed more distally than the T-28 stems in the middle third of the component. Charnley prostheses failed in both the proximal and middle third of the stem with the majority present in the middle third. Two T-28 stems failed through the femoral neck and one Mueller stem had a double fracture (mid and distal stem).

In 51 hips, serial films were available to evaluate the mechanism leading to stem failure. Forty-two

TABLE 29–6. *Distribution of Radiographic Variables Present in Patients With Fractured Femoral Components**

Radiographic Findings	Percent Occurrence
Cement defects	
Proximal medial	31
Proximal lateral	9
Mid medial	16
Mid lateral	10
Distal medial	22
Distal lateral	29
Cement voids	53
Stems in varus	69
Trochanteric nonunion	10
Limb length discrepancy	9
Neck cement build-up	35
Calcar cancellous bone not removed	62
Cancellous bone at greater trochanter not removed	26
Complete acetabular radiolucencies	44
Acetabular wear	19
Calcar resorption 5 mm	43
Calcar resorption 10 mm	16

*Only 68 radiographs available.

hips (82%) failed by cantilever bending with initial proximal cement loosening. Four hips (8%) failed by cantilever beam bending without proximal cement loosening, but with loss of proximal cortical bone. Finally, 5 stems (10%) failed by Chao's stem overstress mechanism[5] with no cement loosening or loss of cortical support noted.

Results

Followup radiographs were compared to initial postoperative radiographs to determine acetabular migration and femoral subsidence using the criteria

TABLE 29–7.   *Location of Stem Fracture*

Fracture Distance From Neck-Stem Junction Recorded as Percentage of Entire Stem Length	All Prostheses (%)	T-28 (%)	Mueller (%)	Charnley (%)
10	1.4	—	—	—
10–19	24.6	50	—	5
20–29	17.4	35	5	21
30–39	14.5	11	—	5
40–49	15.9	4	32	21
50–59	14.5	—	21	16
60–69	8.7	—	32	32
70–79	2.9	—	10.5	—
80–89	—	—	—	—
90–100	—	—	—	—

previously described by Callaghan, et al.,[3] (Fig. 29–3). Progressive radiolucencies also were noted from these serial radiographs. Femoral bone quality at the time of revision was considered good or poor by comparing the radiographs taken immediately after primary arthroplasty with those made before revision. The quality of the femoral bone at the time of revision was rated poor if the thickness of either aspect of the cortex as seen on the anteroposterior radiograph had decreased by 50% (compared with the thickness seen immediately after the original arthroplasty) along a 10 cm segment of the femoral stem, or if the thickness of both aspects of the cortex had decreased by this amount along a 5 cm segment. Similarly, if there was a 75% decrease in the thickness of one aspect of the cortex along a 5 cm segment, the rating was poor. Finally, if both aspects together measured less than 4 mm in thickness at a point 1 cm distal to the inferior aspect of the lesser trochanter and this decrease was not

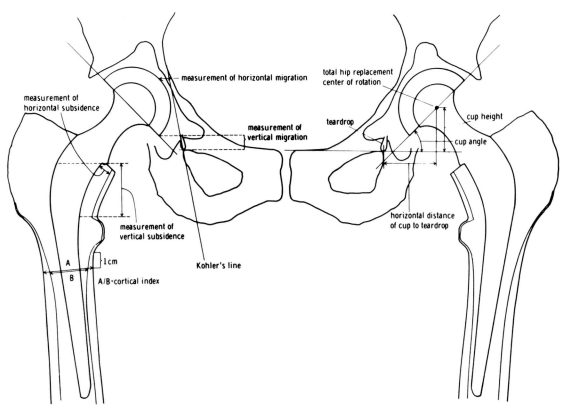

FIG. 29–3. Illustration of the measurements for acetabular migration, femoral subsidence, and cortical index.

caused by local radiologic scalloping of cortex, the bone quality was designated as poor. In addition, the width of the medullary canal and the outside diameter of the femoral shaft were measured separately at a point 1 cm distal to the inferior margin of the lesser trochanter. The cortical index was computed as the ratio of the width of the medullary canal to the outside diameter of the shaft. For example, a small ratio identifies a patient with relatively thick cortical bone in the femoral diaphysis.

We used a rating scale of excellent, good, fair, and poor according to a method described by Pellicci,[15] which considers both radiographic and clinical results. An excellent result is one in which the components are well fixed roentgenographically (nonprogressive radiolucent lines) and the patient is asymptomatic. In a good result the components are well fixed and the patient has mild symptoms that interfere little, if any, with function. In a fair result the patient has no symptoms of loosening, but radiographs show progressive radiolucent lines. Poor results include mechanical failure, infection, and pain that limits function.

Forty-five hips (85%) had good bone quality at the time of revision and 8 hips had bone quality that was considered poor. The average cortical index ratio was 0.62 with only 7 cases greater than 0.7 and 19 cases had a ratio less than 0.6. Hence, on the average, the patients' cortex occupied 38% of the entire diaphyseal diameter. These 2 findings are significantly different from those seen in mechanical failures for other problems. In that review, when bone quality was determined,[3] if femoral stem fractures were excluded, the bone quality was good in 41 hips (40%) and poor in 62 hips (60%). The average cortical index in that study was 0.8 (i.e., the patients' cortical bone occupied only 20% of the entire diaphyseal diameter).

The roentgenographic followup evaluation revealed femoral subsidence in 4 hips (7.5%), acetabular migration in 1 hip (1.8%), progressive femoral radiolucencies in 8 hips (8%) and progressive acetabular radiolucent lines in 3 hips (5.7%). There was nonunion of the greater trochanter in 6 hips (11.3%) with 2 of these hips having a proximal trochanteric migration greater than 1 cm. Five other hips have undergone revision for mechanical failure (9.5%) 3 for femoral loosening and 2 for femoral

fracture (both could have been prevented if intraoperative femoral defects had been bypassed). One fracture occurred 6 weeks after revision at the site of a distal cortical window that was created at the time of revision of the femoral stem fracture to push out the distal stem proximally. The window was replaced but not bypassed at that time. The patient slipped and fractured the femur 6 weeks postoperatively and required a subsequent revision. The second fracture occurred in a patient 2 years after the initial revision when again a lateral perforation was not bypassed. The patient slipped on the ice and sustained a femoral fracture that required revision. One patient had a single nonrecurrent dislocation and one patient had a sciatic nerve palsy, which resolved. There were no infections.

After an average followup of 5.2 years, using the previously mentioned rating scale, excellent results were obtained in 34 hips (64%), good in 10 (19%), fair in 3 (5.7%) and poor in 6 (11.3%). Mechanical failure subsequently occurred in 6 hips (11.3%), 5 of which have been revised (Table 29–8). This can be compared to the average 5 year followup of 194 hips revised for mechanical failures for reasons other than stem fracture (Table 29–9). In those patients results were excellent in 97 (50%) good in 8 (4.1%), fair in 35 (18%) and poor in 54 (27.9%). Subsequent mechanical failure occurred in 45 hips in that group (23.2%), 29 (14.9%) of which required revision. The results of revision for fracture of femoral stems appear significantly better than those seen for other modes of mechanical failure (p < .009 on Kruskal-Wallis, Wilcoxon 2 sample rank sum test).

Technical Considerations

Before embarking on revision of a fractured femoral stem the surgeon must perform an adequate preoperative workup of the patient's hip condition. Sepsis should be ruled out by performing a preoperative aspiration of the hip, preferably, with fluoroscopic assistance so that one is absolutely certain that the specimen has been obtained from the hip joint. The femoral prosthesis head design should be known. This is especially important if the surgeon

TABLE 29–8. *Results of Revision for Femoral Component Fracture*

Hips	Excellent	Good	Fair	Poor	Revision	Mechanical Failure	Follow-up (years)
53	34 (64%)	10 (19%)	3 (5.79%)	6 (11.3%)	5 (9.5%)	6 (11.3%)	5.2 (2–14)

TABLE 29–9.   *Results of Revision for Mechanical Failure Other Than Femoral Component Fracture*

	Hips	Excellent	Good	Fair	Poor	Revision	Mechanical Failure	Follow-up (average in years)
Pellicci	86	37	1	17	31	19	25	8.1
Callaghan	108	60	7	18	23	10	16	3.6
Total	194	97	8	35	54	29	45	5.5
		(50%)	(4.1%)	(18%)	(28%)	(14.9%)	(23.29%)	

is contemplating revising only the femoral component. For example, the Bechtol prosthesis has the same appearance as the Charnley prosthesis but it has a 25 mm head diameter rather than the 22 mm head diameter that is found with the Charnley prosthesis. Thus, a potential mismatch in femoral head component size could occur at the time of surgery and the surgeon must adequately plan to have a prosthesis with the identical head size. During the time of the study of revision arthroplasties done at The Hospital for Special Surgery, modular components were not yet available for implantation. However, at present most modern implant systems have a modular head size that can be placed on the neck of the prosthesis with a Morris taper. These femoral head sizes range from 22 mm to 32 mm to account for various sizes of prostheses that were made over the last 2 decades. One case in the present series did have a preoperative infection in addition to fracture of the femoral stem and a two-stage reimplantation of the hip was performed.

Operative findings were assessed for 53 fracture femoral components that were followed up in this series. All revisions were performed with the patient in a lateral position through a transtrochanteric approach. During extraction of the femoral stem, there were 9 femoral perforations (19%). All but one perforation occurred on the anterior or lateral femoral cortex. After removing the proximal stem and cement, the distal stem was usually found to be well secured by distal cement. This was extracted by making a window distal to the stem in 11 cases (21%), a window proximal to the stem tip in 20 cases (38%), using a Midas Rex extractor from the proximal end of the bone in 21 cases (39%) with the William Harris instruments, and a forceps from the proximal aspect of the femur in 1 case (2%). Even though the Midas Rex equipment was available in the last half of the study, the distal stem could not always be extracted with the William Harris device (about one-fifth of the cases). When using this device the surgeon should first loosen the proximal aspect of the distal cement mantle by using a TU 10 Midas Rex instrument. In addition, precise undercutting of the hole created in the proximal aspect of the distal stem allows the extraction device to engage without fear of its slipping out of the hole. Operative time averaged 4 hours (range 2.5 to 9 hours). Blood loss averaged 1000 ml. The acetabular component was revised for loosening in 9 cases (17%). Long stems were used to bypass defects in 12 cases.

During revision of a fractured femoral stem, it is usually easy to remove the proximal portion of the femoral component because this is usually found to be grossly loose.[17] Frequently, the distal aspect of the stem is securely embedded in acrylic cement. There are numerous ways to extract this compo-

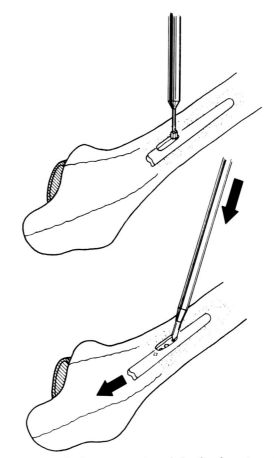

FIG. 29–4. To facilitate extraction of the distal portion of the component, a cortical window is made in the lateral femoral cortex. The stem is driven out of the proximal femur by a thin osteotome or pointed extraction instrument.

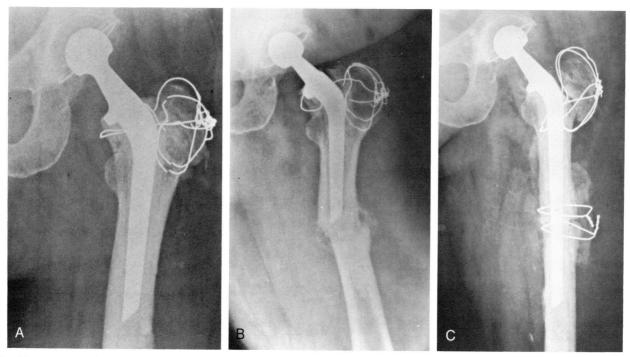

Fɪɢ. 29–5. **A.** Immediate postrevision radiograph with perforation site distal to implant. **B.** Radiograph two years postrevision when the patient fell and fractured the femur through the perforation site. **C.** Femoral revision with long stem and bone graft at the fracture site.

nent. If the femoral shaft is fairly straight and not significantly bowed, then the use of the Midas Rex WH instruments may be satisfactory in extracting the stem. However, it is important to make sure that the surrounding cement mantle in the proximal aspect of the femur should be disrupted as completely as possible using the TU 10 instrument.[17] Only in this way will the surgeon have success in using this instrumentation system for extracting the distal aspect of the stem. It is helpful for the surgeon, when using this instrumentation, to wear an overhead fiberoptic light so that the proximal portion of the component can be better seen. If this instrumentation is unavailable or the femoral shaft is bowed, then one can make a cortical window on the lateral aspect of the femur distal or proximal to the distal tip of the stem (Fig. 29–4). We usually create a cortical window by drilling the margins of a rectangular space approximately one-half cm by 2 cm in dimension. The rectangular shape is outlined by numerous drill holes and then the window is removed after the drill holes are connected by osteotomes, which is done to minimize stress risers. The osteotome may be used to push the stem proximally, and the cement may be removed by using instruments inserted through the window. The reason for placing the cortical window proximal to the stem tip is to enable a standard sized component to be inserted into the femoral

shaft which obviates the need of a long-stemmed component. However, if the surgeon decides that a distal cortical window is most appropriate for extraction, a long-stemmed femoral component must be used so that the stem tip is positioned distal to the cortical window at least twice the distance of the diameter of the femoral shaft. (Fig. 29–5) The cortical window is replaced and if cement is used a rubber glove is placed over it, temporarily, to prevent extrusion of cement during the insertion of the femoral component. Autogenous bone graft or femoral allograft should be used at the site of the cortical window to assist healing. If cementless fixation of a long-stemmed component is chosen, the cortical window should be replaced and autogenous bone graft or allograft should be placed between the prosthesis and bone, and surrounding the cortical window and the femoral cortex. Collis, alternatively, uses an extracting device that is used for fractures that occur in the proximal one-third of the stem. (Fig. 29–6) If there is cortical reaction around the distal aspect of the stem tip, the patient may be at risk of femoral fracture if a standard size stem is replaced into the femoral canal. Therefore the surgeon should opt in this situation to use a long-stemmed prosthesis.

At the time of surgery, the acetabulum is generally tested to ascertain if it is loose. If it is not loose and the polyethylene appears not significantly

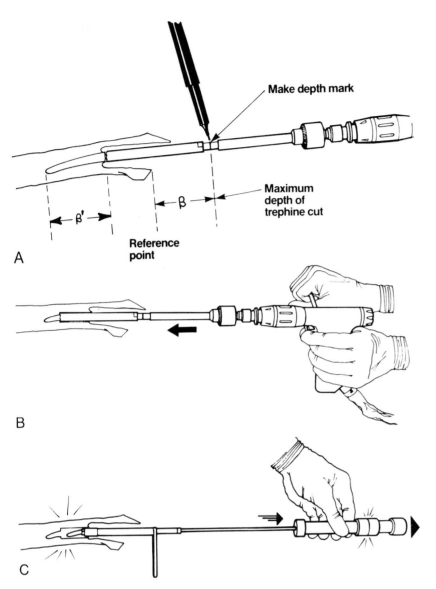

Make depth mark

Maximum
depth of
trephine cut

β

β'

Reference
point

A

B

C

FIG. 29–6. **A.** A trephine is mounted onto a reamer with a size that approximates that of the remaining portion of the femoral stem. **B.** The trephine is advanced to the desired depth. **C.** The implant and trephine are removed using a reverse impact hammer.

worn, then it can remain in place and the femoral component only requires revision. If there is excessive wear on the acetabulum or if it appears grossly loose, then an entire revision of the prosthesis should be performed.

Evaluation of the fractured femoral components that were revised at The Hospital for Special Surgery suggests that the causes of failure are multifactorial. Patients on the average were male, taller, and heavier than those patients who presented to our institution with other modes of mechanical failure, for example, loosening. Contralateral hip disease or hip replacement also was more common in the fractured stem population suggesting that there may be greater weight born on the ipsilateral hip in certain situations of contralateral hip pain or weakness. Roentgenographically, varus position and inadequate cancellous calcar bone removal were frequent findings in the stems that fractured.

Because most specimens are only grossly studied we cannot comment on metallurgic defects seen in the stems by microscopic analysis.

Cantilever bending failure with proximal loosening and distal cement fixation was the predominant mechanism of failure. The secure distal fixation may be accounted for by the thick diaphyseal cortex as noted by the low cortical index seen in these patients (Fig. 29–7). Proximal loosening could be attributed to inadequate cancellous bone removal (62%) acetabular wear debris (circumferential acetabular radiolucencies in 44% and acetabular cup wear in 19%) causing calcar resorption (43%). In addition, the varus position (69%) may cause proximal loosening because of the increased proximal medial loads that this position generates.

The most important operative consideration no matter what method of distal stem extraction is used is to bypass any cortical defects (perforations

FIG. 29–7. **A.** Radiograph of fractured stem previous to revision. Note secure distal fixation. **B.** Seven-year followup radiograph illustrating no lucencies around the femoral component.

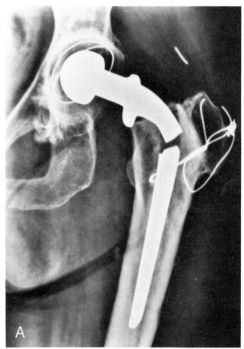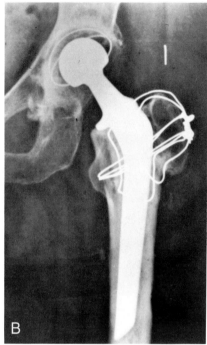

or windows) by 2 or 3 shaft diameters to avoid disastrous postoperative femoral fractures caused by these stress risers. Two of our 6 mechanical failures occurred because this principle was violated.

The long-term results of revision of fractured cemented femoral stem components appear superior to those of cemented revision for other modes of mechanical failure (p < 0.009). We believe that the quality of bone at the time of revision (including a strong diaphyseal cortical support) accounts for this success.

References

1. ANDRIACCHI TP, et al.: A stress analysis of the femoral stem in total hip prostheses. J Bone Joint Surg, 58A:618, 1976.
2. BURSTEIN AH, WRIGHT TM: Neck fractures of femoral prostheses. J Bone Joint Surg, 67A:497, 1985.
3. CALLAGHAN JJ, et al.: Results of revision for mechanical failure after cemented total hip replacement, 1979 to 1982. J Bone Joint Surg, 67A:1074, 1985.
4. CARLSSON AS, GENTZ CF, STENPORT J: Fracture of the femoral prosthesis in total hip replacement according to Charnley. Acta Orthop Scand, 48:650, 1977.
5. CHAO EY, COVENTRY MB: Fracture of the femoral component after total hip replacement. J Bone Joint Surg, 63A:1078, 1981.
6. CHARNLEY J: Fracture of femoral prostheses in total hip replacement: a clinical study. Clin Orthop, 11:105, 1975.
7. COLLIS DK: Femoral stem failure in total hip replacement. J Bone Joint Surg, 59A:1033, 1977.
8. GALANTE JO: Causes of fractures of the femoral component in total hip replacement. J Bone Joint Surg, 62A:670, 1980.
9. GALANTE JO: Metals used in orthopaedic surgery. *In* Orthopaedic Knowledge Update-I. Chicago, American Academy of Orthopaedic Surgeons, 1984.
10. GALANTE JO, ROSTOKER W, DOYLE JM: Failed femoral stems in total hip prostheses. J Bone Joint Surg, 57A:230, 1975.
11. GRUEN TA, McNEICE GM, AMSTUTZ HC: Modes of failure of cemented stem-type femoral components. Clin Orthop, 141:17, 1979.
12. LORD G, BANCEL P: The madreporic cementless total hip arthroplasty: new experimental data and a seven-year clinical follow-up study. Clin Orthop, 176:67, 1983.
13. MARTENS M, et al.: Factors in the mechanical failure of the femoral component in total hip prosthesis. Acta Orthop Scand, 45:693, 1974.
14. MILLER EH, SHASTRI R, CHUN-I S: Fracture failure of a forged vitallium prosthesis. J Bone Joint Surg, 64A:1359, 1982.
15. PELLICCI P, et al: Revision total hip arthroplasty. Clin Orthop, 170:34, 1982.
16. PELLICCI P, et al.: Long-term results of revision total hip replacement. J Bone Joint Surg, 67A:513, 1985.
17. TURNER RH, SCHELLER A (eds): Revision Total Hip Arthroplasty. New York, Grune and Stratton, 1982.
18. WROBLEWSKI BM: Fractured stem in total hip replacement. Acta Orthop Scand, 53:279, 1982.

CHAPTER THIRTY

Infections in Total Hip Replacement

NEAL L. ROCKOWITZ
RICHARD H. ROTHMAN

For the informed patient and surgeon, deep sepsis continues to be the most dreaded complication in total hip arthroplasty . Treatment of the infected patient may require long hospitalization, many weeks of intravenous antibiotic therapy, and multiple surgical procedures. Prolonged patient morbidity and even death resulting from infection have been reported. The economic implications to both the patient and society are immense.

Despite the introduction of prophylactic antibiotics, improved sterile technique, and the use of laminar flow operating rooms, the infection rate subsequent to hip arthroplasty ranges from 0.2 to 2.3% (Table 30–1).[23,57,64] If we accept the current estimates of over 100,000 total hip replacements performed yearly in the United States, then the orthopaedic surgical community must confront at least 1000 new infected total hip patients annually.

Classification
Early Infection

Early wound infection has a wide spectrum of clinical appearances that are often difficult to categorize and separate. The differentiation of sterile clear drainage in a seemingly benign wound from an early superficial infection rests more on clinical judgement in appearance than on bacteriologic data. Contamination of cultures is so common that results of superficial swab samples are more often confusing than helpful.

Likewise, the differentiation between early superficial infection and early deep infection is also a difficult line to draw. If one eliminates the issue of the draining hematoma, which is discussed later, then the patients with sterile drainage and early superficial infections do not appear to be predisposed to late deep infection, the most dreaded specter of this category of complications. In our series, none of the patients with early superficial problems proceeded to late deep sepsis. Other authors dissent from this position. Of course, this is not true with the draining hematomas—they are a definite negative predictive factor in regard to late deep infection.

Sterile Wound Drainage

A fairly large percentage (10.5% of the 2368 postoperative patients) in the Pennsylvania Hospital series had at least one episode of clear serous drainage from an apparently benign wound. (Table 30–1) These patients had no pain, no changes in the appearance of the wound margins, and no temperature elevation. Their wound cultures were negative. None of these patients later developed deep sepsis. It is the authors' policy to obtain a wound culture, preferably by aspiration of the subcutaneous tissues rather than by a skin swab. Superficial skin swabs are often erroneous and subject to contamination by nonpathogenic organisms. The patient is then started on prophylactic antibiotics in the form of cephalexin (Keflex) 500 mgs qid until the drainage stops. If within 48 hours this drainage has not ceased, then the patient is placed at bedrest to further hasten the wound healing. These patients are not regarded as infected, but more accurately as experiencing delayed healing of wounds. This situation is seen more commonly in obese patients and in those in whom the subcutaneous fat was traumatized. Atraumatic technique and meticulous skin closure helps to avoid this type of complication.

Early Superficial Infection

This type of complication is defined as a superficial inflammatory reaction in the wound, usually about a suture or a drain site, characterized by localized swelling and redness of the wound with or without purulent drainage. Culture samples taken

497

TABLE 30–1. *Infection*

Incidence	Number	Percentage
Early Superficial Infection		
Primary	18	1.03
Conversion	6	1.34
Revision	2	1.16
Overall	26	1.1
Early Deep Infection		
Primary	6	.34
Conversion	0	0
Revision	2	1.16
Overall	8	.34
Sterile Drainage		
Primary	187	10.7
Conversion	44	9.8
Revision	19	11.0
Overall	250	10.5
Late Deep Infection (In 1687 cases with followup)		
Primary	7	.40
Conversion	2	.45
Revision	3	1.74
Overall	12	.73

from the area reveal a mixed array of organisms usually associated with skin contamination. These wounds are not painful and not associated with temperature elevations. The wounds respond to local care and systemic antibiotics and in our experience, do not proceed to deep late infection. The recommended treatment at Pennsylvania Hospital is to remove the local suture material, debride any necrotic tissue, and continue twice daily applications of povidone solution (as with all surgical wounds). No effort is made to resuture or close these wounds secondarily. Cultures are taken routinely and the patient placed on cephalexin (Keflex) 500 mgs qid for a period of 10 days. The the antibiotic regimen may be altered depending on the results of the cultures.

Early Deep Infection

This category of early infection has a more significant and ominous implication. In the Pennsylvania Hospital experience, these were individuals who had hematomas that became secondarily infected. During their surgical evacuation, culture samples were found to be positive in five patients. Out of these five, three ultimately progressed to late deep infection. There is also the rare patient who develops hematogenous seeding of his arthroplasty in the early postoperative period.

This diagnosis can only be made with surgical inspection and culture samples of the deep tissues beneath the fascia. At the time of surgery, debridement of all hematoma and infected necrotic tissue is performed with copious irrigation with antibiotic solutions. Invariably, the prosthetic components remain well anchored at this early juncture and the long-term prognosis remains indeterminate. There is no rationale or data to support resection of the components at this early stage (Fig. 30–1). The wounds are closed in a routine fashion over suction drainage and the patient is maintained on 6 weeks of intravenous antibiotics, followed by oral antibiotics for a varying period of time.

It is strongly felt by the authors that aggressive early intervention in the face of a draining hematoma would have lowered the frequency of late deep sepsis and improve the prognosis in these patients.

Since 1972, all hematomas that drained for more than 24 hours have been radically debrided and in these individuals no cases of late deep sepsis have resulted. This is also true of cases of early hematogenous sepsis, which received early aggressive debridement without resection of the prosthesis.

Late Deep Infection

Late deep sepsis remains a dreaded complication of total hip arthroplasty. The apprehension this diagnosis engenders is based on the inability to eliminate the sequelae of the infection and the inability to uniformly retain the prosthetic joint. The situa-

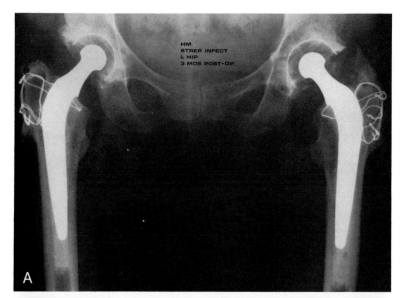

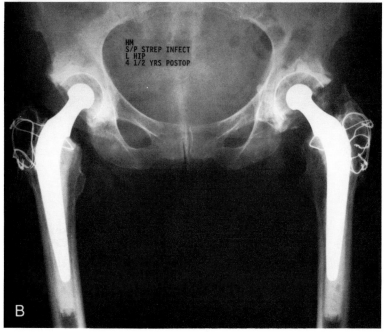

Fig. 30–1. A 60-year-old female with bilateral total hip replacement developed acute onset of fever, chills, and pain in the left hip 2.5 months postoperatively. **A.** Within 24 hours the patient underwent arthrotomy, debridement, and irrigation of the left hip. Operative cultures grew a streptococcus species sensitive to penicillin. The patient was placed on intravenous penicillin for 6 weeks. Clinically she defervesced and her wound went on to uneventful healing. Her preoperative sedimentation rate was 43 and returned to normal postoperatively. **B.** Four and one-half years postoperatively the patient was totally asymptomatic and fully functional. She continued to take penicillin twice a day.

tion is further compounded by the persistent lack of certainty of diagnosis in many situations.

Predisposing Factors and Cause

The sources of sepsis are varied and include (1) contamination during surgery (2) a draining hematoma (3) distant focus of infection (4) prior surgery, and (5) joint injection. Contamination during the surgical procedure may occur either through a break in the surgical sterility or from airborne contamination. Since the early 1960s, many authors have demonstrated that the use of a clean air enclo-

sure (which utilizes a vertical laminar flow system) and a body exhaust system reduces the rates of late deep infection.[12,23,55,57,64] Lidwell[55] reported on a multicenter study of more than 8000 cases. With air contamination rates of 50 to 500 particle forming units/meters^3 (PFU/M^3) in conventionally ventilated rooms, there was a 1.5% sepsis rate; in ultra clean air with less than 10 PFU/M^3, there was a 0.6% sepsis rate. On the other hand, Marotte[64] in 1987 concluded that there was no statistical difference in wound contamination rates between *modern* conventional ventilation and true laminar flow units.

The direction of the flow seems to be as important as its sterility. Salvati, et al.,[88] and Ritter, et al.,[84] have shown that a significant reduction in bacterial counts at the wound site can be obtained using horizontal laminar flow systems. Salvati, however, noted a paradoxical increase in infection rates during total knee replacements performed in horizontal laminar flow rooms. He concluded that the rate of contamination depended on the positioning of personnel about the operating field.

The administration of antibiotic prophylaxis is now a widely accepted practice in most surgical procedures. In 1973, Boyd, et al.,[11] demonstrated a sixfold decrease in infection rate in patients with hip fractures who were treated with prophylactic antibiotics. With respect to total hip replacement, Nelson[75] and Marotte[64] demonstrated a fourfold and fivefold decrease, respectively, in infection rates after the advent of antibiotic prophylaxis. Moreover, both of these studies clearly demonstrated the additive effect of combining clean air enclosures and antibiotic prophylaxis by reporting infection rates as low as 0.5 to 0.6% in both series.

Goldner[37] at Duke University used ultraviolet light in the orthopaedic operating rooms to lower infection rates. The patients and personnel in the operating room must have appropriate skin covering and special glasses to protect them from the potentially harmful UV rays. Clearly, any mechanism that decreases the delivery of bacteria to the open surgical wound is both sensible and prudent.

Draining hematoma during the postoperative course is the second major source of sepsis. Of the 7 late deep infections noted in the Pennsylvania Hospital series, 3 were associated with draining hematomas. None of these had been evacuated surgically during the first 48 hours. Since a more aggressive position has been assumed in regard to surgical evacuation of draining hematomas, none have progressed to late sepsis. This association between draining hematomas and infection has been noted by others.[34,73]

A significant increase in both superficial and deep infections have been shown in diabetic patients.[67,94] Likewise, patients with rheumatoid arthritis have a higher risk of sepsis.[82]

Hematogenous spread from a distant source, such as dental infections, pneumonia, or urinary tract infections, has been well described.[17,27,29,34,60,94] Sepsis also has been noted by spread from a focus distal in the extremity.[97]

Patients who have had prior surgery also constitute an increased risk of late deep infection. Nelson[75] and Fitzgerald[34] report a twofold increase in late deep sepsis in patients who have had hip surgery prior to their index arthroplasty. This may occur because of possible pre-existing subclinical sepsis, decreased local host resistance because of scarring and reduced vascularity, prolonged operating time, and difficulty of surgery. Tietjen[98] in a careful study of the significance of intraoperative intracapsular cultures demonstrated that cultures obtained from previously operated hips are of predictive value in terms of late sepsis. In the absence of previous surgery, these cultures are not of predictive value. Kanner, Steinberg, and Balderston, in reviewing their experience with infected total hip arthroplasties, noted that 48% of the infected hips had undergone an operation prior to the index arthroplasty.[19]

Diagnosis
Clinical Presentation

The history, in patients suspected of late deep sepsis, should include a search for the potential etiologic factors as noted above. Details of the operation and the postoperative course should be sought. Was there evidence of hematoma or drainage? Was the operation conducted in a clean air enclosure and were prophylactic antibiotics used? Has there been a septic focus elsewhere in the body and if so, was it adequately treated? Did the teeth, urinary tract, or gastrointestinal tract undergo a manipulation that might have provoked bacteremia?

In those cases of deep sepsis related to surgical contamination or a draining hematoma, the quality of result usually was impaired soon after surgery. Pain may have been evident to the patient throughout his recovery period and slowly had become progressive in intensity and relentless in nature. Unlike the intermittent mechanical pain of loosening, the pain of sepsis is more persistent and may occur at night as well as during periods of rest. A history of chills, fever, and malaise is generally absent except in the rare acute infectious processes. Persistent drainage, wound inflammation and swelling is unusual, but helpful diagnostically when present.

In the absence of acute inflammatory changes or drainage about the wound, the physical examination is similar to those performed on the patient with nonseptic loosening, and therefore of limited help. Subsidence of the femoral component causes shortening and a limp may be evident. Pain may be provoked at the extremes of rotation.

Laboratory Studies

Most commonly, only the sedimentation rate is abnormal in late deep sepsis. The white blood count (WBC) is usually normal and, therefore, not helpful. Aalto, et al.,[1] has observed that the ESR rises to a peak at approximately 6 days postoperatively and then slowly decreases over the ensuing year, remaining slightly elevated at the end of 1 year. Carlsson[20] noted similar findings but added that in patients with delayed infections the ESR was significantly increased during the first postoperative months and never returned to normal levels. They concluded that an ESR of 40 mm or more noted later than 3 months postoperatively strongly indicates deep infection even if the patient is still free from symptoms. Of course, this statement only holds true when other diseases with elevated ESR and complications such as urinary tract infections or pneumonia are excluded. The results of this study imply that the pathogenesis of deep infections is caused by bacterial contamination during the operation rather than hematogenous spread from a distant focus, which they admit occurs in rare cases.

The authors reviewed their data on sedimentation rates in 57 patients at Pennsylvania Hospital who underwent revision total hip arthroplasty. The patients were divided into 3 groups graded as definite infection (21 patients), probable infection (17 patients), or uninfected (19 patients), using clinical and microbiologic criteria. These criteria are discussed in detail in the section on The Results of Surgery for Infection. The prevalence of hip sepsis in this group was 37%.

Statistical analysis using receiver operating characteristic (ROC) curve analysis indicated that when an ESR of 30 is used as a cut off, 77% of sample patients were correctly classified as definitely infected vs. probably infected or uninfected. (Fig. 30–2) As such, the test had a sensitivity of 66%, a specificity of 84%, a predictive value of 70%, and a negative predictive value of 81%. Thirteen patients misclassified, 6 were false positives, and 7 were false negatives. It thus appears that the erythrocyte sedimentation rate is a useful clinical adjunct to the diagnosis of hip sepsis with an optimal cutoff at 30.

Aspiration of the Hip

Aspiration of the hip joint whether performed in the x-ray department or operating room adds substantially to the diagnostic accuracy. Phillips[80] has reviewed the data from Massachusetts General Hospital and found that they were able to accurately diagnose 10 of 11 deep infections. The sensitivity was 88% and the specificity 83%. The author concluded that there were substantial advantages to aspiration in the department of radiology including lower cost, shorter hospitalization, and simultaneous performance of arthrography if necessary. They emphasized the need for a meticulous aseptic preparation, the avoidance of local anesthetics, and the prompt transportation of the specimen to the laboratory. If no fluid is obtained, *a nonbacteriostatic* saline flush is performed.

Fitzgerald[34] indicated an ability to accurately diagnose deep sepsis in 11 of 15 aspirations. In previ-

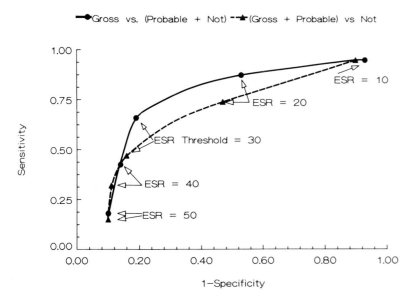

FIG. 30–2. Receiver operating characteristic (ROC) curves for the erythrocyte sedimentation rate (ESR). The specificity of the ESR in predicting infection versus no infection increases linearly until the ESR rate is 30. Beyond 30 only minimal increases in specificity are obtained. At 30 the ESR had a sensitivity of 60% and a specificity of 84% (circles).

ous years it was the policy of the Pennsylvania Hospital to perform needle biopsies of the bone surrounding the prosthetic components in addition to aspiration of the joint. Retrospective review of these data did not reveal a significant advantage to this more formidable procedure.

Radiographic Evaluation

For the most part, the radiographic stigmata noted in patients with deep late sepsis cannot be differentiated from aseptic loosening (Fig. 30–3). In the occasional patient, evidence of periosteal reaction and frank osteomyelitis is seen, but this is not common (see Fig. 30–8). In patients who have had trochanteric osteotomy and wiring, lucent demarcation about the wire tracts is suggestive of sepsis and helpful if seen (see Fig. 30–10 C–G). For the most part the radiographic stigmata of loosening are found: migration of components, fracture of the cement, and demarcation and radiolucent lines between the bone and cement as well as between cement and prosthesis. These signs are not specific. Therefore, every patient who has a radiographically loose total hip arthroplasty must be considered potentially infected and studied with sedimentation rates and preoperative aspiration to further illuminate the possibility of sepsis.

Bone Scanning

Technetium bone scans are helpful in the evaluation of a painful total hip replacement and although sensitive, do not differentiate between the loose and infected total hip prosthesis.[8,83,96,106,107] Freiberger, et al.,[96] and other authors[70,106] have stated that the characteristics noted on the technetium scan including the intensity and isotope distribution may differentiate septic from nonseptic loosening. The Pennsylvania Hospital data have indicated that this is the exception rather than the rule. At our institution, the three-phase bone scan, as well, has proven to be an inaccurate test in differentiating between the septic and nonseptic total hip replacement (Fig. 30–4).

Gallium scans may improve the physician's ability to differentiate the septic from the nonseptic hip. Reing[83] has shown that of 19 patients with definite infections, all had a positive gallium scan. Based on this data, he felt that the combination of a technetium-99 and gallium-67 citrate scan could differentiate between the loose and infected prosthesis. He also emphasized that a negative technetium scan should mitigate against surgical exploration of a painful hip arthroplasty because of the sensitivity of this study in detecting either loosening or sepsis. Williams,[107] commenting on the gallium-67 scan, noted that 13 of 14 patients with definite hip infections also had a positive gallium scan. Newman[76] reviewed the data in 46 gallium scans performed in Auckland, New Zealand. There was a 10% false positive rate and a 21% false negative rate when correlated with the final diagnosis. He concluded that the high instance of false negatives limited the clinical usefulness of gallium-67 scanning. Our own early experience with this study tends to support this data.

More recently Lyons and coauthors,[59] in reviewing their radiographic data from the Mayo clinic, found that gallium scans had an accuracy rate of 77% with regard to infected hip prostheses, with a specificity of 100%, and a relatively low sensitivity of 67%. The authors emphasized that the relative lack of gallium scan sensitivity confirms the need for hip aspiration in the appropriate clinical setting.

A recent study by Mountford, et al.,[70] compared the roles of technetium bone scan, gallium scan, and indium-111 leucocyte scan in identifying infected hip prostheses. They found that the indium-111 leucocyte scan had a lower sensitivity but a higher specificity than gallium for locating infection. They proposed an algorithm for the workup of a patient with a painful hip prosthesis. A bone scan should be conducted first: if a normal or focal pattern is obtained, infection could be excluded and further scanning with other agents is not indicated; if there was a diffuse distribution, infection is almost certainly present. In the rare instance of a diffuse distribution pattern caused by nonseptic synovitis, then neither gallium nor indium leucocyte scan will distinguish this cause from infection. Focal uptake superimposed on the diffuse distribution pattern on a bone scan can be obtained with both infected and noninfected hips and it provides the strongest reason for proceeding to an indium leucocyte scan or gallium scan. This study noted that the indium leucocyte scan was slightly more accurate than the gallium scan. However, convincing data to favor one test over the other was not presented.

When correlating all of the data available on any particular patient, it will be found that certain patients are clearly infected and others are clearly noninfected. Unfortunately, a substantial portion falls into an intermediate category of possible infection. The surgeon's treatment plan must take into consideration this large group of patients in a gray zone of certainty in regard to sepsis (Fig. 30–4).

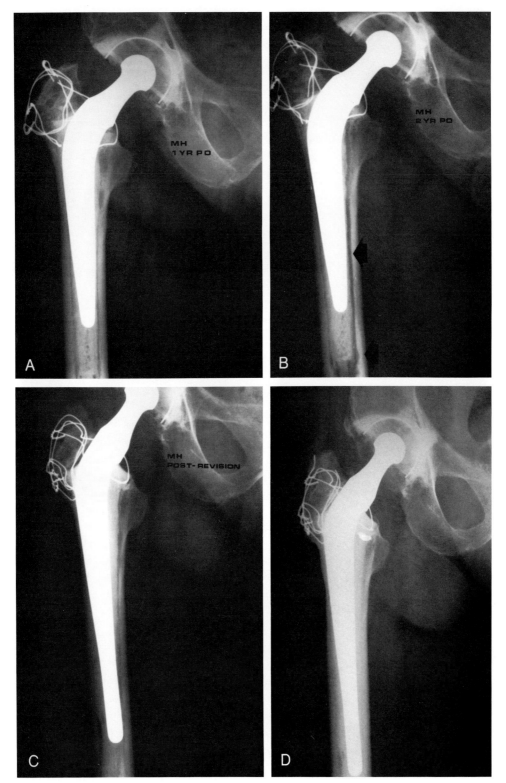

FIG. 30–3. A. A 70-year-old male one year after right total hip arthroplasty with an excellent result. **B.** Six months prior to this x-ray, the patient had developed an abdominal abscess requiring surgery and a colostomy. Subsequently the patient developed pain in the right thigh, which was initially mild but eventually became severe. Radiographic examination revealed a lucency about the femoral component with some scalloping about the tip of the prosthesis (arrows). In the absence of periosteal reaction, a differentiation between aseptic and septic loosening cannot be made based on this x-ray. **C.** The patient underwent a right total hip revision with gentamicin-impregnated cement with an excellent result. In spite of the suggestive history, repeated aspirations and multiple intraoperative cultures failed to identify an infecting organism. Intravenous antibiotics were stopped after the first week. **D.** At 4.3 years postoperative, the patient was totally asymptomatic and fully functional.

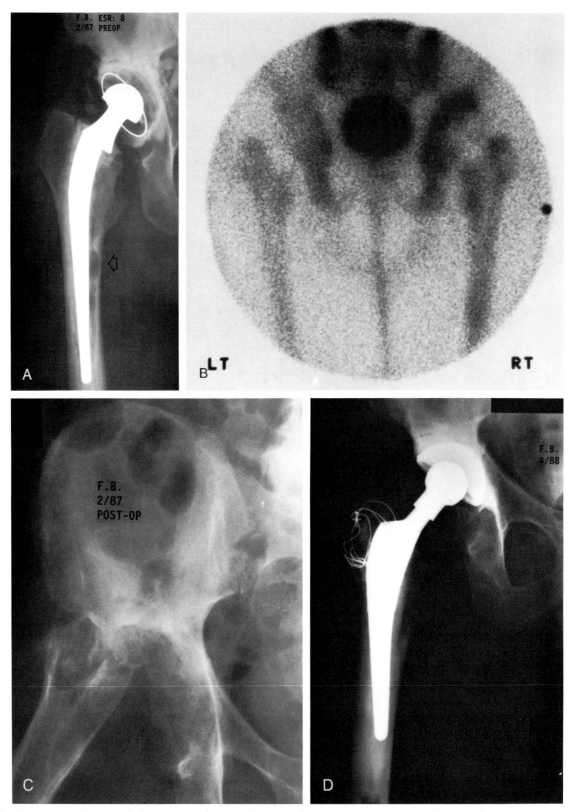

Fɪɢ. 30–4. This case illustrates the importance of performing a *complete* preoperative septic workup. As illustrated in this example, each test by itself is clearly unreliable when one is attempting to differentiate between a septic and nonseptic total hip replacement. **A.** This 64-year-old male had a right total hip replacement performed 1.5 years prior to this x-ray. He presented with an 8-month history of activity-related right thigh pain. Laboratory studies included a normal white blood cell count and an erythrocyte sedimentation rate of 8. Though infection could not be ruled out, it was felt that these x-rays were consistent with loosening secondary to cement-related granulomatous reaction. **B.** This three-phase bone scan was read by the nuclear radiologist as "low probability of infection." Right hip aspirate grew staphylococcus epidermidis, which was interpreted by the infectious disease consultant as a probable contaminant. **C.** Because of the patient's continued complaint of thigh pain, a right total hip revision was planned. During arthrotomy, however, several hundred (milliliters) of gross pus was encountered and a Girdlestone procedure was performed. Intraoperative cultures were positive for staphylococcus epidermidis. **D.** Five months later, the second stage reimplantation was performed with gentamicin-impregnated cement. Intraoperative cultures were negative. At followup 9 months later, the patient was asymptomatic with no signs of infection.

The Surgical Treatment of Sepsis
Diagnostic Definitions

Definite infection is defined as unequivocal microbiology and gross sepsis at surgery. Gross sepsis is defined as purulent material or abundant granulation tissue. Unequivocal microbiology requires either abundant growth of one organism or multiple cultures of the same organism.

Probable Infection is defined as either unequivocal microbiology or gross sepsis at surgery.

Cultures are performed preoperatively by aspiration under the guidance of an image intensifier. At surgery, a minimum of six cultures are obtained with two specimens taken from the capsule, two specimens from the acetabular area, and two specimens from the femur. Whenever possible, the acetabular and femoral specimens are taken from tissue at the bone acrylic interface. All tissues are cultured for aerobic and anaerobic organisms and all appropriate specimens gram-stained. Frozen sections are not routinely performed.

Treatment Options
Girdlestone Resection

In the past, the classical surgical treatment of severe hip sepsis has been Girdlestone resec-

tion.[9,10,35,61,66,74,78,79] Clegg,[25] in 1977, reviewed infected total hip patients treated in this manner and found that although infection was suppressed and pain partially alleviated, the patients remained functionally incapacitated. Traditionally, it has been felt that resection arthroplasty yielded less than desirable functional results but significant pain relief.[3,10,66,78] Kantor, et al.,[52] from Rancho Los Amigos Hospital, reported their results in 41 hips and noted that 93% of the patients had pain in their hips. They performed gait and physiologic analysis on these patients and found that their functional level was inferior to that of an above knee amputee. Eighty-three percent of the patients were minimal community ambulators or nonambulators. They also concluded, interestingly, that postoperative traction did not influence ultimate leg length and thus patients are placed in Bucks traction for pain relief only. Ambulation and transfer training are begun on the second postoperative day.

The overall poor satisfaction obtained by patients receiving Girdlestone resection has been noted by the authors, as well, and for this reason we reserve Girdlestone resection for those patients with fulminant infections, draining sinuses, osteomyelitis, inadequate bone stock for reimplantation, and soft tissues that cannot be adequately debrided at surgery (Figs. 30–5, 30–6)

Although it is our policy to close most Girdle-

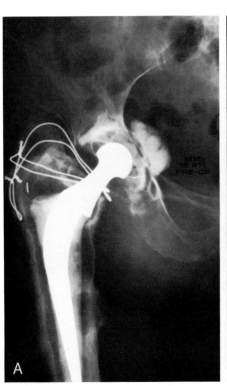
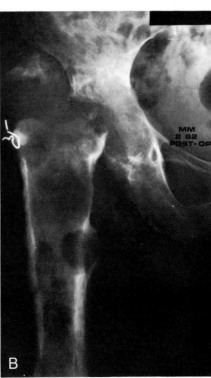

Fig. 30–5. **A.** This patient had an overwhelming pseudomonas infection. **B.** In such cases, Girdlestone resection sacrifices considerable bone stock in both femur and acetabulum. The patient was satisfied with her function and pain relief in spite of a gross limp, severe leg shortening, and instability of the hip.

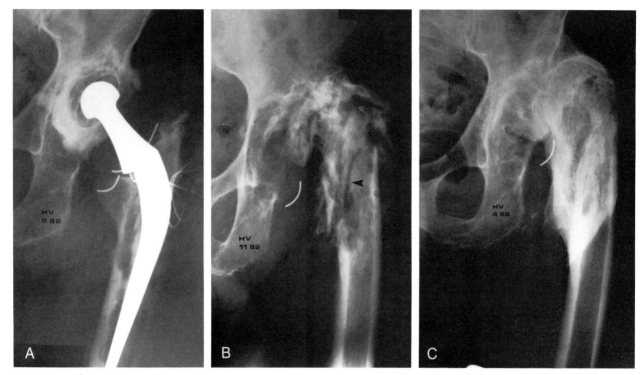

Fig. 30–6. A. This patient was diagnosed as having a staphylococcus epidermidis infection about his left total hip prosthesis in 1979 but refused any treatment until the pain became increasingly severe in 1982. At that time extensive osteolysis of the proximal femur was noted with marked scalloping and destruction of bone about the femoral cortex in the area of the prosthesis. **B.** A resection arthroplasty was performed because of gross sepsis present at surgery. Postoperatively, the patient suffered a fall in a nursing home while ambulating with a walker. A fracture of the proximal femur was noted (arrow). **C.** Fortuitously, the patient went on to spontaneous fusion and is totally asymptomatic. He discontinued antibiotics and his sedimentation rate was 28. The patient uses no ambulatory aids and is satisfied with his result.

stone resections primarily, usually over suction drains, occasionally a wound infection will appear too virulent and complete debridement of infected tissues cannot be assured. In addition, if the patient is toxic, then it may be more prudent to pack the wound open and then perform a delayed closure.

Radical Debridement and Reimplantation

More recently, some centers have proposed radical debridement followed by reimplantation in one or two stages.[47,50,51,68,89,108] Supplemental antibiotic programs have been proposed. A wide spectrum of clinical results have been obtained with this approach. Hunter and Dandy[47] conducted a review of 137 infected total hip arthroplasties and found that only 33% (10 of 30) of the total hip arthroplasties revised for sepsis were successful.

Salvati[89] reported a 91% success rate in 32 one-stage operations and 89% success with 28 two-stage total hip arthroplasties done for sepsis. Jupiter, et al.,[51] reviewed their results in 18 patients with active infection who had total hip arthroplasty. Fourteen of the 18 reconstructions were successful at a mean followup of 42 months. Two of

the four failures were patients with gram negative organisms. Cherney and Amstutz[24] reviewed their results of total hip replacement performed in either one or two stages in 33 hips with active sepsis. Twenty-three of 33 patients (70%) revealed no signs of infection at 3 to 9 years of followup. The success rate when the original organism was gram positive was 78%; the success with gram negative organisms, however, was only 58%. Recently, Harris[42] reported a 78% prosthetic survival at 4 years (14 of 18 patients) for one-stage exchange arthroplasty for septic total hip replacement. They also noted that all 4 failures grew out gram negative rods or mixed flora. Aside from the use of antibiotic cement in 2 cases from Harris' study, antibiotic impregnated bone cement was not used in any of these series.

Radical Debridement with Reimplantation Using Antibiotic-Loaded Cement

The first widely recognized application of a concept that a solution of bone cement could serve as a source of antibiotic in patients with a total joint arthroplasty was reported in the German literature by Bucholz and Engelbrecht in 1970.[15] Now over 2 decades later this concept is the subject of a sizeable literature composed of both laboratory and clinical studies.[6,14,31,45,54,63,69,81,90,92,99-103,110] Despite this widespread attention, the principle continues to be controversial. At standard doses several antibiotics including gentamicin, penicillin, clindamycin and some cephalosporins appear to be released in potentially efficacious amounts. The duration for which these antibiotics continue to be released is extremely uncertain. Reported values for the release of gentamicin from Palacos range from 13 days[6] to five years.[102] Most studies have agreed, however, that the period of maximum antibiotic release is limited to the first few hours or days after implantation. Therefore, it must be assumed that the maximum clinical effectiveness of the released antibiotic might be expected to occur during this period.

The issue of alteration of the biomechanical properties of bone cement by adding antibiotic powder has been addressed by several authors. Bucholz and Engelbrecht[15] reported a reduction in the breaking strength of Palacos of 10 to 15% under static bending loads when gentamicin was added. Marks, et al.,[63] noted that the addition of antibiotics to acrylic cement had no influence on the compressive and diametrical tension strengths of bone cement. It has been clearly shown that antibiotics must only be added to cement in powdered form because aqueous antibiotic solutions will clearly diminish the mechanical strength of bone cement. An excellent review of the literature concerning the use of antibiotic-impregnated cement was presented by Trippel in the Journal of Bone and Joint Surgery in 1986.[100]

In Europe, extensive experience has been gained with the use of antibiotic-loaded acrylic cement. Josefsson, et al.,[50] as well as Bucholz and Engelbrecht[15] have recommended the use of gentamicin containing bone cement in the prophylaxis of postoperative infections in total hip arthroplasty. Although valuable these studies lack appropriate controls and adequate criteria for diagnosis of infection.

Bucholz has reported on 583 infected total hip patients treated with gentamicin-impregnated cement.[14] His revision arthroplasty comprised in one stage: excision of soft tissue, removal of the implant and cement, and replacement with an appropriate implant using Palacos R acrylic cement loaded with an appropriate antibiotic. Systemic antibiotics were rarely used early in the study and are now advocated by Bucholz. He described a 77% success rate for initial one-stage revisions with a 90%

success rate with multiple reoperations. Carlsson[21] noted a 78% (60 of 77) satisfaction rate for one-stage conversions using gentamicin-impregnated cement for infected total hip replacements. The followup in this study, however, was only 1 to 3 years. Soto-Hall[92] has demonstrated in a small series the safety and efficacy of tobramycin in bone cement. The authors now routinely use tobramycin-impregnated cement for reimplantation in cases with probable or definite sepsis (Fig. 30-7).

Suppressive Antibiotics With or Without Debridement

Occasionally a patient with deep sepsis of a total hip arthroplasty has insufficient symptoms to warrant the major reconstructive procedures outlined above. Suppression of the symptoms may be accomplished with antibiotic therapy particularly when a specific organism can be isolated and it is of low virulence and susceptible to antibiotics. This approach also may be used in the extremely elderly and in the patient who cannot tolerate major surgery. These patients must understand that antibiotic therapy is not curative and the results cannot be certain (Fig. 30-8). The treating physician can be somewhat more optimistic if the components appear well fixed radiographically and if the diagnosis is rendered early during the course of the disease. The role of soft tissue debridement and excision of sinus tracts must be individualized. Again it should be emphasized that this program of suppressive antibiotics with or without an associated debridement of soft tissues cannot be looked upon as a definitive approach but rather a compromise that suppresses rather than cures the septic process. (Figs. 30-9, 30-10).

Surgical Treatment Plan

A uniform method of treatment of the infected hip has been used at Pennsylvania Hospital between the years 1970 and 1987. The operative procedure consists of a Charnley approach to the hip with elevation of the trochanter in all cases. Radical debridement is performed with the resection of all infected soft tissue including capsule and scar. All foreign materials including metal, polyethylene, and acrylic cement are painstakingly debrided (Fig. 30-11). A decision is then made regarding the feasibility of reimplantation. This is based on the adequacy of residual bone stock and the appearance of the residual soft tissues. The infecting organism

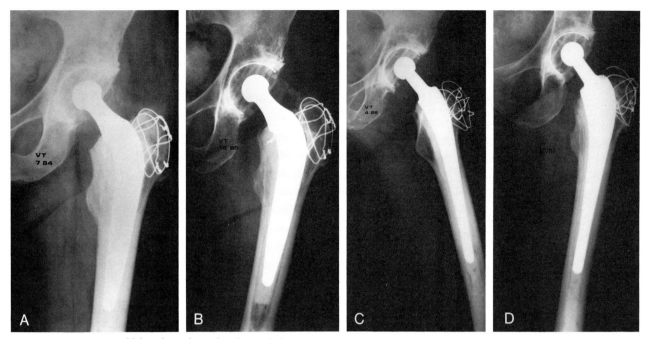

FIG. 30–7. **A.** A 71-year-old female with good early result from total hip replacement for degenerative arthritis of the left hip. Twenty-three years ago the patient underwent a right knee fusion for treatment of osteomyelitis with an unknown organism. There was no evidence of active infection in that knee at the time of arthroplasty. **B.** Within 18 months the patient developed severe and progressive left hip pain with radiographic evidence of loosening shown on this x-ray consisting of a 100% radiolucent line between the cement and bone. Cement prosthesis separation is present in the area of the trochanteric wires. **C.** A one-stage revision using a long-stem prosthesis and gentamicin-impregnated cement was performed with an excellent result at 18 months. Intraoperative cultures identified a streptococcus species, and the patient was placed on intravenous antibiotics for 6 weeks. **D.** At 36 months her left hip was symptom-free, with no signs of infection.

FIG. 30–8. **A.** This 72-year-old female underwent a primary total hip arthroplasty followed by a femoral component revision arthroplasty for aseptic loosening. However, the patient never obtained satisfactory pain relief. Subsequent hip aspiration revealed a streptococcal infection. Suggestive evidence of infection was present in this patient with mild periosteal elevation being present both on the acetabular and femoral components (arrows). The patient was placed on suppressive antibiotics with moderate pain relief. **B.** At last followup the patient noted mild right hip discomfort with a full range of motion. X-ray demonstrates gross loosening of the femoral component.

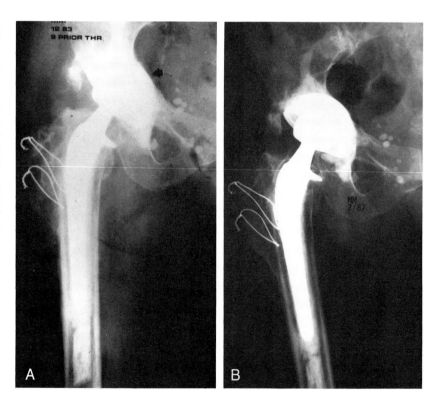

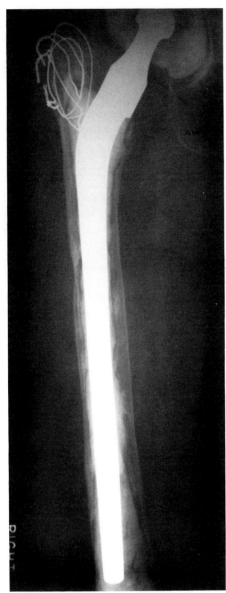

Fig. 30–9. A 68-year-old female who underwent a right revision total hip arthroplasty using a long-stem prosthesis and gentamicin-impregnated cement. Operative cultures grew out streptococcus viridens. Although the patient had 1 year of pain relief after the revision arthroplasty, the pain did reappear and a repeat aspiration revealed the same organism to be present. Because of the frailty of the patient, the length of the prosthesis, and the potential difficulty of further surgery, the patient was placed on intravenous antibiotics. Within 6 weeks her hip pain disappeared. The patient continues on suppressive antibiotics. The prognosis is guarded.

(as identified by preoperative aspiration or gram stain) is not considered.

In marginal situations reimplantation is not undertaken. In fulminant infections, in patients with draining sinuses and in patients with radiographic evidence of osteomyelitis, reimplantation is not performed.

The prosthesis used in most cases is fixed with methylmethacrylate. At the current time the acrylic cement is used with either impregnated gentamicin or tobramycin.

Uncemented porous coated prostheses are used with trepidation in these situations because of the fear of recrudescence of the infection at some time in the future with a biologically well fixed prosthesis (Fig. 30–12).

Postoperatively, ambulation is started as promptly as possible with occasional delays for 3 to 4 weeks because of tenuous trochanteric reattachment.

Supplemental Antibiotics

Once the operative cultures were obtained, all patients received intraoperative antibiotics. Patients with definite infection received 6 weeks of intravenous antibiotics followed by oral antibiotics for life. Patients with probable infections received 3 weeks of intravenous antibiotics followed by oral antibiotics for a period of 1 year. The exact duration of the antibiotic program is difficult to substantiate. It is the authors' feeling that a maximal program of supplemental antibiotics is indicated because of the gravity of these infections and the lack of an effective alternative should the revision surgery fail. The selection of antibiotics is based on the sensitivities obtained from the operative cultures and is made in conjunction with infectious disease consultants.

One-Stage vs. Two-Stage Reimplantation

There is no unanimity of opinion today in the orthopaedic literature with regard to one-stage versus two-stage reimplantation. Bucholz[13] feels that there is no evidence that the delay involved with the two-stage procedure is useful. Certainly there is additional morbidity in the staged procedure and the second operation can be technically difficult. Several authors including Miley, et al.,[68] Wroblewski,[109] Murray,[72] and Harris[42] concur with this opinion and advocate single-stage reimplantation surgery for infected total hip replacements. Salvati[89] and Wilson[108] feel that the reported results favor a two-stage reimplantation. The clinical series reported in the literature to date exhibit insufficient uniformity to allow comparison from one series to the next and this precludes a definitive answer to this question. The authors' data also are in-

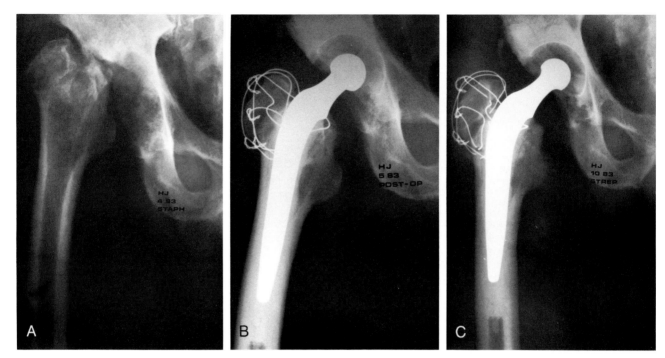

Fig. 30–10. This 77-year-old male with prostatic cancer treated with radiation therapy and orchiectomy developed severe right hip pain initially thought to be radiation necrosis. An erythrocyte sedimentation rate was 115 and a preoperative aspirate grew staphylococcus warneri. **A.** The patient underwent a Girdlestone resection and was placed on intravenous dicloxacillin for 6 weeks. **B.** His ESR dropped to eleven, and 6 months later a conversion total hip arthroplasty was performed with gentamicin-impregnated cement. Operative cultures were negative. The patient was placed on intravenous dicloxacillin for 6 weeks followed by chronic oral dicloxacillin. **C.** Five months postoperatively the patient presented with acute hip pain. The ESR was 107. Questioning of the patient revealed that 3 weeks previously the patient had undergone removal of an infected tooth. The following day the patient underwent incision and drainage of the hip with removal of wires. Operative cultures at that time revealed streptococcus viridens and the patient was then placed on intravenous penicillin.

sufficient to be definitive in this regard. The timing of the second stage reimplantation is difficult as well. The range varies from 3 weeks to 1 year and depends on the virulence of the organism involved, the appearance of the soft tissues, and the sedimentation rate (Fig. 30–13).

Current Policy Regarding Antibiotic-Impregnated Cement

Gentamicin-impregnated cement has had the greatest clinical use and study for the septic total hip arthroplasty. This treatment modality appears both safe and effective. At Pennsylvania Hospital the authors currently utilize tobramycin-impregnated cement in all patients with probable or definite infection who undergo cemented reimplantation whether this is undertaken in one or two stages. At the time of publication gentamicin cement is available only as part of a research protocol. Tobramycin is, therefore, an acceptable alternative. We have also used erythromycin or colistin in appropriate circumstances.

Total Hip Replacement for the Septic Hip (Pennsylvania Hospital Series)

Materials

Patients with sepsis treated between the years 1970 and 1982 were reviewed and evaluated. Fifty patients met the criteria established for the study; 7 of these patients were dead or lost to followup, leaving 43 infected patients. As a control group, the authors reviewed 21 uninfected revision patients who had undergone primary total hip arthroplasty during these years, as well as a random selection of 20 uninfected primary total hip arthroplasty patients. Of the 84 patients in this study group, 50 were women (60%) and 34 were men (40%). The mean age for females was 64 years (range 46 to 88 years) and 63 years for males (range 40 to 81 years). The followup range was from 6 to 118 months with an average of 38.0 months. The diagnoses are shown in Table 30–2.

The authors defined definite infection (25 opera-

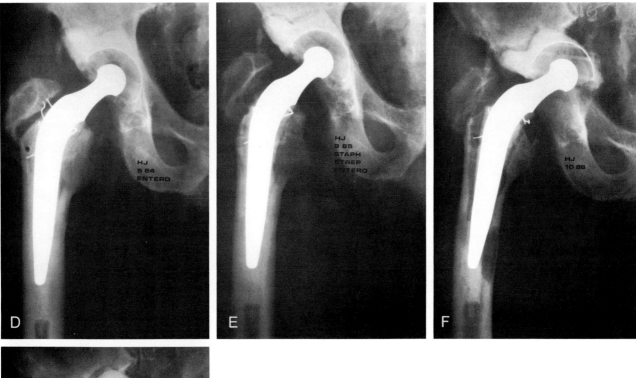

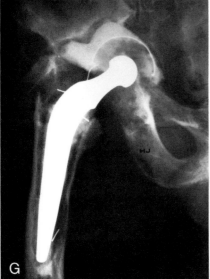

FIG. 30–10 *(continued).* **D.** The patient had acute recurrence of symptoms 7 months later. The ESR was 112, and an aspiration revealed enterococcus. At this point the patient was treated with intravenous vancomycin followed by oral dicloxacillin and ampicillin. **E.** His symptoms abated for 15 months but then because of increasing pain, the patient was taken back to the operating room. Operative cultures at that time revealed enterococcus, staphylococcus epidermidis, and streptococcus. Intravenous treatment included tobramycin, ampicillin, and dicloxacillin. This was followed by oral ampicillin and dicloxacillin. **F, G.** At followups 1 and 2 years postoperatively, the patient had a Charnley rating of A, 5-3-5. His components were grossly loose and there was progressive protrusion of the acetabular component. Furthermore, there was advancing osteolysis of the distal-medial femoral cortex. The patient refused surgery.

TABLE 30-2. *Results of Pennsylvania Hospital Series*

Infected Patients	Preoperative Diagnoses
Total hip arthroplasty for degenerative joint disease	22
Endoprosthesis for trauma	12
Open reduction internal fixation for trauma	4
Total hip arthroplasty for avascular necrosis	3
Fusion for sepsis	2

tions in 23 patients) as unequivocal microbiology *and* gross sepsis at surgery, with probable infection (20 cases) as either unequivocal microbiology *or* gross sepsis at surgery.

The 43 patients in the infected group underwent 45 operative procedures: 8 Girdlestone resections, 12 revisions of septic total hips (termed revision total hip arthroplasty), and 25 conversions of other septic procedures (e.g., internal fixation, Austin-Moore) to total hip arthroplasty (termed conversion total hip arthroplasties). Two of the failed definitively infected revision total hip arthroplasty patients later underwent Girdlestone resections. The results of each procedure at followup are included in the appropriate group.

Our uninfected comparison group consisted of 21 revision total hip arthroplasties (performed for aseptic loosening) and 20 primary total hip arthroplasties selected at random from our total hip arthroplasty data set. We felt that a control group of noninfected total hip arthroplasties performed by the same surgeons using the same prosthesis was necessary to determine the impact of sepsis. Within the control group we felt it essential to separate the revision and primary total hip arthroplasties because of the obvious potential difference in the quality of the results.

Methods

Evaluation: The Charnley "One through Six" Grading System

The Charnley "1 through 6" grading was used to evaluate pain, intensity, function, and range of motion preoperatively and at follow-up (Table 30-3).[111]

Analysis of Data

Analysis of variance, Kruskal-Wallis, and nonparametic analysis of variance tests were used, and all data were analyzed using the statistical analysis system on an IBM 4341 computer.

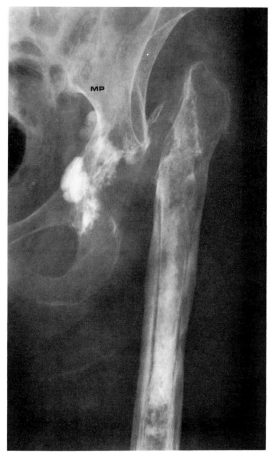

Fig. 30-11. Failure to remove all foreign material, including cement, can be detrimental to the final result. This patient has persistent pain and purulent wound drainage.

Followup

All patients were interviewed by a surgeon other than the operating surgeon.

Results

Intensity of Pain

All groups experienced significant pain relief postoperatively. In general, uninfected patients fared better than patients with probable infections. Patients with definite sepsis who had Girdlestone resections had the worst results (p = 0.0075) (Table 30-4) (Figs. 30-14, 30-15). Revision total hip arthroplasty offered less pain relief than did primary or conversion total hip arthroplasty in each infection category by an average of 0.6 Charnley units (SEM = 0.3, p < 0.01).

Function

All groups except Girdlestone resections improved significantly postoperatively (Table 30-4)

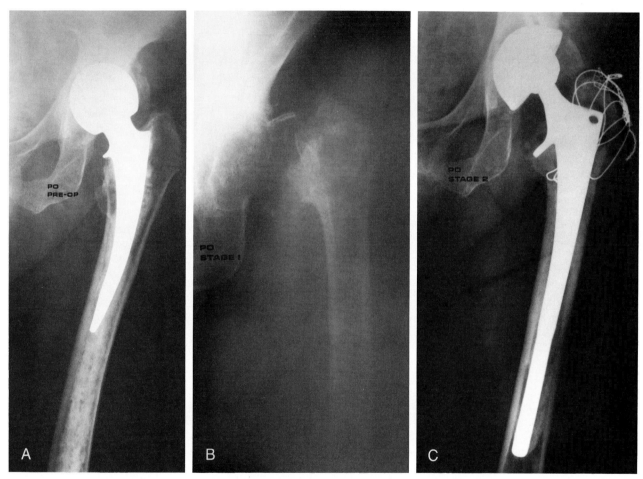

FIG. 30–12. Two-stage revision total hip arthroplasty for infection in a 74-year-old female. **A.** Preoperative x-ray showing an endoprosthesis fixed with cement with the cement extending a long distance past the tip of the prosthesis. The patient was in severe pain with any motion and the preoperative aspirate revealed gross pus. **B.** Stage 1—Resection arthroplasty. A trochanteric osteotomy was performed and it was reattached with suture. Exuberant granulation tissue and purulent exudate was encountered at the time of resection arthroplasty so that a delayed reimplantation was planned. The patient was placed in 5 lbs of Bucks traction. She experienced immediate and dramatic pain relief postoperatively. She underwent a 6-week course of intravenous antibiotic therapy. Cement removal was performed proximally using the Midas-Rex instrumentation. **C.** Stage 2—Noncemented reimplantation. A universal cup (Biomet) and a bias femoral stem (Zimmer) were used. The patient is totally asymptomatic and is walking without ambulatory aids.

514 • Total Hip

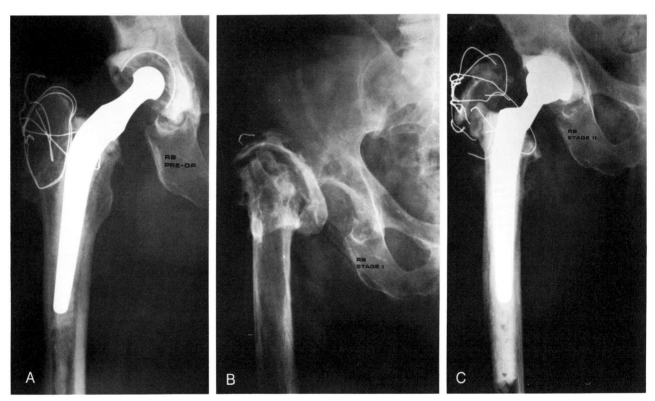

FIG. 30–13. Two-stage revision total hip arthroplasty for infection using gentamicin-impregnated cement. **A.** A 64-year-old male who developed increasing pain in his right hip five years after implantation. Hip aspiration yielded staphylococcus aureus species. Radiographic evaluation reveals loosening of the acetabular component but the femoral component appears to be intact. **B.** Stage 1—A resection arthroplasty was performed and after 6 weeks of intravenous antibiotic therapy the patient was placed on oral cephalexin (Keflex). The patient refused to continue his medication after 1 year and at that time had only intermittent disability in the right hip and moderate pain. He required at least one crutch for ambulation and the leg was shortened by one inch. **C.** Stage 2—Reimplantation of cemented total hip replacement using gentamicin-impregnated cement. The ESR was 8, the preoperative aspiration was negative, there was no gross evidence of infection at the time of reimplantation, and the operative cultures were negative. The patient is pain-free but has a slight Trendelenburg gait because of the trochanteric separation.

TABLE 30–3. *Charnley 1 through 6 Grading System*

Pain
1—Severe, spontaneous.
2—Severe on attempting to walk, prevents all activity.
3—Pain is tolerable, permitting limited activity, night pain, or pain with examination motion.
4—Pain following activity, decreased with rest.
5—Pain is slight or intermittent. Pain when starting to walk, which decreases with an increase in activity.
6—No pain.
Function of Walking
1—Bedridden or chair bound.
2—Time and distance very limited, one or two assistive devices always needed for ambulation.
3—One assistive device usually required, without gross limp, is noticeable for longer distances.
4—Long distances with one cane, limited distances without a cane, moderate limp.
5—Walks with a slight limp, without an assistive device.
6—Normal gait.

Range of Motion
(Sum of all range in degrees)

Grade	1	2	3	4	5	6
Total	0–30	30–60	60–100	100–160	160–210	over 210

(Figs. 30–16, 30–17). Revision total hip arthroplasty fared worse than conversion total hip arthroplasty by an average of 0.6 Charnley units (p < 0.05). The preoperative Charnley score of 2.9 for Girdlestone resections decreased to 2.4 at followup, representing a functional failure of treatment. A striking difference is observed when the followup

Girdlestone scores are compared to those of the infected revision total hip arthroplasties: 2.4 vs. 4.7 (p < 0.001) (Fig 30–17).

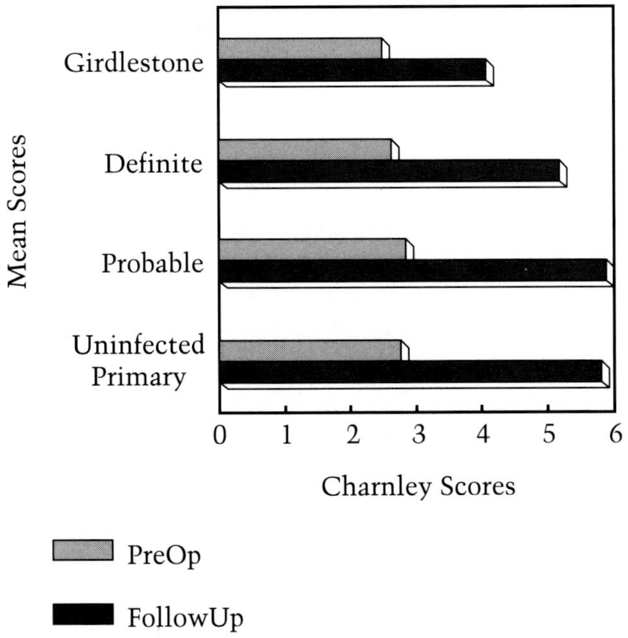

Range of Motion

In general, all groups had an adequate range of motion postoperatively. (No functional difference exists between scores of 5 and 6). Girdlestone resection with a mean 3.9 Charnley score had the lowest range of motion when compared to all other groups (p = 0.006) (Table 30-4) (Figs. 30–18, 30–19).

Microbiology

Among those patients with unequivocally positive microbiology, 30 (70%) had gram positive cocci, 1 (2%) had gram negative rods, 12 (28%) had mixed flora, and one patient had a tuberculous infection of the hip (Fig. 30–20). We found no correlation between type of organism and survival rate of prosthesis, recurrence of infection, or Charnley grade at followup.

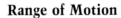

■ PreOp

■ FollowUp

FIG. 30–14. Charnley pain intensity for conversion total hip arthroplasty. Pain relief from conversion total hip arthroplasty is excellent for all grades of infection and is significantly better than the pain relief obtained from a Girdlestone resection.

Radiology

A review of preoperative and followup x-rays revealed no changes pathognomonic for infection as opposed to aseptic loosening.

TABLE 30–4. *Charnley Grades Preoperatively and At Followup*

Surgical Category	Pain Intensity		Function		ROM	
	Preoperative	Followup	Preoperative	Followup	Preoperative	Followup
N						
8 Girdlestone	2.6	4.3	2.9	2.4	4.6	3.9
(SEM)		(0.5)		(0.2)		(0.8)
Definitely Infected:						
7 Revision THA	3.2	4.3	2.8	4.7	4.0	5.0
(SEM)		(0.6)		(0.6)		(0.4)
10 Conversion THA	2.7	5.4	2.3	5.2	3.3	5.2
(SEM)		(0.3)		(0.4)		(0.3)
Probably Infected:						
5 Revision THA	2.4	4.8	2.4	4.8	4.6	5.8
(SEM)		(0.6)		(0.6)		(0.2)
15 Conversion THA	2.9	5.9	2.6	5.6	3.3	5.8
(SEM)		(0.1)		(0.2)		(0.1)
Not Infected:						
21 Revision THA	2.7	5.5	2.8	5.0	4.5	5.7
(SEM)		(0.2)		(0.3)		(0.1)
20 Conversion THA	2.8	5.8	2.5	5.7	3.0	4.8
(SEM)		(0.1)		(0.2)		(0.1)

Gross Sepsis at Surgery

Within the infected group, the finding of frankly purulent material at surgery was a negative predictor for followup pain intensity (p = 0.003), function (p < 0.0001), and range of motion (p < 0.0001). One hundred percent of patients with frank purulence and 60% of patients with only granulation material had unequivocally positive cultures. Granulation tissue alone did not correlate with outcome.

Number of Operations Prior to Index Total Hip Arthroplasty

There is an average decrease in function of 0.3 units at followup for each operation performed prior to the index arthroplasty (SEM = 0.11, p < 0.003)

One- Versus Two-Stage Procedures

Three of the 5 definitely infected revision total hip arthroplasties were done in one stage, and all 5 of the probably infected revision total hip arthroplasties were done in one stage. Twenty-two of the 25 conversion arthroplasties were done in one stage. Therefore there is insufficient data to comment on the efficacy of one- versus two-stage procedures.

Survival Rate

Eighty-three percent of the total hip arthroplasties revised for sepsis (revision total hips) were in place without signs of infection at followup. One hundred percent of the conversion total hips retained their prosthesis. Twenty-four of the 25 pa-

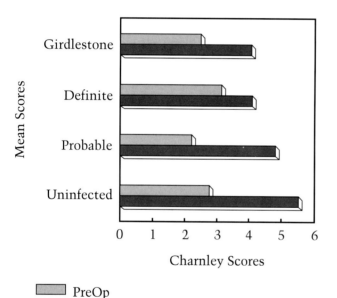

FIG. 30–15. Charnley pain intensity for revision total hip arthroplasty. Pain relief from revision total hip arthroplasty is significant, however, it is not as great as that obtained for conversion total hip arthroplasty. This difference is not statistically significant. Pain relief from revision total hip arthroplasty for definitely infected hips is not better than the pain relief from Girdlestone resection. However, function and range of motion are significantly improved (see Figures 30–17 and 30–19).

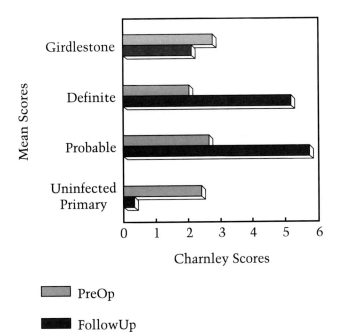

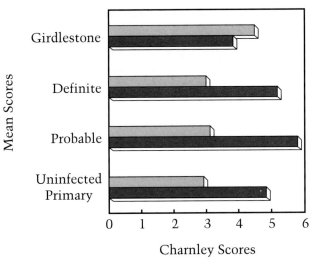

Fig. 30–16. Charnley function after conversion total hip arthroplasty. Function is greatly improved for all grades of infection and is significantly better than function obtained from Girdlestone resection.

Fig. 30–18. Charnley range of motion for conversion total hip arthroplasty. Range of motion is significantly worse with a Girdlestone resection. There is no significant difference between the three grades of infection for conversion hip replacement.

tients (96%) in this group are without signs or symptoms of infection. The patient with persistent symptoms of infection was not considered a candidate for resection because of insufficient disability.

Conclusions

The authors undertook this study in order to clarify the decision-making process for surgeons confronted with the dilemma of the infected total hip. A practical system of definitions was used for

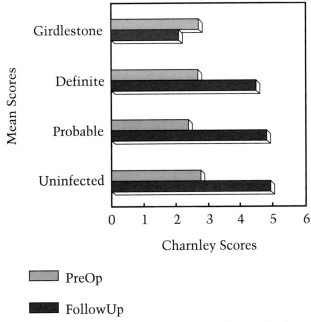

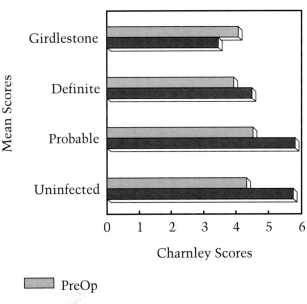

Fig. 30–17. Charnley function for revision total hip arthroplasty. Functional improvement is not as great as obtained with conversion total hip arthroplasty (see Figure 30–16), but again is significantly greater for all grades of infection than Girdlestone resection.

Fig. 30–19. Charnley range of motion (ROM) for revision total hip arthroplasty. Again Girdlestone resection is significantly worse in terms of range of motion than is a revision total hip arthroplasty.

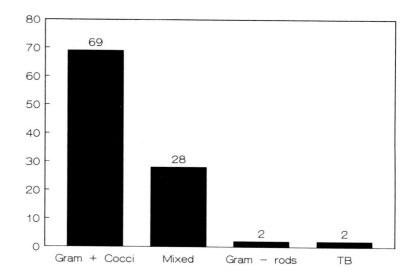

Fig. 30-20. Microbiology of infected total hip arthroplasty. Gram positive cocci were identified in 69% of those cases with positive cultures. There was no correlation between type of organism and survival rate of prosthesis, recurrence of infection, or Charnley grade at followup.

diagnosis and a surgical treatment plan undertaken based on the clinical appearance of the tissues at surgery, rather than bacteriologic data.

Basically, the surgeon decides in the operating room whether to resect alone, or to resect and reimplant a new prosthesis, either in one or two stages. The treatment plan used here was to radically debride, and then, if bone stock permitted, and the remaining tissues were clean, to reimplant a new total hip prosthesis using antibiotic-impregnated cement. Long-term systemic antibiotics were used and chosen on the basis of sensitivity test results.

Using the above plan, 83% of revision total hip arthroplasties and 100% of conversion total hip arthroplasties survived (i.e., prosthesis survival, not patient survival).

At followup, the quality of result and degree of improvement were satisfactory both for the conversion total hip arthroplasty patients and the revision total hip arthroplasty patients. Although pain improved with both total hip arthroplasty and Girdlestone arthroplasty, far better function was obtained with total hip arthroplasty. This finding is in agreement with a recent review by Cherney and Amstutz and with a preponderance of evidence presented in the literature. In general, definite infections fared worse than probable infections, and both of these groups fared worse than the noninfected control groups. Revision total hip arthroplasty did more poorly than conversion total hip arthroplasty at followup in terms of pain intensity. From this study, a conclusion could not be made regarding one- versus two-stage reimplantation.

The authors' system of definitions appears validated because the quality of result at followup related well to the intensity of infection. The system also takes into account the probability that a certain portion of clinically infected hip patients do not have a positive bacteriologic infection.

References

1. AALTO K et al: Changes in erythrocyte sedimentation rate and C-reactive protein after total hip arthroplasty. Clin Orthop, 184:118–120, 1984.
2. AHLBERG A, CARLSSON AS, LINDBERG L: Hematogenous infection in total joint replacement. Clin Orthop, 137:69–75, 1978.
3. AHLGREN S, et al.: Function after removal of a septic total hip prosthesis. Acta Orthop Scand, 51:541–545, 1980.
4. AINSCOW DA: The risk of hematogenous infection in total joint replacements. J Bone Joint Surg, 66B:580–582, 1984.
5. BALDERSTON RA, et al.: Treatment of the septic hip with total hip arthroplasty. Clin Orthop, 221:231–237, 1987.
6. BAYSTON R, MILNER RD: The sustained release of antimicrobial drugs from bone cement. J Bone Joint Surg, 64B:460–464, 1982.
7. BENJAMIN J, VOLZ R: Efficacy of a topical antibiotic irrigant in decreasing or eliminating bacterial contamination in surgical wounds. Clin Orthop, 184:114–117, 1984.
8. BERGSTROM B, et al.: Radiographic abnormalities caused by postoperative infection following total hip arthroplasty. Clin Orthop, 99:95–102, 1974.
9. BITTAR ES, PETTY W: Girdlestone arthroplasty for infected total hip arthroplasty. Clin Orthop, 170:83–87, 1982.
10. BOURNE RB, et al.: A six year follow-up of infected total hip replacements managed by Girdlestone's arthroplasty. J Bone Joint Surg, 66B:340–343, 1984.
11. BOYD RJ, BURKE JF, COLTON T: A double blind clinical trial of prophylactic antibiotics in hip fractures. J Bone Joint Surg 55A:11251–1258, 1973.
12. BRADY LP, ENNEKING WF, FRANCO JA: The effect of operating room environment on the infection rate after Charnley low

friction total hip replacement. J Bone Joint Surg 57A:80–83, 1975.

13. BUCHOLZ HW, et al.: Management of deep infection of total hip replacement. J Bone Joint Surg, 63B:342–353, 1981.

14. BUCHOLZ HW, ELSON RA, HEINERT K: Antibiotic-loaded acrylic cement: current concepts. Clin Orthop, 190:96–108, 1984.

15. BUCHOLZ HW, ENGELBRECHT H: Uber die Depotwirkung einiger Antibiotica bei Vermischung mit dem Kunstharz Palacos. Chirurg, 41:511–515, 1970.

16. BUCHOLZ HW, VON FOERSTER G, HEINERT K: Management of infected prostheses. Orthopedics, 7:1620–1625, 1984.

17. BURTON DS, SCHURMAN DJ: Hematogenous infection in bilateral total hip arthroplasty. J Bone Joint Surg, 57A:1004–1005, 1975.

18. CALLAGHAN JJ, et al.: Reimplantation for salvage of the infected hip: rationale for the use of gentamicin impregnated cement and beads. *In* Proceedings of the Hip Society. St. Louis, Mosby pp. 65–94, 1985.

19. CANNER GC, STEINBERG ME, BALDERSTON RA, HEPPENSTALL RB: The infected hip after total hip arthroplasty. J Bone Joint Surg, 66A:1393–99, 1984.

20. CARLSSON AS, et al.: Erythrocyte sedimentation rate in infected and non-infected total hip replacements. Acta Orthop Scand, 49:287–290, 1978.

21. CARLSSON AS, et al.: Revision with gentamicin-impregnated cement for deep infections in total hip arthroplasties. J Bone Joint Surg, 60A:1069–74, 1978.

22. CARLSSON AS, et al.: Radiographic loosening after revision with Gentamicin-containing cement for deep infection in total hip arthroplasties. Clin Orthop, 194:271–279, 1985.

23. CHARNLEY J: Postoperative infection after total hip replacement with special reference to air contamination in the operating room. Clin Orthop, 87:167–187, 1972.

24. CHERNEY D, AMSTUTZ H: Total hip replacement in the previously septic hip. J Bone Joint Surg, 65A:1256–1265, 1983.

25. CLEGG J: The results of pseudoarthrosis after removal of an infected total hip prosthesis. J Bone Joint Surg, 59B:298–301, 1977.

26. COVENTRY MB: Treatment of infections occurring in total hip surgery. Orthop Clin North Am, 6:991–1003, 1975.

27. CRUESS RL, BICKEL WS, VON KESSLER KLC: Infections in total hips secondary to a primary source elsewhere. Clin Orthop, 106:99–101, 1975.

28. DEL SEL HJ, CHARNLEY J: Total hip replacement following infection in the opposite hip. Clin Orthop, 141: 138–142, 1979.

29. DOWNES EM: Late infection after total hip replacement. J Bone Joint Surg, 59B:42–44, 1977.

30. DUPONT JA: Significance of operative cultures in total hip arthroplasty. Clin Orthop, 211:122–127, 1986.

31. ELSON RA, et al.: Antibiotic loaded acrylic cement. J Bone Joint Surg, 59B:200–205, 1977.

32. FERRARI A, CHARNLEY J: Conversion of hip joint pseudarthrosis to total hip replacement. Clin Orthop, 121:12–19, 1976.

33. FITZGERALD RH, et al: Bacterial colonization of wounds and sepsis in total hip arthroplasty. J Bone Joint Surg, 55A:1242–1250, 1973.

34. FITZGERALD RH, NOLAN DR, et al.: Deep wound sepsis following total hip arthroplasty. J Bone Joint Surg, 59A:847–855, 1977.

35. GIRDLESTONE GR: Acute pyogenic arthritis of the hip, An operation giving free access and effective drainage. Lancet, 1:419–421, 1943.

36. GLYNN MK, SHEEHAN JM: An analysis of the causes of deep

infection after hip and knee arthroplasties. Clin Orthop, 178:202–206, 1983.

37. GOLDNER JL, et al.: Ultraviolet light for the prevention of airborne infection in the operating room—2064 total hip arthroplasty procedures 1969–1983, personal communication.

38. GREENOUGH CG: An investigation into contamination of operative suction. J Bone Joint Surg, 68B:151–153, 1986.

39. GRISTINA AG, KOLKIN J: Total joint replacement and sepsis. J Bone Joint Surg, 65A:128–134, 1983.

40. GRISTINA AG, COSTERTON JW: Bacterial adherence to biomaterials and tissue. J Bone Joint Surg, 67A:264–273, 1985.

41. HARDINGE K, CLEARY J, CHARNLEY J: Low friction arthroplasty for healed septic and tuberculous arthritis. J Bone Joint Surg, 61B:144–147, 1979.

42. HARRIS WH: One-staged exchange arthroplasty for septic total hip replacement. *In* AAOS Instructional Course Lectures. St. Louis, Mosby, 226–228, 1985.

43. HARRIS WH, WHITE RE, 3RD: Resection arthroplasty for non-septic failure of total hip arthroplasty. Clin Orthop, 171:62–67, 1982.

44. HEROLD RA, LOTKE PA, MACGREGOR RR: Prosthetic joint infections secondary to rapidly growing mycobacterium fortuitum. Clin Orthop, 216:183–186, 1987.

45. HOFF SF, FITZGERALD RH, KELLY PJ: The depot administration of Penicillin G and Gentamicin in acrylic bone cement. J Bone Joint Surg. 63A:798–804, 1981.

46. HUGHES PW, et al.: Treatment of subacute sepsis of the hip by antibiotics and joint replacement criteria for diagnosis with evaluation of twenty-six cases. Clin Orthop, 141:143–157, 1979.

47. HUNTER G, DANDY D: The natural history of the patient with an infected total hip replacement. J Bone Joint Surg, 59B:293–297, 1977.

48. HUNTER GA: The results of reinsertion of a total hip prosthesis after sepsis. J Bone Joint Surg, 61B:422–423, 1979.

49. JAMES ETR, HUNTER GA, CAMERON HU: Total hip revision arthroplasty: Does sepsis influence the results? Clin Orthop, 170:88–94, 1982.

50. JOSEFSSON G, LINDBERG L, WIKLANDER B: Systemic antibiotics and Gentamicin-containing bone cement in the prophylaxis of postoperative infections in total hip arthroplasty. Clin Orthop, 159:194–200, 1981.

51. JUPITER JB, KARCHMER AW, LOWELL JD, HARRIS WH: Total hip arthroplasty in the treatment of adult hips with current or quiescent sepsis. J Bone Joint Surg, 63A:194–200, 1981.

52. KANTOR GS, et al.: Resection arthroplasty following infected total hip replacement arthroplasty. J Arthroplasty, 1:83–89, 1986.

53. KIM YY, et al.: Arthroplasty using the Charnley prosthesis in old tuberculosis of the hip. Clin Orthop, 211:116–121, 1986.

54. LEVIN PD: The effectiveness of various antibiotics in Methylmethacrylate. J Bone Joint Surg, 57B:234–237, 1975.

55. LIDWELL OM, et al.: Effect of ultraclean air in operating rooms on deep sepsis in the joint after total hip or knee replacement: a randomized study. Br Med J 285:10, 1982.

56. LIDWELL OM: Sepsis after total hip or knee joint replacement in relation to airborne contamination. Phil Trans R Soc Lond B, 302:583–592, 1983.

57. LIDWELL OM: Clean air at operation and subsequent sepsis in the joint. Clin Orthop, 211:91–101, 1986.

58. LINDGREN U, et al.: Bacteria in hip surgery. Acta Orthop Scand 47:320–323, 1976.

59. LYONS CW, et al.: Evaluation of radiographic findings in

painful hip arthroplasties. Clin Orthop, 195:239–251, 1985.

60. MALLORY TH: Sepsis in total hip replacement following pneumococcal pneumonia. J Bone Joint Surg, 55A:1753–1754, 1973.

61. MALLORY TH: Excision arthroplasty with delayed wound closure for the infected total hip replacement. Clin Orthop, 137:106–111, 1978.

62. MARCHETTI PG, et al.: Clinical evaluation of 104 hip resection arthroplasties after removal of a total hip prosthesis. J Arthroplasty, 2:37–41, 1987.

63. MARKS KE, NELSON CL, LAUTENSCHLAGER EP: Antibiotic impregnated acrylic bone cement. J Bone Joint Surg, 58A:358–364, 1976.

64. MAROTTE JH, et al.: Infection rate in total hip arthroplasty as a function of air cleanliness and antibiotic prophylaxis. J Arthroplasty, 2:77–82, 1987.

65. McCUE SF, BERG EW, SAUNDERS EA: Efficacy of double-gloving as a barrier to microbial contamination during total joint arthroplasty. J Bone Joint Surg, 63A:811–813, 1981.

66. McELWAINE JP, COLVILLE J: Excision arthroplasty for infected total hip replacements. J Bone Joint Surg, 66B:168–171, 1984.

67. MENON T, et al.: Charnley low friction arthroplasty in diabetic patients. J Bone Joint Surg, 65B:580–581, 1983.

68. MILEY GB, SCHELLER AD JR, TURNER RH: Medical and surgical treatment of the septic hip with one-stage revision arthroplasty. Clin Orthop, 170:76–82, 1982.

69. MORAN JM, GREENWALD AS, MATEJCZYK M: Effect of gentamicin on shear and interface strengths of bone cement. Clin Orthop, 141:96–101, 1979.

70. MOUNTFORD PJ, et al.:^{99}Tc^m-MDP, ^{67}Ga-Citrate and ^{111}In-leucocytes for detecting prosthetic hip infection. Nucl Med Commun 7:113–120, 1986.

71. MURRAY WR: Use of antibiotic containing bone cement. Clin Orthop, 190:89–95, 1984.

72. MURRAY WR: Treatment of the infected total hip arthroplasty. *In* AAOS Instructional Course Lectures. St. Louis, Mosby, 229–233, 1968.

73. NELSON JP: Deep infection following total hip arthroplasty. J Bone Joint Surg, 59A:1042–1044, 1977.

74. NELSON CL, BERGMAN BR: Femoral head and neck excision arthroplasty. *In* Surgery of the Musculoskeletal System. New York, Churchill Livingstone, pp. 91–98, 1983.

75. NELSON JP, et al.: The effect of previous surgery, operating room environment, and preventive antibiotics on postoperative infection following total hip arthroplasty. Clin Orthop, 147:167–169, 1980.

76. NEWMAN EF: Gallium-67 citrate scanning in orthopaedics. J Bone Joint Surg, 65B:517, 1983.

77. O'NEILL DA, HARRIS WH: Failed total hip replacement: assessment by plain radiographs, arthrograms, and aspiration of the hip joint. J Bone Joint Surg, 66A:540–546, 1984.

78. PARR PL, et al.: Resection of the head and neck of the femur with and without angulation osteotomy. J Bone and Joint Surg, 53A:935–944, 1971.

79. PETTY W, GOLDSMITH S: Resection arthroplasty following infected total hip arthroplasty. J Bone Joint Surg, 62A:889–896, 1980.

80. PHILLIPS WC, KATTAPURAN SV: Efficacy of preoperative hip aspiration performed in the radiology department. Clin Orthop, 179:141–146, 1983.

81. PICKNELL B, MIZEN L, SUTHERLAND R: Antibacterial activity of antibiotics in acrylic bone cement. J Bone Joint Surg, 59B:302–307, 1977.

82. POSS R, et al.: Factors influencing the incidence and outcome of infection following total joint arthroplasty. Clin Orthop, 182:117–126, 1984.

83. REING CM, RICHIN PF, KENMORE PI: Differential bone-scanning in the evaluation of painful total joint arthroplasty. J Bone Joint Surg, 61A: 933–936, 1979.

84. RITTER MA, FRENCH ML, HART JB: Microbiological studies in a horizontal wall-less laminar air-flow operating room during actual surgery. Clin Orthop, 97:16–18, 1973.

85. RITTER M, et al.: The surgeon's garb. Clin Orthop, 153:204–209, 1980.

86. RITTER MA, STRINGER EQ: Intraoperative wound cultures: their value and long term effect on the patient. Clin Orthop, 155:180–185, 1981.

87. RITTER MA, MISAMORE HEW: Incidence of infection in total joint replacement arthroplasty. Contemp Orthop 7:29–35, 1983.

88. SALVATI EA, et al.: Infection rates after 3175 total hip and total knee replacements performed with and without a horizontal unidirectional filtered air flow system. J Bone Joint Surg, 64A:525–535, 1982.

89. SALVATI EM, et al.: Reimplantation in infection: a 12 year experience. Clin Orthop, 170:62–75, 1982.

90. SALVATI EA, et al.: Reimplantation in infection, elution of gentamicin from cement and beads. Clin Orthop, 207:83–93, 1986.

91. SCHURMAN DJ, et al.: Antibiotic-acrylic bone cement composites, studies of Gentamicin and Palacos. J Bone Joint Surg, 60A:978–984, 1978.

92. SOTO-HALL R, et al.: Tobramycin in bone cement. Clin Orthop, 175:60–64, 1983.

93. SOUTHWOOD RT, et al.: Infection in experimental hip arthroplasties. J Bone Joint Surg, 67B:229–231, 1985.

94. STINCHFIELD RE: Late Hematogenous infection of total joint replacement. J Bone Joint Surg, 62A:1345–1350, 1980.

95. SURIN VV, SUNDHOLM K, BACKMAN L: Infection after total hip replacement. J Bone Joint Surg, 65B:412–418, 1983.

96. TEHRANZADEH J, SCHNEIDER R, FREIBERGER RH: Radiologic evaluation of painful total hip replacement. Radiology, 141:355–362, 1981.

97. THOMAS B, et al: Infection of total hip arthroplasty from distal extremity sepsis. Clin Orthop, 181:121–125, 1983.

98. TIETJEN R, STINCHFIELD FE, MICHELSEN CB: The significance of intracapsular cultures in total hip operations. Surg Gynecol Obstet, 144:699–702, 1977.

99. TORHOLM C, et al.: Total hip joint arthroplasty with Gentamicin impregnated cement. Clin Orthop, 181:99–105, 1983.

100. TRIPPEL SB: Antibiotic-impregnated cement in total joint arthroplasty. J Bone Joint Surg, 68A:1297–1302, 1986.

101. WAHLIG H, et al.: The release of Gentamicin from Polymethylmethacrylate beads. J Bone Joint Surg, 60B:270–275, 1978.

102. WAHLIG H, et al.: Pharmacokinetic study of Gentamicin-loaded cement in total hip replacements. J Bone Joint Surg, 66B:175–179, 1984.

103. WALENKAMP GH, VREE TB, VAN RENS TJ: Gentamicin-PMMA beads, pharmacokinetic and nephrotoxicological study. Clin Orthop, 206:171–183, 1986.

104. WEBER FA, LAUTENRACH EE: Revision of infected total hip arthroplasty. Clin Orthop, 211:108–115, 1986.

105. WHYTE W, et al.: A bacteriologically occlusive clothing system for use in the operating room. J Bone Joint Surg, 65B:502–506, 1983.

106. WILLIAMS ED, et al.: 99 Tc^m-diphosphonate scanning as an

aid to diagnosis of infection in total hip joint replacements. Br J Radiology, 50:562–566, 1977.

107. Williams F, et al.: Gallium-67 Scanning in the painful total hip replacement. Clin Radiology 32:431–439, 1981.

108. Wilson PD, Aglietti P, Salvati EA: Subacute sepsis of the hip treated by antibiotics and cemented prosthesis. J Bone Joint Surg, 56A:879–898, 1974.

109. Wroblewski BM: One-stage revision of infected cemented total hip arthroplasty. Clin Orthop, 211:103–107, 1986.

110. Wroblewski BM, Esser M, Srigley DW: Release of Gentamicin from bone cement, an in-vivo study. Acta Orthop Scand, 57:413–414, 1986.

111. Merle D'Aubigne R, Postel M: Functional results of hip arthroplasty with acrylic prosthesis. J Bone Joint Surg, 36A:451, 1954.

Index

Page numbers in italics indicate illustrations; numbers followed by "t" indicate tables.

Aluminum
  systemic effects of, 416
Ambulation. *See also* Gait; Limp(s)
  after hip surgery, 228
Amish people
  chondroectodermal dysplasia and, 173, *174*
Anatomy, of hip, 1–40. *See also* names of specific
    structures
Anesthesia
  and patient position, 71
  damage to cervical cord and, 427–428
  for elderly patient, 231, 393
  for rheumatoid hip surgery
    spinal/epidural, 427–428
  for total hip arthroplasty, 393
    spinal/epidural, 393
  support personnel for, 71
Aneurysm, aortic
  differential diagnosis of, 296
Ankylosis, hip joint
  rheumatoid arthritis and, 430, *436*, 437
"Antalgic" gait
  hip pain and, 256
  in rheumatoid arthritis, 260
Antibiotics
  cement-loaded
    for reimplantation, 506–507
    for total hip arthroplasty, 49
  for septic arthritis of hip, 164
  predisposing to septic arthritis, 289
  preoperative use, 229, 231–232
    for arthroplasty, 393, 500
    for biopsy, 357
    for "revision," 476, 500
  suppressive, in hip infections, 507, *509*, *510*
Anti-inflammatory (non-steroidal) drugs
  for Legg-Calve-Perthes disease, 143
  in uncemented total hip arthroplasty, 412
Aortic aneurysm
  differential diagnosis of, 296
Arcades of Benninghof, 13
Arcuate line, *4–5*, 7
Artery(ies). *See also* names of specific arteries about the
    hip joint, 72–73
Arthritis. *See* Osteoarthritis; Rheumatoid arthritis;
    Septic arthritis
Arthrodesis, hip, 308–346
  for diseases/disorders
    osteonecrosis, femoral head, 384
    rheumatoid arthritis, 433
    slipped capital femoral epiphysis, 157
    tubercular hip, 310, 312–313, 325, 344–347,
      345
    vs. arthroplasty, 308, 313
    vs. osteotomies, 313–314
  gait after, 310, 311–312, *312*
  history of, 308, 310, 312–313
  in child, 309, 312–313, 333–334
  indications for, 313
    for failed arthroplasty, 313–314

  in child, 313
  in young adult, 313–314
  pain and, 314
  position of, *309*, 309–310, *310*
  postoperative care of, 311
  surgical techniques for, 74, 315–346
    Abbot and Lucas, *316*, *317*, 342–344, *343*
    Barmada, 340–342, *341*, 342
    Brittain, *318*, 326, *327*
    Charnley, 338–340, *339*, *341*
    combined intra- and extra-articular, 315, 320, *321*
    DePalma, 330–332, *331–333*
    extra-articular, 309
    femoroischial transplantation, 344–347
    Ghormley, 321, *321*
    Henderson, 321, *321*
    intra-articular, 315
    ischiofemoral, 324–325
    Kirkaldy-Willis, *316–317*, 326–327, 328
    Lam, 328, 330
    muscle tension type, 342–344, *343*
    Ranawat, Jordan, Wilson, Jr., 321–323, *322–324*
    Schneider, 335–338, *336*, *337*
    Stewart and Coker, 330, *330*
    Thompson, *316–317*, 323, *324*
    Trumble, *319*, 325–326, *326*
    Watson-Jones-Robinson, *316–317*, 328, *329*
    White, 332–335, *334*, *335*
Arthrography
  for diagnosis, congenital dislocation of hip, 111–112,
    118, *118*
Arthroplasty, cup, 349–354
  complications of, 353–354
  for osteonecrosis, femoral head, 380, 381
  history of, 349
  indications for, 349–351
  rehabilitation regimen, 353
  results of, 380–381
  revision of, 449–451, *450*
  technique of, *350–352*, 351–353, *354*
Arthroplasty, hemi-
  for osteonecrosis, femoral head, 381–382
    indications for, 221
    results of, 219
  for rheumatoid arthritis, 432–433
Arthroplasty, revision
  acetabular, 452–469, 493t
    acetabular component position and, 465–469
    bone grafting and, 412, *453–456*, 459, 460,
      462–469, 463–469
    bone stock quality and, 457–459
    component design and, 449–451, *450*, 459–462,
      461, *462*. *See also* Prosthesis(es), design of, for
      acetabulum
    deficiencies, classification of, 452, 452t *453–455*
    failure of, 457–460
    "high hip" position, 466, *468*
    indications for, 452t, *453–456*, 458
    preoperative planning, 452–455
    prosthesis removal, 456–457